From the publisher of *Nursing* journal

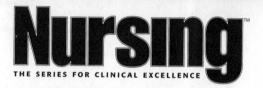

THE SERIES FOR CLINICAL EXCELLENCE

Understanding Diseases

DISCARD

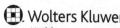

Wolters Kluwer | Lippincott Williams & Wilkins
Health

Philadelphia · Baltimore · New York · London
Buenos Aires · Hong Kong · Sydney · Tokyo

Staff

Executive Publisher
Judith A. Schilling McCann, RN, MSN

Editorial Director
H. Nancy Holmes

Clinical Director
Joan M. Robinson, RN, MSN

Art Director
Elaine Kasmer

Editorial Project Manager
Ann E. Houska

Clinical Manager
Collette Bishop Hendler, RN, BS, CCRN

Clinical Project Manager
Kathryn Henry, RN, BSN, CCRC

Editors
Linda Hager, Elizabeth Jacqueline Mills

Clinical Editors
Joanne M. Bartelmo, RN, MSN;
Anita Lockhart, RN, MSN

Copy Editors
Kimberly Bilotta (supervisor), Scotti Cohn,
Tom DeZego, Jen Fielding, Amy Furman,
Elizabeth Mooney, Dona Perkins,
Irene Pontarelli, Pamela Wingrod

Designer
Linda Franklin (project manager),
Lynn Foulk (book design),
Joseph John Clark (cover design)

Digital Composition Services
Diane Paluba (manager), Joyce Rossi Biletz,
Donna S. Morris

Manufacturing
Beth J. Welsh

Editorial Assistants
Megan L. Aldinger, Karen J. Kirk,
Linda K. Ruhf

Design Assistant
Georg W. Purvis IV

Indexer
Barbara Hodgson

ACC Library Services
Austin, Texas

NSDIS010407

Library of Congress
Cataloging-in-Publication Data

Nursing. Understanding diseases.
    p. ; cm.
  Includes bibliographical references and index.
  1. Diseases—Handbooks, manuals, etc. 2. Nursing—Handbooks, manuals, etc. I. Lippincott Williams & Wilkins.
  [DNLM: 1. Nursing Care—Handbooks. 2. Disease—Handbooks. 3. Nursing Process—Handbooks. WY 49 N9759 2008]
  RT65.N826 2008
  610.73—dc22   2006101878
  ISBN-13: 978-1-58255-665-9 (alk. paper)
  ISBN-10: 1-58255-665-2 (alk. paper)

Contents

Contributors and consultants

Pamela C. Anania, APRN, MSN
Nursing Lab Instructor/Adjunct Faculty
Brookdale Community College
Lincroft, N.J.

Julie A. Calvery, RN, MSN
Instructor
University of Arkansas
Fort Smith

Lillian Craig, RN, MSN, FNP-C
Family Nurse Practitioner
Adjunct Faculty
Oklahoma Panhandle State University
Goodwell

Vivian C. Gamblian, RN, MSN
Professor of Nursing
Collin County Community College
McKinney, Tex.

Kay L. Luft, RN, MN, CCRN
Assistant Professor
Saint Luke's College
Kansas City, Mo.

Monica Narvaez Ramirez, RN, MSN
Nursing Instructor
University of the Incarnate Word School of
    Nursing & Health Professions
San Antonio, Tex.

Ruthie Robinson, RN, PhD, FAEN
Director Clinical Research
Christus Hospital
Beaumont, Tex.

Lisa Salamon, APRN-BC, MSN, WOCN
Clinical Nurse Specialist
Aurora Healthcare
St. Luke's Medical Center
Milwaukee

Bruce Austin Scott, APRN-BC, MSN
Nursing Instructor
San Joaquin Delta College
Staff Nurse
St. Josephs Medical Center
Stockton, Calif.

Kimberly Such-Smith, RN, BSN, LNC
Nurse Case Manager/Legal Nurse
    Consultant
Nursing Analysis & Review, LLC
Byron, Minn.

Allison J. Terry, RN, PhD
Director, Center for Nursing
Alabama Board of Nursing
Montgomery

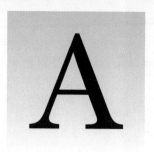

Acne vulgaris

An inflammatory disorder of the sebaceous glands, acne vulgaris is the most common skin problem in adolescents, although lesions can appear as early as age 8. Although acne is more common and more severe in boys than girls, it usually occurs in girls at an earlier age and tends to last longer, sometimes into adulthood. The prognosis is good with treatment.

Causes
- Exact cause unknown
- Possible primary causes: follicular occlusion, androgen-stimulated sebum production, and *Propionibacterium acnes*

Flare-ups
- Certain drugs, including corticosteroids, glucocorticoids, halogens, phenobarbital, phenytoin (Dilantin), isoniazid (Laniazid), and lithium
- Cosmetics
- Emotional stress
- Exposure to industrial compounds
- Trauma or rubbing from tight clothing
- Unfavorable climate

Signs and symptoms
- Closed comedo, or whitehead (if it doesn't protrude from the follicle and is covered by the epidermis)
- Open comedo, or blackhead (if it does protrude and isn't covered by the epidermis)
- Inflammation and characteristic acne pustules, papules or, in severe forms, cysts or abscesses
- Scarring, if chronic recurring lesions

Diagnostic tests
- Results of culture and sensitivity testing of pustules show causative organism of secondary bacterial infection.

Treatment
- A topical antibacterial (such as benzoyl peroxide, clindamycin [Cleocin], or erythromycin) is prescribed, alone or with tretinoin (Avita), a keratolytic, or salicylic acid.
- A systemic antibiotic, usually tetracycline (Sumycin), decreases bacterial growth until the patient is in remission; then a lower dose is used for long-term maintenance. Tetracycline is contraindicated during pregnancy and childhood because it discolors developing teeth. Erythromycin is an alternative for these patients.
- Because of its severe adverse effects, a 16- to 20-week course of oral isotretinoin (Accutane) is limited to those with severe papulopustular or cystic acne who don't respond to conventional therapy. (See *Avoiding risks of isotretinoin therapy,* page 2.)

Avoiding risks of isotretinoin therapy

Because isotretinoin is known to cause birth defects, the manufacturer, with approval of the Food and Drug Administration, recommends the following precautions:
- Pregnancy testing before dispensing
- Effective contraception during treatment
- Dispensing only a 30-day supply
- Repeat pregnancy testing throughout the treatment period
- Informed consent of the patient or parents regarding the drug's adverse effects.

- Oral hormonal contraceptives (such as Ortho Tri-Cyclen) or spironolactone (Aldactone) may be prescribed for female patients because these drugs have anti-androgenic effects.
- Intralesional corticosteroid injections may be ordered.
- Exposure to ultraviolet light may be ordered (but never when a photosensitizing agent, such a tretinoin, is being used).
- Cryotherapy may be ordered.
- Additional treatments include comedo extraction, dermabrasion, or acne surgery, which involves drainage and extraction of larger cysts.

Nursing considerations

- Check the patient's drug history because certain drugs may cause an acne flare-up.
- Try to identify predisposing factors that may be eliminated or modified.
- Explain to the patient and his family that the prescribed treatment is more likely to improve acne than a strict diet and fanatic scurbbing with soap and water. Provide written instructions regarding treatment.
- Instruct the patient using tretinoin to apply it at least 30 minutes after washing the face and at least 1 hour before bedtime. Warn against using it around the eyes or lips. After treatments, the skin should look pink and dry. If it appears red or starts to peel, the preparation may have to be weakened or applied less often. Advise the patient to avoid exposure to sunlight or to use a sunscreen.
- If the prescribed regimen includes tretinoin and benzoyl peroxide, avoid skin irritation by using one preparation in the morning and the other at night.

DRUG CHALLENGE

 Instruct the patient to take tetracycline on an empty stomach and not to take it with an antacid or milk.

- f the patient is taking isotretinoin, tell him to avoid vitamin A supplements, which can worsen any adverse reactions.
- Warn the female patient taking isotretinoin about the severe risk of teratogenesis associated with the use of this drug.
- Monitor the patient's liver function and lipid levels when isotretinoin is used.
- Offer emotional support.

Acromegaly and gigantism

Acromegaly and gigantism are chronic, progressive diseases marked by hormonal dysfunction and startling skeletal overgrowth. Acromegaly occurs after epiphyseal closure, causing bone thickening and transverse growth and visceromegaly. Gigantism begins before epiphyseal closure and causes proportional overgrowth of all body tissues.

Acromegaly develops slowly, whereas gigantism develops abruptly. Although the prognosis depends on the causative factor, these disorders usually reduce life expectancy unless treated in a timely way.

Causes
- Extrapyramidal pituitary lesions or other tumors that cause oversecretion of hGH
- Oversecretion of human growth hormone (hGH) that produces changes throughout the entire body, resulting in acromegaly and, when oversecretion occurs before puberty, gigantism
- Possible genetic cause
- Somatotropic adenomas

Signs and symptoms
Acromegaly
- Arthropathy
- Carpal tunnel syndrome
- Proximal muscle weakness
- Fatigue
- Acanthosis nigricans (an eruption of velvet warty benign growths and hyperpigmentation occurring in the skin of the axillae, neck, anogenital area)
- Skin tags
- Oily skin
- Cartilaginous and connective tissue overgrowth
- Enlarged supraorbital ridge and thickened ears and nose
- Marked projection of the jaw, which may interfere with chewing
- Voice sounds deep and hollow
- Thickened fingers
- Coronary artery disease
- Cardiomyopathy with arrhythmias, left ventricular hypertrophy, and decreased diastolic function
- Hypertension
- Upper airway obstruction with sleep apnea
- Generalized visceromegaly, including cardiomegaly, macroglossia, and thyroid gland enlargement
- Barrel chest and kyphosis
- Signs of diabetes mellitus and glucose intolerance

Gigantism
- Same skeletal abnormalities and signs of glucose intolerance seen in acromegaly
- Pituitary tumor enlargement (causing loss of other trophic hormones, such as thyroid-stimulating hormone, luteinizing hormone, follicle-stimulating hormone, and corticotropin)

Diagnostic tests
- Serum hGH levels measured by radioimmunoassay typically are elevated.
- Glucose suppression test fails to suppress the hormone level to below the accepted normal value of 2 ng/ml.
- Skull X-rays, a computed tomography scan, arteriography, and magnetic resonance imaging determine the presence and extent of the pituitary lesion.
- Bone X-rays show a thickening of the cranium (especially of frontal, occipital, and parietal bones) and of the long bones as well as osteoarthritis in the spine.

Treatment
- Cranial or transsphenoidal hypophysectomy or pituitary radiation therapy is ordered to remove the underlying tumor.
- Replacement of thyroid and gonadal hormones and cortisone are ordered, postoperatively.
- Bromocriptine (Parlodel) and octreotide (Sandostatin) are used to inhibit hGH synthesis.

Nursing considerations

- Provide the patient with emotional support to help him cope with an altered body image.
- Assess the patient for skeletal changes and muscle weakness.
- Perform or assist with range-of-motion exercises.

Keep the patient's skin dry. Avoid using an oily lotion because the skin is already oily.

- Monitor the patient's blood glucose level. Check for signs and symptoms of hyperglycemia, including fatigue, polyuria, and polydipsia.
- Reassure the patient and his family that the disease causes mood changes, which can be managed with treatment.
- Before surgery, reinforce what the surgeon has told the patient and try to allay the patient's fear.
- After surgery
  - Diligently monitor the patient's vital signs and neurologic status. Be alert for signs of increased intracranial pressure.
  - Check blood glucose levels frequently. Remember, hGH levels usually fall rapidly after surgery, removing an insulin antagonist effect in many patients and possibly precipitating hypoglycemia.
  - Measure intake and output hourly and watch for large increases in urine output. Transient diabetes insipidus, which sometimes occurs after surgery for hyperpituitarism, can cause such increases in urine output.
  - If the transsphenoidal approach is used, the surgical site is packed with a piece of tissue usually taken from a midthigh donor site. Watch for cerebrospinal fluid leaks from the packed site. Look for increased external nasal drainage or drainage into the nasopharynx.
  - Help the patient get out of bed and walk on the first or second day after surgery, per prescribed level of activity.
- Make sure the patient and his family understand which hormones are to be taken and why, as well as the correct times and dosages.

▌Acute coronary syndromes

Acute myocardial infarction (MI), including ST-segment elevation MI (STEMI) and non–ST-segment elevation MI (NSTEMI), and unstable angina are now recognized as part of a group of clinical diseases called acute coronary syndromes (ACSs). Rupture or erosion of plaque—an unstable and lipid-rich substance—initiates almost all coronary syndromes. The rupture results in platelet adhesions, fibrin clot formation, and activation of thrombin.

Mortality is high when treatment is delayed, and almost one-half of sudden deaths caused by an MI occur before hospitalization or within 1 hour of the onset of symptoms. The prognosis improves if vigorous treatment begins immediately.

Causes
- Atherosclerosis
- Embolus

Risk factors
- Diabetes
- Elevated homocysteine, C-reactive protein, and fibrinogen levels
- Excessive alcohol consumption
- Family history of heart disease
- High-fat, high-carbohydrate diet
- Hyperlipoproteinemia
- Hypertension
- Obesity
- Postmenopausal status

- Sedentary lifestyle
- Smoking
- Stress

Signs and symptoms
Angina
- Burning, squeezing, and a crushing tightness in the substernal or precordial chest that may radiate to the left arm or shoulder blade, the neck, or the jaw
- Pain after physical exertion, emotional excitement, exposure to the cold or consumption of a large meal

MI
- Uncomfortable pressure, squeezing, burning, severe persistent pain or fullness in the center of the chest lasting several minutes (usually longer than 15 minutes)
- Pain radiating to the shoulders, neck, arms, or jaw or pain in the back between the shoulder blades
- Lightheadedness or fainting
- Sweating
- Nausea
- Shortness of breath
- Anxiety or a feeling of impending doom

Diagnostic tests
- Electrocardiography helps determine which area of the heart and which coronary arteries are involved.
- Serial cardiac enzymes and protein levels may show a characteristic rise in CK-MB, the proteins troponin T and I, and myoglobin.
- Laboratory testing may reveal elevated white blood cell count and erythrocyte sedimentation rate and changes in electrolyte levels.
- Echocardiography may show ventricular wall motion abnormalities and may detect septal or papillary muscle rupture.

- Transesophageal echocardiography may reveal areas of decreased heart muscle wall movement, indicating ischemia.
- Chest X-rays may show left-sided heart failure, cardiomegaly, or other noncardiac causes of dyspnea and chest pain.
- Nuclear imaging scanning using thallium 201 or technetium 99m can be used to identify areas of infarction and areas of viable muscle cells.
- Cardiac catheterization may be used to identify the involved coronary artery as well as to provide information on ventricular function and pressures and volumes within the heart. (See *Viewing the coronary arteries,* page 6.)

Treatment
- Supplemental oxygen is used to increase oxygen supply to the heart.
- Nitroglycerin is ordered to relieve chest pain.
- Morphine is prescribed to relieve pain.
- Aspirin is used to inhibit platelet aggregation.
- Low-cholesterol, low-sodium, low-fat, high-fiber diet is ordered.
- For the patient with unstable angina and NSTEMI, treatment also includes:
  - a beta-adrenergic blocker to reduce the heart's workload and oxygen demands.
  - heparin and a glycoprotein IIb/IIIa inhibitor to minimize platelet aggregation and the danger of coronary occlusion with high-risk patients (patients with planned catheterization and positive troponin).
  - nitroglycerin I.V. to dilate coronary arteries and relieve chest pain.
  - percutaneous transluminal coronary angioplasty (PTCA) or coronary artery bypass graft (CABG) surgery for obstructive lesions.
  - an antilipemic to reduce elevated serum cholesterol or triglyceride levels.

Viewing the coronary arteries

Acute coronary syndrome commonly results when a thrombus progresses and occludes blood flow through a coronary artery. This illustration shows the major coronary vessels that may be involved.

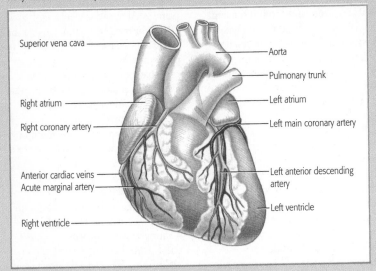

- For the patient with STEMI, treatment includes the above initial interventions and also:
  - thrombolytic therapy (unless contraindicated) within 12 hours of onset of symptoms to restore vessel patency and minimize necrosis.
  - heparin I.V. to promote patency in the affected coronary artery.
  - a glycoprotein IIb/IIIa inhibitor to minimize platelet aggregation.
  - an angiotensin-converting enzyme (ACE) inhibitor to reduce afterload and preload and prevent remodeling (begin 6 hours after admission or when the patient's condition is stable)
  - PTCA, stent placement, or CABG surgery to open blocked or narrowed arteries.

Nursing considerations

- Institute continuous cardiac monitoring and frequently monitor the electrocardiogram (ECG) to detect rate changes or arrhythmias. Place rhythm strips in the patient's chart periodically according to your facility's policy.
- Monitor and record the patient's blood pressure, temperature, and heart and breath sounds.
- Explain the importance of reporting pain immediately.
- Obtain a 12-lead ECG during episodes of chest pain.
- Assess and record location, severity, and duration of pain.
- Give prescribed analgesics and other medications.
- Check the patient's blood pressure after giving nitroglycerin, especially after the first dose.
- Monitor intake and output closely.

- Monitor the patient for crackles, cough, tachypnea, and edema, which may indicate impending left-sided heart failure.
- If the patient has undergone PTCA, provide sheath care. Maintain strict bed rest and keep the leg with the sheath insertion site immobile. Monitor the site closely for bleeding. Check peripheral pulses in the affected leg frequently.
- Provide emotional support, and help to reduce stress and anxiety.
- Initiate cardiac rehabilitation, according to your facility's protocol.
- Review dietary restrictions with the patient. If he must follow a low-cholesterol, low-sodium, low-fat, high-fiber diet, provide a list of foods that he should avoid. Ask the dietitian to speak to the patient and his family.
- Refer the patient to a smoking-cessation program, if needed.
- Thoroughly explain the patient's treatment regimen. Warn the patient about adverse reactions to drugs, and advise him to report them to his practitioner.
- Refer the patient to a weight-reduction program, if needed.
- Counsel the patient to resume sexual activity progressively.

Acute respiratory distress syndrome

A form of pulmonary edema that causes acute respiratory failure, acute respiratory distress syndrome (ARDS) results from increased permeability of the alveolocapillary membrane. Fluid accumulates in the lung interstitium, alveolar spaces, and small airways, causing the lung to stiffen. This stiffening impairs ventilation, prohibiting adequate oxygenation of pulmonary capillary blood. Severe ARDS can cause intractable and fatal hypoxemia, but patients who recover may have little or no permanent lung damage.

Causes
- Aspiration of gastric contents
- Cardiopulmonary bypass
- Drug overdose (barbiturates, glutethimide, opioids) or blood transfusion
- Microemboli (fat or air emboli or disseminated intravascular coagulation)
- Near drowning
- Oxygen toxicity
- Pancreatitis
- Sepsis (primarily gram-negative)
- Smoke or chemical inhalation (nitrous oxide, chlorine, ammonia)
- Trauma (lung contusion, head injury, long bone fracture with fat emboli)
- Viral, bacterial, or fungal pneumonia

Signs and symptoms
Early
- Rapid, shallow breathing and dyspnea (within hours to days of the initial injury)
- Intercostal and suprasternal retractions
- Crackles and rhonchi on auscultation
- Hypoxemia causes restlessness, apprehension, mental sluggishness, motor dysfunction, and tachycardia

Late
- Overwhelming hypoxemia
- Hypotension
- Decreased urine output
- Respiratory and metabolic acidosis
- Ventricular fibrillation or standstill

Diagnostic tests
- Arterial blood gas (ABG) analysis first shows a decreased partial pressure of arterial oxygen (Pa_{O_2})—less than 60 mm Hg—and a decreased partial pressure of arterial carbon dioxide (Pa_{CO_2})—less than 35 mm Hg. pH usually shows respiratory alkalosis. As ARDS becomes more severe, ABG levels indicate respiratory acidosis (a Pa_{CO_2} greater than 45 mm Hg) and metabolic acidosis (a bicarbonate level less than 22 mEq/L) as

well as a decreasing PaO_2, despite oxygen therapy.

- Pulmonary artery (PA) catheterization helps identify the cause of pulmonary edema by allowing evaluation of pulmonary artery wedge pressure (PAWP) (normal PAWP values in ARDS are 12 mm Hg or less) and collection of PA blood (shows decreased oxygen saturation, indicating tissue hypoxia).
- Serial chest X-rays initially show bilateral infiltrates; in later stages, the X-rays show ground-glass appearance and, eventually (as hypoxemia becomes irreversible), "whiteouts" of both lung fields.
- Gram stain and sputum culture and sensitivity test results show infectious organism (if infection is the cause).
- Blood cultures reveal the infectious organism.
- Serum amylase levels increase if the patient has underlying pancreatitis.
- Toxicology test identifies the drug ingested in ARDS caused by a drug overdose.

Treatment

- Treatment of the underlying cause is started.
- Humidified oxygen is given through a tight-fitting mask, which allows for the use of continuous positive airway pressure.
- For hypoxemia that doesn't respond adequately to this treatment, the following may be ordered: ventilatory support with intubation, volume ventilation, and positive end-expiratory pressure (PEEP); pressure-controlled inverse ratio ventilation to reverse the conventional inspiration-to-expiration ratio and minimize the risk of barotrauma.
- When a patient with ARDS needs mechanical ventilation, an opioid, sedative, or neuromuscular blocker may be ordered to ease ventilation and decrease oxygen consumption.

- High-dose steroids may be prescribed for ARDS caused by fat emboli or chemical injury.
- Diuretics are ordered.
- Correction of electrolyte and acid-base abnormalities is ordered.
- I.V. fluids and a vasopressor may be needed to maintain blood pressure.
- Antimicrobial is prescribed if the patient has a treatable infection.

Nursing considerations

- Frequently assess the patient's respiratory status. Be alert for retractions on inspiration. Note rate, rhythm, and depth of respirations, and watch for dyspnea and the use of accessory muscles of respiration. On auscultation, listen for adventitious or diminished breath sounds. Check for clear, frothy sputum that may indicate pulmonary edema.
- Observe and document the patient's neurologic status, including level of consciousness and mental sluggishness.
- Maintain a patent airway by suctioning, using sterile, nontraumatic technique. Ensure adequate humidification to help liquefy tenacious secretions.
- Closely monitor heart rate and blood pressure. Watch for arrhythmias that may result from hypoxemia, acid-base disturbances, or electrolyte imbalance.
- Give medications as prescribed.
- With PA catheterization, know the desired PAWP level. Watch for decreasing mixed venous oxygen saturation.
- Monitor serum electrolyte levels, and report any imbalances immediately. Measure intake and output, and weigh the patient daily.
- Check ventilator settings frequently. Monitor ABG levels; check for metabolic and respiratory acidosis and PaO_2 changes.
- If the patient has severe hypoxemia, he may need controlled mechanical ventilation with PEEP and inverse ratio ventila-

tion. Give sedatives, as needed, to reduce restlessness.

- Because PEEP may decrease cardiac output, check for hypotension, tachycardia, and decreased urine output. Suction only as needed to maintain PEEP.
- Reposition the patient frequently, and note any increase in secretions, temperature, or hypotension, which may indicate a deteriorating condition.
- Accurately record caloric intake. Give tube feedings and parenteral nutrition, if required.
- Perform passive range-of-motion exercises, or help the patient perform active exercises, if possible. Provide meticulous skin care. Allow periods of uninterrupted sleep.
- Provide the patient and his family with emotional support.

Acute respiratory failure

In patients with essentially normal lung tissue, acute respiratory failure (ARF) usually means a partial pressure of arterial carbon dioxide ($Paco_2$) greater than 50 mm Hg and a partial pressure of arterial oxygen (Pao_2) less than 50 mm Hg. These limits, however, don't apply to patients with chronic obstructive pulmonary disease (COPD), who commonly have a consistently high $Paco_2$ and low Pao_2. In COPD patients, ARF is indicated only by acute deterioration in arterial blood gas (ABG) levels and corresponding clinical deterioration.

Causes

- Airway irritants—smoke or fumes
- Any condition that increases the work of breathing and decreases the respiratory drive of patients with COPD
- Chest trauma
- Head trauma
- Heart failure

- Injudicious use of sedatives, opioids, tranquilizers, or oxygen
- Metabolic acidosis
- Myocardial infarction
- Myxedema
- Pneumothorax
- Pulmonary emboli
- Thoracic or abdominal surgery

Signs and symptoms

- Increased, decreased, or normal respiratory rate, depending on the cause; shallow or deep respirations, or respirations that alternate between the two; and air hunger
- Cyanosis of the oral mucosa, lips, and nail beds possible, depending on the hemoglobin (Hb) level and arterial oxygenation
- Crackles, rhonchi, wheezes, or diminished breath sounds
- Restlessness, confusion, loss of concentration, irritability, tremulousness, diminished tendon reflexes, and papilledema; possible coma
- Tachycardia, with increased cardiac output and mildly elevated blood pressure (occurs early in response to a low Pao_2)
- Arrhythmias
- Pulmonary hypertension
- Accessory muscle use
- Tachypnea
- Cold, clammy skin

Diagnostic tests

- Pulse oximetry may show decreased arterial oxygen saturation.
- ABG analysis reveals hypercapnia and hypoxemia; bicarbonate levels are increased, indicating metabolic alkalosis or metabolic compensation for chronic respiratory acidosis.
- Hb levels and hematocrit are abnormally low, possibly due to blood loss, indicating decreased oxygen-carrying capacity.

- Serum electrolyte levels may indicate hypokalemia, which may result from compensatory hyperventilation—an attempt to correct alkalosis; hypochloremia is common with metabolic alkalosis.
- White blood cell count is elevated if ARF is due to bacterial infection; in certain cases of profound septicemia, the leukocyte count may be decreased.
- Gram stain and sputum culture results can identify pathogens.
- Chest X-rays reveal pulmonary pathology, such as emphysema, atelectasis, lesions, pneumothorax, infiltrates, or effusions.
- Electrocardiography reveals arrhythmias, which commonly suggest cor pulmonale and myocardial hypoxia. Large P waves ("p pulmonale") may indicate a history of right-sided heart failure.

Treatment

- Oxygen therapy using nasal prongs or a Venturi mask to raise the patient's PaO_2 (if the patient has COPD) is used cautiously to promote oxygenation.
- Bidirectional positive-pressure airway mask is used over the oronasal region or mechanical ventilation through an endotracheal or a tracheostomy tube is ordered (if significant respiratory acidosis persists).
- High-frequency ventilation is instituted (if the patient doesn't respond to conventional mechanical ventilation).
- Antibiotics are prescribed for infection.
- Bronchodilator is used to maintain airway patency.
- Anxiolytic is ordered to promote relaxation and reduce anxiety.
- Corticosteroids are prescribed to decrease inflammation.
- Histamine-receptor antagonist may be ordered to prevent ulcer formation.

Nursing considerations

- Assess the patient's respiratory status frequently (pulse oximetry, breath sounds, and ABG results) and report changes immediately.
- Give enough oxygen to maintain a PaO_2 of at least 50 to 60 mm Hg. Patients with COPD usually require only small amounts of supplemental oxygen.
- Maintain a patent airway. If the patient is retaining carbon dioxide, encourage him to cough and to breathe deeply with pursed lips.
- If the patient is alert, have him use an incentive spirometer.
- Keep the head of the bed elevated to at least 30 degrees.
- If the patient is intubated and lethargic, turn him every 1 to 2 hours.
- Use postural drainage and chest physiotherapy to help clear the patient's secretions.
- Monitor and record serum electrolyte levels carefully, and correct imbalances; monitor fluid balance by recording the patient's intake and output or daily weight.
- Monitor the patient for cardiac arrhythmias.
- Give prescribed medications.

For mechanical ventilation

- Check ventilator settings, cuff pressures, and ABG values frequently because the fraction of inspired oxygen (FIO_2) setting depends on ABG levels. Draw a blood sample for ABG analysis 20 to 30 minutes after every FIO_2 change, or check ABG levels with oximetry, as ordered.
- Change ventilator circuits every 24 to 48 hours, per your facility's policy.
- Suction the trachea, after hyperoxygenation, as needed. Observe for a change in the quantity, consistency, or color of secretions. Provide humidification to liquefy the secretions.

▪ Keep the nasotracheal tube midline within the nostrils, and provide good hygiene. Loosen tape periodically to prevent skin breakdown. Avoid excessive movement of any tubes, and make sure the ventilator tubing is adequately supported.

▪ Provide an alternate means of communication.

▪ Provide emotional support to the patient and his family.

Acute tubular necrosis

Acute tubular necrosis (ATN) is the most common cause of acute renal failure in critically ill patients, and it accounts for about 75% of all cases of acute renal failure. ATN injures the tubular segment of the nephron, causing renal failure and uremic syndrome. Mortality can be as high as 70%, depending on complications from underlying diseases. Patients with nonoliguric forms of ATN have a better prognosis.

Causes

▪ Diseased tubular epithelium
▪ Ischemic injury to glomerular epithelial cells
▪ Ischemic injury to vascular endothelium
▪ Obstruction of urine flow

Signs and symptoms

▪ Bleeding abnormalities (petechiae and ecchymosis)
▪ Decreased urine output
▪ Dry mucous membranes and skin
▪ Hyperkalemia
▪ Lethargy
▪ Twitching or seizures
▪ Uremic odor of the breath
▪ Uremic syndrome with oliguria (or, rarely, anuria) and confusion, which may progress to uremic coma

Diagnostic tests

▪ Urinalysis reveals urinary sediment containing red blood cells (RBCs) and casts and diluted urine with a low specific gravity (1.010), low osmolality (less than 400 mOsm/kg), and a high sodium level (40 to 60 mEq/L).

▪ Blood studies reveal elevated blood urea nitrogen and serum creatinine levels, anemia, defects in platelet adherence, metabolic acidosis, and hyperkalemia.

▪ Electrocardiography may show arrhythmias (from electrolyte imbalances) and, with hyperkalemia, a widening QRS complex, disappearing P waves, and tall, peaked T waves.

Treatment

▪ Administration of diuretics and infusion of a large volume of fluids flush tubules of cellular casts and debris and replace fluid loss. Long-term fluid management requires daily replacement of projected and calculated losses (including insensible loss).

▪ Transfusion of packed RBCs is ordered for anemia.

▪ An antibiotic is prescribed to treat infection.

▪ Emergency I.V. administration of 50% glucose, regular insulin, and sodium bicarbonate is ordered to treat hyperkalemia.

▪ Sodium polystyrene sulfonate with sorbitol may be given orally or by enema to reduce extracellular potassium levels.

▪ Peritoneal dialysis or hemodialysis may be needed if the patient is catabolic.

Nursing considerations

▪ Assess cardiovascular and respiratory status frequently and report changes immediately.

▪ Accurately record intake and output, including wound drainage, nasogastric output, and peritoneal dialysis and hemodialysis balances. Weigh the patient daily. Watch for fluid overload.

- Monitor hemoglobin level and hematocrit, and give blood products as prescribed. Watch for early signs and symptoms of a transfusion reaction (such as fever, rash, and chills). If the patient develops such signs and symptoms, stop the transfusion immediately and notify the practitioner.
- Give prescribed medications.
- Monitor laboratory results, and be alert for evidence of electrolyte imbalances.
- Enforce dietary restriction of foods containing sodium and potassium, such as bananas, orange juice, and baked potatoes.
- To maintain an anabolic state, provide adequate calories and essential amino acids, while restricting protein intake. Total parenteral nutrition may be indicated if the patient is severely debilitated or catabolic.
- Watch for signs of diminishing renal perfusion, including hypotension and decreased urine output.
- Encourage coughing and deep breathing to prevent pulmonary complications.
- Perform passive range-of-motion exercises. Help the patient to walk as soon as possible, but guard against exhaustion.
- Provide good skin care; apply lotion or bath oil for dry skin.
- Provide reassurance and emotional support. Encourage the patient and his family to express their fears.

Adrenal hypofunction

Primary adrenal hypofunction or insufficiency (Addison's disease) originates within the adrenal gland itself and is characterized by decreased mineralocorticoid, glucocorticoid, and androgen secretion. Secondary adrenal hypofunc-

tion is due to impaired pituitary secretion of corticotropin and is characterized by decreased glucocorticoid secretion. Secretion of aldosterone, the major mineralocorticoid, is typically unaffected.

Addison's disease is relatively uncommon, though it can occur at any age, in either sex. Secondary adrenal hypofunction occurs when a patient abruptly stops taking an exogenous steroid after long-term therapy or when the pituitary is injured by a tumor or by infiltrative or autoimmune processes. With an early diagnosis and adequate replacement therapy, the prognosis for the person with adrenal hypofunction is good.

Adrenal crisis (addisonian crisis), a critical deficiency of mineralocorticoids and glucocorticoids, generally follows acute stress, sepsis, trauma, surgery, or omission of steroid therapy in patients who have chronic adrenal insufficiency. A medical emergency, adrenal crisis necessitates immediate, vigorous treatment.

Causes
Primary hypofunction
- Autoimmune process in which circulating antibodies react specifically against the adrenal tissue
- Bilateral adrenalectomy
- Hemorrhage into the adrenal gland
- Infections (histoplasmosis, cytomegalovirus)
- Neoplasms
- Tuberculosis

Secondary hypofunction
- Abrupt withdrawal of long-term corticosteroid therapy
- Hypopituitarism (causing decreased corticotropin secretion)
- Removal of a corticotropin-secreting tumor

Adrenal crisis

- Exhausted body stores of glucocorticoids in a patient with adrenal hypofunction after trauma, surgery, or other physiologic stress

Signs and symptoms
Primary hypofunction

- Anorexia
- Areas of vitiligo (absence of pigmentation)
- Asthenia (constant fatigue) is the cardinal symptom, most evident in times of stress
- Bronzed color of the skin
- Craving for salty food
- Darkening of scars
- Decreased tolerance for even minor stress
- Fatigue or asthenia (constant fatigue); asthenia is the cardinal symptom most evident in times of stress
- Increased pigmentation of the mucous membranes, especially the buccal mucosa
- Nausea
- Orthostatic hypotension
- Vomiting
- Weak, irregular pulse
- Weakness
- Weight loss

Secondary hypofunction

- Similar to those of primary hypofunction but without hyperpigmentation because corticotropin and melanocyte-stimulating hormone levels are low

Adrenal crisis

- Coma and death (if untreated)
- Dehydration
- High fever followed by hypothermia (occasionally)
- Hypotension
- Nausea
- Profound weakness and fatigue
- Vomiting

Diagnostic tests

- The corticotropin stimulation test demonstrates plasma cortisol response to corticotropin (administered I.V. over 6 to 8 hours), and may be used to distinguish primary from secondary adrenal insufficiency.
  - With primary adrenal insufficiency (Addison's disease), plasma and urine cortisol levels fail to rise normally in response to corticotropin.
  - With secondary adrenal insufficiency, repeated doses of corticotropin over successive days produce a gradual increase in cortisol levels until normal values are reached. In secondary insufficiency, the aldosterone level is also normal.
- The following laboratory findings strongly suggest acute adrenal insufficiency in a patient with typical symptoms of Addison's disease:
  - Plasma cortisol level is decreased (less than 10 µl/dl in the morning, with a lower level in the evening).
  - Serum sodium level is reduced.
  - Serum potassium, serum calcium, and blood urea nitrogen levels are increased.
  - Hematocrit and lymphocyte and eosinophil counts are elevated.

Treatment

- Lifelong corticosteroid replacement is ordered, usually with cortisone or hydrocortisone.
- For patients with Addison's disease, treatment with oral fludrocortisone (Florinef) is necessary to prevent dangerous dehydration, hypotension, and electrolyte disturbances with hyponatremia and hyperkalemia. (See *Avoiding adrenal crisis,* page 14.)

For adrenal crisis

- Initially, hydrocortisone 100 mg I.V. bolus administration is followed by 50- to 100-mg doses given I.M. or diluted

Avoiding adrenal crisis

A patient with adrenal hypofunction requires lifelong corticosteroid therapy. To help him comply with the prescribed treatment, be sure to incorporate the following into your patient teaching:

■ Teach the patient to recognize the symptoms of too great or too little a dose.

■ Tell the patient that the dose may need to be increased during times of stress (when he has a cold, for example).

■ Teach the patient how to give himself an injection of hydrocortisone.

■ Advise the patient to keep an emergency kit available containing hydrocortisone in a prepared syringe for use in times of stress.

■ Warn that any stress may require additional cortisone to prevent adrenal crisis.

■ Warn that infection, injury, or profuse sweating in hot weather may precipitate adrenal crisis.

■ Instruct the patient to always carry a medical identification card stating that he takes a steroid and giving the name of the drug and the dosage.

with dextrose in normal saline solution and given I.V. until the patient's condition stabilizes; up to 300 mg/day of hydrocortisone and 3 to 5 L of I.V. normal saline solution are required during the acute stage of adrenal crisis.

■ Maintenance doses of hydrocortisone are needed after an adrenal crisis.

Nursing considerations

■ If the patient is experiencing adrenal crisis, monitor vital signs carefully, especially for hypotension, volume depletion, and other signs of shock (decreased level of consciousness and urine output). Watch for hyperkalemia before

treatment and for hypokalemia after treatment.

■ Check the blood glucose level in the patient with diabetes periodically because steroid replacement may necessitate adjustment of the insulin dosage.

■ Carefully record weight and intake and output. While waiting for the mineralocorticoid to take effect, make sure the patient gets plenty of fluids to compensate for excessive fluid loss.

■ If the patient also has an acute medical illness or is undergoing a surgical procedure, he'll require additional steroids to cover these stressful periods.

For maintenance therapy

■ Advise the patient to watch for symptoms of adrenal crisis, and tell him how to provide the necessary self-care when he's discharged from the facility.

■ Arrange for a diet that maintains a balance of sodium and potassium.

■ If the patient is receiving a steroid, monitor him for cushingoid signs such as fluid retention around the eyes and face. Watch for fluid and electrolyte imbalance, especially if the patient is receiving a mineralocorticoid. Monitor his weight and blood pressure to assess body fluid status.

■ If the patient receives only a glucocorticoid, observe him for orthostatic hypotension or electrolyte abnormalities, which may indicate a need for mineralocorticoid therapy.

▌Allergic purpura

Allergic purpura, or anaphylactoid purpura, is a type of nonthrombocytopenic purpura characterized by allergy symptoms and acute or chronic vascular inflammation affecting the skin, joints, or GI or genitourinary (GU) tract. When allergic purpura primarily affects the GI tract with accompanying joint pain, it's called *Henoch-Schönlein syndrome* or *ana-*

phylactoid purpura. However, the term *allergic purpura* applies to purpura associated with many other conditions such as erythema nodosum. An acute attack of allergic purpura can last for several weeks and is potentially fatal (usually from renal failure), although most patients recover.

Fully developed allergic purpura is persistent and debilitating, possibly leading to chronic glomerulonephritis (especially after a streptococcal infection). Allergic purpura affects more males than females and is most prevalent in children ages 3 to 7. The prognosis is more favorable for children than for adults.

Causes
- Allergy to some drugs and vaccines, to insect bites, or to some foods (such as wheat, eggs, milk, and chocolate)
- Autoimmune reaction directed against vascular walls, triggered by a bacterial infection (particularly streptococcal infection)

Signs and symptoms
- Angioneurotic edema (occasionally)
- Anorexia
- Bleeding from the mucosal surfaces of the ureters, bladder, or urethra
- Glomerulonephritis (occasionally)
- Headache
- Henoch-Schönlein syndrome
- Localized edema of the hands, feet, or scalp
- Moderate and irregular fever
- Nephritis
- Paresthesia
- Periarticular effusion
- Pruritus
- Renal hemorrhages
- Rheumatoid pain
- Skin lesions that are purple, macular, ecchymotic, and varying in size, usually appearing in symmetrical patterns on the arms and legs; in children they usually expand and become hemorrhagic

Diagnostic tests
- White blood cell count and erythrocyte sedimentation rate are elevated.
- Tourniquet test result is positive.
- Coagulation test results are normal.
- X-rays of the small bowel may reveal areas of transient edema.
- Test results for blood in the urine and stool are usually positive.
- Increased blood urea nitrogen and serum creatinine levels may indicate renal involvement.

Treatment
- A corticosteroid may be given to relieve edema from severe allergic purpura.
- An analgesic may be given to relieve joint and abdominal pain.
- Some patients with chronic renal disease may benefit from immunosuppression with azathioprine (Imuran) or a corticosteroid, along with identification of the provocative allergen.

Nursing considerations
- Encourage the patient to maintain an elimination diet to help identify specific allergenic foods so that these foods can be eliminated from his diet.
- Monitor skin lesions and assess level of pain. Provide an analgesic, if needed.
- Watch carefully for complications: GI and GU tract bleeding, edema, nausea, vomiting, headache, hypertension (with nephritis), abdominal rigidity and tenderness, and absence of stool (with intussusception).
- Help with passive or active range-of-motion exercises if the patient is bedridden.
- After the acute stage, stress the need for the patient to *immediately* tell the practitioner if symptoms recur and to

return for follow-up urinalysis as scheduled.

Allergic rhinitis

An immune disorder, allergic rhinitis is a reaction to airborne (inhaled) allergens. Depending on the allergen, the resulting rhinitis and conjunctivitis may be seasonal (hay fever) or year-round (perennial allergic rhinitis). Allergic rhinitis is the most common atopic allergic reaction, affecting more than 20 million U.S. residents.

Causes
- Immunoglobulin (Ig) E–mediated, type I hypersensitivity response to an environmental antigen (allergen) in a genetically susceptible individual

Signs and symptoms
- Dark circles under the eyes (allergic shiners)

Seasonal allergic rhinitis
- Excessive lacrimation
- Headache or sinus pain

- Itching in the throat
- Malaise
- Nasal obstruction or congestion
- Paroxysmal sneezing
- Profuse watery rhinorrhea
- Pruritus of the nose and eyes, usually accompanied by pale, cyanotic, edematous nasal mucosa; red and edematous eyelids and conjunctivae

Perennial allergic rhinitis
- Chronic nasal obstruction or stuffiness extending to eustachian tube obstruction, particularly in children
- Nasal polyps
- Conjunctivitis and other extranasal effects (rare)

Diagnostic tests
- Microscopic examination of sputum and nasal secretions reveals excessive eosinophils.
- Blood chemistry studies show normal or elevated IgE levels.
- Skin testing, paired with tested responses to environmental stimuli, can help pinpoint the responsible allergens.

Treatment
- Eliminate the environmental antigen, if possible.
- Immunotherapy or desensitization with injections of extracted allergens may be indicated.
- Antihistamines, such as fexofenadine (Allegra), loratadine (Claritin), and cetirizine (Zyrtec), may be prescribed.
- Inhaled intranasal steroids, such as flunisolide (Aerobid) and beclomethasone (Qvar), may be indicated.

Nursing considerations
- When caring for the patient with allergic rhinitis, monitor his compliance with the prescribed drug regimen. Also, carefully note any changes in the control of his symptoms or any signs of drug misuse.

Avoiding bouts of allergic rhinitis

If the patient has allergic rhinitis, advise him to reduce environmental exposure to airborne allergens by:
- sleeping with windows closed
- avoiding the outdoors during high-pollen seasons
- using room air conditioners and air filtration devices to filter allergens and minimize moisture and dust
- eliminating dust-collecting items (such as wool blankets, deep-pile carpets, and heavy drapes) from the home
- removing pets, if animal dander is the suspected allergen.

- Before giving allergen injections, assess the patient's symptoms. Afterward, watch for adverse reactions, including anaphylaxis and severe localized erythema.
- Keep epinephrine and emergency resuscitation equipment available, and observe the patient for 30 minutes after the injection. Instruct the patient to call the practitioner if a delayed reaction occurs.
- Teach the patient how to reduce environmental exposures. (See *Avoiding bouts of allergic rhinitis.*)
- If the patient's condition is severe or resistant to conventional treatment, he may have to consider a drastic change in lifestyle, such as relocation to a pollen-free area, either seasonally or year-round.

Alzheimer's disease

Also known as *primary degenerative dementia,* Alzheimer's disease accounts for more than half of all dementias. An estimated 5% of people older than age 65 have a severe form of this disease, and 12% suffer from mild to moderate dementia. The signs and symptoms of Alzheimer's disease have an insidious onset. Because this is a primary progressive dementia, the prognosis is poor.

Causes
- Exact cause unknown
- Environmental factors, such as aluminum and manganese
- Genetic immunologic factors
- Neurochemical factors, such as deficiencies in acetylcholine (a neurotransmitter), somatostatin, substance P, and norepinephrine
- Trauma
- Viral factors such as slow-growing central nervous system viruses

Signs and symptoms
- Forgetfulness
- Recent memory loss
- Difficulty learning and remembering new information
- Deterioration in personal hygiene and appearance
- Inability to concentrate
- Difficulty in performing tasks that require abstract thinking and activities that require judgment
- Progressive and severe deterioration in memory, language, and motor function
- Loss of coordination
- Inability to write or speak
- Personality changes (restlessness, irritability)
- Nocturnal awakenings
- Disorientation
- Emotional lability

Diagnostic tests
The diagnosis is based on an accurate history from a reliable family member, mental status and neurologic examinations, and psychometric testing.
- Positron emission tomography scan measures the metabolic activity of the cerebral cortex and may help in reaching an early diagnosis.
- Computed tomography scan may show progressive brain atrophy in excess of that which occurs during normal aging.
- Magnetic resonance imaging may rule out intracranial lesions as the source of dementia.
- Various tests are performed to rule out other disorders. Ultimately, however, the disease can't be confirmed until death, when an autopsy reveals pathologic findings.

Treatment
- Centrally acting anticholinesterases—donepezil (Aricept), rivastigmine (Exelon), and galantamine (Razadyne)—are used to treat memory deficits and potentially delay the onset of Alzheimer's disease.

- Memantine (Namenda) is an N-methyl-D-aspartic acid (NMDA) receptor antagonist prescribed to treat moderate to severe disease.
- A psychostimulator (such as methylphenidate) may be ordered to enhance the patient's mood.
- Other drugs may be prescribed to treat specific behavioral symptoms, such as anxiety, depression, agitation, and sleeplessness.

Nursing considerations

- Focus on supporting the patient's abilities and teach him to compensate for the abilities he has lost.
- Establish an effective communication system with the patient and his family to help them adjust to the patient's altered cognitive abilities.
- Offer emotional support to the patient and his family. Teach them about the disease, and refer them to social service and community resources for legal and financial advice and support.
- Provide the patient with a safe environment. Encourage him to exercise to help maintain mobility.

Amyotrophic lateral sclerosis

Commonly called *Lou Gehrig disease,* after the New York Yankee first baseman who died of this disorder, amyotrophic lateral sclerosis (ALS) is the most common motor neuron disease causing muscular atrophy. Onset occurs between ages 40 and 70. A chronic, progressively debilitating disease, ALS is invariably fatal.

Causes

- Exact cause unknown; genetic component in about 10% of patients
- Autoimmune disorder that affects immune complexes in the renal glomerulus and basement membrane
- Metabolic interference in nucleic acid production by nerve fibers
- Nutritional deficiency related to a disturbance in enzyme metabolism
- Virus that creates metabolic disturbances in motor neurons

Signs and symptoms

- Fasciculations, accompanied by atrophy and weakness, especially in the muscles of the forearms and the hands
- Impaired speech
- Difficulty chewing, swallowing, and breathing
- Choking
- Excessive drooling

Diagnostic tests

- Electromyography shows electrical abnormalities in involved muscles.
- Muscle biopsy may disclose atrophic fibers interspersed among normal fibers.
- Protein content of cerebrospinal fluid is increased in one-third of patients, but this finding alone doesn't confirm ALS.

Treatment

- Symptoms are supported, and emotional, psychological, and physical support is given.
- Riluzole (Rilutek), a neuroprotector, may improve signs and symptoms, increasing survival time and quality of life.
- Baclofen (Kemstro) or diazepam (Valium) may be prescribed to control spasticity that interferes with activities of daily living.

Nursing considerations

- Care begins with a complete neurologic assessment—a baseline for future evaluations of progressing disease.
- Implement a rehabilitation program designed to help the patient maintain independence for as long as possible.
- Help the patient obtain equipment, such as a walker and a wheelchair. Arrange for a visiting nurse to monitor

the patient's status, provide support, and teach the family about the illness.

■ Depending on the patient's muscular capacity, assist with bathing, personal hygiene, and transfers from wheelchair to bed. Help the patient establish a regular bowel and bladder routine.

■ To help the patient handle increased accumulation of secretions and dysphagia, teach him to suction himself.

■ Teach the patient's family which signs and symptoms of aspiration pneumonia are important to report (fever, increased respiratory rate, increased or colored secretions, difficulty breathing).

■ To prevent skin breakdown, provide good skin care when the patient is bedridden. Turn him frequently, keep his skin clean and dry, and use sheepskins or pressure-relieving devices.

■ If the patient has trouble swallowing, give him soft, solid foods and position him upright during meals. Gastrostomy and nasogastric tube feedings may be necessary if he can no longer swallow.

■ Teach the patient (if he's still able to feed himself) or family members how to give gastrostomy feedings.

■ Provide emotional support. Prepare the patient and his family for his eventual death. Patients with ALS may benefit from a hospice program.

Anaphylaxis

Anaphylaxis is a dramatic and widespread acute atopic reaction marked by the sudden onset of rapidly progressive urticaria and respiratory distress. A severe anaphylactic reaction may precipitate vascular collapse, leading to systemic shock and, sometimes, death.

Causes

■ Ingestion of or other systemic exposure to a sensitizing drug or other substance

■ Sensitizing substances include:

–Allergen extracts
–Diagnostic chemicals (sodium dehydrocholate and radiographic contrast media)
–Foods (legumes, nuts, berries, seafood, and egg albumin)
–Enzymes (such as L-asparaginase)
–Hormones
–Insect venom (honeybees, wasps, hornets, yellow jackets, fire ants, mosquitoes, and certain spiders)
–Local anesthetics
–Penicillin and other antibiotics
–Polysaccharides
–Salicylates
–Serums (usually horse serum)
–Sulfite-containing food additives
–Sulfonamides
–Vaccines

Signs and symptoms

■ Angioedema
■ Cardiac arrhythmias
■ Diarrhea
■ Dyspnea
■ Feeling of impending doom or fright
■ Hoarseness
■ Hypotension
■ Nasal mucosal edema and congestion
■ Nasal pruritus
■ Nausea
■ Profuse watery rhinorrhea
■ Severe stomach cramps
■ Shock
■ Shortness of breath
■ Sneezing
■ Stridor
■ Sudden sneezing attacks
■ Sweating
■ Urinary urgency and incontinence
■ Urticaria
■ Weakness

Diagnostic tests

■ Anaphylaxis can be diagnosed by the rapid onset of severe respiratory or cardiovascular symptoms after ingestion or injection of a drug, vaccine, diagnostic

Showing patients how to use an anaphylaxis kit

If the practitioner has prescribed an anaphylaxis kit for the patient to use in an emergency, explain that the kit contains everything that he needs to treat an allergic reaction: two epinephrine autoinjectors, alcohol swabs, a tourniquet, and antihistamine tablets.

Instruct the patient to notify the practitioner at once if anaphylaxis occurs (or to ask someone else to call him) and to use the anaphylaxis kit as follows:

Getting ready
- Take the epinephrine autoinjector from the kit. Don't remove the cap until ready to use.
- Next, clean about 4" (10 cm) of the skin on your arm or thigh with an alcohol swab. (If you're right-handed, clean your left arm or thigh; if you're left-handed, clean your right arm or thigh.)

Injecting the epinephrine
- Position the black tip of the epinephrine autoinjector over the injection site.
- Firmly push the device into the injection site. A loud clicking sound indicates that the device is injecting the medication, so hold the injector in place for 10 seconds.
- Remove the autoinjector, and dispose of it properly.
Note: The practitioner can determine the correct dosage and administration for infants and children younger than age 12.

Removing the insect's stinger
- Quickly remove the insect's stinger if it's visible. Use a dull object, such as a fingernail or tweezers, to pull it straight out. If the stinger can't be removed quickly, stop trying. Go on to the next step.

Applying the tourniquet
- If you were stung on an arm or a leg, apply a tourniquet between the sting site and your heart. Tighten the tourniquet by pulling the string.
- After 10 minutes, release the tourniquet by pulling on the metal ring.

Taking the antihistamine tablets
- Chew and swallow the antihistamine tablets. (Children ages 12 and younger should follow the directions supplied by the practitioner or provided in the kit.)

Following up
- Apply ice packs—if available—to the sting site. Avoid exertion, keep warm, and see a practitioner or go to a facility immediately.
- *Important:* If you don't notice an improvement within 10 minutes, give yourself a second injection by following the directions in the kit. Proceed as before, following the injection instructions.

Special instructions
- Keep the kit handy for emergency treatment at all times.
- Ask the pharmacist for storage guidelines.
- Periodically check the epinephrine in the preloaded syringe. A pinkish brown solution needs to be replaced.
- Note the kit's expiration date, and replace the kit before that date.

agent, food, or food additive or after an insect sting.

Treatment
- Give an immediate injection of 0.1 to 0.5 ml of epinephrine 1:1,000 aqueous solution, repeated every 5 to 20 minutes as needed.
- Epinephrine can be given by I.M. or subcutaneously, if the patient is still normotensive and hasn't lost consciousness.

- Cardiopulmonary resuscitation should be performed if the patient is in cardiac arrest.
- Endotracheal intubation or tracheotomy and mechanical ventilation are used to maintain airway potency and oxygenation.
- Vasopressors, such as norepinephrine, dopamine, or phenylephrine, may be ordered.
- Corticosteroids are prescribed to reduce inflammation.
- Diphenhydramine is prescribed for long-term management.
- A bronchodilator, such as aminophylline I.V., is used to control bronchospasm.
- Volume expanders, such as normal saline solution or albumin, are given to support blood pressure.

Nursing considerations

- Assess respiratory status and maintain airway patency. Observe the patient for early signs and symptoms of laryngeal edema (stridor, hoarseness, and dyspnea).
- If the patient is experiencing cardiac arrest, begin cardiopulmonary resuscitation, including chest compressions and assisted ventilation; further therapy depends on the patient's response.
- Give volume expanders and I.V. vasopressors norepinephrine and dopamine to support blood pressure, as prescribed. Monitor blood pressure, central venous pressure, and urine output as a response index.
- To prevent anaphylaxis, teach the patient to avoid exposure to known allergens. If the patient has an allergy to insect stings, he should carry an anaphylaxis kit whenever he goes outdoors. Show him how to use the kit. (See *Showing patients how to use an anaphylaxis kit.*) In addition, if the patient is prone to anaphylaxis, he should wear a medical

identification bracelet identifying his allergies.
- If a patient must receive a drug to which he's allergic, prevent a severe reaction by making sure he receives careful desensitization with gradually increasing doses of the antigen or advance administration of steroids. Make sure he receives each dose under close medical observation.

Aneurysm, abdominal

With abdominal aneurysm, an abnormal dilation in the arterial wall generally occurs in the aorta between the renal arteries and iliac branches. Such aneurysms are seven times more common in hypertensive men than in women and are most prevalent in white patients ages 50 to 80. More than 50% of all people with untreated abdominal aneurysms die within 2 years of diagnosis, primarily from hemorrhage and shock from the aneurysm's rupture; more than 85%, within 5 years.

Causes

- Arteriosclerosis or atherosclerosis (in about 95% of cases)
- Cystic medial necrosis
- Syphilis and other infections
- Trauma

Signs and symptoms

- Diminished peripheral pulses or claudication (rarely unless embolization occurs)
- Hypotension
- Lumbar pain that radiates to the flank and groin may signify enlargement and imminent rupture
- Pulsating mass in the periumbilical area
- Severe, persistent abdominal and back pain with rupture into the peritoneal cavity
- Shock

Endovascular grafting for repair of an abdominal aortic aneurysm

Endovascular grafting is a minimally invasive procedure for the patient who requires repair of an abdominal aortic aneurysm. Endovascular grafting reinforces the walls of the aorta to prevent rupture and prevents expansion of the aneurysm.

The procedure is performed with fluoroscopic guidance, whereby a delivery catheter with an attached compressed graft is inserted through a small incision into the femoral or iliac artery over a guide wire. The delivery catheter is advanced into the aorta, where it's positioned across the aneurysm. A balloon on the catheter expands the graft and affixes it to the vessel wall. The procedure generally takes 2 to 3 hours to perform. Patients are instructed to walk the first day after surgery and are discharged from the facility in 1 to 3 days.

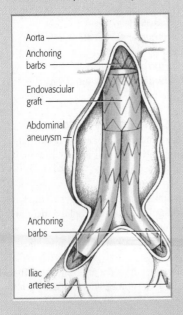

- Aorta
- Anchoring barbs
- Endovasciular graft
- Abdominal aneurysm
- Anchoring barbs
- Iliac arteries

- Sweating
- Systolic bruit over the aorta
- Tachycardia
- Tenderness may be present on deep palpation
- Weakness
- Death

Diagnostic tests
- X-ray shows an aneurysm.
- Abdominal ultrasonography or echocardiography allows determination of aneurysm size, shape, and location.
- Anteroposterior and lateral X-rays of the abdomen outline the mass 75% of the time.
- Aortography shows the condition of vessels proximal and distal to the aneurysm and the extent of the aneurysm, but usually underestimates the diameter.

Treatment
- The aneurysm is resected and the damaged section replaced with a Dacron graft prevents rupture. (See *Endovascular grafting for repair of an abdominal aortic aneurysm.*)
- In asymptomatic patients, surgery is advised when the aneurysm is 5 to 6 cm in diameter.
- In patients with poor perfusion distal to the aneurysm, external grafting may be done.
- Beta-adrenergic blockers are prescribed to decrease the rate of growth of the aneurysm.

Nursing considerations
- Monitor vital signs and type and cross-match blood.
- Obtain ordered kidney function tests (blood urea nitrogen, creatinine, and electrolyte levels), blood samples (complete blood count with differential), an electrocardiogram and cardiac evaluation, baseline pulmonary function tests, and arterial blood gas (ABG) analysis.

- Be alert for signs of rupture, which may be immediately fatal. Watch closely for any signs of acute blood loss (decreasing blood pressure; increasing pulse and respiratory rates; cool, clammy skin; restlessness; and decreased sensorium).

ACTION STAT!

 If rupture does occur, the first priority is to get the patient to surgery immediately. Medical antishock trousers may be used while transporting him to surgery. Surgery allows direct compression of the aorta to control hemorrhage. Large amounts of blood may be needed during the resuscitative period to replace blood loss. In such a patient, renal failure due to ischemia is a major postoperative complication, possibly requiring hemodialysis.

- Before elective surgery, weigh the patient, insert an indwelling urinary catheter and an I.V. line, and assist with insertion of an arterial line and a pulmonary artery catheter to monitor fluid and hemodynamic balance. Also, give him a prophylactic antibiotic.
- If the patient is undergoing complex abdominal surgery (that is, with I.V. lines, endotracheal [ET] and nasogastric [NG] intubation, and mechanical ventilation), explain the surgical procedure and the expected postoperative care in the intensive care unit.
- After surgery, closely monitor vital signs, intake and hourly output, neurologic status (level of consciousness, pupil size, and sensation in arms and legs), and ABG levels.
- Assess the depth, rate, and character of respirations and breath sounds at least every hour.
- Watch for signs of bleeding (such as increased pulse and respiratory rates and hypotension), which may occur retroperitoneally from the graft site.

Check abdominal dressings for excessive bleeding or drainage.
- Be alert for fever and other signs of infection.
- After NG intubation for intestinal decompression, irrigate the tube frequently to ensure patency. Record the amount and type of drainage.
- Suction the ET tube often. If the patient can breathe unassisted and has good breath sounds, adequate ABG levels, tidal volume, and vital capacity 24 hours after surgery, he'll be extubated and require oxygen by mask. Weigh the patient daily to evaluate fluid balance.
- Help the patient walk as soon as he's able (usually the 2nd day after surgery).
- Provide psychological support for the patient and family.

Aneurysm, cerebral

With cerebral aneurysm, localized dilation of a cerebral artery results from a weakness in the arterial wall. Its most common form is the saccular (berry) aneurysm, a saclike outpouching in a cerebral artery. Cerebral aneurysms usually arise at an arterial junction in the circle of Willis, the circular anastomosis forming the major cerebral arteries at the base of the brain. Cerebral aneurysms usually rupture, causing subarachnoid hemorrhage. About half of all patients who suffer a subarachnoid hemorrhage die immediately. In about 20% of patients, multiple aneurysms occur. With new and better treatment, the prognosis is improving.

Causes

- Combination of congenital defect and degenerative process
- Congenital defect such as weak arterial wall
- Degenerative process, such as hypertension and atherosclerosis

Danger signals in cerebral aneurysm

You must act quickly if you notice danger signals in the patient with a cerebral aneurysm. Watch for an enlarging aneurysm, rebleeding, intracranial clot, vasospasm, and other complications. These complications may be heralded by:
- decreased level of consciousness
- unilateral enlarged pupil
- onset or worsening of hemiparesis or motor deficit
- increased blood pressure
- slowed pulse rate
- worsening of headache or sudden onset of a headache
- renewed or worsened nuchal rigidity
- renewed or persistent vomiting.
   Intermittent signs, such as restlessness, extremity weakness, and speech alterations, can also indicate increasing intracranial pressure.

Signs and symptoms
- Bleeding into the brain tissues, causing hemiparesis, hemisensory defects, dysphagia, and visual defects
- Bleeding, causing nuchal rigidity, back and leg pain, fever, restlessness, irritability, occasional seizures, and blurred vision
- Complications include increased intracranial pressure (ICP), rebleeding episode, vasospasm, acute hydrocephalus (due to abnormal accumulation of cerebrospinal fluid [CSF] within the cranial cavity because of CSF blockage by blood or adhesions), and pulmonary embolism (an adverse effect of deep vein thrombosis [DVT] or aneurysm treatment) (see *Danger signals in cerebral aneurysm*)
- If aneurysm is near internal carotid artery, diplopia, ptosis, dilated pupil, and inability to rotate the eye

- Rupture, causing sudden severe headache, nausea, vomiting, and altered level of consciousness (LOC), including a deep coma

Degrees of severity
The severity of symptoms varies from patient to patient, depending on the site and amount of bleeding. Patients with ruptured cerebral aneurysms are grouped as follows:
- Grade I: minimal bleeding. The patient is alert with no neurologic deficit; slight headache and nuchal rigidity.
- Grade II: mild bleeding. The patient is alert, with a mild to severe headache, nuchal rigidity and, possibly, third-nerve palsy.
- Grade III: moderate bleeding. The patient is confused or drowsy, with nuchal rigidity and, possibly, a mild focal deficit.
- Grade IV: severe bleeding. The patient is stuporous, with nuchal rigidity and, possibly, mild to severe hemiparesis.
- Grade V: moribund (commonly fatal). If nonfatal, the patient is decerebrate or in a deep coma.

Diagnostic tests
- Computed tomography (CT) scan reveals subarachnoid or ventricular blood.
- Magnetic resonance imaging or magnetic resonant angiography can identify a cerebral aneurysm as a "flow void" or by computer reconstruction of cerebral vessels.
- Cerebral angiography confirms the aneurysm's location and displays the vessel's condition.
- Lumbar puncture may be used to identify blood in CSF when the CT scan is normal; it's contraindicated when there are signs of increased ICP.

Treatment
- Oxygenation and ventilation are the initial emergency treatments.

- Surgical repair (by clipping, ligating, or wrapping the aneurysm neck with muscle) is usually done as soon as the patient's condition allows it after the initial bleeding.

When surgical correction is risky, when the aneurysm is in a dangerous location, or when surgery is delayed because of vasospasm, treatment includes:
- bed rest in a relaxing environment (if immediate surgery isn't possible, bed rest may continue for 4 to 6 weeks)
- avoidance of coffee, other stimulants, and aspirin
- codeine or another analgesic as needed
- avoiding constipation; a stool softener is crucial to prevent straining and resultant rebleeding
- hydralazine or another antihypertensive if the patient is hypertensive
- nimodipine, a calcium channel blocker to decrease cerebral vessel vasospasm
- a corticosteroid to reduce edema
- phenytoin or another anticonvulsant
- phenobarbital or another sedative
- aminocaproic acid, a fibrinolytic inhibitor, to minimize the risk of rebleeding by delaying blood clot lysis.

Nursing considerations
- During initial treatment after a hemorrhage, establish and maintain a patent airway because the patient may need supplemental oxygen. Position the patient to promote pulmonary drainage and prevent upper airway obstruction. If he's intubated, preoxygenation with 100% oxygen before suctioning to remove secretions will prevent hypoxia and vasodilation from carbon dioxide accumulation.
- Institute aneurysm precautions to minimize the risk of rebleeding and to avoid increased ICP. Such precautions include bed rest in a quiet, darkened room (keeping the head of the bed flat or under 30 degrees); limited visits; avoidance of caffeine, other stimulants, and strenu-

ous physical activity; and restricted fluid intake. Be sure to explain to the patient why these restrictive measures are necessary.
- Turn the patient often when ICP is stable. Encourage deep breathing and leg movement. Warn the patient to avoid all unnecessary physical activity. Assist him with active range-of-motion (ROM) exercises (unless the practitioner has forbidden them); if the patient is paralyzed, perform regular passive ROM exercises.
- Monitor arterial blood gas (ABG) levels, LOC, and vital signs often, and accurately measure intake and output. Avoid taking the patient's temperature rectally because vagus nerve stimulation may cause cardiac arrest.
- Give fluids and monitor I.V. infusions to avoid increased ICP.
- Assess the patient for dysphagia: gurgling voice, coughing, pulmonary secretions, delayed swallowing, food pocketing, and cranial nerve dysfunction (V, VII, IX, X, or XII).
- Initiate a speech evaluation and give recommendations for maximum safety during feeding, such as positioning, food consistency, and strategies for swallowing. If the patient is at risk for aspiration, insert a nasogastric or gastric tube.
- If the patient can eat, provide a high-bulk diet (bran, salads, and fruit) to prevent straining during defecation, which can increase ICP.

D o ' s   &   d o n ' t s

 Give a prescribed stool softener or a mild laxative as needed. Don't force fluids. Implement a bowel elimination program based on previous habits. If the patient is receiving a steroid, check the stool for blood.

- If the patient is experiencing weakness of cranial nerve III (impaired lid closure), V (impaired sensation), or VII (impaired tearing), give artificial tears or ophthalmic ointment to minimize corneal damage. An occlusive metal eye patch may also be needed.

■ Give the patient a sedative to help minimize stress. Be alert for signs of oversedation. Raise the side rails to help protect him from injury. If possible, avoid using restraints because they can cause agitation and raise ICP.

■ Give antihypertensives if necessary. Carefully monitor blood pressure, and be alert for any significant change, especially a rise in systolic pressure. Be careful to avoid activities that may suddenly increase blood pressure.

DRUG CHALLENGE

Give aminocaproic acid (Amicar) I.V. in dextrose 5% in water or orally at least every 2 hours to maintain therapeutic blood levels. (Renal insufficiency may necessitate a dosage adjustment.) Monitor the patient for adverse reactions, such as nausea and diarrhea (most common with oral administration) and phlebitis (most common with I.V. administration).

■ Reduce the risk of DVT by applying antiembolism stockings or sequential compression devices.

■ If the patient can't speak, establish a simple means of communication, or use cards or a slate. Try to limit conversation to topics that won't further frustrate him. Encourage his family to speak to him in a normal tone, even if he doesn't seem to respond.

■ Provide the patient with emotional support, and include his family in his care as much as possible. Encourage family members to adopt a realistic attitude, but don't discourage hope.

■ Before discharge, refer the patient to a visiting nurse or a rehabilitation center, if necessary, and teach the patient and

his family how to recognize signs of rebleeding.

■ Aneurysm, thoracic aortic

Thoracic aortic aneurysm is characterized by an abnormal widening of the ascending, transverse, or descending part of the aorta. Aneurysm of the ascending part of the aorta is the most common type—and is usually fatal. The aneurysm may be dissecting, a hemorrhagic separation in the aortic wall, usually within the medial layer; saccular, an outpouching of the arterial wall, with a narrow neck; or fusiform, a spindle-shaped enlargement encompassing the entire aortic circumference. Some aneurysms progress to serious and, eventually, lethal complications, such as rupture of an untreated thoracic dissecting aneurysm into the pericardium, with resulting tamponade.

Causes
■ Atherosclerosis
■ Congenital disorders such as coarctation of the aorta
■ Fungal infection (mycotic aneurysms) of the aortic arch and descending segments
■ History of traumatic chest injury
■ Hypertension (in dissecting aneurysm)
■ Intimal tear in the ascending aorta initiates a dissecting aneurysm (60% of patients)
■ Syphilis, usually of the ascending part of the aorta (uncommon because of antibiotics)
■ Trauma, usually of the descending part of the aorta around the thorax, from an accident that shears the aorta transversely (acceleration-deceleration injuries)

Signs and symptoms
■ Abrupt onset of neurologic deficits if dissection involves the carotid arteries

- Aortic insufficiency
- Bradycardia
- Difference in blood pressure between the right and left arms
- Pain described as severe, boring, and ripping and extends to the neck, shoulders, lower back, and abdomen but rarely radiates to the jaw and arms; more severe on the right side
- Pericardial friction rub caused by a hemopericardium
- Sharp, tearing pain that usually starts suddenly between shoulder blades and may radiate to chest, with an aneurysm of the descending part of the aorta
- Sudden, sharp, tearing pain that radiates to the shoulders, also causing hoarseness, dyspnea, dysphagia, and dry cough, with an aneurysm of the transverse part of the aorta
- Unequal intensities of the right and left carotid pulses and radial pulses

Diagnostic tests

- Aortography, the most definitive test, shows the lumen of the aneurysm, its size and location, and the false lumen in a dissecting aneurysm.
- Electrocardiography helps distinguish a thoracic aneurysm from a myocardial infarction.
- Echocardiography may help identify a dissecting aneurysm of the aortic root.
- Hemoglobin level may be normal or low because of blood loss from a leaking aneurysm.
- Computed tomography scan and magnetic resonance imaging can confirm and locate the aneurysm and may be used to monitor its progression.
- Transesophageal echocardiography is used to measure the aneurysm in both the ascending and the descending aorta.

Treatment

- An antihypertensive, such as nitroprusside (Nitropress), may be given.

- A negative inotropic that decreases contractility force, such as propranolol (Inderal), may be given.
- Oxygen is administered for respiratory distress.
- An opioid is given for pain.
- I.V. fluids and blood transfusions may be needed.
- Surgery consists of resecting the aneurysm, restoring normal blood flow through a Dacron or Teflon graft replacement and, with aortic valve insufficiency, replacing the aortic valve.

Nursing considerations

- Monitor the patient's blood pressure, pulmonary artery wedge pressure (PAWP), and central venous pressure (CVP). Also, evaluate the patient's pain, breathing, and carotid, radial, and femoral pulses.
- Review laboratory test results, which must include a complete blood count with differential, electrolyte levels, typing and crossmatching for whole blood, arterial blood gas analysis, and urinalysis.
- Insert an indwelling urinary catheter. Give dextrose 5% in water or lactated Ringer's solution and an antibiotic as needed. Carefully monitor nitroprusside I.V. infusion rate; use a separate I.V. line for infusion. Adjust the dose by slowly increasing the infusion rate. Meanwhile, check blood pressure every 5 minutes until it stabilizes.
- If bleeding from an aneurysm is suspected, give a whole blood transfusion.
- Explain diagnostic tests. If surgery is scheduled, explain the procedure and expected postoperative care (I.V. lines, endotracheal and drainage tubes, cardiac monitoring, ventilation).
  After repair of a thoracic aneurysm:
- Evaluate the patient's level of consciousness. Monitor vital signs; pulmonary artery pressure, PAWP, and CVP; pulse rate; urine output; and pain.

- Check respiratory function. Carefully observe and record type and amount of chest tube drainage, and frequently assess heart and breath sounds.
- Monitor I.V. therapy.
- Give medications as appropriate.
- Watch for signs of infection, especially fever, and excessive wound drainage.
- Assist the patient with range-of-motion exercises for the legs, to prevent thromboembolism due to venostasis during prolonged bed rest.
- After vital signs and respiration have been stabilized, encourage and assist the patient in turning, coughing, and deep breathing. If necessary, provide intermittent positive-pressure breathing to promote lung expansion.
- Help the patient walk as soon as he's able.
- Before discharge, ensure adherence to antihypertensive therapy by explaining the need for such drugs as well as their adverse effects. Teach the patient how to monitor his blood pressure.
- Throughout hospitalization, offer the patient and family psychological support.

Aneurysm, ventricular

Ventricular aneurysm is marked by an outpouching (almost always of the left ventricle) that produces ventricular wall dysfunction in 10% to 20% of patients after a myocardial infarction (MI). A ventricular aneurysm may develop within days to weeks after an MI, or may be delayed for years. An untreated ventricular aneurysm can lead to arrhythmias, systemic embolization, or heart failure and may cause sudden death. Resection improves the prognosis in patients with heart failure or refractory ventricular arrhythmias.

Causes

- MI destroying a large muscular section of the left ventricle; necrosis reducing the ventricular wall to a thin sheath of fibrous tissue, which stretches under intracardiac pressure to form a separate noncontractile sac (aneurysm)

Signs and symptoms

- Arrhythmias (such as premature ventricular contractions and ventricular tachycardia)
- Chronic heart failure (characterized by dyspnea, fatigue, edema, crackles, gallop rhythm, and jugular vein distention)
- Left ventricular dysfunction
- Palpitations
- Pulmonary edema
- Pulsus alternans with left-sided heart failure
- Signs and symptoms of cardiac dysfunction (weakness on exertion, fatigue, angina)
- Systemic embolization
- Visible or palpable systolic precordial bulge

Diagnostic tests

- Left ventriculography reveals left ventricular enlargement with an area of akinesia or dyskinesia (during cineangiography) and diminished cardiac function.
- Electrocardiography may show persistent ST-T wave elevations after an MI.
- Chest X-ray may demonstrate an abnormal bulge distorting the heart's contour if the aneurysm is large; the X-ray may be normal if the aneurysm is small.
- Noninvasive nuclear cardiology scan may indicate the site of infarction and suggest the area of aneurysm.
- Echocardiography shows abnormal motion in the left ventricular wall.

Treatment

- Treatment may require only routine medical examination to follow the patient's condition or aggressive measures for intractable ventricular arrhythmias, heart failure, and emboli.

■ I.V. antiarrhythmics are ordered, followed by oral maintenance (procainamide [Procanbid], quinidine, or disopyramide [Norpace]).

■ Cardioversion is performed.

■ Emergency treatment for heart failure with pulmonary edema includes oxygen, I.V. digoxin (Lanoxin), I.V. furosemide, I.V. morphine sulfate, I.V. nitroprusside (Nitropress), and intubation (if needed); maintenance therapy includes an oral nitrate and an angiotensin-converting enzyme inhibitor (captopril [Capoten] or enalapril [Vasotec]).

■ Systemic embolization requires anticoagulation therapy or embolectomy.

■ Refractory ventricular tachycardia, heart failure, recurrent arterial embolization, and persistent angina with coronary artery occlusion may require surgery (aneurysmectomy with myocardial revascularization).

Nursing considerations

■ If ventricular tachycardia occurs, monitor blood pressure and heart rate. If sustained ventricular tachycardia occurs, give I.V. lidocaine.

ACTION STAT!

 If cardiac arrest occurs, start cardiopulmonary resuscitation (CPR) and call for assistance, resuscitative equipment, and medication.

■ If the patient is experiencing heart failure, closely monitor vital signs, heart sounds, intake and output, fluid and electrolyte balances, and blood urea nitrogen and creatinine levels.

■ Because of the threat of systemic embolization, frequently check peripheral pulses and the color and temperature of extremities. Be alert for sudden changes in sensorium that indicate cerebral em-

bolization and for any signs that suggest renal failure or a progressive MI.

■ If the patient is conscious and requires cardioversion, give diazepam I.V. as needed before cardioversion. Explain to him that cardioversion is a lifesaving procedure that provides brief electric shocks to the heart.

DRUG CHALLENGE

 If the patient is receiving an antiarrhythmic, check appropriate laboratory tests. For instance, if he takes procainamide, check his antinuclear antibodies because this drug may induce symptoms that mimic those of lupus erythematosus.

If the patient is scheduled to undergo resection, perform the following:

■ Before surgery, explain expected postoperative care in the intensive care unit (including use of such things as endotracheal tube, ventilator, hemodynamic monitoring, chest tubes, and drainage bottle).

■ After surgery, monitor vital signs, intake and output, heart sounds, and pulmonary artery pressures. Watch for signs of infection, such as fever and purulent drainage.

■ Teach the patient to report light-headedness or dizziness, which may indicate arrhythmia. Encourage him to follow his prescribed drug regimen—even during the night—and to watch for adverse reactions.

■ Because arrhythmias can cause sudden death, refer the family to a community-based CPR training program.

■ Provide psychological support for the patient and his family.

▌Aneurysms, femoral and popliteal

Femoral and popliteal aneurysms result from progressive atherosclerotic changes occurring in the walls (medial layer) of the major peripheral arteries. Aneurysmal formations may be fusiform (spindle-shaped) or saccular (pouchlike), with the fusiform type being three times more common. These formations may be single or multiple segmental lesions, in many cases affecting both legs, and may accompany other arterial aneurysms located in the abdominal aorta or iliac arteries. The clinical course is usually progressive, eventually ending in thrombosis, embolization, and gangrene. Elective surgery before complications arise greatly improves the prognosis.

Causes
- Atherosclerosis
- Bacterial infection
- Congenital weakness in the arterial wall (rarely)
- Peripheral vascular reconstructive surgery (causes "suture line" aneurysms, whereby a blood clot forms a second lumen, also called *false aneurysms*)
- Trauma (blunt or penetrating)

Signs and symptoms
- Popliteal aneurysms, which may cause pain in popliteal space, edema, and venous distention
- Femoral and popliteal aneurysms, which can produce symptoms of severe ischemia in leg or foot, due to acute thrombosis
- Acute aneurysmal thrombosis symptoms, including severe pain, loss of pulse and color, coldness in affected leg or foot, and gangrene
- Distal petechial hemorrhages, which may develop from aneurysmal emboli

Diagnostic tests
- With femoral aneurysm, diagnosis is confirmed by bilateral palpation that reveals a pulsating mass above or below the inguinal ligament.

- When thrombosis has occurred, palpation detects a firm, nonpulsating mass.
- Arteriography may also detect associated aneurysms, especially those in the abdominal aorta and the iliac arteries.
- Ultrasonography may be helpful in determining the size of the femoral or popliteal aneurysm.

Treatment
- Surgical bypass and reconstruction of the artery is indicated, usually with an autogenous saphenous vein graft replacement.
- Arterial occlusion that causes severe ischemia and gangrene may require leg amputation.

Nursing considerations
Before corrective surgery, perform the following:
- Evaluate circulatory status, noting the location and quality of peripheral pulses in the affected arm or leg.
- Give a prophylactic antibiotic or anticoagulant as needed.
- Discuss expected postoperative procedures with the patient, and review the surgical procedure.

ACTION STAT!
 Carefully monitor the patient for early signs and symptoms of thrombosis or graft occlusion (loss of pulse, decreased skin temperature or sensation, or severe pain) and infection (fever).

After arterial surgery, perform the following:
- Palpate distal pulses at least every hour for the first 24 hours, then as frequently as needed. Correlate these findings with preoperative circulatory assessment. Mark the sites on the patient's skin where pulses are palpable, to facilitate repeated checks.

■ Help the patient walk soon after surgery, to prevent venostasis and thrombus formation.

■ Tell the patient to immediately inform the practitioner of any recurrence of symptoms because the saphenous vein graft replacement can fail or another aneurysm may develop.

■ If the patient has undergone a popliteal artery resection, explain to him that swelling may persist for some time. If antiembolism stockings are prescribed, make sure they fit properly, and teach the patient how to apply them. Warn against wearing constrictive apparel.

DRUG CHALLENGE

 Explain the importance of follow-up blood studies to monitor anticoagulant therapy. Warn the patient to avoid trauma, tobacco, and aspirin. Suggest measures to prevent bleeding such as using an electric razor. Tell the patient to report signs of bleeding immediately (bleeding gums, easy bruising, or black, tarry stools).

▌ Ankylosing spondylitis

A chronic, usually progressive inflammatory disease, ankylosing spondylitis primarily affects the sacroiliac, apophyseal, and costovertebral joints and adjacent soft tissue. Generally, the disease begins in the sacroiliac joints and gradually progresses to the lumbar, thoracic, and cervical regions of the spine. Deterioration of bone and cartilage can lead to fibrous tissue formation and eventual fusion of the spine or peripheral joints.

Causes
■ Exact cause unknown
■ Familial tendency
■ Histocompatibility antigen HLA-B27 (positive in more than 90% of patients with this disease) and circulating immune complexes suggesting immunologic activity
■ Underlying infection

Signs and symptoms
■ These signs and symptoms progress unpredictably, and the disease can go into remission, exacerbation, or arrest at any stage.
 – Intermittent lower back pain that's usually most severe in the morning or after a period of inactivity (first sign)
 – Stiffness and limited motion of the lumbar spine
 – Pain and limited expansion of the chest due to involvement of the costovertebral joints
 – Peripheral arthritis involving shoulders, hips, and knees
 – Kyphosis in advanced stages, caused by chronic stooping to relieve symptoms, and hip deformity and associated limited range of motion (ROM)
 – Tenderness over the site of inflammation
 – Pain or tenderness at tendon insertion sites (enthesitis), especially the Achilles' or patellar tendon
 – Mild fatigue, fever, anorexia, or loss of weight; unilateral acute anterior uveitis; aortic insufficiency and cardiomegaly; upper lobe pulmonary fibrosis (mimics tuberculosis)
 – Severe neurologic complications, such as cauda equina syndrome and paralysis, which can occur secondary to fracture of a rigid cervical spine or C1-C2 subluxation.

Diagnostic tests
■ Typical symptoms, a family history, and the presence of HLA-B27 strongly suggest ankylosing spondylitis, but confirmation of the diagnosis requires these characteristic X-ray findings:
 – blurring of the bony margins of joints in the early stage

– bilateral sacroiliac involvement
– patchy sclerosis with superficial bony erosions
– eventual squaring of vertebral bodies
– "bamboo spine" with complete ankylosis.

Treatment

■ No treatment reliably stops disease progression, so treatment aims to delay further deformity.
■ Anti-inflammatory analgesics (indomethacin [Indocin] and sulfasalazine [Azulfidine]) may be prescribed to control pain and inflammation.
■ Severe hip involvement usually necessitates surgical hip replacement.
■ Severe spinal involvement may require a spinal wedge osteotomy to separate and reposition the vertebrae.

DO'S & DON'TS

 To minimize deformities, advise the patient to:
■ avoid physical activity that places undue stress on the back such as lifting heavy objects
■ stand upright; sit upright in a high, straight chair; and avoid leaning over a desk
■ sleep in a prone position on a hard mattress and avoid using pillows under the neck or knees
■ avoid prolonged walking, standing, sitting, and driving
■ perform regular stretching and deep-breathing exercises and swim regularly, if possible
■ have height measured every 3 to 4 months to detect tendency toward kyphosis
■ use braces of lightweight supports
■ seek vocational counseling if work requires standing or prolonged sitting at a desk
■ contact the local Arthritis Foundation chapter for a support group.

Nursing considerations

■ Ankylosing spondylitis can be an extremely painful and crippling disease, so the caregiver's main responsibility is to promote the patient's comfort while preserving as much mobility as possible. Keep in mind that his limited ROM makes simple tasks difficult. Offer support and reassurance.
■ Apply local heat and provide massage to relieve pain. Assess mobility and degree of discomfort frequently.
■ Teach and assist with daily exercises as needed to help the patient maintain strength and function. Stress the importance of maintaining good posture.
■ If treatment includes surgery, provide postoperative care.

■ Anthrax

Anthrax is an acute bacterial infection that most commonly occurs in grazing animals, such as cattle, sheep, goats, and horses. It can also affect people who come in contact with contaminated animals or their hides, bones, fur, hair, or wool. It's also used as an agent for bioterrorism and biological warfare. Anthrax infection occurs worldwide but is most common in developing countries. In humans, anthrax occurs in three forms, depending on the mode of transmission: cutaneous, inhalational, and GI.

Causes

■ *Bacillus anthracis,* which exists in the soil as spores that can live for years. Transmission to humans usually occurs through:
– exposure to or handling of infected animals or animal products
– ingestion of undercooked meat from an infected animal (GI anthrax)
– inhalation (inhalational anthrax)
– spores entering body through abraded or broken skin (cutaneous anthrax)

Signs and symptoms

■ Signs and symptoms usually occur within 1 to 7 days of exposure but may take as long as 60 days to appear. The signs and symptoms of anthrax depend on the form acquired:

– *Cutaneous anthrax:* begins as small, elevated, itchy lesion that resembles an insect bite, develops into a vesicle in 1 to 2 days, and finally becomes a small, painless ulcer with a necrotic (black) center; commonly accompanied by enlarged lymph glands in the surrounding area; mortality of 20% without treatment and less than 1% with treatment

– *Inhalational anthrax:* flulike signs and symptoms—malaise, fever, headache, myalgia, and chills—progressing to severe respiratory difficulties with dyspnea, stridor, chest pain, and cyanosis, followed by shock; usually fatal, even with treatment

– *GI anthrax:* acute inflammation of the intestinal tract, with nausea, vomiting, decreased appetite, and fever, progressing to abdominal pain, vomiting blood, and severe diarrhea; 25% to 60% fatal, even with treatment

Diagnostic tests

■ Anthrax can be diagnosed through *B. anthracis* cultures of the blood, skin lesions, or sputum of an exposed patient. Additionally, specific antibodies may be detected in the blood.

Treatment

■ Antibiotics (penicillin, ciprofloxacin, and doxycycline) are effective against anthrax.

■ Treatment is started immediately after exposure, to prevent anthrax infection.

Nursing considerations

■ Any case of anthrax in either livestock or a person must be reported to the appropriate public health office.

■ Supportive measures are geared toward the type of anthrax exposure.

DRUG CHALLENGE

 An anthrax vaccine is available but, due to limited supplies, it's now given only to U.S. military personnel and isn't for routine civilian use.

Aplastic and hypoplastic anemias

Aplastic and hypoplastic anemias result from injury to or destruction of stem cells in bone marrow or the bone marrow matrix, causing pancytopenia (anemia, granulocytopenia, thrombocytopenia) and bone marrow hypoplasia. Although commonly used interchangeably with other terms for bone marrow failure, *aplastic anemias* properly refer to pancytopenia resulting from the decreased functional capacity of a hypoplastic, fatty bone marrow. These disorders usually produce fatal bleeding or infection, particularly when they're idiopathic or stem from the use of chloramphenicol or from infectious hepatitis. Mortality for patients who have aplastic anemia with severe pancytopenia is 80% to 90%.

Causes

■ Congenital (congenital hypoplastic anemia or Blackfan-Diamond anemia, which develops between ages 2 months and 3 months, and Fanconi's syndrome, which develops between birth and age 10) due to consistent familial (genetic) history or from an induced change in the development of the fetus

■ Damaged bone marrow microvasculature creates an unfavorable environment for cell growth and maturation

■ Damaged or destroyed stem cells inhibit red blood cell (RBC) production

- Drugs (antibiotics, anticonvulsants)
- Immunologic factors (unconfirmed)
- Preleukemic and neoplastic infiltration of bone marrow
- Radiation
- Severe disease (especially hepatitis)
- Toxic agents (such as benzene and chloramphenicol)

Signs and symptoms

- Ecchymosis and petechiae, if thrombocytopenia present
- Headache
- Heart failure
- Neutropenia, possibly leading to infection (with fever, oral and rectal ulcers, and sore throat) but without characteristic inflammation
- Pallor
- Progressive weakness and fatigue
- Shortness of breath
- Tachycardia
- Thrombocytopenia (easy bruising and bleeding, especially from the mucous membranes [nose, gums, rectum, and vagina]) or bleeding into the retina or central nervous system

Diagnostic tests

Confirmation of aplastic anemia requires a series of laboratory tests:

- RBCs are usually normochromic and normocytic (although macrocytosis [larger-than-normal erythrocytes] and anisocytosis [excessive variation in erythrocyte size] may exist), with a total count of 1 million/µl or less. Absolute reticulocyte count is very low.
- Serum iron level is elevated (unless bleeding occurs), but total iron-binding capacity is normal or slightly reduced. Hemosiderin is present, and tissue iron storage is visible microscopically.
- Platelet, neutrophil, and white blood cell counts fall.
- Coagulation test results (bleeding time), reflecting decreased platelet count, are abnormal.

- Bone marrow aspiration from several sites may yield a "dry tap," and a biopsy will show severely hypocellular or aplastic marrow, with varied amounts of fat, fibrous tissue, or gelatinous replacement; absence of tagged iron (because iron is deposited in the liver rather than in bone marrow) and megakaryocytes; and depression of erythroid elements.

Treatment

- Identifiable causes must be eliminated.
- Transfusions of packed RBCs and platelets are given.
- Human leukocyte antigen–matched leukocytes or antithymocyte globulin are used alone or with cyclosporine (for children and severely neutropenic patients).
- Bone marrow transplantation is indicated in severe aplasia and for patients who need constant RBC transfusions.
- An antibiotic specific to infection is prescribed.
- Respiratory support with oxygen is given.
- A corticosteroid is used to stimulate erythroid production (tends to be successful in children but not adults).
- A marrow-stimulating agent, such as an androgen (which is controversial), may be ordered.
- An antilymphocyte globulin may be ordered.
- An immunosuppressant may be given (if the patient doesn't respond to other therapy).
- Colony-stimulating factor is used to encourage the growth of specific cellular components.

Nursing considerations

DO'S & DON'TS

 If the platelet count is low (less than 20,000/µl), prevent hemorrhage by avoiding I.M. injections, suggesting the use of an electric razor and a soft toothbrush, humidifying oxygen to prevent drying of mucous membranes, and promoting regular bowel movements through the use of a stool softener and a proper diet to prevent constipation.

- Apply pressure to venipuncture sites until bleeding stops. Detect bleeding early by checking for blood in the urine and stool and assessing the skin for petechiae.
- Help prevent infection by performing meticulous hand hygiene before entering the patient's room, by making sure the patient is receiving a nutritious diet (high in vitamins and proteins) to improve his resistance, and by encouraging meticulous mouth and perianal care.
- Watch for life-threatening hemorrhage, infection, adverse reactions to drug therapy, and blood transfusion reaction.
- Make sure throat, urine, nasal, rectal, and blood cultures are done regularly and correctly to check for infection. Teach signs of infection, and tell him to report them immediately.
- If the patient's hemoglobin level is low, which causes fatigue, schedule frequent rest periods.
- If blood transfusions are necessary, be alert for a transfusion reaction by checking the patient's temperature and watching for other signs and symptoms, such as rash, hives, itching, back pain, restlessness, and shaking chills.
- Reassure and support the patient and his family by explaining the disease and its treatment, particularly if the patient has recurring acute episodes. Explain the purpose of all prescribed drugs, and discuss possible adverse reactions, including which ones should be reported promptly.
- If the patient is receiving an anemia-inducing drug, monitor the results of his blood chemistry studies carefully to prevent aplastic anemia.

- Support efforts to educate the public about the hazards of toxic agents. Tell parents to keep toxic agents out of the reach of children.
- Encourage people who work with radiation to wear protective clothing and a radiation-detecting badge and to observe plant safety precautions.

DRUG CHALLENGE

 Those who work with the solvent benzene should know that 10 parts/million is the highest safe environmental level and that a delayed reaction to benzene may develop.

Appendicitis

The most common abdominal surgical disease, appendicitis is inflammation of the vermiform appendix due to an obstruction. Although appendicitis may occur at any age and affects both sexes equally, it's most common between puberty and age 30. Since the advent of antibiotics, the incidence and the death rate of appendicitis have declined. If left untreated, this disease is fatal.

Causes
- Obstruction of the intestinal lumen caused by a fecal mass, stricture, barium ingestion, or viral infection

Signs and symptoms
Early
- Generalized or localized colicky periumbilical or epigastric pain, anorexia, nausea, and vomiting
- Pain localized in the right lower quadrant of the abdomen (McBurney's point)
- Abdominal "boardlike" rigidity
- Retractive respirations
- Increasing tenderness
- Increasingly severe abdominal spasms
- Rebound tenderness (rebound tenderness on the opposite side of the ab-

domen suggests peritoneal inflammation)
- Minimal, vague symptoms and mild abdominal tenderness in elderly patients

Later
- Constipation (although diarrhea is also possible)
- Temperature of 99° to 102° F (37.2° to 38.9° C)
- Tachycardia
- Perforation or infarction of appendix, indicated by sudden cessation of abdominal pain

Diagnostic tests
- The white blood cell count will be moderately elevated (12,000 to 20,000/µl), with increased numbers of immature cells.
- Imaging studies are unnecessary in patients with a typical presentation of appendicitis.

Treatment
- Appendectomy is the only effective treatment.
- If peritonitis develops, treatment involves GI intubation, parenteral replacement of fluids and electrolytes, and administration of an antibiotic.

Nursing considerations
- Give I.V. fluids to prevent dehydration.

Do's & don'ts

Never give a cathartic or an enema, and never apply heat to the right lower quadrant of the patient's abdomen; these actions may cause the appendix to rupture.

- Restrict the patient to nothing by mouth until surgery is performed.
- Give a systemic antibiotic to reduce postoperative wound infection.
- To minimize pain, place the patient in Fowler's position.

- Following appendectomy, monitor vital signs and intake and output.
- Teach the patient to cough, breathe deeply, and turn frequently to prevent pulmonary complications.
- Document bowel sounds, passing of flatus, and bowel movements. In a patient whose nausea and abdominal rigidity have subsided, these signs indicate that he may resume oral fluids.
- Watch closely for surgical complications. Continuing pain and fever may signal an abscess. The complaint that "something gave way" may mean wound dehiscence. If an abscess or peritonitis develops, incision and drainage may be necessary. Monitor wound drainage.
- Help the patient ambulate as soon as possible after surgery (within 24 hours).
- With appendicitis complicated by peritonitis, a nasogastric tube may be needed to decompress the stomach and reduce nausea and vomiting.

Arterial occlusive disease

With arterial occlusive disease, the obstruction or narrowing of the lumen of the aorta and its major branches causes an interruption of blood flow, usually to the legs and feet. Arterial occlusive disease may affect the carotid, vertebral, innominate, subclavian, mesenteric, or celiac artery. Occlusions, which may be acute or chronic, commonly cause severe ischemia, skin ulceration, and gangrene. The prognosis depends on the location of the occlusion, the development of collateral circulation to counteract reduced blood flow and, if the patient has acute disease, the time elapsed between occlusion and its removal.

Causes
- Atherosclerosis
- Endogenous, from embolus formation or thrombosis

- Exogenous, from trauma or fracture

Predisposing factors
- Aging
- Conditions such as hypertension, hyperlipidemia, and diabetes
- Family history of vascular disorders, myocardial infarction, or stroke
- Smoking

Signs and symptoms
- Vary widely, according to the occlusion site (see *Clinical features of arterial occlusive disease,* page 38)

Diagnostic tests
- Arteriography demonstrates the type (thrombus or embolus), location, and degree of obstruction and collateral circulation. Arteriography is particularly useful in patients with chronic disease or for evaluating candidates for reconstructive surgery.
- Doppler ultrasonography and plethysmography are noninvasive tests that, in acute disease, show decreased blood flow distal to the occlusion.
- Ophthalmodynamometry helps determine the degree of obstruction in the internal carotid artery by comparing ophthalmic artery pressure with brachial artery pressure on the affected side. A more than 20% difference between pressures suggests insufficiency.
- EEG and a computed tomography scan may be necessary to rule out brain lesions.

Treatment
- Effective treatment depends on the cause, location, and size of the obstruction.
- For mild chronic disease, supportive measures include elimination of smoking, control of hypertension, and initiation of a walking program.
- For carotid artery occlusion, antiplatelet therapy may begin with dipyridamole (Persantine) and aspirin or clopidogrel (Plavix).
- For intermittent claudication of chronic occlusive disease, pentoxifylline (Trental) may improve blood flow through the capillaries, particularly in patients who are poor candidates for surgery.
- Acute arterial occlusive disease usually requires surgery to restore circulation to the affected area. Possible procedures include embolectomy, thromboendarterectomy, patch grafting, bypass graft arthrectomy.
- Thrombolytic therapy with urokinase (Abbokinase), streptokinase (Streptase), or alteplase (Activase) may be given.
- Balloon angioplasty compresses the obstruction.
- Laser angioplasty may be ordered (excision and hot-tip lasers vaporize the obstruction).
- Stent placement prevents reocclusion.
- Any of the above treatments may be used concurrently.
- Lumbar sympathectomy may be considered as adjunct to surgery, depending on condition of the sympathetic nervous system.
- Amputation may be necessary with failure of surgery or development of gangrene, persistent infection, or intractable pain.
- Heparin may be given to prevent embolus formation (for embolic occlusion).
- Bowel resection may be done after restoration of blood flow (for mesenteric artery occlusion).

Nursing considerations
- Provide comprehensive patient teaching, such as proper foot care. Explain all diagnostic tests and procedures. Advise the patient to stop smoking and to follow the prescribed medical regimen.

Clinical features of arterial occlusive disease

A patient with arterial occlusive disease may have a wide variety of signs and symptoms depending on which portion of the vasculature is affected by the disorder.

Site of occlusion	Signs and symptoms
Aortic bifurcation (saddle block occlusion, an emergency associated with cardiac embolization)	Sensory and motor deficits (muscle weakness, numbness, paresthesia, paralysis) and signs of ischemia (sudden pain; cold, pale legs with decreased or absent peripheral pulses) in both legs
Carotid arterial system ■ Internal carotid arteries ■ External carotid arteries	Neurologic dysfunction (transient ischemic attacks [TIAs] due to reduced cerebral circulation produce unilateral sensory or motor dysfunction [transient monocular blindness, hemiparesis], possible aphasia or dysarthria, confusion, decreased mentation, and headache; these recurrent clinical features usually last 5 to 10 minutes but may persist up to 24 hours and may herald a stroke); absent or decreased pulsation with an auscultatory bruit over the affected vessels
Femoral and popliteal arteries (associated with aneurysm formation)	Intermittent claudication of the calves on exertion; ischemic pain in feet; pretrophic pain (heralds necrosis and ulceration); leg pallor and coolness; blanching of feet on elevation; gangrene; no palpable pulses in ankles and feet
Iliac artery (Leriche's syndrome)	Intermittent claudication of lower back, buttocks, and thighs relieved by rest; absent or reduced femoral or distal pulses; possible bruit over femoral arteries; impotence
Innominate brachiocephalic artery	Neurologic dysfunction (signs and symptoms of vertebrobasilar occlusion); indications of ischemia (claudication) of right arm; possible bruit over right side of neck
Mesenteric artery ■ Superior (most commonly affected) ■ Celiac axis ■ Inferior	Bowel ischemia, infarct necrosis, and gangrene; sudden, acute abdominal pain; nausea and vomiting; diarrhea; leukocytosis; and shock due to massive intraluminal fluid and plasma loss
Subclavian artery	Subclavian steal syndrome (characterized by the backflow of blood from the brain through the vertebral artery on the same side as the occlusion, into the subclavian artery distal to the occlusion); clinical effects of vertebrobasilar occlusion and exercise-induced arm claudication; possible gangrene, usually limited to the digits
Vertebrobasilar system ■ Vertebral arteries ■ Basilar arteries	Neurologic dysfunction (TIAs of brain stem and cerebellum produce binocular visual disturbances, vertigo, dysarthria, and "drop attacks" [falling down without loss of consciousness]); less common than carotid TIA

Preoperatively (during an acute episode)

▪ Assess the patient's circulatory status by checking for the most distal pulses and by inspecting his skin color and temperature.

▪ Provide pain relief as needed.

▪ Give heparin by continuous I.V. drip as needed. Use an infusion monitor or pump to ensure the proper flow rate.

▪ Reposition the leg frequently to prevent pressure; avoid elevating or applying heat.

▪ Watch for signs of fluid and electrolyte imbalance, and monitor intake and output for signs of renal failure (urine output less than 30 ml/hour).

▪ If the patient has a carotid, innominate, vertebral, or subclavian artery occlusion, monitor him for signs and symptoms of stroke, such as numbness in an arm or a leg and intermittent blindness.

Postoperatively

▪ Monitor the patient's vital signs. Continuously assess his circulatory function by inspecting skin color and temperature and by checking for distal pulses. In charting, compare earlier assessments and observations. Watch closely for signs of hemorrhage (including tachycardia and hypotension), and check dressings for excessive bleeding.

▪ If the patient has a carotid, innominate, vertebral, or subclavian artery occlusion, assess neurologic status frequently for changes in level of consciousness, muscle strength, and pupil size.

▪ If the patient has mesenteric artery occlusion, connect a nasogastric tube to low intermittent suction. Monitor intake and output (low urine output may indicate damage to renal arteries during surgery). Check bowel sounds for the return of peristalsis. Increasing abdominal distention and tenderness may indicate extension of bowel ischemia with resulting gangrene, necessitating further excision, or they may indicate peritonitis.

▪ If the patient has aortic bifurcation, also known as *saddle-block occlusion,* check distal pulses for adequate circulation. Watch for indications of renal failure and mesenteric artery occlusion (such as severe abdominal pain) and for cardiac arrhythmias, which may precipitate embolus formation.

▪ If the patient has iliac artery occlusion, monitor urine output for signs of renal failure from decreased perfusion to the kidneys as a result of surgery. Provide meticulous catheter care.

▪ If the patient has femoral or popliteal artery occlusion, discourage prolonged sitting.

▪ After amputation, check the patient's stump carefully for drainage, and record its color and amount and the time. Elevate the stump and give an analgesic. Because phantom limb pain is common, explain this phenomenon to the patient.

▪ When preparing the patient for discharge, instruct him to watch for signs and symptoms of recurrence (such as pain, pallor, numbness, paralysis, and absence of pulse), which can result from graft occlusion or occlusion at another site. Warn him against wearing constrictive clothing.

▌Ascariasis

Also known as *roundworm infection,* ascariasis is caused by the parasitic worm *Ascaris lumbricoides.* After ingestion, *A. lumbricoides* ova hatch and release larvae, which penetrate the intestinal wall and reach the lungs through the bloodstream. After about 10 days in pulmonary capillaries and alveoli, the larvae migrate to the bronchioles, bronchi, trachea, and epiglottis. There, they're swallowed and return to the intestine to mature into worms. It occurs worldwide but is most common in tropical areas with poor sanitation and in Asia, where farmers use human stool as fertilizer. In the United States, it's more prevalent in the South, particularly among children younger than age 12.

Causes
■ *A. lumbricoides,* a large roundworm transmitted by ingestion of soil contaminated with human stool that harbors ova; ingestion occurs directly (by eating contaminated soil) or indirectly (by eating poorly washed raw vegetables grown in contaminated soil)

Signs and symptoms
■ Larvae migrating by the lymphatic and the circulatory systems cause various symptoms—for example, when they invade the lungs, pneumonitis may result
■ No symptoms in established infection
■ Severe disease causes stomach pain, vomiting, restlessness, disturbed sleep, and intestinal obstruction
■ Vague stomach discomfort
■ Vomiting a worm or passing a worm in the stool

Diagnostic tests
■ Microscopic identification of ova in the stool or observation of adult worms, which may be passed rectally or by mouth, confirms the diagnosis.
■ When migrating larvae invade the alveoli, X-rays show characteristic bronchovascular markings: infiltrates, patchy areas of pneumonitis, and widening of hilar shadows.
■ A complete blood count shows eosinophilia.

Treatment
■ Anthelmintic (pyrantel or piperazine) temporarily paralyzes the worms, permitting peristalsis to expel them.

■ Mebendazole (Vermox) and albendazole (Albenza) block the worms' nutrition.

DRUG CHALLENGE

 The benzimidazoles are contraindicated in pregnant patients and in patients with severe infections because they may cause ectopic migration.

■ In intestinal obstruction, nasogastric suctioning controls vomiting; when suctioning can be stopped, piperazine is instilled and the tube clamped; a second dose of oral piperazine is given 24 hours later.
■ Surgery is indicated if treatment is ineffective.

Nursing considerations
■ Isolation is unnecessary; proper disposal of stool and soiled linen, using standard precautions, should be adequate.
■ Teach the patient that he can prevent reinfection by washing his hands thoroughly, especially before eating and after defecating, and by bathing and changing his underwear and bed linens daily.
■ Inform the patient about the adverse effects of drugs prescribed for him.

DRUG CHALLENGE

 Be aware that piperazine is contraindicated in a patient with a seizure disorder and that it may cause stomach upset, dizziness, and urticaria. Pyrantel produces red stool and vomitus and may cause stomach upset, headache, dizziness, and rash; albendazole and mebendazole may cause abdominal pain and diarrhea.

Aspergillosis

Aspergillosis is an opportunistic, sometimes life-threatening infection caused by fungi of the genus *Aspergillus,* usually *A. fumigatus, A. flavus,* or *A. niger.* It produces infection only in vulnerable persons, such as those with excessive or prolonged use of antibiotics, glucocorticoids, or other immunosuppressants; from radiation; from such conditions as acquired immunodeficiency syndrome, Hodgkin's disease, leukemia, azotemia, alcoholism, sarcoidosis, bronchitis, or bronchiectasis; from organ transplants; and, in aspergilloma, from tuberculosis or another cavitary lung disease.

It occurs in four major forms:
- *Aspergilloma,* which produces a fungus ball in the lungs (called a *mycetoma*)
- *Allergic aspergillosis,* a hypersensitive asthmatic reaction to *Aspergillus* antigens
- *Aspergillosis endophthalmitis,* an infection of the anterior and posterior chambers of the eye that can lead to blindness
- *Disseminated aspergillosis,* an acute infection that produces septicemia, thrombosis, and infarction of virtually any organ but especially the heart, lungs, brain, and kidneys.

Aspergillus may cause infection of the ear (otomycosis), cornea (mycotic keratitis), or prosthetic heart valve (endocarditis); pneumonia (especially in those receiving an immunosuppressant, such as an antineoplastic drug or high-dose steroid therapy); sinusitis; and brain abscesses.

The prognosis varies with each form. Occasionally, aspergilloma causes fatal hemoptysis.

Causes

- *Aspergillus,* commonly found in fermenting compost piles and damp hay, transmitted by inhalation of fungal spores or, in aspergillosis endophthalmitis, by the invasion of spores through a wound or other tissue injury

Signs and symptoms

- Colonization of the bronchial tree with *Aspergillus,* producing plugs and atelectasis and forming a tangled ball of hyphae (fungal filaments), fibrin, and exudate in a cavity left by a previous illness such as tuberculosis (TB); symptoms absent or mimicking those of TB (productive cough and purulent or blood-tinged sputum, dyspnea, empyema, and lung abscesses)
- *Allergic aspergillosis:* wheezing, dyspnea, cough with some sputum production, pleural pain, and fever
- *Aspergillosis endophthalmitis (2 to 3 weeks after eye injury or surgery):* clouded vision, eye pain, and reddened conjunctivae; after infecting the anterior and posterior chambers, purulent exudate
- *Disseminated aspergillosis:* thrombosis, infarctions, and the typical signs and symptoms of septicemia (such as chills, fever, hypotension, and delirium), with azotemia, hematuria, urinary tract obstruction, headaches, seizures, bone pain and tenderness, and soft-tissue swelling; rapidly fatal

Diagnostic tests

- In patients with aspergilloma, a chest X-ray reveals a crescent-shaped radiolucency surrounding a circular mass, but this isn't definitive for aspergillosis.
- In patients with aspergillosis endophthalmitis, a history of ocular trauma or surgery and a culture or exudate showing *Aspergillus* supports the diagnosis.
- In patients with allergic aspergillosis, sputum examination shows eosinophils.
- Culture of mouth scrapings or sputum showing *Aspergillus* is inconclusive because even healthy persons harbor this fungus.
- In patients with disseminated aspergillosis, culture and microscopic ex-

amination of affected tissue can confirm the diagnosis, but this form is usually diagnosed at autopsy.

Treatment

- Patients with aspergillosis don't have to be isolated.
- Treatment of aspergilloma necessitates local excision of the lesion and supportive therapy, such as chest physiotherapy and coughing, to improve pulmonary function. Those with severe hemoptysis due to fungus ball of the lung may benefit from lobectomy.
- Allergic aspergillosis requires desensitization and, possibly, a steroid.
- Disseminated aspergillosis and aspergillosis endophthalmitis require a 2- to 3-week course of I.V. amphotericin B (Fungizone) (as well as prompt cessation of immunosuppressant therapy).

DRUG CHALLENGE

 The disseminated form of aspergillosis commonly resists amphotericin B therapy and rapidly progresses to death.

DRUG CHALLENGE

 Itraconazole (Sporanox) may be useful in slowing the progression of the disease in patients with immunocompetency.

Nursing considerations

- Help with chest physiotherapy, and instruct the patient to cough effectively.
- Monitor the patient's vital signs, intake and output, and diagnostic test results.
- Provide emotional support for the patient and his family. Be prepared to help the family with grief counseling if the patient has disseminated aspergillosis that isn't responding to therapy.

Asphyxia

A condition of insufficient oxygen and accumulating carbon dioxide in the blood and tissues due to interference with respiration, asphyxia results in cardiopulmonary arrest. Without prompt treatment, it's fatal.

Causes

- Condition or substance that inhibits respiration:
  - Extrapulmonary obstruction, as in tracheal compression from a tumor, strangulation, trauma, or suffocation
  - Hypoventilation as a result of opioid abuse, medullary disease or hemorrhage, pneumothorax, respiratory muscle paralysis, or cardiopulmonary arrest
  - Inhalation of toxic agents, as in carbon monoxide poisoning, smoke inhalation, and excessive oxygen inhalation
  - Intrapulmonary obstruction, as in airway obstruction, severe asthma, foreign-body aspiration, pulmonary edema, pneumonia, and near drowning

Signs and symptoms

- Agitation and confusion leading to coma
- Altered respiratory rate (apnea, bradypnea, or occasional tachypnea)
- Anxiety
- Central and peripheral cyanosis (cherry-red mucous membranes in late-stage carbon monoxide poisoning)
- Decreased breath sounds
- Dyspnea
- Fast, slow, or absent pulse
- Seizures

Diagnostic tests

- Arterial blood gas analysis indicates decreased partial pressure of arterial oxygen (less than 60 mm Hg) and in-

A close look at atelectatic alveoli

Normally, air-filled alveoli exchange oxygen and carbon dioxide with capillary blood. However, in atelectasis, airless, shrunken alveoli can't accomplish gas exchange.

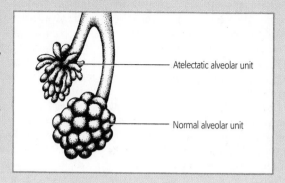

— Atelectatic alveolar unit

— Normal alveolar unit

creased partial pressure of carbon dioxide (greater than 50 mm Hg).

▪ Chest X-rays may show a foreign body, pulmonary edema, or atelectasis.

▪ Toxicology tests may show drugs or chemicals.

▪ A complete blood count may detect abnormal hemoglobin levels.

▪ Pulmonary function tests may indicate respiratory muscle weakness.

Treatment

▪ Immediate respiratory support, with cardiopulmonary resuscitation, endotracheal intubation, and supplemental oxygen is ordered as needed. Then the underlying cause is treated, such as:

– bronchoscopy for extraction of a foreign body

– an opioid antagonist, such as naloxone (Narcan), for opioid overdose

– gastric lavage for poisoning

– limited, graded use of supplemental oxygen for carbon dioxide narcosis caused by excessive oxygen therapy.

Nursing considerations

▪ Respiratory distress is frightening, so reassure the patient during treatment.

▪ Suction carefully, as needed, and encourage deep breathing.

▪ Closely monitor vital signs and laboratory test results.

DRUG CHALLENGE

 To prevent drug-induced asphyxia, warn patients about the danger of taking alcohol with other central nervous system depressants.

▊ Atelectasis

Atelectasis is incomplete expansion of lobules (clusters of alveoli) or lung segments, which may result in partial or complete lung collapse. The collapsed areas are unavailable for gas exchange; unoxygenated blood passes through these areas unchanged, thereby producing hypoxia. Atelectasis may be chronic or acute and occurs to some degree in many patients undergoing upper abdominal or thoracic surgery. The prognosis depends on prompt removal of any airway obstruction, relief of hypoxia, and reexpansion of the collapsed lung. (See *A close look at atelectatic alveoli.*)

Causes

- Bronchial occlusion by mucus plugs, as in patients with chronic obstructive pulmonary disease, bronchiectasis, or cystic fibrosis and in those who smoke heavily
- Bronchogenic carcinoma
- Central nervous system depression (as in drug overdose)
- Condition that makes deep breathing painful (rib fractures, upper abdominal incisions, pleuritic chest pain)
- External compression, which inhibits full lung expansion (tight dressings, obesity)
- Inflammatory lung disease
- Mechanical ventilation using constant small tidal volumes without intermittent deep breaths
- Occlusion by foreign bodies
- Oxygen toxicity
- Prolonged immobility, which causes preferential ventilation of one area of the lung over another
- Pulmonary edema
- Respiratory distress syndrome of the neonate (hyaline membrane disease)

Signs and symptoms

- Anxiety
- Auscultation revealing diminished or bronchial breath sounds
- Compensatory hyperinflation of unaffected areas of the lung
- Cyanosis
- Diaphoresis
- Dyspnea
- Elevation of the ipsilateral hemidiaphragm
- Mediastinal shift to the affected side
- Percussion reveals dullness (when much of lung is collapsed)
- Peripheral circulatory collapse
- Substernal or intercostal retraction
- Tachycardia

Diagnostic tests

- Extensive areas of "microatelectasis" may exist without abnormalities on the chest X-ray. In widespread atelectasis, the chest X-ray shows characteristic horizontal lines in the lower lung zones and, with segmental or lobar collapse, characteristic dense shadows commonly associated with hyperinflation of neighboring lung zones.
- Chest computed tomography is used to confirm findings.
- If the cause is unknown, bronchoscopy is ordered to rule out an obstructing neoplasm or a foreign body.

Treatment

- Incentive spirometry, chest percussion, postural drainage, and frequent coughing and deep-breathing exercises may improve oxygenation.
- Bronchoscopy may help remove secretions.
- Humidity and bronchodilators can improve mucociliary clearance and dilate airways; they may be used with a nebulizer.
- Atelectasis secondary to an obstructing neoplasm may require surgery or radiation therapy.
- Postoperative thoracic and abdominal surgery patients require an analgesic to facilitate deep breathing, which minimizes the risk of atelectasis.

Nursing considerations

- Encourage postoperative and other high-risk patients to cough and deep-breathe every 1 to 2 hours to prevent atelectasis.
- To minimize pain during coughing exercises in postoperative patients, hold a pillow tightly over the incision; teach the patient this technique as well. *Gently* reposition these patients often, and help them walk as soon as possible.
- Give adequate analgesics to control pain.

- During mechanical ventilation, maintain tidal volume at 10 to 15 ml/kg of the patient's body weight to ensure adequate lung expansion. Use the sigh mechanism on the ventilator, if appropriate, to intermittently increase tidal volume at the rate of 3 to 4 sighs per hour.
- Use an incentive spirometer to encourage deep inspiration through positive reinforcement. Teach the patient how to use the spirometer, and encourage him to use it every 1 to 2 hours.
- Humidify inspired air and encourage adequate fluid intake to mobilize secretions. To promote loosening and clearance of secretions, use postural drainage and chest percussion.
- If the patient is intubated or uncooperative, provide suctioning as needed. Use sedatives with discretion because they depress respirations and the cough reflex and suppress sighing.
- Assess breath sounds and ventilatory status frequently, and be alert for any changes.
- Teach the patient about respiratory care, including postural drainage, coughing, and deep breathing.
- Encourage the patient to stop smoking, to lose weight, or both, as needed. Refer him to appropriate support groups for help.
- Provide reassurance and emotional support because the patient may be frightened by his limited breathing capacity.

■ Avian influenza

Avian influenza is a flu infection in birds, but it's of concern to humans, who have no immunity against it. The virus that causes this infection in birds can mutate, easily infecting humans, and potentially starting a deadly worldwide epidemic. Highly infective avian flu viruses, such as H5N1, can survive in the environment for long periods, and infection may be spread simply by touching contaminated surfaces. Birds who recover from the flu can continue to shed the virus in their feces and saliva for as long as 10 days.

The first avian influenza virus to infect humans directly occurred in Hong Kong in 1997 and has since spread across Asia. In October 2005, it was discovered in Turkey and Romania. More than 161 people have been infected with the avian influenza virus A, the "bird flu" virus, designated H5N1, and the current death rate with confirmed infection is more than 50%. The H7N7 avian flu outbreak in the Netherlands resulted in 89 confirmed cases but only one death; the H9N2 avian flu infected three children in Asia and all three recovered. Prognosis depends on the severity of infection and the type of avian influenza virus that caused it.

Causes

- Viral infection with H5N1. Those at risk include:
  - Farmers and other people who work with poultry
  - Health care workers and household contacts of patients with avian influenza
  - People who eat raw or undercooked poultry meat
  - People who handle an infected bird
  - Travelers visiting affected countries

Signs and symptoms

Symptoms of avian flu infection in humans depend on the particular strain of virus. In the H5N1 virus, infection causes classic flulike symptoms, which might include:

- Headache
- Malaise
- Cough (dry or productive)
- Sore throat

- Temperature higher than 100.4° F (38° C)
- Runny nose
- Difficulty breathing
- Diarrhea
- Muscle aches
- Complications including pneumonia, acute respiratory distress, sepsis, and organ failure

Diagnostic tests

- Influenza A/H5 (Asian lineage) Virus Real-time RT-PCR Primer and Probe Set gives preliminary results within 4 hours; older tests required 2 to 3 days.
- Results of chest X-ray, nasopharyngeal culture, and blood differential also help confirm the diagnosis.

Treatment

- The antiviral medication oseltamivir (Tamiflu), and perhaps zanamivir (Relenza), may decrease the severity of the disease, if started within 48 hours after symptoms begin.
- Oseltamivir may also be prescribed for household contacts of people diagnosed with avian flu.

Drug challenge

Samples of H5N1 from human infections proved resistant to the antiviral medications amantadine and rimantadine, so these medications can't be used if an H5N1 outbreak occurs.

- Supportive treatment with mechanical ventilation, I.V. fluids, and symptomatic treatment may be ordered.
- People diagnosed with H5N1 infection should be put in isolation.
- No vaccine against avian influenza is yet available, but a vaccine against H5N1 is being tested in clinical trials.
- An influenza (flu) shot should be given to reduce the chance of an avian flu virus mixing with a human flu virus, which would create a new virus that may easily spread.

Nursing considerations

- Tell patients to call their practitioners if they develop flulike symptoms within 10 days of handling infected birds or traveling to an area with a known avian flu outbreak.
- Travelers shouldn't visit live-bird markets in areas with an avian flu outbreak.
- Those who work with birds that might be infected should use protective clothing and special breathing masks.
- Tell the patient that avoiding undercooked or uncooked meat reduces the risk of exposure to avian flu and other food-borne diseases.
- Teach the patient about proper disposal of tissues and proper hand-washing technique.
- Watch for signs and symptoms of complications.

B

Basal cell epithelioma

A slow-growing, destructive skin tumor, basal cell epithelioma or carcinoma usually occurs in persons older than age 40; it's more prevalent in blond, fair-skinned men and is the most common malignant tumor affecting whites. Changes in epidermal basal cells can diminish maturation and normal keratinization. Continuing division of basal cells leads to mass formation. The three types are noduloulcerative lesion, superficial basal cell epithelioma, and sclerosing basal cell epithelioma.

Causes

- Arsenic ingestion
- Burns
- Immunosuppression
- Prolonged sun exposure (most common)
- Radiation exposure
- Vaccinations (rare)

Signs and symptoms
Noduloulcerative lesions

- Occur most commonly on the face, particularly the forehead, eyelid margins, and nasolabial folds
- Early lesions: small, smooth, pinkish, and translucent papules; telangiectatic vessels crossing the surface; occasionally pigmented
- Later lesions: centers depressed; borders firm and elevated
- Result in ulceration and local invasion (known as *rodent ulcers;* rarely metastasize but, if untreated, can spread to vital areas and become infected; can cause massive hemorrhage if they invade large blood vessels)

Superficial basal cell epitheliomas

- Numerous; commonly on chest and back
- Oval or irregularly shaped, lightly pigmented plaques, with sharply defined, slightly elevated threadlike borders
- Appear scaly with small atrophic areas in center that resemble psoriasis or eczema; usually chronic, but don't tend to invade other areas
- Related to ingestion of or exposure to arsenic-containing compounds

Sclerosing basal cell epitheliomas

- Waxy, sclerotic, yellow to white plaques without distinct borders occurring on the head and neck that look like small patches of scleroderma

Diagnostic tests

- Incisional or excisional biopsy and histologic study may help to determine the tumor type and histologic subtype.

Treatment

- Curettage and electrodesiccation offer good cosmetic results for small lesions.
- Topical fluorouracil is commonly used for superficial lesions. This medication produces marked local irritation or inflammation in the involved tissue but no systemic effects.
- Microscopically controlled surgical excision carefully removes recurrent lesions until a tumor-free plane is achieved. After removal of large lesions, skin grafting may be required.
- Irradiation is used if the tumor location requires it or if the patient is elderly or debilitated and might not withstand surgery.
- Cryotherapy with liquid nitrogen freezes and kills the cells.
- Chemosurgery may be necessary for persistent or recurrent lesions. Chemosurgery consists of periodic applications of a fixative paste (such as zinc chloride) and subsequent removal of fixed pathologic tissue. Treatment continues until the tumor has been completely removed.

Nursing considerations

- Instruct the patient to eat frequent small meals that are high in protein. Suggest eggnog, pureed foods, or liquid protein supplements if the lesion has invaded the oral cavity and is causing eating problems.
- Tell the patient that to prevent the disease from recurring, he needs to avoid excessive sun exposure and use a strong sunscreen or sunshade to protect his skin from damage by ultraviolet rays.
- Advise the patient to relieve local inflammation from topical fluorouracil with cool compresses or corticosteroid ointment.
- Instruct the patient with noduloulcerative basal cell epithelioma to wash his face gently when ulcerations and crust-

ing occur; scrubbing too vigorously may cause bleeding.

Bell's palsy

Bell's palsy is a neurologic disorder that affects the seventh cranial (facial) nerve, producing unilateral facial weakness or paralysis. Onset is rapid. Although it affects all age-groups, it's most common in people ages 20 to 60. In 80% to 90% of patients, it subsides spontaneously, with complete recovery in 1 to 8 weeks; however, recovery may be delayed in older adults. If recovery is partial, contractures may develop on the paralyzed side of the face. Bell's palsy may recur on the same or opposite side of the face.

Causes

- Ischemia, tumor, meningitis, or local trauma
- Seventh cranial nerve blocked by an inflammatory reaction
- Viral disease (most likely herpes simplex or herpes zoster)

Signs and symptoms

- Bell's phenomenon: incomplete eye closure on weak side shows eye movement that's normally covered by eyelid—eye rolls upward when attempt made to close it, with excessive tearing
- Hypersensitivity to sound
- Unilateral facial weakness, occasionally with aching pain around the angle of the jaw or behind the ear
- Weak side characterized by drooping mouth (causing the patient to drool saliva from the corner of his mouth), impaired ability to close the eye, and distorted taste perception over the affected anterior portion of the tongue

Diagnostic tests

- After 10 days, electromyography helps predict the level of expected recovery by distinguishing temporary conduction defects from a pathologic interruption of nerve fibers.

Treatment
- Corticosteroids reduce facial nerve edema and improve nerve conduction and blood flow.
- After the 14th day of corticosteroid therapy, electrotherapy may help prevent atrophy of facial muscles.

Nursing considerations

DRUG CHALLENGE

 If the patient is being treated with corticosteroids, watch for adverse reactions, especially GI distress and fluid retention. If GI distress is troublesome, the patient may benefit from an antacid. If the patient has diabetes, corticosteroids must be used with caution and serum glucose levels frequently monitored.

- To reduce pain, apply moist heat to the affected side of the face, taking care not to burn the skin. If the patient is given an analgesic, monitor him for therapeutic effect of the drug.
- To help maintain muscle tone, massage the patient's face with a gentle upward motion two or three times daily for 5 to 10 minutes, or have him massage his face himself. When he's ready for active exercises, teach him to exercise by grimacing in front of a mirror.
- Advise the patient to protect his eye by covering it with an eye patch, especially when outdoors. Tell him to keep warm, to avoid exposure to dust and wind, and to cover his face when exposure is unavoidable.
- To prevent complications related to swallowing difficulty (aspiration and weight loss), instruct the patient to always sit up straight when eating, chew on the unaffected side, take small bites, and eat nutritionally balanced meals,

while avoiding foods that are hard to chew.
- Arrange for privacy at mealtimes to reduce embarrassment.
- Apply a facial sling to improve lip alignment.
- Give the patient frequent and complete mouth care, being careful to remove residual food that collects between the cheeks and gums.
- Offer psychological support. Reassure the patient that recovery is likely within 1 to 8 weeks.

▌ Benign prostatic hyperplasia

Although most men older than age 50 have some prostatic enlargement, with benign prostatic hyperplasia (BPH), the prostate gland enlarges sufficiently to compress the urethra and cause some overt urinary obstruction. Depending on the size of the enlarged prostate, the age and health of the patient, and the extent of obstruction, BPH is treated symptomatically or surgically.

Whatever the cause, BPH begins with changes in periurethral glandular tissue. As the prostate enlarges, it may extend into the bladder and obstruct urinary outflow by compressing or distorting the prostatic urethra. BPH may also cause a pouch to form in the bladder that retains urine when the rest of the bladder empties. This retained urine may lead to calculus formation or cystitis.

Causes
- Arteriosclerosis
- Imbalance in androgen and estrogen levels and high levels of dihydrotestosterone
- Inflammation
- Metabolic or nutritional disturbance
- Neoplasm

Combating septic shock after prostate surgery

If the postsurgical patient develops severe chills, sudden fever, tachycardia, hypotension, or other signs or symptoms of shock, immediately do the following:
- Notify other care team members.
- Start a rapid I.V. infusion of an antibiotic as needed.

- Watch for pulmonary embolism, heart failure, and renal shutdown.
- Monitor vital signs, central venous pressure, and arterial pressure continuously.

The patient may need supportive care in the intensive care unit.

Signs and symptoms

- Group of symptoms called *prostatism:* reduced urinary stream caliber and force, difficulty starting micturition (straining), feeling of incomplete voiding and, occasionally, urine retention
- Enlarged prostate upon rectal palpation
- Urination more frequent, with nocturia, incontinence and, possibly, hematuria; may result eventually in infection followed by complete urinary obstruction
- Visible midline mass (distended bladder) that represents an incompletely emptied bladder
- Complications that include infection, renal insufficiency, hemorrhage, anemia, and shock

Diagnostic tests

- Excretory urography may indicate urinary tract obstruction, hydronephrosis, calculi or tumors, and filling and emptying defects in the bladder.
- Elevated blood urea nitrogen and serum creatinine levels suggest impaired renal function.
- Urinalysis and urine culture show hematuria, pyuria and, when the bacterial count exceeds 100,000/μl, urinary tract infection (UTI).
- With severe symptoms, a cystourethroscopy is definitive, but this test is performed only immediately before surgery to help determine the best proce-

dure. It can show prostate enlargement, bladder wall changes, and a raised bladder.

Treatment

- Conservative therapy includes prostate massages, sitz baths, short-term fluid restriction for bladder distention, and an antimicrobial for infection. Regular ejaculation may help relieve prostatic congestion.
- Urine flow rates can be improved with alpha-adrenergic blockers, such as doxazosin (Cardura), terazosin (Hytrin), tamsulosin (Flomax), and prazosin (Minipress). These drugs relieve bladder outlet obstruction by preventing contractions of the prostatic capsule and bladder neck. Finasteride (Proscar) may also reduce the size of the prostate in some patients.
- Surgery is the only effective therapy to relieve acute urine retention, hydronephrosis, severe hematuria, recurrent UTIs, and other intolerable signs and symptoms. (See *Combating septic shock after prostate surgery.*)
- A transurethral resection may be performed if the prostate weighs less than 2 oz (56.7 g). In this procedure, a resectoscope removes tissue with a wire loop and electric current. In high-risk patients, continuous drainage with an indwelling urinary catheter alleviates urine retention.

- Alternatively, large prostates can be removed by one of three surgical approaches:
  – *Suprapubic (transvesical) resection:* most common and useful when prostatic enlargement remains within the bladder
  – *Perineal resection:* usually performed for a large gland in older patients and commonly results in impotence and incontinence
  – *Retropubic (extravesical) resection:* allows direct visualization; potency and continence are usually maintained.
- Transurethral microwaves (heat therapy) are now being used in some patients. Their efficacy lies between that of the use of an alpha$_1$-adrenergic blocker and surgery.

Nursing considerations

- Monitor and record the patient's vital signs, intake and output, and daily weight. Watch closely for signs of postobstructive diuresis (such as increased urine output and hypotension), which may lead to serious dehydration, lowered blood volume, shock, electrolyte loss, and anuria.
- Give a prescribed antibiotic, as needed, for UTI, urethral instrumentation, and cystoscopy.
- If urine retention is present, insert an indwelling urinary catheter (usually difficult to do in a patient with BPH). If the catheter can't be passed transurethrally, assist with suprapubic cystostomy (under local anesthetic). Watch for rapid bladder decompression.

After prostate surgery

- Maintain patient comfort, and watch for and prevent postoperative complications.
- Observe the patient for immediate dangers of prostatic bleeding (shock and hemorrhage). Check the catheter frequently (every 15 minutes for the first

2 to 3 hours) for patency and urine color; check the dressings for bleeding.
- Many urologists insert a three-way catheter and establish continuous bladder irrigation. Keep the catheter open at a rate sufficient to maintain returns that are clear and light pink.
- Watch for fluid overload from absorption of the irrigating fluid into systemic circulation. If a regular catheter is being used, observe it closely. If drainage stops because of clots, irrigate the catheter, usually with 80 to 100 ml of normal saline solution, while maintaining strict aseptic technique.
- Also watch for septic shock, the most serious complication of prostate surgery.
- Give belladonna and an opium suppository or another anticholinergic, as needed, to relieve painful bladder spasms that can occur after transurethral resection.
- After an open procedure, provide suppositories (except after perineal prostatectomy), an analgesic to control incisional pain, and frequent dressing changes.
- Continue infusing fluids I.V. until the patient can drink a sufficient amount (2 to 3 qt [2 to 3 L] per day) to maintain adequate hydration.
- Give a stool softener and a laxative, as ordered, to prevent straining. *Don't* check for fecal impaction: A rectal examination could precipitate bleeding.
- After the catheter is removed, the patient may experience urinary frequency, dribbling, and occasional hematuria. Reassure him that he'll gradually regain urinary control. Explain this to the patient's family so they can also reassure the patient.
- Reinforce prescribed limits on activity. Warn the patient against lifting, strenuous exercise, and long automobile rides because these increase bleeding tendency. Also, caution him to restrict sexual

activity for at least several weeks after discharge.

■ Instruct the patient to follow the prescribed oral antibiotic regimen, and tell him the indications for using gentle laxatives. Urge him to seek medical care immediately if he can't void, if he passes bloody urine, or if he develops a fever.

Bladder cancer

Bladder tumors can develop on the surface of the bladder wall (benign or malignant papillomas) or grow within the bladder wall (generally more virulent) and quickly invade underlying muscles. Most bladder tumors (90%) are transitional cell carcinomas, arising from the transitional epithelium of mucous membranes. Less common are adenocarcinomas, epidermoid carcinomas, squamous cell carcinomas, sarcomas, tumors in bladder diverticula, and carcinoma in situ. Bladder tumors are most prevalent in men older than age 50 and are more common in densely populated industrial areas, but women are diagnosed at more advanced stages. (See *Women and bladder cancer.*)

Causes
■ Environmental carcinogens, such as 2-naphthylamine, benzidine, tobacco, and nitrates
■ Squamous cell carcinoma of the bladder is most common in geographic areas where schistosomiasis is endemic

Signs and symptoms
■ In early stages, symptomless in about 25% of patients with bladder tumors
■ First sign is gross, painless, intermittent hematuria (typically with clots in the urine)
■ With invasive lesions, usually suprapubic pain after voiding
■ Other symptoms: bladder irritability, urinary frequency, nocturia, and dribbling

Diagnostic tests
■ Cystoscopy confirms bladder cancer and should be performed when hematuria first appears. When it's performed under anesthesia, a bimanual examination is usually done to determine if the bladder is fixed to the pelvic wall.
■ Biopsy is positive for cancer.
■ Urinalysis can detect blood in the urine and malignant cytology.
■ Excretory urography can identify a large, early-stage tumor or an infiltrating tumor, delineate functional problems in the upper urinary tract, assess hydronephrosis, and detect rigid deformity of the bladder wall.
■ Retrograde cystography evaluates bladder structure and integrity. Test results help to confirm the diagnosis.
■ Pelvic arteriography can reveal tumor invasion into the bladder wall.

Women and bladder cancer

A greater percentage of women are diagnosed with bladder cancer at more advanced stages than men, which may contribute to the higher mortality in women. (Women are about twice as likely to die from the disease as men.) Contributing factors include a higher proportion of nontransitional cell cancer histologies (rare cell types) that occur in women (adenocarcinoma, small cell carcinoma, squamous cell carcinoma); the relative thinness of an elderly woman's bladder (perhaps permitting more rapid extravesical spread); and the older median age at presentation in women. Even higher incidences of bladder cancer were found in women who smoked, used hair dye, or drank tap water containing nitrates.

- Computed tomography scan reveals the thickness of the involved bladder wall and detects enlarged retroperitoneal lymph nodes.
- Ultrasonography can detect metastasis beyond the bladder and can distinguish a bladder cyst from a tumor.

Treatment
Superficial bladder tumors

- These are removed by transurethral (cystoscopic) resection and fulguration (electrical destruction). This procedure is adequate when the tumor hasn't invaded the muscle.
- Intravesicular chemotherapy is used for tumors that occur in many sites and to prevent recurrence. This treatment involves washing the bladder directly with an antineoplastic—most commonly, thiotepa, doxorubicin (Rubex), or mitomycin (Mutamycin).
- Intravesical administration of the live, attenuated bacille Calmette-Guérin (BCG) vaccine has been successful in treating superficial bladder cancers.
- For additional tumors, fulguration may have to be repeated every 3 months for years. However, if the tumors penetrate the muscle layer or recur frequently, cystoscopy with fulguration is no longer appropriate.
- Tumors too large to be treated through a cystoscope require segmental bladder resection to remove a full-thickness section of the bladder. This procedure is feasible only if the tumor isn't near the bladder neck or ureteral orifices. Bladder instillations of thiotepa after transurethral resection may also help control such tumors.
- Immunotherapy may be used to fight cancer. BCG is an immunomodulating agent commonly used following surgery to remove the tumor. Biologic response modifiers—such as interferons, interleukins, colony-stimulating factors, monoclonal antibodies, and vaccines—

may also be used to alter the interaction between the body's immune defenses and the cancer cells. The goal is to boost, direct, or restore the body's ability to fight the disease.

Infiltrating bladder tumors

- Radical cystectomy is the treatment of choice. Surgery involves removal of the bladder with perivesical fat, lymph nodes, urethra, the prostate and seminal vesicles (in males), and the uterus and adnexa (in females). The surgeon forms a urinary diversion, usually an ileal conduit. The patient must then continuously wear an external pouch. (See *Caring for a urinary stoma,* page 54.) Other diversions include ureterostomy, nephrostomy, vesicostomy, ileal bladder, ileal loop, and sigmoid conduit.
- The week before cystectomy, treatment may include external beam therapy to the bladder.
- Males may become impotent following radical cystectomy and urethrectomy because these procedures damage the sympathetic and parasympathetic nerves that control erection and ejaculation. At a later date, the patient may desire a penile implant to make sexual intercourse (without ejaculation) possible.

Advanced bladder cancer

- Cystectomy, radiation therapy, and systemic chemotherapy with such drugs as cyclophosphamide, fluorouracil (Efudex), doxorubicin, and cisplatin (Platinol-AQ) are used in combination and are sometimes successful in arresting bladder cancer.
- Cisplatin is the single most effective agent.

Nursing considerations
- Before surgery, assist in selecting a stoma site that the patient can see (usually in the rectus muscle to minimize the

Caring for a urinary stoma

If your patient has a urinary stoma, be sure to review the following patient-teaching points:

■ First, show the patient how to prepare and apply the pouch, which may be reusable or disposable. If he chooses the reusable type, he'll need at least two.

■ To select the right-sized pouch, teach the patient to measure the stoma and order a pouch with an opening that clears the stoma with a ⅛" margin. Instruct him to remeasure the stoma after he goes home, in case the size changes. The pouch should have a drainage valve at the bottom. Tell him to empty the pouch when it's one-third full or every 2 to 3 hours.

■ To ensure a good skin seal, advise the patient to select a skin barrier that contains synthetics and little or no karaya (which urine tends to destroy). Check the pouch frequently to make sure that the skin seal remains intact. A good skin seal with a skin barrier may last for 3 to 6 days, so change the pouch only that often. Tell the patient that he can wear a loose-fitting elastic belt to help secure the pouch.

■ The ileal conduit stoma reaches its permanent size 2 to 4 months after surgery. Because the intestine normally produces mucus, tell the patient not to be alarmed by mucus that appears in the draining urine.

■ Instruct the patient to keep the skin around the stoma clean and free from irritation, as follows:

  − After removing the pouch, wash the skin with water and mild soap. Rinse well with clear water to remove soap residue, and then gently pat the skin dry; don't rub.

  − Place a gauze sponge soaked with vinegar-water (1 part to 3 parts) over the stoma for a few minutes to prevent buildup of uric acid crystals. While preparing the skin, place a rolled-up dry sponge over the stoma to collect draining urine.

  − Coat the skin with a silicone skin protector, and cover with the collection pouch. If skin irritation or breakdown occurs, apply a layer of antacid precipitate to the clean, dry skin before coating with the skin protector.

■ Advise the patient that he can level uneven surfaces on his abdomen—such as gullies, scars, or wedges—with various specially prepared products or skin barriers.

risk of herniation). Do so by assessing the abdomen in various positions.

■ After surgery, encourage the patient to look at the stoma. Provide a mirror to make viewing easier.

■ To obtain a specimen for culture and sensitivity testing, catheterize the patient using sterile technique. Insert the lubricated tip of the catheter into the stoma about 2" (5 cm). In many facilities, a double telescope-type catheter is available for ileal conduit catheterization.

■ Advise the patient with a urinary stoma that he may participate in most activities, except for heavy lifting and contact sports.

■ When a patient with a urinary diversion is discharged, arrange for follow-up home health care or refer him to an enterostomal therapist, who will help coordinate the patient's care.

■ Teach the patient about his urinary stoma. Encourage appropriate relatives or other caregivers to attend the teaching session. Advise this person beforehand that a negative reaction to the stoma can impede the patient's adjustment.

■ All high-risk people—for example, chemical workers and people with a history of benign bladder tumors or persistent cystitis—should have periodic cytologic examinations and learn about the dangers of disease-causing agents.

■ Refer the patient to such resources as the American Cancer Society and the United Ostomy Association.

Blastomycosis

Also called *Gilchrist's disease,* blastomycosis is caused by the yeastlike fungus *Blastomyces dermatitidis,* which usually infects the lungs and produces bronchopneumonia. Less commonly, this fungus may disseminate through the blood and cause osteomyelitis and central nervous system (CNS), skin, and genital disorders.

Untreated blastomycosis is slowly progressive and usually fatal; however, spontaneous remissions occasionally occur. With antifungal therapy and supportive treatment, the prognosis for patients with blastomycosis is good.

Blastomycosis is generally found in North America (where *B. dermatitidis* normally inhabits the soil) and is endemic to the southeastern United States. Sporadic cases have also been reported in Africa. Blastomycosis usually infects men between ages 30 and 50, but no occupational link has been found.

Causes

■ *B. dermatitidis* probably inhaled by people in close contact with soil

Signs and symptoms

■ Initial signs and symptoms of pulmonary blastomycosis mimic those of a viral upper respiratory tract infection. These findings typically include pleuritic chest pain, fever, shaking, chills, night sweats, malaise, anorexia, weight loss, and a dry, hacking, or productive cough (occasionally hemoptysis).

■ Cutaneous blastomycosis causes small, painless, nonpruritic, and nondistinctive macules or papules on exposed body parts. These lesions become raised and reddened and occasionally progress to draining skin abscesses or fistulas.

■ Skeletal involvement causes soft-tissue swelling, tenderness, and warmth over bony lesions, which generally occur in the thoracic, lumbar, and sacral regions; long bones of the legs; and, in children, the skull.

■ Genital involvement produces painful swelling of the testes, the epididymis, or the prostate; deep perineal pain; pyuria; and hematuria.

■ CNS involvement causes meningitis or cerebral abscesses, resulting in a decreased level of consciousness (LOC), lethargy, and change in mood or affect.

■ Other dissemination may result in Addison's disease (adrenal insufficiency), pericarditis, and arthritis.

Diagnostic tests

■ Culture of *B. dermatitidis* is taken from skin lesions, pus, sputum, or pulmonary secretions.

■ Biopsy of tissue from the skin or lungs or of bronchial washings, sputum, or pus is ordered as appropriate.

■ Immunodiffusion testing detects antibodies for the A and B antigen of blastomycosis.

■ Chest X-ray may show pulmonary infiltrates in pulmonary blastomycosis.

■ Blood tests show an increased white blood cell count and erythrocyte sedimentation rate.

■ Other blood studies show slightly increased serum globulin levels, mild normochromic anemia and, with bone lesions, an increased alkaline phosphatase level.

Treatment

- All forms of blastomycosis respond to I.V. amphotericin B. Therapy is 8 to 10 weeks for skin and noncavitary lung lesions and 10 to 12 weeks for cavitary lesions or infection extending beyond lung and skin.
- Oral itraconazole (Sporanox) may be used as an alternative, especially for monomeningeal blastomycosis patients who can take the drug reliably (6 to 12 months).

Nursing considerations

- If the patient has severe pulmonary blastomycosis, check for hemoptysis. If he's febrile, provide a cool room, and give tepid sponge baths.
- If blastomycosis causes joint pain or swelling, elevate the joint and apply heat.
- If the patient has a CNS infection, watch him carefully for decreasing LOC and unequal pupillary response.
- If the patient is a male with disseminated disease, watch for hematuria.

DRUG CHALLENGE

 Infuse I.V. amphotericin B slowly (a too-rapid infusion may cause circulatory collapse). During the infusion, monitor vital signs. (Temperature may rise but should subside within 1 to 2 hours.) Watch for decreased urine output, and monitor laboratory test results for increased blood urea nitrogen and serum creatinine levels and hypokalemia, which may indicate renal toxicity. Immediately report any hearing loss, tinnitus, or dizziness.

- To relieve adverse reactions to amphotericin B, give antiemetics, antihistamines, and antipyretics, as needed.

Blepharitis

A common inflammation, blepharitis produces a red-rimmed appearance of the margins of the eyelids. In many cases, it's chronic and bilateral and affects upper and lower lids. *Seborrheic blepharitis* is characterized by waxy scales and is common in older adults and in those with red hair. *Staphylococcal (ulcerative) blepharitis* is characterized by tiny ulcerated areas along the lid margins. Both types may coexist.

Blepharitis tends to recur and become chronic. It can be controlled if treatment begins before the onset of ocular involvement.

Causes

- Seborrheic blepharitis: results from seborrhea of scalp, eyebrows, or ears
- Ulcerative blepharitis: results from *Staphylococcus aureus* infection

Signs and symptoms

- Itching, burning, foreign-body sensation, and sticky, crusted eyelids on waking
- Constant irritation results in unconscious rubbing of eyes (causing reddened rims) or continual blinking
- Waxy scales in seborrheic blepharitis
- Flaky scales on lashes, loss of lashes, and ulcerated areas on lid margins in ulcerative blepharitis

Diagnostic tests

- With ulcerative blepharitis, a culture of the ulcerated lid margin shows *S. aureus.*

Treatment

Early treatment is essential to prevent recurrence or complications. In addition to warm compresses, treatment depends on which type of blepharitis the patient has.

• Seborrheic blepharitis: Eyelashes may be shampooed daily (using a mild shampoo on a damp applicator stick or a washcloth) to remove scales from the lid margins; also, the scalp and eyebrows should be frequently shampooed.
• Ulcerative blepharitis: Warm compresses may be applied and an appropriate antibiotic ointment may be used at bedtime; additionally, a combination antibiotic and steroid, such as prednisolone may be used; inflammation of the conjunctiva or cornea may be treated orally with tetracycline or doxycycline.
• Blepharitis resulting from pediculosis: Nits should be removed (with forceps) or ophthalmic physostigmine or other insecticidal ointment may be applied. (This may cause pupil constriction and, possibly, headache, conjunctival irritation, and blurred vision from the film of ointment on the cornea.)

Nursing considerations
• Instruct the patient to gently remove scales from the lid margins daily with an applicator stick or a clean washcloth.
• Teach the patient the following method for applying warm compresses: First, run warm water into a clean bowl. Then immerse a clean cloth in the water, and wring it out. Place the warm cloth against the closed eyelid. (Be careful not to burn the skin.) Hold the compress in place until it cools. Continue this procedure for 15 minutes.
• Antibiotic ophthalmic ointment should be applied after a 15-minute application of warm compresses.
• Treatment of seborrheic blepharitis also requires attention to the face and scalp.

Bone tumors, primary malignant

A rare type of bone cancer, primary malignant bone tumors (sarcomas of the bone) constitute less than 1% of all malignant tumors. Most malignant bone tumors are secondary, caused by seeding from a primary site. Primary malignant bone tumors are more common in males, especially in children and adolescents, although some types do occur in patients between ages 35 and 60.

The tumors may originate in osseous or nonosseous tissue. Osseous bone tumors arise from the bony structure itself and include osteogenic sarcoma (the most common), parosteal osteogenic sarcoma, chondrosarcoma (chondroblastic), and malignant giant cell tumor. Together they make up 60% of all malignant bone tumors. Nonosseous tumors arise from hematopoietic, vascular, and neural tissues and include Ewing's sarcoma, fibrosarcoma (fibroblastic), and chordoma. Osteogenic and Ewing's sarcomas are the most common bone tumors in childhood. (See *Types of primary malignant bone tumors,* pages 58 and 59.)

Causes
• Characteristic translocation of genetic material from chromosome 22 to chromosome 11 (in Ewing's sarcoma cells)
• Genetic abnormalities (retinoblastoma, Rothmund Thomson syndrome) or exposure to carcinogens (such as ingested radium in watch dial painters) (most cases have no immediately apparent cause)
• Heredity, trauma, and excessive radiation therapy (theoretical)

Signs and symptoms
• Limb pain and refusal to walk with limited range of motion common findings in children with bone tumors
• Bone pain: the most common indication of a primary malignant bone tumor; usually more intense at night and not associated with mobility; dull and usually localized, although may be referred

Types of primary malignant bone tumors

Type	Clinical features	Treatment
Osseous origin		
Chondro-sarcoma	▪ Develops from cartilage ▪ Painless; grows slowly but is locally recurrent and invasive ▪ Occurs most often in the pelvis, proximal femur, ribs, and shoulder girdle ▪ Usually occurs in males ages 30 to 50	▪ Wide surgical resection if possible; amputation if necessary
Malignant giant cell tumor	▪ Arises from benign giant cell tumor ▪ Found most often in long bones, especially in knee area ▪ Usually occurs in females ages 18 to 50	▪ Total excision ▪ Radiation for recurrent disease ▪ Chemotherapy
Osteogenic sarcoma	▪ Osteoid tumor present in specimen ▪ Tumor arises from bone-forming osteoblast ▪ Occurs most commonly in the femur but also in the tibia and the humerus and, occasionally, the fistula, ileum, vertebra, or mandible ▪ Most common bone cancer; usually occurs in males ages 10 to 30 ▪ May metastasize to the lungs	▪ Preoperative chemotherapy ▪ Surgery (wide resection or amputation) ▪ Postoperative chemotherapy
Parosteal osteogenic sarcoma	▪ Develops on surface of bone instead of interior ▪ Progresses slowly ▪ Occurs most often in the distal femur but also in the tibia, humerus, and ulna ▪ Usually occurs in females ages 30 to 40	▪ Surgery (tumor resection, possible amputation, interscapulothoracic surgery, hemipelvectomy)
Nonosseous origin		
Chordoma	▪ Derived from embryonic remnants of notochord ▪ Progresses slowly ▪ Usually found at end of vertebral column and in sphenooccipital, sacrococcygeal, and vertebral areas ▪ Characterized by constipation and visual disturbances ▪ Usually occurs in males ages 50 to 60 ▪ Originates in bone marrow and invades shafts of long and flat bones	▪ Surgical resectioning (commonly resulting in neural defects) ▪ Radiation (palliative, or when surgery isn't applicable, as in occipital area)

Types of primary malignant bone tumors *(continued)*

Type	Clinical features	Treatment
Nonosseous origin *(continued)*		
Ewing's sarcoma	▪ Originates in bone marrow and invades shafts of long and flat bones ▪ Usually affects lower extremities, most often the femur, innominate bones, ribs, tibia, humerus, vertebra, and fibula; may metastasize to the lungs ▪ Patients may present with systemic symptoms suggesting infection (fever, local tenderness, warmth, swelling) ▪ Pain increasingly severe and persistent ▪ Usually occurs in males ages 10 to 20 ▪ Prognosis has improved dramatically with effective chemotherapy	▪ High-voltage radiation (Tumor is very radiosensitive.) ▪ Chemotherapy to slow growth ▪ Amputation only if there's no evidence of metastasis
Fibrosarcoma	▪ Relatively rare ▪ Originates in fibrous tissue of bone ▪ Invades long or flat bones (femur, tibia, mandible) but also involves the periosteum and overlying muscle ▪ Usually occurs in males ages 30 to 40	▪ Amputation ▪ Radiation ▪ Chemotherapy ▪ Bone grafts (with low-grade fibrosarcoma)

from the hip or spine, which results in weakness or a limp

▪ A mass or tumor that may be tender and swell; typically palpable

▪ Pathologic fractures

▪ Late stages: patient may be cachectic, with fever and impaired mobility

Diagnostic tests

▪ A biopsy (by incision or by aspiration) confirms a primary malignant bone tumor.

▪ Bone X-rays, radioisotope bone and computed tomography (CT) scans, and magnetic resonance imaging are all useful in assessing tumor size.

▪ Serum alkaline phosphatase levels are usually elevated in patients with sarcoma.

▪ Bone scans and CT scans of the lungs are important in checking for metastatic disease.

Treatment

▪ Excision of the tumor along with a 3″ (7.6 cm) margin is the treatment of choice. It may be combined with preoperative chemotherapy.

▪ In some patients, radical surgery (such as hemipelvectomy or interscapulothoracic amputation) is necessary. However, surgical resection of the tumor (commonly with preoperative *and* postoperative chemotherapy) has saved limbs from amputation.

▪ Intensive chemotherapy includes administration of doxorubicin (Rubex), ifosfamide, cisplatin (Platinol-AQ), and high doses of methotrexate (Trexall), alone or in various combinations for osteosarcomas. Additionally, vincristine, etoposide, and dactinomycin (Cosmegen) may be added if the patient has Ewing's sarcoma. Chemotherapy may be infused intra-arterially into the long bones of the legs.

Nursing considerations

- Be sensitive to the emotional strain caused by the threat of amputation. Encourage communication, and help the patient set realistic goals.
- If the surgery will affect the patient's lower extremities, have a physical therapist teach him how to use assistive devices (such as a walker) preoperatively.
- Teach the patient how to readjust his body weight so that he can get into and out of the bed and wheelchair.
- Before surgery, start I.V. infusions to maintain fluid and electrolyte balance and to have an open vein available if blood or plasma is needed during surgery.
- After surgery, check vital signs and circulation to the extremities every 15 minutes for the first hour, every 30 minutes for the next 2 hours, every hour for the next 4 hours, every 2 hours for the next 4 hours, and then every 4 hours when the patient's condition is stable.
- Check the dressing periodically for oozing.
- Elevate the foot of the bed or place the stump on a pillow for the first 24 hours. (Be careful not to leave the stump elevated for more than 48 hours because this may lead to contractures.)
- To ease the patient's anxiety, give him an analgesic for pain before morning care. If necessary, brace him with pillows, keeping the affected part at rest.
- Urge the patient to eat foods high in protein and vitamins and to get plenty of rest and sleep to promote recovery.

DRUG CHALLENGE

 If the patient is receiving methotrexate, dietary folate should be avoided.

- Encourage some physical exercise. Give a stool softener, as prescribed, to maintain proper elimination.
- Encourage the patient to drink plenty of fluids to prevent dehydration. Accurately record intake and output. After a hemipelvectomy, insert a nasogastric tube to prevent abdominal distention. Continue low gastric suction for 2 days after surgery or until bowel sounds return and the patient can tolerate a liquid diet. Give an antibiotic to prevent infection. Perform a transfusion, if necessary, and provide pain relievers. Keep drains in place to facilitate wound drainage and prevent infection. Use an indwelling urinary catheter until the patient can void voluntarily.
- Keep in mind that rehabilitation programs after limb salvage surgery vary, depending on the patient, the body part affected, and the type of surgery performed. For example, one patient may have a surgically implanted prosthesis (for example, after joint surgery), whereas another may have reconstructive surgery requiring an allograft (such as bone from a bone bank) or an autograft (bone from the patient's own body).

Encourage early rehabilitation for amputees as follows:
- Start physical therapy 24 hours postoperatively. Pain usually isn't severe after amputation. If it is, watch for a wound complication, such as hematoma, excessive stump edema, or infection.
- Be aware of the "phantom limb" syndrome, in which the patient "feels" an itch or tingling in an amputated extremity. This can last for several hours or persist for years. Explain that this sensation is normal and usually subsides.

■ To avoid contractures and ensure the best conditions for wound healing, warn the patient that he shouldn't:
– hang the stump over the edge of the bed
– sit in a wheelchair with the stump flexed
– place a pillow under his hip, knee, or back or between his thighs
– lie with knees flexed
– rest an above-the-knee stump on the crutch handle
– abduct an above-the-knee stump.
■ Wash the stump, massage it gently, and keep it dry until it heals. Make sure the bandage is firm and worn day and night. Know how to reapply the bandage to shape the stump for a prosthesis.
■ To help the patient select a prosthesis, consider his needs and the types of prostheses available. The rehabilitation staff will help him make the final decision, but because most patients are uninformed about choosing a prosthesis, give some guidelines. Keep in mind the patient's age and any neurosensory problems. Generally, children need relatively simple devices, whereas older adults may need prostheses that provide more stability. Consider finances, too. Children outgrow prostheses, so advise parents to plan accordingly.
■ The same points are applicable for an interscapulothoracic amputee, but losing an arm causes a greater cosmetic problem. Consult an occupational therapist, who can teach the patient how to perform daily activities with one arm.
■ Try to instill a positive attitude toward recovery. Urge the patient to resume an independent lifestyle.

<u>DO'S & DON'TS</u>

 Refer older patients to community health services, if necessary. Suggest tutoring for children to help them keep up with schoolwork.

■ Urge patients to immediately report any new pain or masses.
■ Patients with large bone grafts or prosthetic implants require antibiotic prophylaxis when undergoing dental procedures.

▌Botulism

A paralytic illness, botulism results from an exotoxin produced by the gram-positive, anaerobic bacillus *Clostridium botulinum*. It occurs as botulism food poisoning, wound botulism, and infant botulism. Mortality from botulism is about 5% to 10%, with death usually caused by respiratory failure during the first week of illness. Botulism occurs worldwide and affects more adults than children.

Causes
■ Food poisoning: ingesting inadequately cooked contaminated foods
■ Infant botulism: GI tract becomes colonized with *C. botulinum* from some unknown source, then exotoxin is produced within the intestine
■ Wound botulism: open areas infected with *C. botulinum* that secretes toxin (rare)

Signs and symptoms
Food poisoning
■ Onset from 12 to 36 hours (range, 6 hours to 8 days) after the ingestion of contaminated food; severity varying with the amount of toxin ingested and the patient's degree of immunocompetence (onset within 24 hours signaling critical and potentially fatal illness)
– Acute symmetrical cranial nerve impairment (characterized by ptosis, diplopia, and dysarthria), followed by descending weakness or paralysis of

muscles in the extremities or trunk and dyspnea from respiratory muscle paralysis; such impairment doesn't affect mental or sensory processes and isn't associated with fever
– Diarrhea
– Dry mouth
– Sore throat
– Vomiting
– Weakness

Infant botulism
■ Usually afflicts infants ages 3 to 20 weeks; can produce hypotonic (floppy) infant syndrome, characterized by:
– Areflexia
– Constipation
– Cranial nerve deficits including flaccid facial expression, ptosis, and ophthalmoplegia
– Depressed gag reflex
– Feeble cry
– Generalized muscle weakness
– Hypotonia
– Inability to suck
– Loss of head control
– Respiratory arrest

Diagnostic tests
■ Identification of the exotoxin in the patient's serum, stool, or gastric content or in the suspected food confirms the diagnosis.
■ Electromyogram shows diminished muscle action potential after a single supramaximal nerve stimulus.
■ Diagnosis must rule out conditions commonly confused with botulism, such as Guillain-Barré syndrome, myasthenia gravis, stroke, staphylococcal food poisoning, tick paralysis, chemical intoxication, carbon monoxide poisoning, fish poisoning, trichinosis, and diphtheria.

Treatment
■ With botulism food poisoning, the treatment of choice is administration of *botulinum* antitoxin, available through the Centers for Disease Control and Prevention.
■ Infant botulism requires supportive care because neither antitoxin nor antibiotics are beneficial; human botulism immune globulin is experimental.

DRUG CHALLENGE

 Antibiotics and aminoglycosides shouldn't be given because they increase the risk of neuromuscular blockade. They should be used only to treat secondary infections.

Nursing considerations
To help prevent botulism
■ Encourage patients to observe proper techniques in processing and preserving foods.
■ Warn them to avoid even tasting food from a bulging can or one with a peculiar odor and to sterilize by boiling any utensil that comes in contact with food that may be contaminated with botulism toxin. Remember: Ingestion of even a small amount of the food can prove fatal.

If you suspect ingestion of contaminated food
■ Obtain a careful history of the patient's food intake for the past several days. Check to see if other family members exhibit similar symptoms and share a common food history.
■ Observe the patient carefully for abnormal neurologic signs. If he returns home, tell his family to watch for signs of weakness, blurred vision, and slurred speech and to return the patient to the facility immediately if such signs appear.
■ If ingestion occurred within the past several hours, induce vomiting, begin gastric lavage, and give a high enema to purge any unabsorbed toxin from the bowel.

If signs and symptoms of botulism appear

▪ Bring the patient to the intensive care unit, and monitor cardiac and respiratory function carefully.

▪ Give *botulinum* antitoxin, as ordered, to neutralize any circulating toxin. Before giving antitoxin, obtain an accurate patient history of allergies, especially to horses, and perform a skin test.

▪ Collect serum samples to identify the toxin before giving antitoxin.

▪ After giving antitoxin, watch for anaphylaxis or other hypersensitivity and serum sickness. Keep epinephrine 1:1,000 (for subcutaneous administration) and emergency airway equipment available.

▪ Closely observe and accurately record neurologic function, including bilateral motor status (including reflexes and ability to move arms and legs).

▪ Give I.V. fluids as needed. Turn the patient often, and encourage deep-breathing exercises. Assisted respiration may be required.

▪ The patient needn't be isolated.

▪ Because botulism is sometimes fatal, keep the patient and his family informed about the course of the disease.

▪ Immediately notify local public health authorities of all cases of botulism.

Brain abscess

Brain abscess is a free or encapsulated collection of pus that usually occurs in the temporal lobe, cerebellum, or frontal lobes. It can vary in size and may present singly or multilocularly. Brain abscess has a relatively low occurrence. Although it can occur at any age, it's most common in people ages 10 to 35 and is rare in older adults.

An untreated brain abscess is usually fatal; with treatment, the prognosis is only fair. About 30% of patients develop focal seizures. Multiple metastatic abscesses secondary to systemic or other infections have the poorest prognosis.

A brain abscess usually begins with localized inflammatory necrosis and edema, septic thrombosis of vessels, and suppurative encephalitis. This is followed by thick encapsulation of accumulated pus, and adjacent meningeal infiltration by neutrophils, lymphocytes, and plasma cells. Increasing pressure in the brain results in more damage.

Causes

▪ Bacteremia

▪ Bacterial endocarditis

▪ Cranial trauma, such as a penetrating head wound or compound skull fracture; penetrating head trauma or bacteremia usually leads to staphylococcal infection; pulmonary disease, to streptococcal infection

▪ Human immunodeficiency virus infection

▪ Occurs in about 2% of children with congenital heart disease, possibly because hypoxic brain is good culture medium for bacteria (commonly pyogenic bacteria, such as *Staphylococcus aureus* and *Streptococcus viridans*)

▪ Pelvic, abdominal, and skin infections

▪ Pulmonary or pleural infection

▪ Subdural empyema

▪ Usually other infection, especially otitis media, sinusitis, dental abscess, and mastoiditis

Signs and symptoms

▪ Early signs and symptoms characteristic of a bacterial infection, including headache, chills, fever, malaise, confusion, and drowsiness, with seizures, muscle weakness, and paresthesia

▪ Elevated white blood cell count with a differential indicating infection

▪ Symptoms similar to those of a brain tumor, as lesion enlarges, correlating with a disturbance of function in the invaded lobe

- Other features differ with the site of the abscess:
  - *temporal lobe abscess:* auditory-receptive dysphasia, central facial weakness, hemiparesis
  - *cerebellar abscess:* dizziness, coarse nystagmus, gaze weakness on the lesion side, tremor, ataxia
  - *frontal lobe abscess:* expressive dysphasia, hemiparesis with unilateral motor seizure, drowsiness, inattention, mental function impairment, seizures

Diagnostic tests

- Enhanced computed tomography (CT) scan and, occasionally, arteriography (which highlights the abscess by a halo) help locate the site.
- Examination of cerebrospinal fluid can help confirm infection, but lumbar puncture is too risky because it can release the increased intracranial pressure (ICP) and provoke cerebral herniation.
- A CT-guided stereotactic biopsy may be performed to drain and culture the abscess.
- Culture and sensitivity of drainage identifies the causative organism.
- Skull X-rays and a radioisotope scan show an abscess.

Treatment

- Administration of a penicillinase-resistant antibiotic such as nafcillin for at least 2 weeks before surgery can combat the underlying infection and reduce the risk of spreading the infection.
- Surgical aspiration or drainage of the abscess is done or delayed until the abscess becomes encapsulated (a CT scan helps determine this) and is contraindicated in patients with congenital heart disease or another debilitating cardiac condition.
- Other treatments during the acute phase are palliative and supportive; they include mechanical ventilation and administration of I.V. fluids with a diuretic (urea, mannitol) and a glucocorticoid (dexamethasone) to combat increased ICP and cerebral edema. An anticonvulsant, such as phenytoin or phenobarbital, can help prevent seizures.

Nursing considerations

- The patient with an acute brain abscess requires intensive care monitoring.
- Frequently assess neurologic status, especially cognition and mentation, speech, and sensorimotor and cranial nerve function.
- Early increases in ICP can be detected by using the mini-mental status examination, Glasgow Coma Scale, and National Institutes of Health Stroke Scale. These highly sensitive tools facilitate recognition of early neurologic changes and may assist in retarding the increase of ICP. Once increased, ICP results in abnormal pupils, depressed respirations, widened pulse pressure, and tachycardia or bradycardia; the cycle of increased ICP may be irreversible.
- Assess and record vital signs at least every hour.
- Monitor fluid intake and output carefully because fluid overload could contribute to cerebral edema.
- If surgery is necessary, explain the procedure to the patient and his family and answer their questions.
- After surgery, continue frequent neurologic assessment. Monitor vital signs and intake and output.
- Watch for signs and symptoms of meningitis (including nuchal rigidity, headaches, chills, and sweats), an ever-present threat.
- Change the dressing often. *Never allow bandages to remain damp.* Reinforce the dressing, or change it as ordered. To promote drainage and prevent reaccumulation of the abscess, position the patient on the operative side. Measure drainage from Hemovac or other types of drains as instructed by the surgeon.

■ If the patient remains stuporous or comatose for an extended period, give meticulous skin care to prevent pressure ulcers, and position him to preserve function and prevent contractures.

■ If the patient requires isolation because of postoperative drainage, make sure he and his family understand why.

■ Ambulate the patient as soon as possible to prevent immobility and encourage independence.

■ To prevent brain abscess, stress the need for treatment of otitis media, mastoiditis, dental abscess, and other infections. Give a prophylactic antibiotic, as needed, after a compound skull fracture or penetrating head wound.

Brain tumors, malignant

With an incidence of 4.5 per 100,000 patients, malignant brain tumors (gliomas, meningiomas, and schwannomas) are common (slightly more so in men than in women).

Tumors may occur at any age. In adults, incidence is usually highest between ages 40 and 60. The most common tumor types in adults are gliomas and meningiomas; these tumors are usually supratentorial (above the covering of the cerebellum).

In children, incidence is generally highest before age 1 and then again between ages 2 and 12. The most common tumors in children are astrocytomas, medulloblastomas, ependymomas, and brain stem gliomas. In children, brain tumors are one of the most common causes of death from cancer.

The onset of symptoms is usually insidious, and brain tumors are commonly misdiagnosed.

Causes
■ Unknown
■ Congenital
■ Heredity
■ Ionized radiation exposure

Signs and symptoms
■ Central nervous system changes by invading and destroying tissues and by secondary effect—mainly compression of the brain, cranial nerves, and cerebral vessels; cerebral edema; and increased intracranial pressure (ICP)
■ Vary with the type of tumor, its location, and the degree of invasion (see *Clinical features of malignant brain tumors*, pages 66 to 68)

Diagnostic tests
■ Tissue biopsy performed by stereotactic surgery; in this procedure, a head ring is affixed to the skull, and an excisional device is guided to the lesion by a computed tomography (CT) scan or magnetic resonance imaging (MRI).
■ Skull X-rays, a brain scan, a CT scan, MRI, and cerebral angiography confirm diagnosis and identify location of tumor.
■ Lumbar puncture shows increased pressure and protein levels, decreased glucose levels and, occasionally, tumor cells in cerebrospinal fluid (CSF).

Treatment
■ Remedial approaches include removing a resectable tumor; reducing a nonresectable tumor; relieving cerebral edema, increased ICP, and other signs and symptoms; and preventing further neurologic damage.
■ The mode of therapy depends on the tumor's histologic type, radiosensitivity, and location and may include surgery, radiation, chemotherapy, or decompression of increased ICP with a diuretic, corticosteroid or, possibly, ventriculoatrial or ventriculoperitoneal shunting of CSF.
■ *Astrocytomas.* Surgical resection of low-grade cystic cerebellar astrocytomas brings long-term survival. Treatment of

(*Text continues on page 68.*)

Clinical features of malignant brain tumors

Tumor	Clinical features
Astrocytoma ■ Second most common malignant glioma (about 30% of all gliomas) ■ Occurs at any age; incidence higher in males ■ Occurs most often in white matter of cerebral hemispheres; may originate in any part of the CNS ■ Cerebellar astrocytomas usually confined to one hemisphere	**General** ■ Headache; mental activity changes ■ Decreased motor strength and coordination commonly unilateral ■ Seizures; scanning speech ■ Altered vital signs **Localized** ■ Third ventricle: changes in mental activity and level of consciousness, nausea, pupillary dilation and sluggish light reflex; later—paresis or ataxia ■ Brain stem and pons: early—ipsilateral trigeminal, abducens, and facial nerve palsies; later—cerebellar ataxia, tremors, other cranial nerve deficits ■ Third or fourth ventricle or aqueduct of Sylvius: secondary hydrocephalus ■ Thalamus or hypothalamus: variety of endocrine, metabolic, autonomic, and behavioral changes
Ependymoma ■ Rare glioma ■ Most common in children and young adults ■ Located most often in fourth and lateral ventricles	**General** ■ Similar to oligodendroglioma ■ Increased ICP and obstructive hydrocephalus, depending on tumor size
Glioblastoma multiforme (spongioblastoma multiforme) ■ Peak incidence between ages 50 and 60; twice as common in males; most common glioma ■ Unencapsulated, highly malignant; grows rapidly and infiltrates the brain extensively; may become enormous before diagnosed ■ Occurs most often in cerebral hemispheres, especially frontal and temporal lobes (rarely in brain stem and cerebellum) ■ Occupies more than one lobe of affected hemisphere; may spread to opposite hemisphere by corpus callosum; may metastasize into cerebrospinal fluid (CSF), producing tumors in distant parts of the central nervous system (CNS)	**General** ■ Increased intracranial pressure (ICP), causing nausea, vomiting, headache, papilledema ■ Mental and behavioral changes ■ Altered vital signs (increased systolic pressure, widened pulse pressure, respiratory changes) ■ Speech and sensory disturbances ■ In children, irritability, projectile vomiting **Localized** ■ Midline: headache (bifrontal or bioccipital); worse in morning; intensified by coughing, straining, or sudden head movements ■ Temporal lobe: psychomotor seizures ■ Central region: focal seizures ■ Optic and oculomotor nerves: visual defects ■ Frontal lobe: abnormal reflexes, motor responses

Clinical features of malignant brain tumors *(continued)*

Tumor	Clinical features
Medulloblastoma ■ Rare glioma ■ Incidence highest in children ages 4 to 6 ■ Affects males more than females ■ Frequently metastasizes via CSF	**General** ■ Increased ICP **Localized** ■ Brain stem and cerebrum: papilledema, nystagmus, hearing loss, flashing lights, dizziness, ataxia, paresthesia of face, cranial nerve palsies (V, VI, VII, IX, X, primarily sensory), hemiparesis, suboccipital tenderness; compression of supratentorial area produces other general and focal symptoms
Meningioma ■ Most common nongliomatous brain tumor (15% of primary brain tumors) ■ Peak incidence among 50-year-olds; rare in children; more common in females than in males (ratio 3:2) ■ Arises from the meninges ■ Common locations include parasagittal area, sphenoidal ridge, anterior part of the skull, cerebellopontile angle, spinal canal ■ Benign, well-circumscribed, highly vascular tumors that compress underlying brain tissue by invading overlying skull	**General** ■ Headache ■ Seizures (in two-thirds of patients) ■ Vomiting ■ Changes in mental activity ■ Similar to schwannomas **Localized** ■ Skull changes (bony bulge) over tumor ■ Sphenoidal ridge, indenting optic nerve: unilateral visual changes and papilledema ■ Prefrontal parasagittal: personality and behavioral changes ■ Motor cortex: contralateral motor changes ■ Anterior fossa compressing both optic nerves and frontal lobes: headaches and bilateral vision loss ■ Pressure on cranial nerves causes varying symptoms
Oligodendroglioma ■ Third most common glioma ■ Occurs in middle adult years; more common in women ■ Slow-growing	**General** ■ Mental and behavioral changes ■ Decreased visual acuity and other visual disturbances ■ Increased ICP **Localized** ■ Temporal lobe: hallucinations, psychomotor seizures ■ Central region: seizures (confined to one muscle group or unilateral) ■ Midbrain or third ventricle: pyramidal tract symptoms (dizziness, ataxia, paresthesia of the face) ■ Brain stem and cerebrum: nystagmus, hearing loss, dizziness, ataxia, paresthesia of face, cranial nerve palsies, hemiparesis, suboccipital tenderness, loss of balance

(continued)

Clinical features of malignant brain tumors (continued)

Tumor	Clinical features
Schwannoma ■ Types: (acoustic neurinoma, neurilemoma, cerebellopontile angle tumor) ■ Accounts for about 10% of all intracranial tumors ■ Higher incidence in women ■ Onset of symptoms between ages 30 and 60 ■ Affects the craniospinal nerve sheath, usually cranial nerve VIII; also V and VII and, to a lesser extent, VI and X on the same side as the tumor ■ Benign but often classified as malignant because of its growth patterns; slow-growing—may be present for years before symptoms occur	**General** ■ Stiff neck and suboccipital discomfort ■ Secondary hydrocephalus ■ Ataxia and uncoordinated movements of one or both arms due to pressure on brain stem and cerebellum **Localized** ■ V: early—facial hypoesthesia or paresthesia on side of hearing loss; unilateral loss of corneal reflex ■ VI: diplopia or double vision ■ VII: paresis progressing to paralysis (Bell's palsy) ■ VIII: Unilateral hearing loss with or without tinnitus ■ X: weakness of palate, tongue, and nerve muscles on same side as tumor

other astrocytomas includes repeated surgery, radiation therapy, and shunting of fluid from obstructed CSF pathways. Some astrocytomas are highly radiosensitive, but others are radioresistant.

■ *Gliomas.* Treatment usually requires resection by craniotomy, followed by radiation therapy and chemotherapy. The combination of nitrosoureas (carmustine [BCNU], lomustine [CCNU], or procarbazine) and postoperative radiation is more effective than radiation alone.

■ *Medulloblastomas.* Treatment involves resection and, possibly, intrathecal infusion of methotrexate or another antineoplastic.

■ *Meningiomas.* Treatment requires resection, including dura mater and bone (operative mortality may reach 10% because of large tumor size).

■ *Oligodendrogliomas* and *ependymomas.* Treatment includes resection and radiation therapy.

■ *Schwannomas.* Microsurgical technique allows complete resection of the tumor

and preservation of facial nerves. Although schwannomas are moderately radioresistant, postoperative radiation therapy is necessary.

■ Chemotherapy for malignant brain tumors includes a nitrosourea to help break down the blood-brain barrier and permit other chemotherapeutic drugs to go through as well. Intrathecal and intra-arterial administration of drugs maximizes drug action.

■ Palliative measures for gliomas, astrocytomas, oligodendrogliomas, and ependymomas include dexamethasone for cerebral edema and an antacid and a histamine-receptor antagonist for stress ulcers. These tumors and schwannomas may also require an anticonvulsant.

Nursing considerations

■ Perform a comprehensive assessment (including a complete neurologic evaluation) to provide baseline data and guide subsequent care. Obtain a thorough health history concerning onset of symptoms.

- Help the patient and his family cope with the treatment, potential disabilities, and changes in lifestyle resulting from his tumor.

During hospitalization

- Carefully document seizure activity (occurrence, nature, and duration).
- Maintain airway patency.
- Monitor patient safety.
- Give prescribed anticonvulsants as required.
- Check continuously for changes in neurologic status, and watch for an increase in ICP.
- Watch for and immediately report sudden unilateral pupillary dilation with loss of light reflex; this ominous change indicates imminent transtentorial herniation.
- Carefully monitor respiratory changes.

ALERT

 Abnormal respiratory rate and depth may point to rising ICP or herniation of the cerebellar tonsils from an expanding infratentorial mass.

- Monitor temperature carefully. Fever commonly follows hypothalamic anoxia but might also indicate meningitis. Use hypothermia blankets preoperatively and postoperatively to keep the patient's temperature down and minimize cerebral metabolic demands.
- Give a steroid and an osmotic diuretic, such as mannitol, as needed, to reduce cerebral edema. Fluids may be restricted to 1½ qt (1.4 L) every 24 hours. Monitor fluid and electrolyte balance to avoid dehydration.
- Observe the patient for signs and symptoms of stress ulcers: abdominal distention, pain, vomiting, and black,

tarry stool. Give an antacid and a histamine-2-receptor antagonist as needed.

After surgery

- Continue to monitor general neurologic status and watch for signs of increased ICP, such as an elevated bone flap and typical neurologic changes. To reduce the risk of increased ICP, restrict fluids to 1½ qt every 24 hours.
- Elevate the head of the patient's bed about 30 degrees to promote venous drainage and reduce cerebral edema after supratentorial craniotomy. Position him on his side to allow drainage of secretions and prevent aspiration.
- As appropriate, instruct the patient to avoid Valsalva's maneuver or isometric muscle contractions when moving or sitting up in bed; they can increase intrathoracic pressure and thereby increase ICP.
- Withhold oral fluids as ordered; they may provoke vomiting and, consequently, raise ICP.
- After infratentorial craniotomy, keep the patient flat for 48 hours, but logroll him every 2 hours to minimize complications of immobilization. Prevent other complications by paying careful attention to ventilatory status and to cardiovascular, GI, and musculoskeletal function.
- Observe the wound carefully for infection and sinus formation. Radiation therapy is usually delayed until after the surgical wound heals, but it can induce wound breakdown even then.
- After radiation, watch for signs of rising ICP because radiation may cause brain inflammation.
- Tell the patient to watch for and immediately report signs of infection or bleeding that appear within 4 weeks after the start of chemotherapy because nitrosoureas used as adjuncts to radiotherapy and surgery can cause delayed bone marrow depression.

- Before chemotherapy, give prochlor-perazine (Compazine) or another anti-emetic, as needed, to minimize nausea and vomiting.
- Teach the patient signs of recurrence; urge compliance with the treatment regimen.
- Begin rehabilitation early because brain tumors may cause residual neurologic deficits that handicap the patient physically or mentally.
- Consult with occupational and physical therapists to encourage independence in daily activities.
- As necessary, provide aids for self-care and mobilization such as bathroom rails for wheelchair patients.
- If the patient is aphasic, arrange for consultation with a speech pathologist.

Breast cancer

Along with lung cancer, breast cancer is a leading killer of women ages 35 to 54. It occurs in men, though only rarely. (See *Breast cancer in men.*) The overall breast cancer death rate for American women has fallen. Lymph node involvement is the most valuable prognostic predictor. With adjuvant therapy, 70% to 75% of women with negative nodes will survive 10 years or more, compared with 20% to 25% of women with positive nodes.

Although breast cancer may develop anytime after puberty, it's most common after age 50.

Breast cancer is more common in the left breast than in the right and more common in the upper outer quadrant. Growth rates vary. Theoretically, slow-growing breast cancer may take up to 8 years to become palpable at 1 cm in size. It spreads by way of the lymphatic system and the bloodstream, through the right side of the heart to the lungs and, eventually, to the other breast, the chest wall, liver, bone, and brain.

Classified by histologic appearance and location of the lesion, breast cancer may be:
- *adenocarcinoma*—arising from the epithelium
- *intraductal*—developing within the ducts (includes Paget's disease)
- *infiltrating*—occurring in parenchymatous tissue of the breast
- *inflammatory (rare)*—rapidly growing tumor, in which the overlying skin becomes edematous, inflamed, and indurated
- *lobular carcinoma in situ*—involving lobes of glandular tissue
- *medullary or circumscribed*—a large tumor with a rapid growth rate

Causes
- Unknown; estrogen implicated by high incidence in women

Risk factors
- Endometrial or ovarian cancer
- Estrogen therapy, antihypertensives, high-fat diet, obesity, and fibrocystic dis
- Exposure to low-level ionizing radiation
- Family history of breast cancer
- First pregnancy after age 31
- Long menses; began menses early or menopause late
- Never pregnant
- Unilateral breast cancer

At lower risk
- Pregnant before age 20
- Multiple pregnancies
- Of Indian or Asian nationality

Signs and symptoms
- A lump or mass in the breast (a hard, stony mass is usually malignant)
- A change in symmetry or size of the breast
- A change in breast skin (thickening, scaly skin around the nipple, dimpling, edema [peau d'orange], or ulceration)

▪ A change in skin temperature (a warm, hot, or pink area; suspect cancer in a non–breast-feeding woman past childbearing age until proven otherwise)

▪ Unusual drainage or discharge (a spontaneous discharge of any kind in a non–breast-feeding woman warrants thorough investigation; so does any discharge produced by breast manipulation [greenish black, white, creamy, serous, or bloody]) (If a breast-feeding infant rejects one breast, this may suggest breast cancer.)

▪ A change in the nipple, such as itching, burning, erosion, or retraction

▪ Pain (not usually a symptom of breast cancer unless the tumor is advanced, but it should be investigated)

▪ Bone metastasis, pathologic bone fractures, and hypercalcemia

▪ Edema of the arm

Diagnostic tests

▪ Although not proven to lower mortality, breast self-examination may detect palpable breast lumps, allowing the woman to contact her practitioner for early evaluation.

▪ Mammography is indicated for any woman whose physical examination might suggest breast cancer. It should be done as a baseline on women ages 35 to 39, every 1 to 2 years for women ages 40 to 49, and annually for women older than age 50, women who have a family history of breast cancer, and women who have had unilateral breast cancer, to check for new disease. However, the value of mammography is questionable for women younger than age 35 (because of the density of the breasts), except those who are strongly suspected of having breast cancer. False-negative results can occur in as many as 30% of all tests.

▪ Fine-needle aspiration or surgical biopsy is done if a mass is suspicious and the mammography is negative.

Breast cancer in men

Although breast cancer in men is unusual, unilateral lesions should be evaluated as for women. Gynecomastia in men can begin unilaterally and is typically asymmetric. Treatment is generally the same as for women—surgery, radiation, and chemotherapy as indicated by the extent of the cancer.

▪ Ultrasonography, which can distinguish a fluid-filled cyst from a tumor, can also be used instead of an invasive surgical biopsy.

▪ Bone scan, computed tomography scan, measurement of alkaline phosphatase levels, liver function studies, and a liver biopsy can detect distant metastasis.

▪ A hormonal receptor assay done on the tumor can determine if the tumor is estrogen- or progesterone-dependent. (This test guides decisions to use therapy that blocks the action of the estrogen hormone that supports tumor growth.)

Treatment

▪ In choosing therapy, the patient and practitioner should consider the stage of the disease, the woman's age and menopausal status, and the disfiguring effects of the surgery. Treatment for breast cancer may include one or any combination of the following.

Surgery

▪ A lumpectomy may be done on an outpatient basis and may be the only surgery needed, especially if the tumor is small and there's no evidence of axillary node involvement. Radiation therapy is usually combined with this surgery.

▪ A two-stage procedure, in which the surgeon removes the lump, confirms that it's malignant, and discusses treatment options with the patient, is desirable because it allows the patient to participate in her treatment plan. Sometimes, if the tumor is diagnosed as malignant, such planning can be done before surgery.

■ In lumpectomy and dissection of the axillary lymph nodes, the tumor and the axillary lymph nodes are removed, leaving the breast intact.

■ A simple mastectomy removes the breast but not the lymph nodes or pectoral muscles.

■ A modified radical mastectomy removes the breast and the axillary lymph nodes.

■ A radical mastectomy, the performance of which has declined, removes the breast, the pectoralis major and minor, and the axillary lymph nodes.

■ After a mastectomy, reconstructive surgery can create a breast mound if the patient desires it and doesn't have evidence of advanced disease.

Chemotherapy, tamoxifen, and peripheral stem cell therapy

■ Various cytotoxic drug combinations are used as either adjuvant or primary therapy, depending on several factors, including staging and estrogen receptor status.

■ The most commonly used antineoplastics are cyclophosphamide, fluorouracil, methotrexate, doxorubicin, vincristine, paclitaxel, and prednisone.

■ A common drug combination used in both premenopausal and postmenopausal women is cyclophosphamide, methotrexate, and fluorouracil.

■ Tamoxifen (Nolvadex), an estrogen antagonist, is the adjuvant treatment of choice for postmenopausal patients with positive estrogen receptor status.

■ Peripheral stem cell therapy may be used for patients with advanced breast cancer.

Primary radiation therapy

■ Used before or after tumor removal, it's effective for small tumors in early stages with no evidence of distant metastasis; it's also used to prevent or treat local recurrence.

■ Presurgical radiation to the breast in patients with inflammatory breast cancer helps make tumors more surgically manageable.

Other drug therapy

■ Patients may also receive estrogen, progesterone, androgen, or antiandrogen aminoglutethimide therapy. With growing evidence that breast cancer is a systemic, not a local, disease, the success of these drug therapies has led to a decline in ablative surgery.

Nursing considerations

■ To provide good care for a breast cancer patient, begin with a history; assess the patient's feelings about her illness, and determine what she knows about it and what she expects.

Before surgery

■ Be sure you know what kind of surgery is scheduled so you can prepare the patient. If a mastectomy is scheduled, in addition to the usual preoperative preparation (for example, skin preparations and allowing nothing by mouth), also perform the following:

– Teach the patient how to deep breathe and cough to prevent pulmonary complications and how to rotate her ankles to prevent thromboembolism.

– Tell the patient she can ease her pain by lying on the affected side or by placing a hand or pillow on the incision. Show her where the incision will be. Inform her that she'll receive pain medication and that she needn't fear addiction.

– Explain to the patient that after mastectomy, an incisional drain or suction device (Hemovac) will be used to remove accumulated serous or sanguineous fluid and to keep the tension off the suture line, promoting healing.
– Advise the patient to ask her practitioner about reconstructive surgery or to call the local or state medical society for the names of plastic reconstructive surgeons who regularly perform surgery to create breast mounds. In many cases, reconstructive surgery may be planned before the mastectomy.

After surgery

■ Inspect the dressing anteriorly and posteriorly. Be alert for bleeding.
■ Measure and record the amount and note the color of drainage. Expect drainage to be bloody during the first 4 hours and afterward to become serous.
■ Check circulatory status (blood pressure, pulse rate, respirations, and bleeding).
■ Monitor intake and output for at least 48 hours after general anesthesia.
■ Encourage coughing and turn the patient every 2 hours to prevent complications. (Positioning a small pillow under the patient's arm provides comfort.)
■ Encourage the patient to get out of bed as soon as possible (even as soon as the anesthesia wears off or the first evening after surgery).
■ Prevent lymphedema of the arm, which may be an early complication of any breast cancer treatment that involves lymph node dissection. Help the patient prevent lymphedema by instructing her to exercise her hand and arm regularly and to avoid activities that might cause infection in this hand or arm (infection increases the chance of developing lymphedema). Such prevention is important because lymphedema can't be treated effectively.

■ Inspect the incision. Encourage the patient and her partner to look at her incision as soon as feasible, perhaps when the first dressing is removed.
■ Instruct the patient about breast prostheses. The American Cancer Society's Reach to Recovery program can provide instruction, emotional support and counseling, and a list of area stores that sell prostheses.
■ Provide psychological and emotional support. Many patients fear cancer and possible disfigurement and worry about loss of sexual function. Explain that breast surgery doesn't interfere with sexual function and that the patient may resume sexual activity as soon as she desires after surgery.
■ Explain to the patient that she may experience "phantom breast syndrome" (a phenomenon in which a tingling or a pins-and-needles sensation is felt in the area of the amputated breast tissue) or depression following mastectomy. Listen to the patient's concerns, offer support, and refer her to an appropriate organization, such as the American Cancer Society's Reach to Recovery.

Bronchiectasis

A condition marked by chronic abnormal dilation of bronchi and destruction of bronchial walls, bronchiectasis can occur throughout the tracheobronchial tree or can be confined to one segment or lobe. However, it's usually bilateral and involves the basilar segments of the lower lobes. This disease has three forms: cylindrical (fusiform), varicose, and saccular (cystic).

It affects people of both sexes and all ages. Because of the availability of antibiotics to treat acute respiratory tract infections, the incidence of bronchiectasis has dramatically decreased in the past 20 years. Its incidence is highest among the Inuit of the Arctic and the

Maoris of New Zealand. Bronchiectasis is irreversible once established.

The different forms of bronchiectasis may occur separately or simultaneously. In cylindrical bronchiectasis, the bronchi expand unevenly, with little change in diameter, and end suddenly in a squared-off fashion. In varicose bronchiectasis, abnormal, irregular dilation and narrowing of the bronchi give the appearance of varicose veins. In saccular bronchiectasis, many large dilations end in sacs.

Causes

- Conditions associated with repeated damage to bronchial walls and abnormal mucociliary clearance, which cause a breakdown of supporting tissue adjacent to airways. Such conditions include:
  – Congenital anomalies (uncommon), such as bronchomalacia, congenital bronchiectasis, immotile cilia syndrome, and Kartagener's syndrome, a variant of immotile cilia syndrome characterized by situs inversus viscerum, bronchiectasis, and either nasal polyps or sinusitis
  – Immunologic disorders (agammaglobulinemia, for example)
  – Inhalation of corrosive gas or repeated aspiration of gastric juices into the lungs
  – Mucoviscidosis (cystic fibrosis)
  – Obstruction (by a foreign body, tumor, or stenosis) in association with recurrent infection
  – Recurrent, inadequately treated bacterial respiratory tract infections, such as tuberculosis, and complications of measles, pneumonia, pertussis, or influenza

Signs and symptoms

- Initially, may be asymptomatic
- Frequent bouts of pneumonia or hemoptysis
- The classic sign: chronic cough that produces copious, foul-smelling, mucopurulent secretions, possibly totaling several cupfuls daily
- Coarse crackles during inspiration over involved lobes or segments, occasional wheezes, dyspnea
- Sinusitis
- Weight loss
- Anemia
- Malaise
- Clubbing
- Recurrent fever, chills, and other signs and symptoms of infection
- Chronic malnutrition and amyloidosis as well as right-sided heart failure and cor pulmonale due to hypoxic pulmonary vasoconstriction with advanced bronchiectasis

Diagnostic tests

- Chest X-rays show peribronchial thickening, areas of atelectasis, and scattered cystic changes in the patient with recurrent bronchial infections, pneumonia and hemoptysis.
- Computed tomography scanning's high-resolution techniques determine anatomic changes.
- Bronchoscopy helps to identify the source of secretions and pinpointing the site of bleeding in hemoptysis.
- Sputum culture and Gram stain identify predominant organisms.
- Complete blood count detects anemia and leukocytosis.
- Pulmonary function studies detect decreased vital capacity, expiratory flow, and hypoxemia; these tests also help determine the physiologic severity of the disease and the effects of therapy, as well as help evaluate patients for surgery.
- When cystic fibrosis is suspected as the underlying cause of bronchiectasis, a sweat electrolyte test is useful.

Treatment

■ Oral or I.V. antibiotic is given for 7 to 10 days or until sputum production decreases.

■ For severe cases, several different antibiotics may be used sequentially in a continuous regimen to minimize bacterial resistance.

■ If the patient has bronchospasm and thick, tenacious sputum, a bronchodilator, combined with postural drainage and chest percussion, can help remove secretions. Bronchoscopy may be used to help mobilize secretions.

■ Hypoxia requires oxygen therapy, and severe hemoptysis requires lobectomy, segmental resection, or bronchial artery embolization if pulmonary function is poor.

Nursing considerations

■ Provide supportive care, and help the patient adjust to the permanent changes in lifestyle that irreversible lung damage necessitates. Thorough patient teaching is vital.

■ Give an antibiotic, as needed, and explain all diagnostic tests.

■ Perform chest physiotherapy, including postural drainage and chest percussion designed for involved lobes, several times per day. The best times to do this are early morning and just before bedtime. Instruct the patient to maintain each position for 10 minutes. Then perform percussion, and tell him to cough.

■ To help prevent bronchiectasis, treat bacterial pneumonia vigorously and stress the need for immunization to prevent childhood diseases.

■ Review patient teaching guidelines. (See *Teaching about bronchiectasis*.)

Teaching about bronchiectasis

When teaching a patient and his family about bronchiectasis, be sure to review the following points:

■ Instruct the patient to perform coughing and deep-breathing exercises.

■ Advise the patient to stop smoking.

■ Encourage the patient to get as much rest as possible.

■ Encourage the patient to take in balanced, high-protein meals and fluids.

■ Teach postural drainage, percussion, and mouth care.

■ Teach proper disposal of secretions.

■ Tell the patient to avoid air pollutants and people who have upper respiratory tract infections.

Bronchiolitis obliterans with organizing pneumonia

Idiopathic bronchiolitis obliterans with organizing pneumonia (BOOP), also known as *cryptogenic organizing pneumonia,* is one of several types of bronchiolitis obliterans. *Bronchiolitis obliterans* is a generic term describing an inflammatory disease of the small airways. *Organizing pneumonia* refers to unresolved pneumonia, in which inflammatory alveolar exudate persists and eventually undergoes fibrosis.

BOOP has been diagnosed with increasing frequency since it was first discovered, although much debate still exists about the various pathologies and classifications of bronchiolitis obliterans.

Most patients with BOOP are between ages 50 and 60. Incidence is equally divided between men and women. A smoking history doesn't seem to increase the risk of developing BOOP.

BOOP is responsive to treatment and usually can be completely reversed with corticosteroid therapy. A few deaths have been reported, particularly in patients who had more widespread pathologic changes in the lungs and those who developed opportunistic infections or other complications related to steroid therapy.

Causes

- Unknown
- Other forms of BOOP may be associated with specific diseases or situations, such as:
  - Bacterial, viral, or mycoplasmal respiratory tract infections
  - Bone marrow, heart, or heart-lung transplantation
  - Collagen vascular diseases, such as rheumatoid arthritis or systemic lupus erythematosus
  - Drug therapy with amiodarone, bleomycin, penicillamine, or lomustine
  - Inflammatory diseases, such as Crohn's disease, ulcerative colitis, or polyarteritis nodosa
  - Inhalation of toxic gases

Signs and symptoms

- Anorexia and weight loss
- Dry crackles on chest auscultation
- Dyspnea (especially on exertion)
- Fever
- Flulike syndrome lasting from several weeks to several months
- Malaise
- Persistent and nonproductive cough
- Productive cough, hemoptysis, chest pain, generalized aching, and night sweats (less common)

Diagnostic tests

- Chest X-ray usually shows patchy, diffuse airspace opacities with a ground-glass appearance that may migrate from one location to another. High-resolution computed tomography scans show areas of consolidation. Except for the migrating opacities, these findings are nonspecific and present in many other respiratory disorders.
- Pulmonary function tests may be normal or show reduced capacities. The diffusing capacity for carbon monoxide is generally low.
- Arterial blood gas analysis usually shows mild to moderate hypoxemia at rest, which worsens with exercise.
- Blood tests reveal an increased erythrocyte sedimentation rate, increased C-reactive protein level, and increased white blood cell count with a somewhat increased proportion of neutrophils and a minor rise in eosinophils. Immunoglobulin (Ig) G and IgM levels are normal or slightly increased, and the IgE level is normal.
- Bronchoscopy reveals normal or slightly inflamed airways. Bronchoalveolar lavage fluid obtained during bronchoscopy shows a moderate elevation in lymphocyte levels and, sometimes, elevated neutrophil and eosinophil levels. Foamy-looking alveolar macrophages may also be found.
- Lung biopsy, thoracoscopy, or bronchoscopy is required to confirm the diagnosis of BOOP. Pathologic changes in lung tissue include plugs of connective tissue in the lumen of the bronchioles, alveolar ducts, and alveolar spaces.

These changes may occur in other types of bronchiolitis and in other diseases that cause organizing pneumonia. They also differentiate BOOP from constrictive bronchiolitis, characterized by inflammation and fibrosis that surround and may narrow or completely obliterate the bronchiolar airways. Although the pathologic findings in proliferative and constrictive bronchiolitis are different, the causes and presentations may overlap. Any known cause of bronchiolitis obliterans or organizing pneumonia must be ruled out before the diagnosis of BOOP is made.

Treatment

- Corticosteroids are the treatment of choice for BOOP, although the ideal dosage and duration are controversial. In most cases, treatment begins with 1 mg/kg/day of prednisone for at least several days to several weeks; the dosage is then gradually reduced over several months to a year, depending on the patient's response. Relapse is common when the steroid dosage is tapered off or stopped but usually can be reversed when the dosage is increased or resumed. Occasionally, a patient may need to continue corticosteroid therapy indefinitely.
- Immunosuppressant-cytotoxic drugs, such as cyclophosphamide (Cytoxan), are used when the patient can't tolerate or is unresponsive to corticosteroids.
- Oxygen is used to correct hypoxemia. The patient may need either no oxygen or a small amount of oxygen at rest and a greater amount when he exercises.
- Other treatments vary, depending on the patient's symptoms, and may include an inhaled bronchodilator, a cough suppressant, and bronchial hygiene therapy.

Nursing considerations

- Explain all diagnostic tests. The patient may experience anxiety and frustration because of the length of time and number of tests needed to establish the diagnosis.
- Monitor the patient for adverse reactions to the corticosteroid therapy: weight gain, "moon face," glucose intolerance, fluid and electrolyte imbalance, mood swings, cataracts, peptic ulcer disease, opportunistic infections, and osteoporosis leading to bone fractures. These effects may leave many patients

unable to tolerate the treatment. Teach the patient and his family about these adverse reactions, emphasizing which ones they should report to the practitioner.

- Teach measures that may help prevent complications related to treatment, such as infection control and improved nutrition.
- Teach breathing, relaxation, and energy conservation techniques to help the patient manage symptoms.
- Monitor oxygenation, at rest and with exertion. The practitioner will probably prescribe an oxygen flow rate for use when the patient is at rest and a higher one for exertion. Teach the patient how to increase the oxygen flow rate to the appropriate level for exercise.
- If the patient needs oxygen at home, ensure continuity of care by making appropriate referrals to discharge planners, respiratory care practitioners, and home equipment vendors.

▌Buerger's disease

Buerger's disease, also known as *thromboangiitis obliterans,* is an inflammatory, nonatheromatous occlusive condition that causes segmental lesions and subsequent thrombus formation in small- and medium-sized arteries (and sometimes the veins), resulting in decreased blood flow to the feet and legs. It may produce ulceration and, eventually, gangrene. The incidence is highest among men of Asian and Jewish ancestry, ages 20 to 40, who smoke heavily.

Causes

- Unknown
- Definite link to smoking

Signs and symptoms

- Intermittent claudication (pain in muscles resulting from inadequate blood

supply) of the instep, aggravated by exercise and relieved by rest
- When exposed to low temperatures, the feet initially cold, cyanotic, and numb; later, red, hot, and tingling
- Painful fingertip ulcerations (occasionally)
- Impaired peripheral pulses
- Migratory superficial thrombophlebitis
- Ulceration, muscle atrophy, and gangrene (in later stages)

Diagnostic tests
- Doppler ultrasonography shows diminished circulation in the peripheral vessels.
- Plethysmography helps detect decreased circulation in the peripheral vessels.
- Arteriography locates lesions and rules out atherosclerosis.
- Biopsy of the affected vessel can confirm the diagnosis.

Treatment
- No specific treatment exists, except abstention from tobacco.
- Arterial bypass of larger vessels may be used in some cases, as well as local debridement, depending on symptoms and severity of ischemia.
- An antibiotic may also be useful as well as an exercise program that uses gravity to fill and drain the blood vessels or, in severe disease, a lumbar sympathectomy to increase blood supply to the skin.
- Amputation may be necessary if the patient suffers from nonhealing ulcers, intractable pain, or gangrene.

Nursing considerations
- Strongly urge the patient to permanently stop smoking to enhance the effectiveness of treatment. If necessary, refer him to a self-help group to facilitate the process.

- Warn the patient to avoid precipitating factors, such as emotional stress, exposure to extreme temperatures, and trauma.
- Teach the patient proper foot care, especially the importance of wearing well-fitting shoes and cotton or wool socks. Show him how to inspect his feet daily for cuts, abrasions, and signs and symptoms of skin breakdown, such as redness and soreness. Remind him to seek medical attention immediately after any trauma.
- To minimize discomfort and ulcerations of the feet, use a padded footboard or bed cradle to prevent pressure from bed linens. Protect the feet with soft padding. Wash them gently with a mild soap and tepid water, rinse thoroughly, and pat dry with a soft towel.
- Provide the patient with emotional support. If necessary, refer the patient for psychological counseling to help him cope with restrictions imposed by this chronic disease.
- If the patient has undergone amputation, assess rehabilitative needs, especially regarding changes in body image. Refer him to physical therapists, occupational therapists, and social service agencies as needed.

Burns

A major burn is a horrifying injury, necessitating painful treatment and a long period of rehabilitation. It's typically fatal or permanently disfiguring and incapacitating (emotionally and physically). In the United States, about 2.5 million people annually suffer burns.

The depth of damage to the skin and tissue and the size of the burn are important factors in burn assessment and classification.

Depth of burn

This illustration shows the depth of tissue damage in partial- and full-thickness burns. A partial-thickness burn damages the epidermis and part of the dermis, whereas a full-thickness burn affects the epidermis, dermis, and subcutaneous tissue.

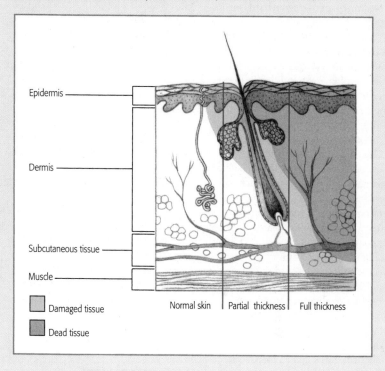

Epidermis

Dermis

Subcutaneous tissue

Muscle

Damaged tissue

Dead tissue

Normal skin | Partial thickness | Full thickness

Depth of skin and tissue damage

A traditional method gauges burn depth by degrees, although most burns are a combination of different degrees and thicknesses. (See *Depth of burn*.)

■ *Superficial partial-thickness (first-degree)*—Damage is limited to the epidermis, causing erythema and pain.

■ *Deep partial-thickness (second-degree)*—The epidermis and part of the dermis are damaged, producing blisters and mild-to-moderate edema and pain.

■ *Full-thickness (third-degree)*—The epidermis and the dermis are damaged with damage extending into the subcu-

taneous tissue layer; may also involve muscle, bone, and interstitial tissues.

Burn size

The size is usually expressed as the percentage of body surface area (BSA) covered by the burn. The Rule of Nines chart most commonly provides this estimate, although the Lund-Browder classification is more accurate because it allows for BSA changes with age. A correlation of the burn's depth and size permits an estimate of its severity.

■ *Major*—third-degree burns on more than 10% of BSA; second-degree burns on more than 25% of adult BSA (more

than 20% in children); burns of hands, face, feet, or genitalia; burns complicated by fractures or respiratory damage; electrical burns; all burns in poor-risk patients
- *Moderate*—third-degree burns on 3% to 10% of BSA; second-degree burns on 15% to 25% of adult BSA (10% to 20% in children)
- *Minor*—third-degree burns on less than 3% of BSA; second-degree burns on less than 15% of adult BSA (10% in children).

Causes
- Chemical burns: contact, ingestion, inhalation, or injection of acids, alkalis, or vesicants that cause tissue injury and necrosis
- Electrical burns: coagulation necrosis caused by intense heat; usually occur after contact with faulty electrical wiring or high-voltage power lines or when electric cords are chewed (by young children)
- Friction or abrasion burns: skin rubbed harshly against a coarse surface
- Sunburn: excessive exposure to sunlight
- Thermal burns: flame, flash, scald or contact with hot objects (for example, residential fires, motor vehicle accidents, playing with matches, improperly stored gasoline, space heater or electrical malfunctions); or improper handling of firecrackers, scalding accidents, and kitchen accidents (such as a child climbing on top of a stove or grabbing a hot iron); in children, burns sometimes caused by parental abuse

Signs and symptoms
- Blisters
- Charred mouth, burned lips, burns on the head, neck, or face; wheezing, change in voice, difficulty breathing and coughing; singed nose hairs or eyebrows; or dark carbon-stained mucus
- Edema
- Pain
- Peeling skin or red skin
- Signs of shock
- White or charred skin

Diagnostic tests
- Urinalysis may reveal myoglobinuria and hemoglobinuria.
- Arterial blood gas levels may reveal hypoxia.
- Fiber-optic bronchoscopy may reveal inhalation injury.
- Carboxyhemoglobin is elevated with smoke inhalation.
- Complete blood count shows elevated white blood cell count.
- Blood urea nitrogen and creatinine levels may be elevated.

Treatment
- Immediate, aggressive burn treatment increases the patient's chance for survival. Later, supportive measures and strict aseptic technique can minimize infection. Meticulous, comprehensive burn care can make the difference between life and death. (See *Fluid replacement: The first 24 hours after a burn.*)

For minor burns
- The burned area is immersed in cool saline solution (55° F [12.8° C]) or cool compresses are applied. Ice should never be applied directly to the wound.
- Pain medication is used as needed.
- Debridement is done to devitalized tissue, taking care not to break any blisters. The wound is covered with an antimicrobial and a bulky, nonstick dressing, and give tetanus prophylaxis as needed.

For moderate and major burns
- The patient's airway, breathing, and circulation are assessed, and signs of smoke inhalation and pulmonary dam-

age: singed nasal hairs, mucosal burns, voice changes, coughing, wheezing, soot in the mouth or nose, and darkened sputum watched for.

- Endotracheal intubation may be necessary with 100% oxygen administration.
- Bleeding is controlled and smoldering clothing, rings, and other constricting items are removed. If clothing is stuck to the patient's skin, soak it first in saline solution.
- Burns are covered with a clean, dry, sterile bed sheet. (Never cover large burns with saline-soaked dressings because they can drastically lower body temperature.)
- I.V. therapy starts immediately to prevent hypovolemic shock and maintain cardiac output. Lactated Ringer's solution or a fluid replacement formula is used.
- When the patient's condition is stable, a brief history of the burn is taken.
- Blood samples taken include a complete blood count; electrolyte, glucose, blood urea nitrogen, and creatinine levels; arterial blood gas analysis; and typing and crossmatching.
- Monitoring of intake and output, and frequent vital signs are done. An arterial line may be inserted if blood pressure is unobtainable with a cuff.
- A central venous pressure line, additional I.V. lines (using venous cutdown, if necessary), and an indwelling urinary catheter may be inserted.
- To combat fluid evaporation through the burn and the release of fluid into interstitial spaces (possibly resulting in hypovolemic shock), fluid therapy is continued as needed.
- A urine specimen to check for myoglobinuria and hemoglobinuria is taken.
- A nasogastric tube is inserted to decompress the stomach and avoid aspiration of stomach contents.
- Electrical and chemical burns demand special attention. Tissue damage from

Fluid replacement: The first 24 hours after a burn

Use the Parkland formula as a general guideline for the amount of fluid replacement. Give 4 ml/kg of crystalloid × % total burn surface area; give half of the solution over the first 8 hours (calculated from time of injury) and the balance over the next 16 hours. Vary the specific infusions according to the patient's response, especially urine output.

electrical burns is difficult to assess because internal destruction along the conduction pathway is usually greater than the surface burn would indicate. Electrical burns that ignite the patient's clothes may cause thermal burns as well. If the electric shock caused ventricular fibrillation and cardiac and respiratory arrest, begin cardiopulmonary resuscitation at once. An estimate of the voltage should be obtained.

- For a chemical burn, the wound is irrigated with copious amounts of water or normal saline solution.

Do's & don'ts

 Using a weak base (such as sodium bicarbonate) to neutralize hydrofluoric acid, hydrochloric acid, or sulfuric acid on skin or mucous membrane is contraindicated because the neutralizing agent can actually produce more heat and tissue damage.

- For a chemical burn of the eyes, flush them with large amounts of water or saline solution for at least 30 minutes; for an alkali burn, irrigate until the pH of the cul-de-sacs returns to normal.
- The patient should close his eyes so they can be covered with a dry, sterile

dressing. The type of chemical causing the burn and the presence of any noxious fumes is noted and the patient is referred for an emergency ophthalmologic examination.

■ If the patient will be transferred to a specialized burn care unit within 4 hours after the burn, the burn wound itself isn't treated in the emergency department. Instead, the patient is prepared for transport by wrapping him in a sterile sheet and a blanket for warmth and elevating the burned extremity to decrease edema. Then the patient is transported immediately. At the burn unit, the patient will receive specialized treatments, including skin grafts of various types.

Nursing considerations

■ When assessing a wound keep the following in mind:

– *Location:* Burns on the face, hands, feet, and genitalia are the most serious because of possible loss of function.

– *Configuration:* Circumferential burns can cause total occlusion of circulation in an extremity as a result of edema. Burns on the neck can produce airway obstruction, whereas burns on the chest can lead to restricted respiratory expansion.

– *History of complicating medical problems:* Note disorders that impair peripheral circulation, especially diabetes, peripheral vascular disease, and chronic alcohol abuse.

– *Other injuries:* Consider injuries sustained at the time of the burn, such as with a blast injury or motor vehicle accident.

ALERT
Victims younger than age 4 or older than age 60 have a higher incidence of complications and, consequently, a higher mortality. Elderly people are at risk for complications

due to preexisting medical conditions and delayed wound healing, as well as being prone to complications from the fluid resuscitation required (heart failure, pulmonary edema).

– Pulmonary injury: Smoke inhalation can cause pulmonary injury.

■ After burn debridement, provide the patient with thorough teaching and complete aftercare instructions. Stress the importance of keeping the dressing dry and clean, elevating the burned extremity for the first 24 hours, taking the prescribed analgesic, and returning for a wound check in 1 to 2 days.

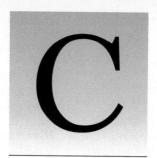

Calcium imbalance

Calcium plays an indispensable role in cell permeability, formation of bones and teeth, blood coagulation, transmission of nerve impulses, and normal muscle contraction. Nearly all (99%) of the body's calcium is found in the bones, with the remaining 1% existing in ionized form in serum. It's the maintenance of the 1% of ionized calcium in the serum that's critical to healthy neurologic function. Severe calcium imbalance requires emergency treatment because a deficiency (hypocalcemia) can lead to tetany and seizures; an excess (hypercalcemia), to cardiac arrhythmias and coma.

Causes
Hypocalcemia
- Burns
- Hypomagnesemia
- Hypoparathyroidism as a result of injury, disease, or surgery
- Inadequate intake of calcium and vitamin D
- Loss of calcium from the GI tract due to severe diarrhea or laxative abuse
- Malabsorption of calcium from the GI tract
- Overcorrection of acidosis
- Pancreatic insufficiency or pancreatitis
- Renal failure
- Severe infections

Hypercalcemia
- Adrenal insufficiency
- Hyperparathyroidism
- Hyperthyroidism
- Hypervitaminosis D
- Milk-alkali syndrome
- Multiple fractures and prolonged immobilization
- Multiple myeloma
- Sarcoidosis
- Thiazide diuretics
- Tumors

Signs and symptoms
Hypocalcemia
- Cardiac arrhythmias
- Carpopedal spasm
- Digital and perioral paresthesia
- Hyperactive reflexes
- Positive Chvostek's sign
- Positive Trousseau's sign
- Seizures
- Tetany
- Twitching

Hypercalcemia
- Anorexia
- Cardiac arrhythmias
- Coma
- Constipation
- Decreased muscle tone
- Dehydration
- Lethargy
- Muscle weakness
- Nausea and vomiting

- Polydipsia
- Polyuria

Diagnostic tests
Hypocalcemia
- Total serum calcium level below 8.5 mg/dl confirms hypocalcemia.
- Ionized serum calcium level less than 4.5 mg/dl also helps confirm the diagnosis.
- Electrocardiogram (ECG) reveals a lengthened QT interval, a prolonged ST segment, and arrhythmias.

Hypercalcemia
- Total serum calcium level above 10.5 mg/dl confirms hypercalcemia.
- Ionized serum calcium level greater than 5.3 mg/dl also helps confirm the diagnosis.
- Urine test results show an increase in urine calcium precipitation.
- ECG reveals a shortened QT interval and heart block.

Treatment
- An acute imbalance requires immediate correction, followed by maintenance therapy and correction of the underlying cause.

Hypocalcemia
- A mild calcium deficit may require adequate intake of calcium, vitamin D, protein and, possibly, oral calcium supplements.

ACTION STAT!
Acute hypocalcemia is an emergency that needs immediate correction by I.V. administration of calcium gluconate or calcium chloride.

- Chronic hypocalcemia also requires vitamin D supplements to facilitate GI absorption of calcium. A mild deficiency is treated with multivitamin preparations;

a severe deficiency is treated with several forms of vitamin D (ergocalciferol [vitamin D_2], cholecalciferol [vitamin D_3], calcitriol, and dihydrotachysterol, a synthetic form of vitamin D_2).

Hypercalcemia
- Ensure adequate hydration with normal saline solution, which promotes calcium excretion in urine.
- Administer loop diuretics, such as ethacrynic acid and furosemide, to promote calcium excretion.

DRUG CHALLENGE

Thiazide diuretics inhibit calcium excretion and are contraindicated in hypercalcemic patients.

- Corticosteroids, such as prednisone and hydrocortisone, are helpful in treating sarcoidosis, hypervitaminosis D, and certain tumors.
- Plicamycin (Mithracin) can lower the serum calcium level and is especially effective against hypercalcemia secondary to certain tumors.
- Calcitonin may also be helpful in certain instances.
- Sodium phosphate solution administered by mouth or by retention enema promotes calcium deposits in bone and inhibits its absorption from the GI tract.

Nursing considerations
- If the patient is receiving massive transfusions of citrated blood or has chronic diarrhea, severe infection, or insufficient dietary intake of calcium or protein (common in elderly patients), monitor him for hypocalcemia.

Hypocalcemia
- Monitor serum calcium levels every 12 to 24 hours, and report any decreases.

■ When giving calcium supplements, frequently check the pH level; an alkalotic state that exceeds 7.45 pH inhibits calcium ionization.

■ Check for Chvostek's and Trousseau's signs.

DRUG CHALLENGE

 Slowly administer I.V. calcium gluconate in dextrose 5% in water (never in saline solution, which encourages renal calcium loss). Don't infuse more than 1 g/hour, except in emergencies. Don't add I.V. calcium gluconate to solutions containing bicarbonate; it will precipitate.

■ When administering calcium solutions, watch for anorexia, nausea, and vomiting, which are signs of overcorrection of hypercalcemia. If the patient is receiving calcium chloride, watch for abdominal discomfort.

DRUG CHALLENGE

 If the patient is receiving a cardiac glycoside with large doses of oral calcium supplements, monitor him closely for a possible drug interaction; also, watch for signs and symptoms of digoxin toxicity, including anorexia, nausea, vomiting, yellow vision, and cardiac arrhythmias.

■ Give an oral calcium supplement 1 to 1½ hours after meals or with milk.

■ Observe seizure precautions for patients with severe hypocalcemia that may lead to seizures.

■ Warn the patient not to overuse antacids because they may aggravate his condition.

■ To prevent hypocalcemia, advise all patients (especially elderly ones) to eat foods rich in calcium, vitamin D, and protein, such as fortified milk and cheese, soybean products, and sardines. Discourage long-term use of laxatives.

Hypercalcemia

■ Monitor serum calcium levels frequently, and report any increases.

■ Increase fluid intake to dilute calcium in serum and urine and to prevent renal damage and dehydration.

■ If the patient is receiving normal saline solution diuresis therapy, monitor him for signs of heart failure.

■ Monitor intake and output, and check the urine for renal calculi and acidity. Provide acid-ash drinks, such as cranberry juice, because calcium salts are more soluble in acid than in alkali.

■ Frequently check the patient's ECG and vital signs.

DRUG CHALLENGE

 If the patient is receiving a cardiac glycoside, watch for signs and symptoms of toxicity.

■ If the patient has chronic hypercalcemia, handle him *gently* to prevent pathologic fractures.

■ If the patient is bedridden, reposition him frequently, and encourage range-of-motion exercises to promote circulation and prevent urinary stasis and calcium loss from bone.

■ To prevent recurrence, suggest a low-calcium diet and increased fluid intake.

▌Candidiasis

Also called *candidosis* and *moniliasis,* candidiasis is usually a mild, superficial fungal infection caused by the *Candida* genus. The infection usually affects the nails (onychomycosis), skin (diaper rash), or mucous membranes, especially the oropharynx (thrush), vagina (candidiasis), esophagus, and GI tract. Rarely, these fungi enter the bloodstream

Identifying thrush

Candidiasis of the oropharyngeal mucosa (thrush) causes cream-colored or bluish white pseudomembranous patches on the tongue, mouth, or pharynx. Fungal invasion may extend to circumoral tissues.

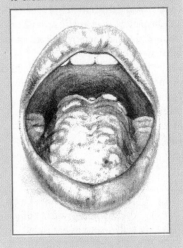

and invade the kidneys, lungs, endocardium, brain, or other structures, causing serious infections. Such systemic infection is most prevalent among drug abusers and patients already hospitalized, particularly patients with diabetes or those in an immunosuppressed state. The prognosis varies, depending on the patient's resistance.

Causes
■ Most cases: *C. albicans.* Also *C. parapsilosis, C. tropicalis,* and *C. guilliermondii*

Risk factors
■ Predominant use of broad-spectrum antibiotics, which decrease the number of normal flora and permits an increase of candidal organisms
■ Diabetes mellitus

■ Lowered resistance from a disease (such as cancer), radiation, aging, human immunodeficiency virus infection, or use of immunosuppressant medications
■ I.V. or urinary catheter use, drug abuse, or surgery
■ Infant exposure while passing through the birth canal
■ Total parenteral nutrition

Signs and symptoms
Superficial candidiasis produces signs and symptoms that correspond to the site of infection.
■ *Esophageal mucosa:* dysphagia, retrosternal pain, regurgitation, and scales in the mouth and throat
■ *Nails:* red, swollen, darkened nail bed; purulent discharge and the separation of a pruritic nail from the nail bed
■ *Oropharyngeal mucosa:* cream-colored or bluish white patches of exudate on the tongue, mouth, or pharynx that reveal bloody engorgement when scraped; possible swelling with resulting respiratory distress in infants; occasionally, pain and a burning sensation in the throats and mouths of adults (see *Identifying thrush*)
■ *Skin:* scaly, erythematous, papular rash, sometimes covered with exudate, appearing below the breast, between the fingers, and at the axillae, groin, and umbilicus; papules at the edges of the rash with diaper rash, papules appear at the edges of the rash
■ *Vaginal mucosa:* white or yellow discharge, with pruritus and local excoriation; white or gray raised patches on vaginal walls, with local inflammation; dyspareunia

Systemic infection produces chills, hypotension, prostration, high, spiking fever and, occasionally, rash. Specific signs and symptoms depend on the site of infection.

- *Brain:* headache, nuchal rigidity, seizures, focal neurologic deficits
- *Endocardium:* systolic or diastolic murmur, fever, chest pain, embolic phenomena
- *Eye:* endophthalmitis, blurred vision, orbital or periorbital pain, scotoma, exudate
- *Pulmonary system:* hemoptysis, fever, cough
- *Renal system:* fever, flank pain, dysuria, hematuria, pyuria

Diagnostic tests

- Gram stain of skin, vaginal scrapings, pus, or sputum or on skin scrapings reveals *Candida*. For systemic infections, blood or tissue culture reveals *Candida*.

Treatment

- Improve the underlying condition (control diabetes, discontinuing catheterization or antibiotic therapy).
- Antifungal therapy may include nystatin (Nilstat) for superficial candidiasis, clotrimazole (Gyne-Lotrimin) and miconazole (Monistat) for mucous membrane and vaginal infections, ketoconazole (Nizoral) or fluconazole (Diflucan) for chronic candidiasis of the mucous membranes, or I.V. amphotericin B with or without 5-fluorocytosine for systemic infections.

Nursing considerations

- If the patient is using nystatin solution, instruct him to swish it around in his mouth for several minutes before swallowing it.
- If the patient is an infant with thrush, swab nystatin on the oral mucosa.
- Provide the patient with a nonirritating mouthwash, to loosen tenacious secretions, and a soft toothbrush.

DRUG CHALLENGE

 Relieve mouth discomfort with a prescribed topical anesthetic, such as lidocaine, at least 1 hour before meals. Be aware that it may suppress the gag reflex and cause aspiration.

- If the patient has severe dysphagia, provide a soft diet. If he has mild dysphagia, tell him to chew his food thoroughly, and make sure he doesn't choke.
- If the patient is obese, use cornstarch or dry padding in intertriginous areas to prevent irritation.
- Assess the patient with candidiasis for underlying causes such as diabetes mellitus.

DRUG CHALLENGE

 If the patient is receiving amphotericin B for systemic candidiasis, he may have severe chills, fever, anorexia, nausea, and vomiting. Administer acetaminophen (Tylenol), an antihistamine, or an antiemetic to help reduce adverse reactions.

- If the patient has renal involvement, carefully monitor intake and output and urine for blood and protein.
- Check high-risk patients daily, especially those receiving an antibiotic, for patchy areas, irritation, sore throat, bleeding of mouth or gums, or other signs and symptoms of superinfection. Check for vaginal discharge; record the color and amount.
- Encourage a pregnant patient in the third trimester of pregnancy to be examined for vaginal candidiasis to protect her child from infection at birth.

Cardiac arrhythmias

Abnormal electrical conduction or automaticity changes heart rate and rhythm in cardiac arrhythmias, also called cardiac dysrhythmias. (See *Types of cardiac arrhythmias.*)

Arrhythmias vary in severity from mild and asymptomatic, requiring no treatment, to catastrophic, necessitating immediate resuscitation. Arrhythmias are generally classified according to their origin (ventricular or supraventricular). Their effect on cardiac output and blood pressure determines their clinical significance.

Causes
- Congenital
- Degeneration of the conductive tissue necessary to maintain normal heart rhythm (such as sick sinus syndrome)
- Drug toxicity
- Myocardial ischemia, infarction, or organic heart disease

Signs and symptoms
- Chest pain
- Cold, clammy extremities
- Dizziness
- Pallor
- Palpitations
- Reduced urine output
- Syncope
- Weakness

Diagnostic tests
- Electrocardiography allows detection and identification of arrhythmias. (See *Types of cardiac arrhythmias.*)

Treatment
- See *Types of cardiac arrhythmias.*

Nursing considerations
- If the patient isn't being monitored, assess him for rhythm disturbances.

- If the patient's pulse is abnormally rapid, slow, or irregular, watch for signs of hypoperfusion, such as hypotension and diminished urine output. If the patient is being monitored, document any arrhythmias and assess him for possible causes and effects.

ACTION STAT!

 When life-threatening arrhythmias develop, rapidly assess the level of consciousness, respirations, and pulse rate. Start cardiopulmonary resuscitation, if indicated. Give medications as needed, and prepare for any necessary medical procedures (for example, cardioversion).

- Monitor the patient for predisposing factors—such as fluid and electrolyte imbalance—and signs of drug toxicity, especially digoxin toxicity. If he's experiencing drug toxicity, the next dose may have to be withheld.
- To prevent arrhythmias in a postoperative cardiac patient, provide adequate oxygen and reduce the heart's workload, while carefully maintaining metabolic, neurologic, respiratory, and hemodynamic status.
- To avoid temporary pacemaker malfunction, install a fresh battery before each insertion. Carefully secure the external catheter wires and the pacemaker box. Assess the threshold daily. Watch closely for premature contractions, a sign of myocardial irritation. To avert permanent pacemaker malfunction, restrict the patient's activity after insertion, monitor the pulse rate regularly, and watch for signs of decreased cardiac output.
- If the patient has a permanent pacemaker, warn him about environmental and electrical hazards, as indicated by the pacemaker manufacturer.

(Text continues on page 98.)

Types of cardiac arrhythmias

This table reviews many common cardiac arrhythmias and outlines their features, causes, and treatments. Use a normal electrocardiogram strip, if available, to compare normal cardiac rhythm configurations with the rhythm strips below. Characteristics of normal rhythm include:

- identical atrial and ventricular rates, with constant PR interval
- PR interval of 0.12 to 0.2 second
- QRS duration less than 0.12 second
- regular and uniform QRS complexes and P waves
- ventricular and atrial rates of 60 to 100 beats/minute.

Arrhythmia and features	Causes	Treatment
Sinus arrhythmia 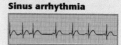 ■ Irregular atrial and ventricular rhythms ■ Normal P wave preceding each QRS complex	■ A normal variation of normal sinus rhythm in athletes, children, and elderly people ■ Also seen in digoxin toxicity and inferior wall myocardial infarction (MI)	■ Atropine if rate decreases below 40 beats/minute and the patient is symptomatic
Sinus tachycardia 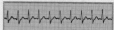 ■ Regular atrial and ventricular rhythms ■ Rate more than 100 beats/minute; rarely, more than 160 beats/minute ■ Normal P wave preceding each QRS complex	■ Normal physiologic response to fever, exercise, anxiety, pain, dehydration; may also accompany shock, left-sided heart failure, cardiac tamponade, hyperthyroidism, anemia, hypovolemia, pulmonary embolism, and anterior wall MI ■ May also occur with atropine, epinephrine, isoproterenol, quinidine, caffeine, alcohol, and nicotine use	■ Correction of underlying cause ■ Beta-adrenergic blockers or calcium channel blockers for symptomatic patients
Sinus bradycardia 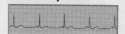 ■ Regular atrial and ventricular rhythms ■ Rate less than 60 beats/minute ■ Normal P waves preceding each QRS complex	■ Normal in a well-conditioned heart, as in an athlete ■ Increased intracranial pressure; increased vagal tone due to straining during defecation, vomiting, intubation, mechanical ventilation; sick sinus syndrome, hypothyroidism; inferior wall MI ■ May also occur with anticholinesterase, beta-adrenergic blocker, digoxin, and morphine use	■ Correction of underlying cause ■ For low cardiac output, dizziness, weakness, altered level of consciousness, or low blood pressure; advanced cardiac life support (ACLS) protocol for administration of atropine ■ Temporary pacemaker or permanent pacemaker ■ Dopamine or epinephrine infusion

(continued)

Types of cardiac arrhythmias *(continued)*

Arrhythmia and features	Causes	Treatment
Sinoatrial (SA) arrest or block 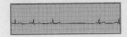 ■ Regular atrial and ventricular rhythms, except for missing complex ■ Normal P waves preceding each QRS complex; missing during pause ■ Pause not equal to a multiple of the previous sinus rhythm	■ Acute infection ■ Coronary artery disease (CAD), degenerative heart disease, acute inferior wall MI ■ Vagal stimulation, Valsalva's maneuver, carotid sinus massage ■ Digoxin, quinidine, or salicylate toxicity ■ Pesticide poisoning ■ Pharyngeal irritation caused by endotracheal (ET) intubation ■ Sick sinus syndrome	■ Correction of underlying cause ■ Atropine I.V. for symptoms ■ Temporary or permanent pacemaker for repeated episodes
Wandering atrial pacemaker 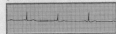 ■ Slightly irregular atrial and ventricular rhythms ■ PR interval varies ■ Irregular P waves with changing configuration, indicating that they aren't all from SA node or single atrial focus; may appear after the QRS complex ■ QRS complexes uniform in shape but irregular in rhythm	■ Rheumatic carditis due to inflammation involving the SA node ■ Digoxin toxicity ■ Sick sinus syndrome	■ No treatment if patient is asymptomatic ■ Treatment of underlying cause if patient is symptomatic

Types of cardiac arrhythmias *(continued)*

Arrhythmia and features	Causes	Treatment
Premature atrial contraction (PAC) 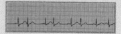 ■ Premature, abnormal-looking P waves that differ in configuration from normal P waves ■ QRS complexes after P waves, except in very early or blocked PACs ■ P wave usually buried in the preceding T wave or identified in the preceding T wave	■ Coronary disease, valvular heart disease, atrial ischemia, coronary atherosclerosis, heart failure, acute respiratory failure, chronic obstructive pulmonary disease (COPD), electrolyte imbalance, hypoxia ■ Digoxin toxicity; use of aminophylline, adrenergics, or caffeine ■ Anxiety	■ Usually no treatment needed ■ Treatment of underlying cause
Paroxysmal supraventricular tachycardia 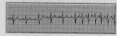 ■ Regular atrial and ventricular rhythms ■ Heart rate more than 160 beats/minute; rarely exceeds 250 beats/minute ■ P waves regular but aberrant; difficult to differentiate from preceding T wave ■ P wave preceding each QRS complex ■ Sudden onset and termination of arrhythmia	■ Intrinsic abnormality of AV conduction system ■ Physical or psychological stress, hypoxia, hypokalemia, cardiomyopathy, congenital heart disease, MI, valvular disease, Wolff-Parkinson-White syndrome, cor pulmonale, hyperthyroidism, systemic hypertension ■ Digoxin toxicity; use of caffeine, marijuana, or central nervous system stimulants	■ If patient is unstable, immediate cardioversion ■ If patient is stable: vagal stimulation, Valsalva's maneuver, and carotid sinus massage ■ Priority if cardiac function is preserved: calcium channel blocker, beta-adrenergic blocker, digoxin, and cardioversion (consider procainamide, amiodarone, or sotalol if each preceding treatment is ineffective in rhythm conversion) ■ If ejection fraction is less than 40% or patient is in heart failure: digoxin, amiodarone, then diltiazem

(continued)

Types of cardiac arrhythmias *(continued)*

Arrhythmia and features	Causes	Treatment
Atrial flutter 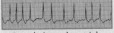 • Regular atrial rhythm; rate 250 to 400 beats/minute • Variable ventricular rate, depending on degree of atrioventricular (AV) block (usually 60 to 100 beats/minute) • Sawtooth P-wave configuration possible (F waves) • QRS complexes uniform in shape but commonly irregular in rate	• Heart failure, tricuspid or mitral valve disease, pulmonary embolism, cor pulmonale, inferior wall MI, carditis • Digoxin toxicity	• If patient is unstable with a ventricular rate more than 150 beats/minute: immediate cardioversion • If patient is stable: calcium channel blockers, beta-adrenergic blockers, or antiarrhythmics • Possibly, anticoagulation therapy (heparin, enoxaparin, or warfarin) • Radiofrequency ablation to control rhythm
Atrial fibrillation • Grossly irregular atrial rhythm; rate exceeding 400 beats/minute • Grossly irregular ventricular rhythm • QRS complexes of uniform configuration and duration • PR interval indiscernible • No P waves, or P waves that appear as erratic, irregular, baseline fibrillatory waves	• Heart failure, COPD, thyrotoxicosis, constrictive pericarditis, ischemic heart disease, sepsis, pulmonary embolus, rheumatic heart disease, hypertension, mitral stenosis, atrial irritation, complication of coronary bypass or valve replacement surgery • Nifedipine and digoxin use	• If patient is unstable with a ventricular rate more than 150 beats/minute: immediate cardioversion • If patient is stable: ACLS protocol for cardioversion and drug therapy (may include calcium channel blockers, beta-adrenergic blockers, or antiarrhythmics) • Anticoagulants, such as heparin, enoxaparin, or warfarin. • Class III antiarrhythmic, dofetilide (Tikosyn) for conversion of atrial fibrillation and atrial flutter to normal sinus rhythm • Radiofrequency catheter ablation to the His bundle to interrupt all conduction between atria and the ventricles (in resistant patients with recurring symptomatic atrial fibrillation) • Maze procedure: sutures placed in strategic places in the atrial myocardium to prevent electrical circuits from developing perpetuating atrial fibrillation

Types of cardiac arrhythmias *(continued)*

Arrhythmia and features	Causes	Treatment
Premature junctional contractions *(junctional premature beats)* 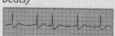 ▪ Irregular atrial and ventricular rhythms ▪ Inverted P waves; may precede, be hidden within, or follow QRS complex ▪ PR interval less than 0.12 second if P wave precedes QRS complex ▪ Normal QRS complex configuration and duration	▪ MI, ischemia ▪ Digoxin toxicity and excessive caffeine or amphetamine use	▪ Correction of underlying cause ▪ Discontinuation of digoxin if appropriate
Junctional rhythm 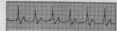 ▪ Regular atrial and ventricular rhythms; atrial rate 40 to 60 beats/minute; ventricular rate usually 40 to 60 beats/minute (60 to 100 beats/minute is accelerated junctional rhythm) ▪ P waves preceding, hidden within (absent), or after QRS complex; inverted if visible ▪ PR interval (when present) less than 0.12 second ▪ QRS complex configuration and duration normal, except in aberrant conduction	▪ Inferior wall MI or ischemia, hypoxia, vagal stimulation, sick sinus syndrome ▪ Acute rheumatic fever ▪ Valve surgery ▪ Digoxin toxicity	▪ Correction of underlying cause ▪ Atropine for symptomatic slow rate ▪ Pacemaker insertion if patient doesn't respond to drugs ▪ Discontinuation of digoxin if appropriate

(continued)

Types of cardiac arrhythmias *(continued)*

Arrhythmia and features	Causes	Treatment
Junctional tachycardia 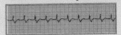 ■ Regular atrial and ventricular rhythms ■ Atrial rate more than 100 beats/minute; however, P waves may be absent, hidden in QRS complex, or preceding T wave ■ Ventricular rate more than 100 beats/minute ■ Inverted P wave; may occur before or after QRS complex, may be hidden in QRS complex, or may be absent ■ Normal QRS complex configuration and duration	■ Myocarditis, cardiomyopathy, inferior wall MI or ischemia, acute rheumatic fever, complication of valve replacement surgery ■ Digoxin toxicity	■ Correction of underlying cause ■ Beta-adrenergic blockers, calcium channel blockers, or amiodarone ■ Discontinuation of digoxin if appropriate
First-degree AV block 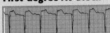 ■ Regular atrial and ventricular rhythms ■ PR interval more than 0.20 second ■ P wave precedes QRS complex ■ Normal QRS complex	■ May be seen in a healthy person ■ Inferior wall MI or ischemia, hypothyroidism, hypokalemia, hyperkalemia ■ Digoxin toxicity; use of quinidine, procainamide, or beta-adrenergic blockers, calcium channel blockers, or amiodarone	■ Correction of underlying cause ■ Possibly atropine (if severe bradycardia develops and patient is symptomatic) ■ Cautious use of digoxin, calcium channel blockers, and beta-adrenergic blockers
Second-degree AV block *Mobitz I (Wenckebach)* 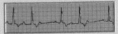 ■ Regular atrial rhythm ■ Irregular ventricular rhythm ■ Atrial rate exceeds ventricular rate ■ PR interval progressively but only slightly longer with each cycle until QRS complex disappears (dropped beat); PR interval shorter after dropped beat	■ Inferior wall MI, cardiac surgery, acute rheumatic fever, vagal stimulation ■ Digoxin toxicity; use of propranolol, quinidine, or procainamide	■ Treatment of underlying cause ■ Atropine or temporary pacemaker for symptomatic bradycardia ■ Discontinuation of digoxin if appropriate

Types of cardiac arrhythmias *(continued)*

Arrhythmia and features	Causes	Treatment
Second-degree AV block *Mobitz II* 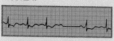 ▪ Regular atrial rhythm ▪ Regular or irregular ventricular rhythm, with varying degree of block ▪ P-P interval constant ▪ QRS complexes periodically absent	▪ Severe CAD, anterior wall MI, acute myocarditis ▪ Digoxin toxicity	▪ Temporary or permanent pacemaker ▪ Atropine, dopamine, or epinephrine for symptomatic bradycardia ▪ Discontinuation of digoxin if appropriate
Third-degree AV block *(complete heart block)* 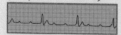 ▪ Regular atrial rhythm ▪ Slow ventricular rate and regular rhythm ▪ No relation between P waves and QRS complexes ▪ No constant PR interval ▪ QRS interval normal (nodal pacemaker) or wide and bizarre (ventricular pacemaker); rates regular ▪ PR interval varies ▪ P wave may be buried in QRS complexes or T wave ▪ Normal QRS complex	▪ Inferior or anterior wall MI, congenital abnormality, rheumatic fever, hypoxia, postoperative complication of mitral valve replacement, Lev's disease (fibrosis and calcification that spreads from cardiac structures to the conductive tissue), Lenegre's disease (conductive tissue fibrosis) ▪ Digoxin toxicity	▪ Atropine, dopamine, or epinephrine for symptomatic bradycardia ▪ Temporary or permanent pacemaker

(continued)

Types of cardiac arrhythmias *(continued)*

Arrhythmia and features	Causes	Treatment

Premature ventricular contraction (PVC)

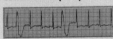

- Regular atrial rhythm
- Irregular ventricular rhythm
- QRS complex premature, usually followed by a complete compensatory pause
- QRS complex wide and distorted, usually more than 0.14 second
- Premature QRS complexes occurring singly, in pairs, or in threes, alternating with normal beats; focus from one or more sites
- Ominous when clustered, multifocal, with R wave on T pattern

- Heart failure, hypercapnia, hypokalemia, hypocalcemia, myocardial irritation by ventricular catheter or a pacemaker, old or acute MI, ischemia, or contusion
- Drug toxicity (cardiac glycosides, aminophylline, tricyclic antidepressants, beta-adrenergic blockers [isoproterenol or dopamine])
- Caffeine, tobacco, or alcohol use
- Psychological stress, anxiety, pain, exercise

- If warranted, procainamide, lidocaine, or amiodarone I.V.
- Treatment of underlying cause
- Discontinuation of drug causing toxicity
- PVC induced by hypokalemia: potassium chloride I.V.
- PVC induced by hypomagnesemia: magnesium sulfate I.V.

Ventricular tachycardia

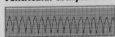

- Ventricular rate 140 to 220 beats/minute, regular or irregular rhythm
- QRS complexes wide, bizarre, and independent of P waves
- P waves not discernible
- May start and stop suddenly

- CAD, rheumatic heart disease, mitral valve prolapse, heart failure, cardiomyopathy, ventricular catheters, hypokalemia, hypercalcemia, pulmonary embolism, myocardial ischemia, infarction, or aneurysm
- Digoxin, procainamide, epinephrine, or quinidine toxicity
- Anxiety

- Pulseless: Initiate cardiopulmonary resuscitation (CPR); follow ACLS protocol for defibrillation, ET intubation, and administration of epinephrine or vasopressin, followed by amiodarone or lidocaine; if ineffective, magnesium sulfate or procainamide
- With pulse: If hemodynamically stable monomorphic ventricular tachycardia (VT), follow ACLS protocol for administration of procainamide, sotalol, amiodarone, or lidocaine; if ineffective, initiate synchronized cardioversion

Types of cardiac arrhythmias *(continued)*

Arrhythmia and features	Causes	Treatment
Ventricular tachycardia *(continued)*		■ If polymorphic VT: follow ACLS protocol for administration of beta-adrenergic blockers, lidocaine, amiodarone, procainamide, or sotalol; if ineffective, initiate synchronized cardioversion ■ If torsades: magnesium, then overdrive pacing; possibly, isoproterenol, phenytoin, or lidocaine (if rhythm persists) ■ Implanted cardioverter defibrillator, if recurrent VT
Ventricular fibrillation 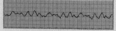 ■ Ventricular rhythm chaotic; rate rapid ■ QRS complexes wide and irregular; no visible P waves	■ Myocardial ischemia or infarction, untreated ventricular tachycardia, R-on-T phenomenon, hypokalemia, hyperkalemia, hypercalcemia, alkalosis, electric shock, hypothermia ■ Digoxin, epinephrine, or quinidine toxicity	■ Pulseless: Initiate CPR; follow ACLS protocol for defibrillation, ET intubation, and administration of epinephrine or vasopressin, lidocaine or amiodarone; if ineffective, magnesium sulfate or procainamide. ■ Implantable cardioverter defibrillator, if risk for recurrent VT
Asystole 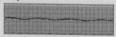 ■ No atrial or ventricular rate or rhythm ■ No discernible P waves, QRS complexes, or T waves	■ Myocardial ischemia or infarction, aortic valve disease, heart failure, hypoxia, hypokalemia, severe acidosis, electric shock, ventricular arrhythmia, AV block, pulmonary embolism, heart rupture, cardiac tamponade, hyperkalemia, electromechanical dissociation ■ Cocaine overdose	■ Continue CPR, follow ACLS protocol for ET intubation, transcutaneous pacing, and administration of epinephrine and atropine

■ Tell the patient to report light-headedness or syncope, and stress the importance of regular checkups.

Cardiac tamponade

With cardiac tamponade, a rapid, unchecked rise in intrapericardial pressure impairs diastolic filling of the heart. The rise in pressure usually results from blood or fluid accumulation in the pericardial sac. If fluid accumulates rapidly, the condition can be fatal, necessitating emergency lifesaving measures. Slow accumulation and rise in pressure may not produce immediate symptoms because the fibrous wall of the pericardial sac can gradually stretch to accommodate 1 to 2 L of fluid.

Causes

■ Acute myocardial infarction (MI)
■ Effusion (from cancer, a bacterial infection, tuberculosis or, rarely, acute rheumatic fever)
■ Hemorrhage from nontraumatic causes (rupture of the heart or great vessels or anticoagulant therapy in a patient with pericarditis)
■ Hemorrhage from trauma (gunshot or stab wounds of the chest, perforation during cardiac or central venous catheterization or, rarely, cardiac surgery)
■ Idiopathic (Dressler's syndrome)
■ Uremia

Signs and symptoms

■ Anxiety, restlessness
■ Diaphoresis
■ Drop in ventricular end-systolic volume due to inadequate preload
■ Dyspnea
■ Hepatomegaly
■ Increase of pericardial pressure transmitting equally across the heart cavities

and causing a matching rise in intracardiac pressure, especially atrial and end-diastolic ventricular pressures
■ Increased venous blood pressure with jugular vein distention
■ Muffled heart sounds on auscultation
■ Narrow pulse pressure
■ Pallor or cyanosis
■ Paradoxical pulse (an abnormal inspiratory drop in systemic blood pressure greater than 15 mm Hg)
■ Reduced arterial blood pressure
■ Tachycardia

Diagnostic tests

■ Chest X-ray shows slightly widened mediastinum and cardiomegaly.
■ Electrocardiography may reveal changes produced by acute pericarditis and rules out other cardiac disorders.
■ Pulmonary artery catheterization indicates increased right atrial pressure, right ventricular diastolic pressure, and central venous pressure (CVP).
■ Echocardiography records pericardial effusion with signs of right ventricular and atrial compression.

Treatment

■ Treatment may include pericardiocentesis (needle aspiration of the pericardial cavity to remove accumulated blood or fluid) or surgical creation of an opening.
■ A pericardial window may be performed (removing a portion of the pericardium to permit excess pericardial fluid to drain into the pleural space) if tamponade, effusions or adhesions from chronic pericarditis recur.
■ In more severe cases, removal of the toughened encasing pericardium (pericardectomy) may be necessary.
■ The patient with hypotension may require trial volume loading with temporary I.V. normal saline solution with albumin.

■ The patient may require an inotropic drug, such as dopamine, to maintain cardiac output.

DRUG CHALLENGE

 Although inotropic drugs normally improve myocardial function, they may further compromise an ischemic myocardium after an MI.

■ For traumatic injury, the patient may require blood transfusion or a thoracotomy to drain reaccumulating fluid or to repair bleeding sites.
■ The patient with heparin-induced tamponade may be given the heparin antagonist protamine sulfate.
■ The patient with warfarin-induced tamponade may require vitamin K administration.

Nursing considerations
For pericardiocentesis

■ Position the patient at a 45- to 60-degree angle. Connect the precordial electrocardiogram lead to the hub of the aspiration needle with an alligator clamp and connecting wire. When the needle touches the myocardium during fluid aspiration, an ST-segment elevation or premature ventricular contraction is seen.
■ Monitor blood pressure, cardiac rhythm, and CVP during and after pericardiocentesis.
■ Infuse I.V. solutions to maintain blood pressure. Watch for a decrease in CVP and a concomitant rise in blood pressure, which indicate relief of cardiac compression.

ALERT

 Watch for complications of pericardiocentesis, such as ventricular fibrillation, vasovagal re-

sponse, or coronary artery or cardiac chamber puncture. Closely monitor the patient for changes in ECG test results, blood pressure, pulse rate, level of consciousness, and urine output.

For thoracotomy

■ Explain the procedure to the patient. Tell him what to expect postoperatively (chest tubes, drainage bottles, administration of oxygen). Teach him how to turn, deep-breathe, and cough.
■ Administer an antibiotic, protamine sulfate, or vitamin K as needed.
■ Postoperatively, monitor critical parameters, such as vital signs and arterial blood gas levels, and assess heart and breath sounds.
■ Give an analgesic as needed.
■ Maintain the chest drainage system, and be alert for complications, such as hemorrhage and arrhythmias.

▮ Cardiogenic shock

Sometimes called *pump failure*, cardiogenic shock is a condition of diminished cardiac output that severely impairs tissue perfusion. It reflects severe left-sided heart failure and occurs as a serious complication in nearly 15% of all patients hospitalized with an acute myocardial infarction (MI). It typically affects patients whose area of infarction exceeds 40% of muscle mass; in such patients, the fatality rate may exceed 85%. (See *What happens in cardiogenic shock,* page 100.)

Causes

■ Cardiac arrest
■ Cardial amyloidosis
■ End-stage cardiomyopathy and other cardiomyopathies (viral, toxic)
■ MI (most common)

What happens in cardiogenic shock

Regardless of the cause, left ventricular dysfunction initiates a series of compensatory mechanisms that attempt to increase cardiac output and, in turn, maintain vital organ function. Compensatory responses increase heart rate, left ventricular filling pressure (preload), and peripheral resistance to flow to enhance venous return to the heart. The action initially stabilizes the patient's condition but later causes deterioration.

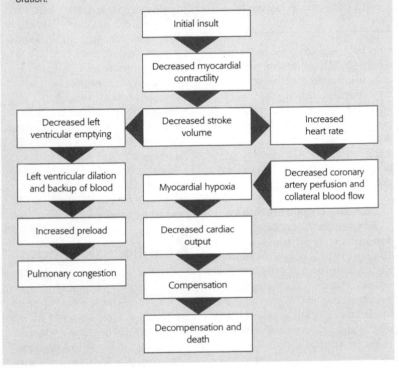

- Myocardial degeneration
- Myocardial ischemia
- Papillary muscle dysfunction
- Ventricular arrhythmias (fibrillation, tachycardia)

Signs and symptoms

- Cold, pale, clammy skin
- Cyanosis
- Drop in systolic blood pressure to 30 mm Hg below baseline or a sustained reading below 80 mm Hg not attributable to medication

- Narrowing pulse pressure
- Oliguria (less than 20 ml of urine/hour)
- Rapid, shallow respirations
- Restlessness, mental confusion, and obtundation
- Tachycardia

Diagnostic tests

- Auscultation detects gallop rhythm and faint heart sounds; if the shock results from rupture of the ventricular septum or papillary muscles, a holosystolic murmur occurs.

- Pulmonary artery pressure (PAP) monitoring reveals increased PAP, increased pulmonary artery wedge pressure (PAWP), reflecting a rise in left ventricular end-diastolic pressure (preload) and increased resistance to left ventricular emptying (afterload) resulting from ineffective pumping and increased peripheral vascular resistance. Thermodilution catheterization reveals a reduced cardiac index (less than 1.8 L/minute/ml).
- Invasive arterial pressure monitoring shows hypotension from impaired ventricular ejection.
- Arterial blood gas (ABG) levels may show metabolic acidosis and hypoxia.
- Electrocardiography may reveal evidence of an acute MI, myocardial ischemia, or ventricular aneurysm.
- Serum enzyme levels show elevated creatine kinase (CK), lactate dehydrogenase (LD), aspartate aminotransferase, and alanine aminotransferase, which point to an MI or myocardial ischemia and suggest heart failure or shock. CK and LD isoenzyme levels may confirm an acute MI.
- Echocardiography (color-flow Doppler) shows left ventricular function, valvular disease, aneurysmal dilation, and ventricular septal defects.

Treatment

- I.V. dopamine is given to increase cardiac output, blood pressure, and renal blood flow; I.V. amrinone or dobutamine is given to increase myocardial contractility.
- Furosemide is used to decrease pulmonary congestion.
- I.V. nitroprusside, a vasodilator, may be used with a vasopressor to further improve cardiac output by decreasing peripheral vascular resistance (afterload)

and reducing left ventricular end-diastolic pressure (preload).

- The intra-aortic balloon pump (IABP) improves coronary artery perfusion and decreases cardiac workload.
- Treatment may include ventricular assist pump or artificial heart in severe intractable cases.
- Percutaneous transluminal coronary angioplasty or coronary artery bypass graft is used to provide immediate reperfusion for treatable lesions.

Nursing considerations

- At the first sign of cardiogenic shock, check the patient's blood pressure and heart rate.

ACTION STAT!

 If the patient is hypotensive or is having difficulty breathing, ensure a patent I.V. line and a patent airway, and provide oxygen to promote tissue oxygenation.

- Monitor ABG levels to measure oxygenation and detect acidosis from poor tissue perfusion. Increase oxygen flow as indicated by ABG measurements. Check complete blood count and electrolyte levels.
- After diagnosis, monitor cardiac rhythm continuously. Frequently assess skin color and temperature and other vital signs. Watch for a drop in systolic blood pressure to less than 80 mm Hg (usually further compromising cardiac output).
- Insert an indwelling urinary catheter to measure output. Watch for an output below 30 ml/hour.
- Using a pulmonary artery catheter, closely monitor PAP, PAWP, and cardiac output. High PAWP indicates heart failure and requires an immediate response.

When a patient requires IABP, reposition him as little as possible. Never flex the patient's "ballooned" leg at the hip because this may displace or fracture the catheter. Assess pedal pulses, skin temperature, and color. Check the dressing on the insertion site frequently for bleeding, and change it according to your facility's policy. Check the insertion site for hematoma or signs of infection, and culture any drainage.

- After the patient's condition becomes hemodynamically stable, gradually reduce the frequency of balloon inflation to wean him from the IABP. During weaning, carefully monitor changes, chest pain, and other signs and symptoms of recurring cardiac ischemia and shock.
- Provide psychological support. The patient and his family may be anxious about the intensive care unit, IABP, and other tubes and devices, so offer reassurance.

Cardiomyopathy, dilated

Resulting from extensively damaged myocardial muscle fibers, dilated cardiomyopathy interferes with myocardial metabolism and grossly dilates all four chambers of the heart, giving the heart a globular appearance. In this disorder, hypertrophy may be present. Dilated cardiomyopathy leads to intractable heart failure, arrhythmias, and emboli. The prognosis for patients without evidence of heart failure varies: some remain stable, some gradually deteriorate, and others rapidly decline.

Causes

- Unknown in most cardiomyopathies
- Antepartum or postpartum cardiomyopathy during the last trimester or within months after delivery, most commonly in multiparous women older than age 30 with malnutrition or preeclampsia
- Complication of alcoholism
- Infiltrative disorders (hemochromatosis, amyloidosis)
- Muscle disorders (myasthenia gravis, progressive muscular dystrophy, myotonic dystrophy)
- Myocardial destruction by toxic, infectious, or metabolic agents, such as certain viruses (after infection with poliovirus, coxsackievirus B, influenza virus, or human immunodeficiency virus), endocrine (hyperthyroidism, pheochromocytoma) and electrolyte disorders, and nutritional deficiencies (beriberi, a thiamine deficiency, or kwashiorkor, a protein deficiency)
- Rheumatic fever, especially among children with myocarditis
- Sarcoidosis

Signs and symptoms

- Cardiomegaly
- Murmur resulting from functional mitral insufficiency
- S_3 and S_4 gallop rhythms
- Signs and symptoms of heart failure—both left-sided (shortness of breath, orthopnea, exertional dyspnea, paroxysmal nocturnal dyspnea, fatigue, and an irritating dry cough at night) and right-sided (edema, liver engorgement, and jugular vein distention)

Diagnostic tests

- Echocardiography confirms the presence of dilated cardiomyopathy.
- Cardiac catheterization may show left ventricular dilation and dysfunction, elevated left ventricular and, sometimes, right ventricular filling pressures, as well as diminished cardiac output.

- Gallium scans may identify patients with dilated cardiomyopathy and myocarditis.
- Electrocardiography may show biventricular hypertrophy, sinus tachycardia, atrial enlargement and, in 20% of patients, atrial fibrillation and bundle-branch heart block.
- Chest X-ray demonstrates cardiomegaly (usually affecting all heart chambers) and may demonstrate pulmonary congestion, pleural or pericardial effusion, or pulmonary hypertension.

Treatment
- Correct the underlying causes.
- Give digoxin, diuretics, and oxygen, as indicated.
- Place the patient on a sodium-restricted diet.
- Enforce bed rest.
- Give steroids, if prescribed.
- Give prescribed vasodilators, such as I.V. nitroprusside (Nitropress), I.V. nitroglycerine, or I.V. nesiritide (Natrecor) to reduce preload and afterload, decreasing congestion and increasing cardiac output.
- Long-term treatment may include prazosin (Minipress), hydralazine, isosorbide dinitrate (Isordil), an angiotensin-converting enzyme inhibitor, and an anticoagulant.
- Some patients may be candidates for heart transplantation if therapies fail.
- Cardiomyoplasty, which wraps the latissimus dorsi muscle around the ventricles, helps the ventricle to effectively pump blood. A cardiomyostimulator delivers bursts of electrical impulses during systole to contract the muscle.

Nursing considerations
- If the patient has acute failure, monitor him for signs of progressive failure (bilateral crackles, increased jugular vein distention) and compromised renal perfusion (oliguria, increased blood urea nitrogen and creatinine levels, electrolyte imbalances). Weigh him daily.

DRUG CHALLENGE

If the patient is receiving a vasodilator, frequently check his blood pressure and heart rate. If he becomes hypotensive, stop the infusion and place him in a supine position, with his legs elevated to increase venous return and to ensure cerebral blood flow.

DRUG CHALLENGE

If the patient is receiving a diuretic, monitor him for signs of resolving congestion (decreased crackles and dyspnea) or too vigorous diuresis. Check the serum potassium level for hypokalemia and renal function for increased creatinine level, especially if therapy includes a cardiac glycoside.

- Before discharge, teach the patient about his illness and its treatment, and encourage family members to learn cardiopulmonary resuscitation.

▌Cardiomyopathy, hypertrophic

A primary disease of the cardiac muscle, previously known as *idiopathic hypertrophic subaortic stenosis,* hypertrophic cardiomyopathy is characterized by disproportionate, asymmetric thickening of the interventricular septum in relation to the free wall of the left ventricle. Cardiac output may be low, normal, or high, depending on whether stenosis is obstructive or nonobstructive. Some patients may remain asymptomatic for years. Sudden death, especially during exercise, may be the initial event (attributed to 36% of athletes who died suddenly).

Causes

- Idiopathic in almost all cases
- Non–sex-linked autosomal dominant trait
- Ventricular septal hypertrophy and the movement of the anterior mitral valve leaflet into the outflow tract during systole, leading to left ventricular dysfunction (from rigidity and decreased diastolic compliance) followed by pump failure

Signs and symptoms

- Exertional dyspnea (90% of patients)
- Angina (75% of patients) at rest and prolonged, unrelieved by nitrates
- Arrhythmias
- Auscultation: harsh systolic murmur along the left sternal border and at the apex, increasing with Valsalva's maneuver and decreasing with squatting
- Heart failure
- Orthopnea
- Palpation: peripheral pulse with a characteristic double impulse (pulsus biferiens) and, with atrial fibrillation, an irregular pulse and loud S_4
- Sudden death (possibly without preceding signs or symptoms)
- Syncope

Diagnostic tests

- Echocardiography (most useful) shows increased thickness of the intraventricular septum and abnormal motion of the anterior mitral leaflet during systole, occluding left ventricular outflow in obstructive disease.
- Cardiac catheterization reveals elevated left ventricular end-diastolic pressure and, possibly, mitral insufficiency.
- Electrocardiography usually demonstrates left ventricular hypertrophy, T-wave inversion, left anterior hemiblock, Q waves in precordial and inferior leads, ventricular arrhythmias and, possibly, atrial fibrillation.

Treatment

- Beta-adrenergic blockers slow the heart rate and increase ventricular filling by relaxing the obstructing muscle, reducing angina, syncope, dyspnea, and arrhythmias. Propranolol (Inderal) is the drug of choice.

DRUG CHALLENGE

 Beta-adrenergic blockers may aggravate symptoms of cardiac decompensation.

- Cardioversion, anticoagulant therapy, and calcium channel blockers (such as verapamil to improve diastolic dysfunction) are used to treat atrial fibrillation.
- Ventricular myotomy (resection of the hypertrophied septum) alone or combined with mitral valve replacement may ease outflow tract obstruction and relieve symptoms. Complications include complete heart block and ventricular septal defect.
- Dual-chamber pacing may prevent progression of hypertrophy and obstruction.
- Implantable defibrillators may be used in patients with malignant ventricular arrhythmias.

Nursing considerations

- Because syncope or sudden death may follow well-tolerated exercise, warn patients against any strenuous physical activity, such as running and weight lifting.

DRUG CHALLENGE

 Avoid nitroglycerin, digoxin, and diuretics because they can worsen obstruction.

▪ If the patient will have dental work or surgery, give prophylaxis for subacute bacterial endocarditis beforehand.

▪ Provide psychological support. If the patient is hospitalized for a long time, be flexible with visiting hours. Refer the patient for psychosocial counseling, as appropriate.

▪ If the patient is a child, have his parents arrange for him to continue his studies in the facility.

▪ Because sudden cardiac arrest is possible, urge the patient's family to learn cardiopulmonary resuscitation.

▪ If propranolol will be discontinued, don't stop the drug abruptly because this could cause rebound effects, resulting in a myocardial infarction or sudden death.

Cardiomyopathy, restrictive

A disorder of the myocardial musculature, restrictive cardiomyopathy is characterized by restricted ventricular filling (the result of left ventricular hypertrophy) and endocardial fibrosis and thickening. The myocardium fails to contract completely during systole, resulting in low cardiac output. If severe, it's irreversible.

Causes
▪ Unknown
▪ Genetic mutations of sarcomere contractile protein gene and cardiac troponin I (TNNI3)
▪ Restrictive cardiomyopathy syndrome: a manifestation of amyloidosis due to infiltration of amyloid into the intracellular spaces in the myocardium, endocardium, and subendocardium

Signs and symptoms
▪ Chest pain

▪ Decreased cardiac output leading to heart failure
▪ Dyspnea
▪ Fatigue
▪ Generalized edema
▪ Liver engorgement
▪ Orthopnea
▪ Pallor
▪ Peripheral cyanosis
▪ S_3 or S_4 gallop rhythms
▪ Systolic murmurs of mitral and tricuspid insufficiency

Diagnostic tests
▪ Chest X-ray shows massive cardiomegaly in advanced stages, affecting all four chambers of the heart; pericardial effusion; and pulmonary congestion.
▪ Echocardiography rules out constrictive pericarditis as the cause of restricted filling by detecting increased left ventricular muscle mass and differences in end-diastolic pressures between the ventricles.
▪ Electrocardiography may show low-voltage complexes, hypertrophy, atrioventricular conduction defects, or arrhythmias.
▪ Arterial pulsation reveals blunt carotid upstroke with small volume.
▪ Cardiac catheterization demonstrates increased left ventricular end-diastolic pressure and rules out constrictive pericarditis as the cause of restricted filling.

Treatment
▪ Cardiac glycoside, a diuretic, and a sodium-restricted diet benefit the patient by easing the symptoms of heart failure.
▪ A vasodilator—such as isosorbide dinitrate (Isordil), prazosin (Minipress), and hydralazine—may be given to control intractable heart failure.
▪ Anticoagulant therapy is provided to prevent thrombophlebitis in a patient on prolonged bed rest.

Nursing considerations

- If the patient is in the acute phase, monitor heart rate and rhythm, blood pressure, urine output, and pulmonary artery pressure readings to help guide treatment.
- Give psychological support. Because a poor prognosis can cause profound anxiety and depression, be especially supportive and understanding, and encourage the patient to express his fears. Refer the patient for psychological counseling, as appropriate.
- Before discharge, teach the patient to watch for and report signs and symptoms of digoxin toxicity (including anorexia, nausea, vomiting, and yellow vision), to record and report weight gain and, if sodium must be restricted, to avoid canned foods, pickles, smoked meats, and table salt.

Carpal tunnel syndrome

The most common of the nerve entrapment syndromes, carpal tunnel syndrome results from compression of the median nerve at the wrist, within the carpal tunnel. This nerve passes through, along with blood vessels and flexor tendons, to the fingers and thumb. (See *Viewing the carpal tunnel.*)

Compression neuropathy causes sensory and motor changes in the median distribution of the hand. Usually occurring in women between ages 30 and 60, it poses a serious occupational health problem, especially in assembly-line workers, packers, secretary-typists, and persons who repeatedly use poorly designed tools. Any strenuous use of the hand—sustained grasping, twisting, or flexing—aggravates this condition.

Causes

- Acromegaly
- Amyloidosis
- Benign tumors
- Damage to the median nerve by dislocation or acute sprain of the wrist
- Diabetes mellitus
- Edema following Colles' fracture
- Hypothyroidism
- Menopause
- Myxedema
- Nerve compression
- Pregnancy
- Renal failure
- Rheumatoid arthritis and flexor tenosynovitis (commonly associated with rheumatic disease)
- Tuberculosis and other granulomatous diseases

Signs and symptoms

- Atrophic nails
- Dry, shiny skin
- Inability to clench hand into a fist
- Paresthesia affecting the thumb, forefinger, middle finger, and half of the fourth finger
- Relief of pain by shaking hands vigorously or dangling arms at his sides
- Weakness, pain (spreading to the forearm and possibly shoulder), burning, numbness, or tingling in the involved hands
- Worsening of symptoms at night and in the morning (due to vasodilation and venous stasis)

Diagnostic tests

- Physical examination reveals decreased sensation to light touch or pinpricks in the affected fingers. Thenar muscle atrophy occurs in about half of all cases of carpal tunnel syndrome.
- The patient exhibits a positive Tinel's sign (tingling over the median nerve on light percussion).
- Positive Phalen's wrist-flexion test (holding the forearms vertically and allowing both hands to drop into com-

plete flexion at the wrists for 1 minute reproduces symptoms of carpal tunnel syndrome).
▪ A compression test supports this diagnosis: A blood pressure cuff inflated above systolic pressure on the forearm for 1 to 2 minutes provokes pain and paresthesia along the distribution of the median nerve.
▪ Electromyography detects a median nerve motor conduction delay of more than 5 msec.
▪ Digital electrical stimulation discloses median nerve compression by measuring the length and intensity of stimulation from the fingers to the median nerve in the wrist.

Treatment
▪ Initially conservative, including resting the hands by splinting the wrist in neutral extension for 1 to 2 weeks.
▪ If a definite link has been established between the patient's condition and his occupation, he may need to seek other work.
▪ Surgical decompression of the nerve by resecting the entire transverse carpal tunnel ligament or by using endoscopic surgical techniques. Neurolysis (freeing of the nerve fibers) may also be necessary.
▪ Oral nonsteroidal anti-inflammatory drugs and injected corticosteroids are the most commonly prescribed medications.

Nursing considerations
▪ Give an analgesic if needed.
▪ Encourage the patient to use his hands as much as possible. If his dominant hand has been impaired, you may need to help him eat and bathe.
▪ Teach the patient how to apply a splint. Tell him not to make it too tight. Demonstrate removal to perform daily gentle range-of-motion exercises. Make

Viewing the carpal tunnel

The carpal tunnel is clearly visible in this palmar view and cross section of a right hand. Note the median nerve, flexor tendons of fingers, and blood vessels passing through the tunnel on their way from the forearm to the hand.

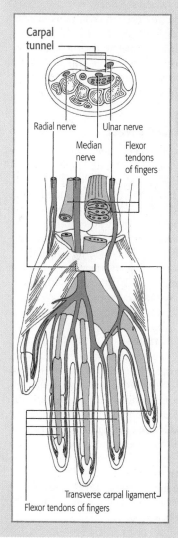

Carpal tunnel

Radial nerve   Ulnar nerve

Median nerve   Flexor tendons of fingers

Transverse carpal ligament
Flexor tendons of fingers

sure the patient knows how to do these exercises before he's discharged.

■ After surgery, monitor vital signs, and regularly check the color, sensation, and motion of the affected hand.

■ Advise the patient who's about to be discharged to occasionally exercise his hands in warm water. If the arm is in a sling, tell him to remove the sling several times per day to do exercises for his elbow and shoulder.

■ Suggest occupational counseling for the patient who has to change jobs because of carpal tunnel syndrome. For those patients who must remain in their current occupation, suggest ergonomic assessment of the work situation.

Cataract

A common cause of vision loss, a cataract is a gradually developing opacity of the lens or lens capsule of the eye. Cataracts commonly occur bilaterally, with each progressing independently. Exceptions are traumatic cataracts, which are usually unilateral, and congenital cataracts, which may remain stationary. A part of aging, they're most prevalent in patients older than age 70. Surgical intervention improves vision in 95% of affected people.

Causes

■ Complicated cataracts: secondary to uveitis, glaucoma, retinitis pigmentosa, and detached retina; systemic diseases, including diabetes, hypoparathyroidism, and atopic dermatitis); or exposure to ionizing radiation or infrared rays

■ Congenital cataracts (neonates): genetic defects or maternal rubella during the first trimester

■ Senile cataracts (elderly patients): degenerative changes in the chemical state of lens proteins

■ Toxic cataracts: prolonged drug or chemical toxicity from prednisone, ergot alkaloids, naphthalene, or phenothiazines; or from excessive exposure to sunlight

■ Traumatic cataracts: foreign-body injury to the lens with sufficient force to allow aqueous or vitreous humors to enter the lens capsule

Signs and symptoms

■ Blinding glare from headlights when driving at night

■ Inability to recognize people or things at a distance

■ Painless, gradual blurring and loss of vision

■ Pupil that progressively turns milky white (in extreme cases)

■ With central opacities, better vision in dim light than in bright light

Diagnostic tests

■ When shining a penlight on the pupil, observation of a white area behind the pupil suggests an advanced cataract.

■ Ophthalmoscopy or slit-lamp examination helps to confirm the diagnosis by revealing a dark area in the normally homogeneous red reflex.

Treatment

■ Extracapsular cataract extraction removes the anterior lens capsule and cortex, leaving the posterior capsule intact. This is done using phacoemulsification equipment, fragmenting the lens with ultrasound, and removal by irrigation and aspiration. A posterior chamber intraocular lens is then implanted.

■ Intracapsular cataract extraction removes the entire lens within the intact capsule by cryoextraction. An extremely cold metal probe is used for gentle traction.

Nursing considerations

- After surgery, the patient is discharged after he recovers from local anesthesia.

Do's & don'ts

 Remind the patient to return for a checkup the day after surgery and to avoid activities that increase intraocular pressure such as straining.

- Urge the patient to protect his eye from accidental injury by wearing his glasses during the day and an eye shield at night. Some patients wear an eye patch for 6 to 8 hours, whereas others may wear a collagen shield (similar to a contact lens) that dissolves in 24 hours.
- Tell the patient he may need either corrective reading glasses or a corrective contact lens, which will be fitted 4 to 8 weeks after surgery.
- If no lens has been implanted, the patient may be given temporary aphakic cataract glasses; in about 4 to 8 weeks, he'll be refracted for his own glasses.
- Administer antibiotic ointment or drops to prevent infection and a steroid to reduce inflammation, or combination steroid-antibiotic eyedrops.
- Monitor the patient for complications, such as a sharp pain in the eye, indicative of increased intraocular pressure, or early signs of infection (such as hyphema or hypopyon).

Cerebral contusion

Acceleration-deceleration or coup-contrecoup injuries to the head can cause cerebral contusion, or bruising of the brain tissue. More serious than a concussion, contusion disrupts normal nerve functions in the bruised area and may cause loss of consciousness, hemorrhage, edema, and even death.

Causes

- Circumstance in which the brain rebounds against the skull, as from a blow from a blunt instrument or a motor vehicle accident

Signs and symptoms

- Decorticate or decerebrate posturing
- Drowsiness, confusion, disorientation, agitation, or violent tendencies
- Hemiparesis
- Labored respirations
- Loss of consciousness for a few minutes or longer
- Lucid period followed by rapid deterioration (possible epidural hematoma)
- Severe scalp wounds
- Temporary aphasia
- Unequal pupillary response
- Unilateral numbness

Diagnostic tests

- An accurate history of the trauma and a neurologic examination are the principal diagnostic tools.
- A computed tomography scan shows ischemic tissue, hematomas, and fractures.

Treatment

- I.V. fluids with lactated Ringer's solution or normal saline solution may be given. Restrict total fluid intake to 1,200 to 1,500 ml/day to reduce volume and intracerebral swelling.
- Dexamethasone may be given I.M. or I.V. for several days to control cerebral edema.
- Mannitol may be given to reduce intracranial pressure (ICP).
- Hyperventilation may be indicated in some patients. If the patient is intubated, a partial pressure of arterial carbon dioxide between 30 and 35 mm Hg is desirable.
- Blood transfusions may be necessary.

- Craniotomy may be used to control bleeding and to aspirate blood.

Nursing considerations

- Maintain a patent airway. Suction as needed, and assist with endotracheal (ET) intubation or a tracheotomy if facial trauma precludes oral ET intubation.
- Perform a neurologic examination, focusing on level of consciousness (LOC), motor responses, and ICP.
- Insert an indwelling urinary catheter as ordered. Monitor intake and output.
- If the patient is unconscious, insert an oral gastric tube to prevent aspiration.
- If spinal injury is ruled out, elevate the head of the bed 30 degrees. Enforce bed rest.
- Carefully observe the patient for leakage of cerebrospinal fluid (CSF) from the nostrils and ear canals. Check bed sheets for a blood-tinged spot surrounded by a lighter ring (halo sign) to determine CSF leakage.

ACTION STAT!

 If CSF leakage develops, raise the head of the bed 30 degrees. If you detect CSF leaking from the patient's nose, place a gauze pad under his nostrils. Be sure to tell him not to blow his nose but to wipe it instead. If CSF leaks from the patient's ear, position him so that the ear drains naturally. Don't pack the ear or nose.

- Monitor respirations and other vital signs regularly (usually every 15 minutes). Abnormal respirations could indicate a breakdown in the respiratory center in the brain stem and a possible impending tentorial herniation—a neurologic emergency.
- Frequently check the patient's neurologic status, including LOC and orientation. Assess him for restlessness.

- After the patient's condition is stabilized, clean and dress any superficial scalp wounds. (If the skin has been broken, tetanus prophylaxis may be necessary.) Assist with suturing if needed.

Cerebral palsy

The most common cause of crippling in children, cerebral palsy is a group of neuromuscular disorders resulting from prenatal, perinatal, or postnatal central nervous system damage. Three major types of cerebral palsy occur—spastic (affects 70%), athetoid (affects 20%), and ataxic (affects 10%)—sometimes in mixed forms. Motor impairment may be minimal (sometimes apparent only during physical activities such as running) or severely disabling. Associated defects—such as seizures, speech disorders, and mental retardation—are common. The prognosis varies. With mild impairment, proper treatment may make a near-normal life possible.

Causes
Prenatal
- Abnormal placental attachment
- Anoxia
- Irradiation
- Isoimmunization
- Malnutrition
- Maternal diabetes
- Maternal infection (especially rubella in the first trimester)
- Rh factor or ABO blood type incompatibility
- Toxemia

Perinatal and birth difficulties
- Abruptio placentae
- Breech presentation
- Depressed maternal vital signs from general or spinal anesthetic
- Forceps delivery
- Inadequate oxygenation of the brain

- Multiple birth (especially infants born last in a multiple birth)
- Placenta previa
- Premature birth
- Prolapsed cord with delay in the delivery of the head
- Prolonged or unusually rapid labor

Infection or trauma during infancy

- Brain infection
- Brain tumor
- Cerebral circulatory anomalies causing blood vessel rupture
- Head trauma
- Kernicterus resulting from erythroblastosis fetalis
- Prolonged anoxia
- Systemic disease resulting in cerebral thrombosis or embolus

Signs and symptoms
Spastic cerebral palsy

- Hyperactive deep tendon reflexes
- Increased stretch reflexes
- Muscle contraction in response to manipulation
- Muscle weakness
- Rapid alternating muscle contraction and relaxation
- Tendency to contractures
- Underdevelopment of affected limbs
- Walking on toes with a scissors gait, crossing one foot in front of the other

Athetoid cerebral palsy

- Athetoid movements: increased during stress, decreased when relaxed, absent during sleep
- Involuntary movements (grimacing, wormlike writhing, dystonia, and sharp jerks) impairing voluntary movement
- Involuntary movements affecting the arms more severely than the legs
- Speech difficulties due to involuntary facial movements

Ataxic cerebral palsy

- Ataxia, making sudden or fine movements almost impossible
- Disturbed balance
- Hypoactive reflexes
- Incoordination (especially of the arms)
- Lack of leg movement during infancy
- Muscle weakness
- Nystagmus
- Tremor (also intention tremor)
- Wide gait as the child begins to walk

Mixed form

- Dental abnormalities
- Impaired motor function leading to difficulties in eating, especially swallowing, thereby inhibiting growth and development
- Impaired speech (about 80%)
- Mental retardation (up to 40% of patients)
- Reading disabilities
- Seizure disorders (about 25%)
- Vision and hearing defects

Diagnostic tests

- An early diagnosis is essential for effective treatment and requires careful clinical observation during infancy and precise neurologic assessment. Suspect cerebral palsy whenever an infant:
  – has difficulty sucking or keeping the nipple or food in his mouth
  – seldom moves voluntarily or has arm or leg tremors with voluntary movement
  – crosses his legs when lifted from behind rather than pulling them up or "bicycling"
  – has legs that are hard to separate, making diaper changing difficult
  – persistently uses only one hand or, as he gets older, uses his hands well but not his legs.
- A computed tomography scan and magnetic resonance imaging may help rule out other problems.

Treatment

- Treatment is primarily supportive and includes:
  - braces or splints and special appliances, such as adapted eating utensils and a low toilet seat with arms, to help the patient perform activities independently
  - an artificial urinary sphincter for the incontinent child who can use hand controls
  - range-of-motion exercises to minimize contractures
  - orthopedic surgery to correct contractures
  - phenytoin (Dilantin), phenobarbital, or another anticonvulsant to control seizures
  - a muscle relaxant or neurosurgery to decrease spasticity.

Nursing considerations

- Provide an adequate diet to meet the child's high-energy needs. Maintain a quiet, unhurried atmosphere with as few distractions as possible. The child may need special utensils and a chair with a solid footrest. Teach him to place food far back in his mouth to facilitate swallowing.
- Encourage the child to chew food thoroughly, drink through a straw, and suck on lollipops to develop the muscle control needed to minimize drooling.
- Allow the child to wash and dress independently, assisting only as needed. The child may need clothing modifications.
- Give all care in an unhurried manner to prevent muscle spasticity from increasing.
- Encourage the child and his family to participate in his care so they can continue it at home.
- Reduce muscle spasms that increase postoperative pain by moving and turning the child carefully after surgery.

- When spasticity occurs, gently rotate the limb inward toward the spasticity and then rotate it outward. Repeating this motion helps relax the spastic extremity. Pressure on the tendons located in the joint socket while rotating increases relaxation. Open a spastic hand by gently grabbing the lateral aspects and moving inward and outward.
- When positioning the child, elongate the down side, making sure that the down shoulder is slightly pulled out and that all limbs are well supported.
- Hand and foot orthotics may be helpful in maintaining mobility. Help the child relax, perhaps by giving a warm bath, before reapplying a bivalved cast.
- Identify and help the family deal with any stress. Parents may feel unreasonable guilt about their child's disability and may need psychological counseling.
- Refer parents to supportive community organizations (local or United Cerebral Palsy Association).

▌Cervical cancer

The third most common cancer of the female reproductive system, cervical cancer is classified as either preinvasive or invasive. Preinvasive cancer is curable 75% to 90% of the time with early detection and proper treatment. If untreated (and depending on the form in which it appears), it may progress to invasive cervical cancer.

With invasive cancer, cancer cells penetrate the basement membrane and can spread directly to contiguous pelvic structures or disseminate to distant sites by lymphatic routes. In 95% of cases, the histologic type is squamous cell carcinoma, which varies from well-differentiated cells to highly anaplastic spindle cells; only 5% are adenocarcinomas. Invasive cancer usually occurs in patients between ages 30 and 50, although in rare cases it can occur in those younger than age 20.

Causes
- Human papillomavirus (HPV)

Risk factors
- Herpesvirus 2 and other bacterial or viral venereal infections
- Intercourse at a young age (younger than age 16)
- Multiple sexual partners

Signs and symptoms
- Early stages: possibly, abnormal vaginal bleeding, persistent vaginal discharge, and postcoital pain and bleeding
- Advanced stages: pelvic pain, vaginal leakage of urine and stool from a fistula, anorexia, weight loss, and anemia

Diagnostic tests
- A cytologic examination (Papanicolaou [Pap] test) can be used to detect cervical cancer before symptoms appear.
- Colposcopy can detect the presence and extent of preclinical lesions requiring a biopsy and histologic examination.
- Staining with Lugol's solution (strong iodine) or Schiller's solution (iodine, potassium iodide, and purified water) may identify areas for a biopsy when the smear shows abnormal cells but there's no obvious lesion. Normal tissues absorb the iodine and turn brown; abnormal tissues are devoid of glycogen and don't change color.
- Cystography, magnetic resonance imaging, computed tomography, and bone scans can be used to detect metastasis.
- Cone biopsy may be performed if endocervical curettage yields a positive result.
- The Vira-Pap test permits examination of the specimen's DNA structure to detect HPV.

Treatment
- Preinvasive lesions may be treated with total excisional biopsy, cryosurgery, laser destruction, conization (and frequent Pap test follow-up) or, rarely, hysterectomy.
- Therapy for invasive squamous cell carcinoma may include radical hysterectomy and radiation therapy (internal, external, or both).

Nursing considerations
- If the patient needs a biopsy, explain to the patient that she may feel pressure, minor abdominal cramps, or a pinch from the punch forceps.
- If the patient is having cryosurgery, explain that a refrigerant will be used to freeze the cervix. Warn the patient that she may experience abdominal cramps, headache, and sweating. Also warn her she'll have profuse, watery discharge for days or weeks.
- If the patient is having laser therapy, explain that the procedure takes about 30 minutes and may cause abdominal cramps.
- Tell the patient to expect a discharge or spotting for about 1 week after an excisional biopsy, cryosurgery, or laser therapy, and advise her not to douche, use tampons, or engage in sexual intercourse during this time. Tell her to watch for and report signs of infection. Stress the need for a follow-up Pap test and a pelvic examination within 3 to 4 months after these procedures and periodically thereafter.
- If the patient is having a hysterectomy, tell her what to expect postoperatively.
- After surgery, monitor vital signs every 15 minutes for 1 hour, every 30 minutes for the next hour, every hour for 2 hours, and then every 4 hours or as per protocol. Watch for signs and symptoms of complications, such as bleeding, ab-

dominal distention, severe pain, and breathing difficulties.

■ Give an analgesic, a prophylactic antibiotic, and subcutaneous heparin, as needed.

■ Explain the internal radiation procedure, as appropriate, and answer the patient's questions. Internal radiation requires a 2- to 3-day facility stay, bowel preparation, a povidone-iodine vaginal douche, a clear liquid diet, and nothing by mouth the night before the implantation; it also requires an indwelling urinary catheter. It's performed in the operating room under general anesthesia, and an applicator containing radioactive material (such as radium or cesium) is implanted.

■ Remember that safety precautions— time, distance, and shielding—begin as soon as the radioactive source is in place. Inform the patient that she'll require a private room. Organize the time you spend with the patient to minimize your exposure to radiation. Inform visitors of safety precautions, and hang a sign listing these precautions on the patient's door.

■ Encourage the patient to lie flat, limit movement (keep objects within reach) and elevate the head of bed slightly while the implant is in place.

■ Check vital signs every 4 hours; watch for skin reaction, vaginal bleeding, abdominal discomfort, or evidence of dehydration.

■ Assist the patient in range-of-motion *arm* exercises (leg exercises and other body movements could dislodge the implant). If needed, give a tranquilizer to help the patient relax and remain still.

■ Explain that external radiation therapy, when necessary, continues for 4 to 6 weeks on an outpatient basis. Teach the patient to watch for and report uncomfortable adverse reactions. Because radiation therapy may increase susceptibility

to infection by lowering the white blood cell count, warn the patient to avoid persons with obvious infections during therapy.

■ Teach the patient to use a vaginal dilator to prevent vaginal stenosis and to facilitate vaginal examinations and sexual intercourse.

■ Reassure the patient that this disease and its treatment shouldn't radically alter her lifestyle or prohibit sexual intimacy.

Chalazion

A common eye disorder, a chalazion is a granulomatous inflammation of a meibomian gland in the upper or lower eyelid. This disorder is characterized by localized swelling and usually develops slowly over several weeks. It may become large enough to press on the eyeball, producing astigmatism, and may have to be incised and curetted surgically. A person susceptible to developing chalazia may have more than one because the upper and lower eyelids contain many meibomian glands. If a chalazion becomes persistent and chronic, meibomian gland cancer should be ruled out by biopsy.

Causes
■ Complication from a hordeolum (stye)
■ Obstruction of the meibomian (sebaceous) gland duct

Signs and symptoms
■ Painless, hard lump that usually points toward the conjunctival side of the eyelid
■ Red elevated area on the conjunctival surface on eversion of the eyelid (see *Identifying a chalazion*)

Identifying a chalazion

A chalazion is a nontender, granulomatous inflammation of a meibomian gland on the eyelid. The swelling may be large enough on the eyeball to cause vision disturbances.

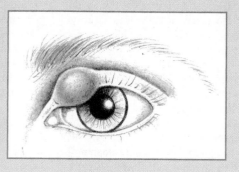

Diagnostic tests
- Visual examination and palpation of the eyelid reveal a small bump or nodule.
- Persistently recurrent chalazia necessitate a biopsy to rule out meibomian cancer.

Treatment
- Warm compresses are applied to open the lumen of the gland.
- Give sulfonamide eyedrops or steroid injection, or both, as prescribed.
- The patient may require incision and curettage under local anesthetic.

Nursing considerations
- Tell the patient to start applying warm compresses at the first sign of lid irritation, to increase the blood supply and keep the lumen open.
- Instruct the patient how to properly apply warm compresses: Tell him to take special care to avoid burning the skin, to always use a clean cloth, and to discard used compresses.
- After surgery, tell the patient that a pressure eye patch will be applied for 8 to 24 hours to control bleeding and swelling. After removal of the patch, treatment consists of warm compresses

applied for 10 to 15 minutes, two to four times per day, and antimicrobial eyedrops or ointment to prevent secondary infection.

◼ Chest injuries, blunt

One-fourth of all trauma deaths in the United States result from chest injuries. Many are blunt chest injuries, which include myocardial contusion and rib and sternal fractures; these may be simple, multiple, displaced, or jagged. Such fractures may cause potentially fatal complications, such as hemothorax, pneumothorax, hemorrhagic shock, and diaphragmatic rupture.

Causes
- Blast injuries
- Fights
- Motor vehicle accidents
- Sports

Signs and symptoms
- Diaphragmatic rupture (usually on the left side): severe respiratory distress
- Flail chest (in which a portion of the chest wall "caves" in): bruised skin, extreme pain, paradoxical chest movements, rapid and shallow respirations,

tachycardia, hypotension, respiratory acidosis, and cyanosis
■ Hemothorax: respiratory distress due to blood pooling in the pleural cavity, compressing the lung and limiting respiratory capacity
■ Large myocardial tears (which can be rapidly fatal) and small myocardial tears (which can cause pericardial effusion)
■ Pneumothorax: severe dyspnea, cyanosis, agitation, extreme pain and subcutaneous emphysema
■ Pulmonary contusion: hemoptysis, hypoxia, dyspnea and, possibly, obstruction
■ Rib fractures: tenderness, slight edema over the fracture site, and pain that worsens with deep breathing and movement causing the patient to hypoventilate.
■ Sternal fractures: persistent chest pain, even at rest
■ Tension pneumothorax: tracheal deviation (away from the affected side), cyanosis, severe dyspnea, absent breath sounds (on the affected side), agitation, jugular vein distention, and shock; life-threatening thoracic pressure buildup, lung collapse, and subsequent mediastinal shift
■ Other signs: cardiac tamponade, pulmonary artery tears, ventricular rupture, and bronchial, tracheal, or esophageal tears or rupture

Diagnostic tests

■ Diagnosis is suggested by a history of trauma with dyspnea, chest pain, and other typical symptoms. A physical examination and diagnostic tests determine the extent of injury.
■ Percussion reveals dullness in hemothorax and tympany in tension pneumothorax.
■ Auscultation may reveal a change in position of the loudest heart sound in

tension pneumothorax or muffled heart tones in cardiac tamponade.
■ Chest X-rays to confirm rib and sternal fractures, pneumothorax, flail chest, pulmonary contusions, lacerated or ruptured aorta, tension pneumothorax, diaphragmatic rupture, lung compression, or atelectasis with hemothorax.
■ With cardiac damage, electrocardiography may show right bundle-branch block. Arrhythmias, conduction abnormalities, and ST-wave changes may occur in myocardial contusions.
■ Serum levels of aspartate aminotransferase, alanine aminotransferase, lactate dehydrogenase, creatine kinase (CK), and the isoenzyme CK-MB levels are elevated.
■ Angiography reveals aortic laceration or rupture.
■ Contrast studies and liver and spleen scans help detect diaphragmatic rupture.
■ Echocardiography, computed tomography scans, and cardiac and lung scans show the extent of the injury.

Treatment
ACTION STAT!

 Blunt chest injuries call for immediate physical assessment, control of bleeding, maintenance of a patent airway, adequate ventilation, and fluid and electrolyte balance.

■ Maintain a patent airway and provide oxygenation; prepare for endotracheal intubation and mechanical ventilation. If the patient has excessive bleeding or hemopneumothorax, intubate him.
■ If the patient has tension pneumothorax, a spinal or 14G to 16G needle must be inserted into the second intercostal space at the midclavicular line, followed by insertion of a chest tube to normalize pressure and reexpand the lung. Give

oxygen under positive pressure, along with I.V. fluids.

■ If the patient has pneumothorax, a chest tube may be placed anterior to the midaxillary line at the fifth intercostal space, to aspirate as much air as possible from the pleural cavity and to reexpand the lungs.

■ If the patient has flail chest, place him in semi-Fowler's position and give him oxygen at a high flow rate under positive pressure.

■ The patient with hemothorax will need insertion of chest tubes in the fifth or sixth intercostal space anterior to the midaxillary line to remove blood. Treat shock with I.V. infusions of lactated Ringer's solution or normal saline solution. Give packed red blood cells for blood losses greater than 1,500 ml or circulating blood volume losses exceeding 30%. Autotransfusion is an option. Give oxygen.

■ For simple rib fractures, give a mild analgesic, encourage bed rest, and apply heat. Don't strap or tape the patient's chest. For more severe fractures, intercostal nerve blocks may be needed. Obtain X-rays before and after the nerve blocks to rule out pneumothorax.

■ For pulmonary contusions, give limited amounts of colloids (for example, salt-poor albumin, whole blood, or plasma) to replace volume and maintain oncotic pressure. Give analgesics, diuretics, and analgesics, if necessary. Steroid use is controversial.

■ For suspected cardiac damage, close intensive care or telemetry may detect arrhythmias and prevent cardiogenic shock. Impose bed rest in semi-Fowler's position (unless the patient requires shock position); as needed, give oxygen, an analgesic, and other supportive drugs to control heart failure or supraventricular arrhythmia.

■ Cardiac tamponade requires pericardiocentesis. Essentially, provide the same care as for a patient who has suffered myocardial infarction.

■ If the patient has myocardial rupture, septal perforation, or another cardiac laceration, immediate surgical repair is mandatory; less severe ventricular wounds require use of a digital or balloon catheter; atrial wounds require a clamp or balloon catheter.

■ For aortic rupture or laceration in patients who reach the facility alive, immediate surgery is mandatory, using synthetic grafts or anastomosis to repair the damage. Give large volumes of I.V. fluids (lactated Ringer's or normal saline solution) and whole blood, along with oxygen at very high flow rates; then transport the patient promptly to the operating room.

■ For a diaphragmatic rupture, insert a nasogastric tube to temporarily decompress the stomach, and prepare the patient for surgical repair.

Nursing considerations

■ Check all pulses and level of consciousness. Evaluate color and temperature of skin, depth of respiration, use of accessory muscles, and length of inhalation compared with exhalation.

■ Check pulse oximetry values for adequate oxygenation. Monitor arterial blood gas values to ensure adequate ventilation; provide oxygen therapy, maintain mechanical ventilation, and provide chest tube care.

■ Observe tracheal position. Look for jugular vein distention and paradoxical chest motion. Listen to heart and breath sounds carefully; palpate for subcutaneous emphysema (crepitation) and a lack of structural integrity in the ribs.

■ Unless severe dyspnea is present, ask the patient to locate the pain, and ask if he's having trouble breathing.

- To prevent atelectasis, instruct the patient on incentive spirometry, deep breathing, coughing, and splinting. Turn the patient frequently and encourage coughing and deep breathing.
- Suction the patient frequently, as indicated.
- Monitor and document vital signs, blood loss, and intake and output.

ACTION STAT!

 Laceration or rupture of the aorta is nearly always immediately fatal. In rare cases, it may develop 24 hours after blunt injury.

ACTION STAT!

 Watch for falling blood pressure, rising pulse rate, and hemorrhage—all require thoracotomy to stop bleeding.

- Give I.V. fluids and transfusions; monitor patient for effects (vital signs, hemodynamic monitoring) and assess laboratory results.
- Watch for complications; prepare for surgery as indicated.
- Provide adequate sedation for pain and monitor for effects.

Chest wounds, penetrating

Depending on their size, penetrating chest wounds may cause varying degrees of damage to bones, soft tissue, blood vessels, and nerves. Mortality and morbidity from a chest wound depend on the size and severity of the wound. Gunshot wounds are usually more serious than stab wounds because they cause more severe lacerations and rapid blood loss and because ricochet commonly damages large areas and multiple organs.

Causes

- Explosions or firearms fired at close range
- Gunshot wounds
- Stab wounds from a knife or ice pick

Signs and symptoms

- Changes in level of consciousness
- Lung lacerations (bleeding and substantial air leakage through the chest tube), arterial lacerations (loss of more than 100 ml of blood/hour through the chest tube), and exsanguination
- Obvious chest injury
- Pneumothorax, tension pneumothorax, and hemothorax
- Sucking sound due to contraction of diaphragm allowing air into the chest cavity
- Tachycardia and a weak, thready pulse from massive blood loss, hypovolemic shock, and anxiety
- Other signs and symptoms: arrhythmias, cardiac tamponade, mediastinitis, subcutaneous emphysema, esophageal perforation, bronchopleural fistula, and tracheobronchial, abdominal, or diaphragmatic injuries

Diagnostic tests

- An obvious chest wound and a sucking sound during breathing confirm the diagnosis. Consider any lower thoracic chest injury a thoracoabdominal injury until proved otherwise.
- Tests to provide baseline data include:
  – pulse oximetry and arterial blood gas analysis to assess respiratory status
  – chest X-rays before and after chest tube placement to evaluate the injury and tube placement

ACTION STAT!

 In an emergency, don't wait for chest X-ray results before inserting the chest tube.

– complete blood count, including hemoglobin (Hb) level, hematocrit, and differential (a low Hb level and hematocrit reflect severe blood loss; in early blood loss, these values may be normal)

– palpation and auscultation of the chest and abdomen to evaluate damage to adjacent organs and structures.

Treatment
ACTION STAT!

 Penetrating chest wounds require immediate support of respiration and circulation, prompt surgical repair, and measures to prevent complications.

- Immediately assess airway, breathing, and circulation. Establish a patent airway, support ventilation, and monitor pulses frequently.
- Place an occlusive dressing (for example, petroleum gauze) over the sucking wound. Monitor patient for signs of tension pneumothorax (tracheal shift, respiratory distress, tachycardia, tachypnea, diminished or absent breath sounds on the affected side); if present, temporarily remove the occlusive dressing to create a simple pneumothorax.
- Control blood loss (also look *under* the patient to estimate loss), type and crossmatch blood, and replace blood and fluids as necessary.
- Prepare the patient for chest X-rays and placement of chest tubes (using water-seal drainage) to reestablish intrathoracic pressure and to drain blood in hemothorax. A second X-ray will evaluate the position of tubes and their functions.
- Emergency surgery may be needed to repair the damage caused by the wound.
- Tetanus and antibiotic prophylaxis may be necessary.

Nursing considerations

- Throughout treatment, monitor central venous pressure and blood pressure to detect hypovolemia, and assess vital signs.
- Maintain patent airway and provide oxygenation; provide chest tube care and maintain mechanical ventilation as indicated.
- Provide pain medication and assess for effect.
- Give I.V. fluids and transfusions; monitor the patient for effects (vital signs, hemodynamic monitoring) and assess laboratory results.
- Watch for complications; prepare for surgery as indicated.
- Reassure the patient, especially if he has been the victim of a violent crime. Report the incident to the police in accordance with local laws. Help contact the patient's family, and offer them reassurance as well.

Chlamydial infections

Urethritis in men and urethritis and cervicitis in women are commonly linked to *Chlamydia trachomatis*. These infections are the most common sexually transmitted diseases in the United States. Trachoma inclusion conjunctivitis (leading cause of blindness in Third World countries) and lymphogranuloma venereum are caused by chlamydial infections. Untreated, chlamydial infections can lead to such complications as acute epididymitis, salpingitis, pelvic inflammatory disease and, eventually, sterility. In pregnant women, spontaneous abortion and premature delivery may occur.

Causes

- *C. trachomatis* due to vaginal or rectal intercourse or oral-genital contact with an infected person

What your patient needs to know about chlamydial infections

Before discharge, teach the patient with a chlamydial infection to:
- continue drug therapy to completion, even if symptoms subside
- practice meticulous personal hygiene
- avoid touching the discharge
- wash and dry his hands before touching his eyes
- abstain from sexual intercourse until he and his partner are treated
- inform sexual contacts of his infection
- return for follow-up testing.

- In neonates: conjunctivitis, otitis media, and pneumonia due to infection during passage through the birth canal

Signs and symptoms
- May be asymptomatic or may show signs of infection on physical examination

Men
- Epididymitis: scrotal swelling and urethral discharge
- Proctitis: diarrhea, tenesmus, pruritus, bloody or mucopurulent discharge, and diffuse or discrete ulceration in the rectosigmoid colon
- Prostatitis: lower back pain, urinary frequency, dysuria, nocturia, and painful ejaculation
- Urethritis: dysuria, erythema, tenderness of urethral meatus, urinary frequency, pruritus, and urethral discharge

Women
- Cervicitis: cervical erosion, mucopurulent discharge, pelvic pain, and dyspareunia
- Endometritis or salpingitis: chills, fever, breakthrough bleeding, bleeding after intercourse, vaginal discharge, dysuria, and pain or tenderness of abdomen, cervix, ureter, or lymph nodes

- Urethral syndrome: dysuria, pyuria, and urinary frequency

Diagnostic tests
- A swab from the infection site (urethra, cervix, or rectum) establishes a diagnosis of urethritis, cervicitis, salpingitis, endometritis, or proctitis.
- A culture of aspirated material establishes a diagnosis of epididymitis.
- Antigen detection methods (enzyme-linked immunosorbent assay, direct fluorescent antibody test) identify chlamydial infection; tissue cell cultures are more sensitive and specific.
- Nucleic acid probes using polymerase chain reactions detect the organism.

Treatment
- Doxycycline and tetracycline are the preferred drugs for treatment of chlamydial infections. Ofloxacin or azithromycin may also be prescribed.
- For pregnant women, azithromycin, in a single 1-g dose for woman and her partner.

Nursing considerations
- Practice standard precautions when caring for a patient with a chlamydial infection.
- Teach the patient about chlamydial infection and its treatment before dis-

charge. (See *What your patient needs to know about chlamydial infections.*)

■ Make sure that the patient fully understands the dosage requirements of any prescribed medications for this infection.

■ If required in your state, report all cases of chlamydial infection to the appropriate local public health authorities, who will then conduct follow-up notification of the patient's sexual contacts.

■ Suggest that the patient and his sexual partners receive testing for human immunodeficiency virus.

■ Check neonates of infected mothers for signs of chlamydial infection. Obtain appropriate specimens for diagnostic testing.

Chloride imbalance

Hypochloremia and *hyperchloremia* are conditions of deficient or excessive serum levels of the anion chloride. A predominantly extracellular anion, chloride accounts for two-thirds of all serum anions. Secreted by stomach mucosa as hydrochloric acid, chloride provides an acid medium conducive to digestion and activation of enzymes. It also participates in maintaining acid-base and body water balances, influences the osmolality or tonicity of extracellular fluid, plays a role in the exchange of oxygen and carbon dioxide in red blood cells, and helps activate salivary amylase (which, in turn, activates the digestive process).

Causes
Hypochloremia
■ Decreased chloride intake or absorption, as in low dietary sodium intake, sodium deficiency, potassium deficiency, metabolic alkalosis, and administration of dextrose I.V. without electrolytes

■ Excessive chloride loss from prolonged diarrhea or diaphoresis, vomiting, gastric suctioning, or gastric surgery

Hyperchloremia
■ Compensatory mechanisms for other metabolic abnormalities, including metabolic acidosis, brain stem injury causing neurogenic hyperventilation, and hyperparathyroidism

■ Excessive chloride intake or absorption from hyperingestion of ammonium chloride, ureterointestinal anastomosis, administering normal saline solution I.V. or by another route (orally, nasogastric tube, saline enema, or irrigation)

■ Hemoconcentration from dehydration

Signs and symptoms
Hypochloremia
■ Muscle hypertonicity, tetany, and shallow, depressed breathing

■ Muscle weakness and twitching when accompanied by sodium loss

Hyperchloremia
■ Agitation
■ Dyspnea
■ Pitting edema
■ Tachycardia, hypertension
■ With metabolic acidosis from excretion of base bicarbonate by the kidneys: weakness, diminished cognitive ability, deep, rapid breathing, and coma

Diagnostic tests
■ A serum chloride level less than 98 mEq/L confirms hypochloremia; supportive values with metabolic alkalosis include a serum pH greater than 7.45 and a serum carbon dioxide level greater than 32 mEq/L.

■ A serum chloride level greater than 106 mEq/L confirms hyperchloremia; with metabolic acidosis, serum pH is less than 7.35 and the serum carbon dioxide level less than 22 mEq/L.

Treatment
- Correct the underlying disorder.

Hypochloremia
- If hypovolemia is present, give the patient I.V. normal saline solution.
- A chloride-containing drug, such as ammonium chloride, may be needed to increase serum chloride levels.
- Potassium chloride may be given for metabolic alkalosis.

Hyperchloremia
- For mild hyperchloremia, give lactated Ringer's solution, which converts to bicarbonate in the liver, increasing base bicarbonate to correct acidosis.
- For severe hyperchloremic acidosis, give I.V. sodium bicarbonate to raise serum bicarbonate level and permit renal excretion of the chloride anion.

Nursing considerations
- Be alert for respiratory difficulty.

Hypochloremia
- Monitor serum chloride levels frequently, particularly during I.V. therapy or in those vulnerable to chloride imbalance (gastric surgery).
- Monitor serum electrolyte levels, arterial blood gas values, and fluid intake and output.
- Watch for excessive or continuous loss of gastric secretions as well as prolonged infusion of dextrose in water without saline.

Hyperchloremia
- Check serum electrolyte levels every 3 to 6 hours.

DRUG CHALLENGE If the patient is receiving high doses of sodium bicarbonate, watch for signs of overcorrection (metabolic alkalosis, respiratory depression) or lingering signs of hyperchloremia, which indicate inadequate treatment.

- To prevent hyperchloremia in a patient receiving an I.V. solution that contains sodium chloride, check laboratory results for elevated serum chloride levels or potassium imbalance and monitor fluid intake and output.
- Watch for signs of metabolic acidosis. When giving I.V. fluids containing lactated Ringer's solution, monitor flow rate according to the patient's age, physical condition, and bicarbonate level, watching for irregularities.

Cholelithiasis, cholecystitis, and related disorders

Diseases of the gallbladder and biliary tract are common, typically painful conditions that usually require surgery and may be life-threatening. In most cases, gallbladder and bile duct diseases occur during middle age. Between ages 20 and 50, they're six times more common in women, but the incidence in men and women becomes equal after age 50. They're commonly associated with deposition of calculi and inflammation. (See *Common sites of calculus formation.*)

Causes
- Vary with the particular disorder

Cholelithiasis
- Commonly occur in periods of gallbladder sluggishness due to pregnancy, use of hormonal contraceptives, diabetes mellitus, Crohn's disease, cirrhosis of the liver, pancreatitis, obesity, and rapid weight loss

Common sites of calculus formation

As depicted below, gallstones vary in size; small stones may travel.

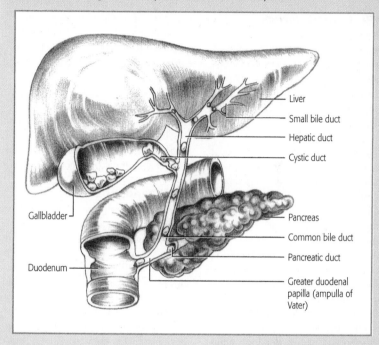

Liver

Small bile duct

Hepatic duct

Cystic duct

Gallbladder

Pancreas

Common bile duct

Pancreatic duct

Duodenum

Greater duodenal papilla (ampulla of Vater)

■ Stones or calculi (gallstones) in the gallbladder, resulting from changes in bile components

Cholecystitis

■ An acute or chronic inflammation of the gallbladder resulting from a gallstone impacted in the cystic duct with inflammation behind the obstruction

Biliary cirrhosis

■ Chronic, progressive disease with autoimmune destruction of the intrahepatic bile ducts and cholestasis

Cholangitis

■ Bacterial or metabolic alteration of bile acids

■ Infection of the bile duct associated with choledocholithiasis and percutaneous transhepatic cholangiography

Choledocholithiasis

■ Lodging of stones in the hepatic and common bile ducts obstructing the flow of bile into the duodenum

Cholesterolosis

■ Cholesterol polyps or crystal deposits in the gallbladder's submucosa resulting from bile secretions containing high concentrations of cholesterol and insufficient bile salts

Gallstone ileus
- Lodging of stones in the terminal ileum

Postcholecystectomy syndrome
- Retained or recurrent common bile duct stones, spasm of the sphincter of Oddi, functional bowel disorder, technical errors, or mistaken diagnoses occurring in those whose gallbladders have been surgically removed

Signs and symptoms
Acute cholelithiasis, acute cholecystitis, choledocholithiasis, and cholesterolosis all produce the symptoms of a classic gallbladder attack, which follow meals rich in fats or may occur at night, suddenly awakening the patient.
- Acute abdominal pain in the right upper quadrant that may radiate to the back, between the shoulders, or to the front of the chest
- Recurring fat intolerance, biliary colic, belching, flatulence, and indigestion
- Diaphoresis, nausea, vomiting, chills, and low-grade fever
- Jaundice (if a stone obstructs the common bile duct)
- Clay-colored stool (with choledocholithiasis)
- Cholangitis: rise in eosinophils, jaundice, abdominal pain, high fever, and chills
- Biliary cirrhosis: jaundice, related itching, weakness, fatigue, slight weight loss, and abdominal pain
- Gallstone ileus: nausea, vomiting, abdominal distention and, possibly, absent bowel sounds if the bowel is completely obstructed
- Complications
  - In cholelithiasis: any disorder associated with gallstone formation (cholangitis, cholecystitis, choledocholithiasis, or gallstone ileus)
  - In cholecystitis: gallbladder complications (empyema, hydrops or mucocele, or gangrene); gangrene may lead to perforation, resulting in peritonitis, fistula formation, pancreatitis, limy bile, and porcelain gallbladder
  - In choledocholithiasis: cholangitis, obstructive jaundice, pancreatitis, and secondary biliary cirrhosis
  - In cholangitis: septic shock and death
  - In gallstone ileus: bowel obstruction, which can lead to intestinal perforation, peritonitis, septicemia, secondary infection, and septic shock

Diagnostic tests
- Ultrasonography and X-rays detect gallstones.
- Percutaneous transhepatic cholangiography allows imaging under fluoroscopic control to help distinguish between gallbladder or bile duct disease and cancer
- Endoscopic retrograde cholangiopancreatography visualizes the biliary tree
- Hepatobiliary iminodiacetic acid analogue scan of the gallbladder helps detect obstruction of the cystic duct.
- Computed tomography scan help distinguish between obstructive and nonobstructive jaundice.
- Oral cholecystography shows stones in the gallbladder and biliary duct obstruction, although this test is gradually being replaced by ultrasonography.
- Elevated icteric index and elevated total bilirubin, urine bilirubin, and alkaline phosphatase levels support the diagnosis.
- White blood cell count is slightly elevated during a cholecystitis attack.
- Serum amylase levels help distinguish gallbladder disease from pancreatitis.
- With suspected heart disease, cardiac enzyme tests and an electrocardiogram

should precede gallbladder and upper GI diagnostic tests.

Treatment

- Surgery is the treatment of choice for gallbladder and bile duct diseases (open or laparoscopic cholecystectomy, cholecystectomy with operative cholangiography, exploration of the common bile duct).
- A low-fat diet prevents attacks.
- Vitamin K treats itching, jaundice, and bleeding tendencies.
- The patient may require insertion of a nasogastric tube, administration of I.V. fluids, and administration of an antibiotic in an acute attack.
- Nonsurgical treatment for choledocholithiasis involves insertion of a flexible catheter, formed around a biliary tube (T tube), through a sinus tract into the common bile duct. Guided by fluoroscopy, the catheter is directed toward the stone. A Dormia basket is threaded through the catheter, opened, twirled to entrap the stone, closed, and withdrawn.

Nursing considerations

- Before surgery, teach the patient to deep breathe, cough, expectorate, and perform leg exercises. Also teach splinting, repositioning, and ambulation techniques. Explain the perioperative procedures to help ease the patient's anxiety and ensure his cooperation.
- After surgery, monitor vital signs for indications of bleeding, infection, or atelectasis.
- If a T tube is surgically placed, maintain tube patency and secure placement. Measure and record bile drainage daily (200 to 300 ml is normal).
- If your patient will be discharged with a T tube, teach him how to perform dressing changes and routine skin care.

- Patients who have had a laparoscopic cholecystectomy may be discharged the same day or within 48 hours after surgery. These patients should have minimal pain, be able to tolerate a regular diet within 24 hours after surgery, and be able to return to normal activity within a week. Food restrictions are unnecessary unless there is an intolerance to a specific food or some underlying condition (such as diabetes, atherosclerosis, or obesity) that requires such restriction.
- Assess the location, duration, and character of any pain. Administer an analgesic, as needed.

▌Chronic fatigue and immune dysfunction syndrome

Chronic fatigue and immune dysfunction syndrome (CFIDS)—also known as *chronic fatigue syndrome, chronic Epstein-Barr virus* [EBV], and *benign myalgic encephalomyelitis*—is typically marked by debilitating fatigue, neurologic abnormalities, and persistent symptoms that suggest chronic mononucleosis. It commonly occurs in adults younger than age 45, and its incidence is highest in women.

Causes

- Possibly human herpesvirus 6 or in other herpesviruses, enteroviruses, or retroviruses
- Reaction to viral illness complicated by dysfunctional immune response, and other factors (sex, age, genetic disposition, prior illness, stress, and environment)

Signs and symptoms

- The Centers for Disease Control and Prevention (CDC) use a "working case

CDC criteria for diagnosing CFIDS

To meet the case definition of the Centers for Disease Control and Prevention (CDC) for chronic fatigue and immune dysfunction syndrome (CFIDS), a patient must fulfill the major criteria plus eight of the symptom criteria, *or* six of the "symptom criteria" and two of the physical criteria.

Major criteria
■ New onset of persistent or relapsing debilitating fatigue in a person without a history of similar symptoms; fatigue that doesn't resolve with bed rest and is severe enough to reduce or impair average daily activity by 50% for 6 months
■ Exclusion of other disorders after evaluation through history, physical examination, and laboratory findings

Symptom criteria
The symptom criteria include the initial development of the main symptom complex over a few hours or days as well as the following other symptoms:
■ Profound or prolonged fatigue, especially after exercise levels that were easily tolerated before
■ Complaints of painful lymph nodes
■ Muscle weakness
■ Sleep disturbances (insomnia or hypersomnia)
■ Migratory arthralgia without joint swelling or redness
■ Photophobia, forgetfulness, irritability, confusion, depression, transient visual scotoma, difficulty thinking, and inability to concentrate.

Physical criteria
These criteria must be recorded on at least two occasions at least 1 month apart.
■ Low-grade fever
■ Nonexudative pharyngitis
■ Palpable or tender nodes

definition" to group symptoms and severity. (See *CDC criteria for diagnosing CFIDS*.)

Diagnostic tests
■ No single test confirms its presence; diagnosis is based on the patient's history and the CDC criteria.

Treatment
■ Treat the underlying cause, if one can be found.
■ Supportive therapy includes:
– anti-inflammatories
– antihistamines
– rest
– tricyclic antidepressant (doxepin [Sinequan])
– histamine-2 blocker (cimetidine [Tagamet])
– anxiolytic (alprazolam [Xanax])
– avoidance of environmental irritants and certain foods
– antiviral (acyclovir [Zovirax])
– immunomodulators (I.V. gamma globulin, Ampligen, and transfer factor).

Nursing considerations
■ Monitor response to treatments.
■ Provide support and assistance as needed. Encourage the patient to perform self-care within confines of the disorder.
■ Pace care activities to provide adequate rest periods.
■ Refer the patient to the CFIDS Association for information as well as to local support groups; supportive contact may benefit the patient.

■ If appropriate, suggest psychological counseling.

Chronic obstructive pulmonary disease

Chronic obstructive pulmonary disease (COPD) is also called *chronic obstructive lung disease.*

It's the most common chronic lung disease, affecting an estimated 17 million U.S. residents, and its incidence is rising. COPD occurs mostly in people older than age 40.

Causes

■ Emphysema, chronic bronchitis, asthma, or any combination of these disorders (see *Understanding chronic obstructive pulmonary disease,* pages 128 to 131)

Risk factors

■ Air pollution
■ Allergies
■ Cigarette smoking
■ Familial and hereditary factors (for example, deficiency of alpha$_1$-antitrypsin)
■ Occupations involving exposure to dusts or noxious gases
■ Recurrent or chronic respiratory tract infections

Signs and symptoms

■ Decreased ability to exercise or do strenuous work (begins in middle age)
■ Productive cough
■ Dyspnea on minimal exertion
■ Frequent respiratory tract infections
■ Intermittent or continuous hypoxemia
■ Grossly abnormal pulmonary function studies
■ Advanced form: thoracic deformities, overwhelming disability, cor pulmonale, severe respiratory failure, and death

Diagnostic tests

■ X-rays rule out associated problems and may show emphysema, hyperinflation, and pulmonary hypertension as the COPD advances.
■ Pulmonary function studies reflect degree of impairment.

Treatment

■ Bronchodilators can help alleviate bronchospasm and enhance clearance of secretions.
■ Inhaled corticosteroids are given as maintenance therapy; oral corticosteroids are helpful for acute worsening.
■ Effective coughing, postural drainage, and chest physiotherapy help to mobilize secretions.
■ Low concentrations of oxygen may be given if arterial blood gas analysis determines need; the oxygen supplementation helps avoid carbon dioxide narcosis.
■ Antibiotics may be given for respiratory tract infections.
■ Pneumococcal vaccination and annual influenza vaccinations are important preventive measures.
■ Lung volume reduction surgery (for carefully selected patients) allows more functional lung tissue to expand and the diaphragm to return to its normally elevated position.

Special considerations

■ Provide comprehensive patient teaching to ensure compliance with therapy. (See *Living with COPD,* page 130.)
■ If the patient is to continue oxygen therapy at home, teach him how to use the equipment correctly. Patients rarely require more than 2 to 3 L/minute.
■ Teach the patient and his family that excessive oxygen therapy may eliminate the hypoxic respiratory drive, causing

(Text continues on page 130.)

Understanding chronic obstructive pulmonary disease

Disease	Causes	Clinical features
Asthma ■ Increased bronchial reactivity to a variety of stimuli producing episodic bronchospasm, airway obstruction, and inflammation ■ Onset in adulthood: commonly without distinct allergies; onset in childhood: typically associated with definite allergens ■ Status asthmaticus: acute asthma attack with severe bronchospasm	■ Possible mechanisms include allergy (resulting in release of mast cell vasoactive and bronchospastic mediators), upper airway infection, exercise, anxiety, coughing or laughing, or a response to aspirin or indomethacin ingestion. ■ Airway obstruction occurs due to spasm of bronchial smooth muscle narrows airways; other causes include inflammatory edema of the bronchial wall and inspissation of tenacious mucoid secretions.	■ History of intermittent attacks of dyspnea and wheezing ■ Mild wheezing progressing to severe dyspnea, audible wheezing, chest tightness (a feeling of being unable to breathe), and a cough that produces thick mucus ■ Other signs and symptoms: prolonged expiration, retraction on inspiration, use of accessory muscles, flaring nostrils, tachypnea, tachycardia, perspiration, and flushing (common symptoms of eczema and allergic rhinitis [hay fever]) ■ Status asthmaticus: prompt treatment to prevent progression to respiratory failure
Chronic bronchitis ■ Excessive mucus production with productive cough for at least 3 months per year for 2 successive years ■ Rarely, significant airway obstruction	■ Severity of disease is related to amount and duration of smoking; respiratory tract infection exacerbates symptoms. ■ Causative mechanisms include hypertrophy and hyperplasia of bronchial mucous glands, increased goblet cells, damage to cilia, squamous metaplasia of columnar epithelium, and chronic leukocytic and lymphocytic infiltration of bronchial walls. Widespread inflammation, distortion, narrowing of airways, and formation of mucus cause ventilation-perfusion imbalance.	■ Insidious onset, with productive cough and exertional dyspnea ■ Other signs and symptoms: colds associated with increased sputum production and worsening dyspnea; copious sputum (gray, white, or yellow); weight gain due to edema; cyanosis; tachypnea; wheezing; prolonged expiratory time; and use of accessory muscles

Confirming diagnostic measures	Management
• Physical examination: rhonchi and wheezing throughout lung fields on expiration and, at times, inspiration; absent or diminished breath sounds during severe obstruction (loud bilateral wheezes; hyperinflated chest) • Chest X-ray: hyperinflated lungs with air trapping during attack; normal during remission • Sputum: presence of Curschmann's spirals (casts of airways), Charcot-Leyden crystals, and eosinophils • Pulmonary function tests: signs of airway obstructive disease, low-normal or decreased vital capacity, and increased total lung and residual capacities (Pulmonary function that may be normal between attacks; partial pressure of arterial oxygen (PaO_2) and partial pressure of arterial carbon dioxide ($PaCO_2$) usually decreased, except in severe asthma, in which $PaCO_2$ may be normal or increased, indicating severe bronchial obstruction) • Serum immunoglobulin E: increased from a possible allergic reaction • Arterial blood gases (ABGs): decreased PaO_2; decreased, normal, or increased $PaCO_2$ (in severe attack) • Electrocardiogram (ECG): sinus tachycardia during an attack; possible signs of cor pulmonale (right axis deviation, peaked P wave) in severe attack (resolves after attack) • Skin tests: may identify allergens • Bronchial challenge testing: evaluates clinical significance of allergens identified by skin testing	• Aerosol containing beta-adrenergic agents (metaproterenol or albuterol); oral beta-adrenergic agents (terbutaline) and oral methylxanthines (theophylline); inhaled, oral, or I.V. corticosteroids • Emergency treatment: Oxygen therapy, corticosteroids, and bronchodilators, such as subcutaneous epinephrine, I.V theophylline, and inhaled agents (such as metaproterenol, albuterol, or ipratropium) • Prevention: Tell the patient to avoid possible allergens. Explain the influence of stress, anxiety, exercise (particularly running), and cold air. Nighttime flare-ups may occur.
• Physical examination: rhonchi and wheezing on auscultation, expiratory prolongation, jugular vein distention, and pedal edema • Chest X-ray: may show hyperinflation and increased bronchovascular markings • Pulmonary function tests: increased residual volume, decreased vital capacity and forced expiratory volumes, and normal static compliance and diffusing capacity • ABGs: decreased PaO_2, normal or increased $PaCO_2$ • Sputum: contains evidence of infection • ECG: may show atrial arrhythmias; peaked P waves in leads II, III, and aV_F; and right ventricular hypertrophy	• Antibiotics for infections • Avoidance of smoking and air pollutants • Bronchodilators to relieve bronchospasm and facilitate mucociliary clearance • Fluid intake, chest physiotherapy, ultrasonic or mechanical nebulizer treatments to loosen secretions and aid in mobilization • Corticosteroids; inhaled corticosteroids for patients with reversibility of hyperactive airways • Diuretics for edema • Oxygen for hypoxia

(continued)

Understanding chronic obstructive pulmonary disease *(continued)*

Disease	Causes	Clinical features
Emphysema ■ Abnormal irreversible enlargement of air spaces distal to terminal bronchioles due to destruction of alveolar walls, resulting in decreased elastic recoil properties of lungs ■ Most common cause of death from respiratory disease in the United States	■ Cigarette smoking or deficiency of alpha$_1$-antitrypsin causes emphysema. ■ Recurrent inflammation associated with release of proteolytic enzymes causes bronchiolar and alveolar wall damage and destruction. Loss of lung-supporting structure results in decreased elastic recoil and airway collapse on expiration; destruction of alveolar walls decreases surface area for gas exchange.	■ Insidious onset, with dyspnea the predominant symptom ■ Other signs and symptoms: chronic cough, anorexia, weight loss, malaise, barrel chest, use of accessory muscles of respiration, prolonged expiratory period with grunting, pursed-lip breathing and tachypnea, and peripheral cyanosis ■ Complications: recurrent respiratory tract infections, cor pulmonale, and respiratory failure

Living with COPD

Review the following points with your patient and his family.
■ Encourage the patient to enroll in available pulmonary rehabilitation programs.
■ Urge him to stop smoking.
■ Encourage the patient to avoid respiratory irritants and install an air conditioner with an air filter in his home.
■ Review the use of any bronchodilators and antibiotics the patient is taking.

■ Review signs of infection, and warn the patient to avoid contact with persons who have a respiratory tract infection.
■ Review deep-breathing, coughing, and chest physiotherapy techniques.
■ Encourage the patient to drink plenty of fluids and to use a humidifier to thin secretions.
■ Emphasize the importance of a balanced diet consisting of small, frequent meals, and the use of nasal oxygen while eating.

confusion and drowsiness, which are symptoms of carbon dioxide narcosis.
■ Help the patient and his family adjust their lifestyles to accommodate the limitations imposed by this debilitating chronic disease. Instruct the patient to allow for daily rest periods and to exercise daily as directed.

 Cirrhosis

A chronic hepatic disease, cirrhosis is characterized by diffuse destruction and fibrotic regeneration of hepatic cells. As necrotic tissue yields to fibrosis, cirrhosis alters liver structure and normal vasculature, impairs blood and lymph flow and, ultimately, causes hepatic insuffi-

Confirming diagnostic measures	Management
■ Physical examination: hyperresonance on percussion, decreased breath sounds, expiratory prolongation, and quiet heart sounds ■ Chest X-ray: in advanced disease, flattened diaphragm, reduced vascular markings at lung periphery, overaeration of lungs, vertical heart, enlarged anteroposterior chest diameter, and large retrosternal air space ■ Pulmonary function tests: increased residual volume, total lung capacity, and compliance; decreased vital capacity, diffusing capacity, and expiratory volumes ■ ABGs: reduced Pao_2 with normal $Paco_2$ ■ ECG: tall, symmetrical P waves in leads II, III, and aV_F; vertical QRS axis; signs of right ventricular hypertrophy late in disease ■ Red blood cells: increased hemoglobin level late in disease	■ Bronchodilators (beta-adrenergics, theophylline) to reverse bronchospasm and promote mucociliary clearance ■ Antibiotics to treat infection; preventive flu and pneumococcal vaccines ■ Mucolytics, fluid intake and, in selected patients, chest physiotherapy to mobilize secretions ■ Oxygen at low-flow settings to treat hypoxia ■ Avoidance of smoking and air pollutants ■ Aerosolized or systemic corticosteroids

ciency. It's a serious, irreversible disease that's the 10th most common cause of death in the United States, usually found in people ages 45 to 75. The prognosis is better in noncirrhotic forms of hepatic fibrosis, which cause minimal hepatic dysfunction and don't destroy liver cells.

Causes
Cholestatic diseases
■ Biliary cirrhosis resulting from bile duct diseases suppressing bile flow
■ Sclerosing cholangitis

Hepatocellular disease
■ Postnecrotic cirrhosis from various types of hepatitis (such as types A, B, C, and D viral hepatitis) or toxic exposures
■ Laënnec's cirrhosis (portal, nutritional, or alcoholic cirrhosis) due to hepatitis C
■ Autoimmune disease (sarcoidosis and chronic inflammatory bowel disease)

Metabolic diseases
■ Wilson's disease, alpha$_1$-antitrypsin deficiency, and hemochromatosis (pigment cirrhosis)

Other types of cirrhosis
■ Budd-Chiari syndrome
■ Cardiac cirrhosis from right-sided heart failure
■ Cryptogenic cirrhosis (unknown cause)

Signs and symptoms
■ Early indications: weakness, fatigue, muscle cramps, weight loss, GI signs and symptoms (anorexia, indigestion, nausea, vomiting, constipation, and diarrhea), and abdominal pain
■ Central nervous system: progressive signs and symptoms of hepatic encephalopathy, such as lethargy, mental changes, slurred speech, asterixis (flapping tremor), peripheral neuritis, para-

noia, hallucinations, extreme obtundation, and coma
- Endocrine: testicular atrophy, menstrual irregularities, gynecomastia, loss of chest and axillary hair, loss of libido, and sterility
- Hematologic: bleeding tendencies, anemia, and hematemesis
- Hepatic: jaundice, hepatomegaly, ascites, edema of the legs, hepatic encephalopathy, and hepatorenal syndrome
- Respiratory: pleural effusion and limited thoracic expansion
- Skin: severe pruritus, extreme dryness, poor tissue turgor, abnormal pigmentation, spider nevi (on upper half of body), palmar erythema, jaundice, and peripheral edema
- Other signs and symptoms: musty breath, enlarged superficial abdominal veins, muscle atrophy, pain in the right upper abdominal quadrant that worsens when the patient sits up or leans forward, splenomegaly, and wasting appearance of chronic illness

Diagnostic tests
- A liver biopsy detects destruction and fibrosis of hepatic tissue.
- A liver scan shows abnormal thickening and, possibly, a liver mass.
- Ultrasonography detects liver enlargement and ascites or hepatic.
- Doppler ultrasonography evaluates patency of the splenic, portal, and hepatic veins.
- Abdominal X-rays show liver size and cysts or gas in the biliary tract or liver, liver calcification, and massive ascites.
- Computed tomography with I.V. contrast or magnetic resonance imaging with serum alpha-fetoprotein levels can help with further assessment of liver nodules.

- Esophagogastroscopy detects causes of bleeding in the esophagus, stomach, and proximal duodenum and confirms the presence of varices.
- Laboratory findings characteristic of cirrhosis include decreased platelet, hematocrit, hemoglobin, albumin, electrolytes (sodium, potassium, chloride, and magnesium), and folate; elevated globulin, serum ammonia, total bilirubin, alkaline phosphatase, serum aspartate aminotransferase, serum alanine aminotransferase, and lactate dehydrogenase; increased thymol turbidity; and coagulation abnormalities characterized by prolonged prothrombin and partial thromboplastin times.

Treatment
- The patient will require a high-calorie and moderate- to high-protein diet; if he develops hepatic encephalopathy, protein intake must be restricted. Sodium is usually restricted to 500 mg/day; fluids, 500 to 1,500 ml/day. If the patient deteriorates, tube feedings or hyperalimentation is needed.
- Supplemental vitamins (A, B complex, D, and K) are given to compensate for the liver's inability to store them; vitamin B, folic acid, and thiamine are administered for deficiency anemia.
- Vitamin K may be prescribed for bleeding tendencies due to hypoprothrombinemia; the patient may also need transfusions of blood and fresh frozen plasma.
- Additional treatment includes rest, moderate exercise, and avoidance of exposure to infections and toxic agents (alcohol, sedatives, and hepatotoxic drugs such as acetaminophen).
- Diuretics (furosemide or spironolactone) are given for edema.

DRUG CHALLENGE

 If the patient receives a diuretic, careful monitoring is necessary; fluid and electrolyte imbalance may precipitate hepatic encephalopathy.

- A beta-adrenergic blocker may be given to decrease pressure from varices.
- Lactulose (orally or rectally) may be given to reduce a high ammonia level. If therapy is inadequate, neomycin may be used.
- Paracentesis and infusions of salt-poor albumin may alleviate ascites.
- Surgical procedures include ligation or banding of varices, splenectomy, esophagogastric resection, and splenorenal or portacaval anastomosis to relieve portal hypertension. Transjugular intrahepatic portosystemic shunt to alleviate severe ascites that is refractory to standard therapy.

Nursing considerations

- Check skin, gums, stool, and vomitus regularly for bleeding. Apply pressure to injection sites to prevent bleeding. Warn the patient against taking aspirin, straining during defecation, and blowing his nose or sneezing too vigorously. Suggest using an electric razor and a soft toothbrush.
- Observe the patient closely for signs and symptoms of behavioral or personality changes—especially increasing stupor, lethargy, hallucinations, and neuromuscular dysfunction—which may indicate increasing ammonia levels. Arouse the patient periodically to determine his level of consciousness. Watch for asterixis, a sign of developing hepatic encephalopathy.
- Monitor ammonia levels to determine effectiveness of lactulose therapy.
- To assess fluid retention, weigh the patient and measure his abdominal girth daily, inspect the ankles and sacrum for dependent edema, and accurately record intake and output. Evaluate the patient before, during, and after paracentesis; this drastic loss of fluid may induce shock.
- To prevent skin breakdown, use lubricating lotion or another moisturizer. Handle the patient gently, and turn and reposition him often to keep skin intact.
- Support the family during this difficult time, and refer the patient to support groups and Alcoholics Anonymous as indicated.

Clostridium difficile infection

Clostridium difficile is a gram-positive anaerobic bacterium usually linked to antibiotic-associated diarrhea. Symptoms may range from asymptomatic carrier states to severe pseudomembranous colitis and are caused by exotoxins produced by the organism: toxin A (an enterotoxin) and toxin B (a cytotoxin). It's more common in patients who have abdominal surgery, patients who are immunocompromised, pediatric patients (especially in day-care centers), and nursing home patients. *C. difficile* may be transmitted directly (contaminated hands) or indirectly (through contaminated equipment, such as bedpans, call bells, rectal thermometers, and nasogastric tubes, and through surfaces, such as bed rails, floors, and toilet seats).

Causes

- Almost any antibiotic that disrupts the intestinal flora (especially clindamycin) or antineoplastics that have antibiotic activity
- Other factors that alter normal intestinal flora (enemas, intestinal stimulants)

Signs and symptoms

- Abdominal pain, cramping, or tenderness
- Electrolyte abnormalities, hypovolemic shock, anasarca (caused by hypoalbuminemia), sepsis, hemorrhage and, possibly, death
- Fever with white blood cell count elevated to 20,000/µl
- In severe cases, toxic megacolon, colonic perforation, and peritonitis
- Soft, unformed stool or watery diarrhea (more than three evacuations in 24 hours) that may be foul-smelling or grossly bloody

Diagnostic tests

- Infection is confirmed by identification of toxins, using cell cytotoxin test (takes 2 days to perform), enzyme immunoassays (less sensitive but results are obtained in a few hours), or stool culture (most sensitive, with 2-day turnaround).
- Endoscopy (flexible sigmoidoscopy) detects pseudomembranes.

Treatment

- Withdraw the causative antibiotic in patients who are mildly symptomatic.
- In more severe cases, metronidazole (Flagyl) or vancomycin (Vancocin) is an effective therapy; metronidazole is the preferred medication. In 10% to 20% of patients, *C. difficile* may recur within 14 to 30 days of treatment. Beyond 30 days, it's questionable whether the recurrence is a relapse or reinfection with *C. difficile.* If metronidazole was the initial treatment, low-dose vancomycin may be effective.
- Give lactobacillus, *Saccharomyces boulardii,* and biological vaccines to restore normal intestinal flora.
- I.V. immunoglobulin may help in relapsing infections.

Nursing considerations

- Risk of infection begins 1 to 2 days after antibiotic therapy is started and persists for as long as 2 to 3 months after the last dose.
- If the patient has or is suspected of having *C. difficile* diarrhea and is unable to practice good hygiene, he should be placed in a single room or with other patients with similar health status.
- If the patient is asymptomatic without diarrhea or fecal incontinence for 72 hours and is able to practice good hygiene, he may be transferred to a single room.
- Standard precautions for contact with blood and body fluids should be used for all direct patient contact and contact with the patient's immediate environment. Use good hand-washing technique with antiseptic soap after direct contact with the patient or the immediate environment.
- Reusable equipment must be disinfected before it's used on another patient.

▌Coal workers' pneumoconiosis

Coal workers' pneumoconiosis (CWP) also called *black lung disease, coal miner's disease, miner's asthma,* and *anthracosis,* is a progressive nodular pulmonary disease that may be simple (characterized by small lung opacities) or complicated (*progressive massive fibrosis* characterized by masses of fibrous tissue in the lungs). The risk of developing CWP depends on the duration of the patient's exposure to coal dust (usually 15 years or longer), intensity of exposure (dust count, particle size), his proximity to the mine site, silica content of the coal (anthracite coal has the highest silica content), and the worker's susceptibility. The prognosis varies. Simple, asymptomatic disease is self-limiting, although it can progress to the complicated form. Complicated CWP may be disabling, resulting in severe ventilatory failure and right-sided heart failure secondary to pulmonary hypertension.

Causes
- Atrophy of supporting tissue, causing permanent dilation of small airways (focal emphysema)
- Inhalation and prolonged retention of respirable coal dust particles (less than 5 microns in diameter) resulting in the formation of macules (accumulations of macrophages laden with coal dust) around the terminal and respiratory bronchioles, surrounded by dilated alveoli
- With lung involvement: gross distortion of pulmonary structures due to enlarging and coalescing fibrous tissue

Signs and symptoms
In complicated CWP only
- Barrel chest (occasionally), hyperresonant lungs with areas of dullness, diminished breath sounds, crackles, rhonchi, and wheezes
- Complications: pulmonary hypertension, right ventricular hypertrophy and cor pulmonale, and pulmonary tuberculosis
- Cough that occasionally produces inky-black, milky, gray, clear, or coal-flecked sputum
- Exertional dyspnea that progresses
- In cigarette smokers: chronic bronchitis and emphysema
- Recurrent bronchial and pulmonary infections producing thick yellow or green sputum

Diagnostic tests
- With simple CWP, chest X-rays show small opacities (less than 10 mm in diameter), which may be present in all lung zones but are more prominent in the upper zones. With complicated CWP, chest X-rays show one or more large opacities ($\frac{1}{2}''$ to $2''$ [1 to 5 cm] in diameter), possibly with cavitation.
- Vital capacity is normal with simple CWP but decreased with complicated CWP.
- Forced vital capacity is decreased in complicated CWP.
- Residual volume and total lung capacity remains normal in simple CWP but is decreased in complicated CWP.
- Diffusing capacity of the lungs for carbon monoxide is significantly decreased in complicated CWP because alveolar septae are destroyed and pulmonary capillaries are obliterated.
- Partial pressure of arterial oxygen is normal in simple CWP but decreased in complicated CWP; partial pressure of arterial carbon dioxide ($Paco_2$) usually remains normal in simple CWP but may decrease because of hyperventilation. $Paco_2$ may also increase if the patient is hypoxic and has severe impairment of alveolar ventilation.

Treatment
- Bronchodilator therapy with theophylline or aminophylline may be used if bronchospasm is reversible.
- The patient may be given oral or inhaled sympathomimetic amines (metaproterenol [Alupent]), corticosteroids (oral prednisone or an aerosol form of a corticosteroid), or cromolyn sodium aerosol.
- Chest physiotherapy (controlled coughing, segmental bronchial drainage) may be combined with chest percussion and vibration to remove secretions.
- Increase the patient's fluid intake (at least 3 qt [3 L] per day).
- Provide respiratory therapy, such as aerosol therapy, an inhaled mucolytic,

and intermittent positive-pressure breathing, as indicated.

■ If the patient has cor pulmonale, a diuretic and a cardiac glycoside might be prescribed and sodium intake may be restricted.

■ In severe cases, oxygen may be administered by cannula or mask (1 to 2 L/minute) if the patient has chronic hypoxia or by mechanical ventilation if partial pressure of arterial oxygen falls below 40 mm Hg.

■ Respiratory tract infections require prompt administration of an antibiotic.

Nursing considerations

■ Watch for signs of developing tuberculosis.

■ Teach the patient to prevent infections by avoiding crowds and persons with respiratory tract infections and by receiving influenza and pneumococcal vaccines.

■ Encourage the patient to stay active to avoid a deterioration in his physical condition but to pace his activities and practice relaxation techniques.

■ Coccidioidomycosis

Also known as *valley fever* and *San Joaquin Valley fever,* coccidioidomycosis is caused by the fungus *Coccidioides immitis.* It occurs primarily as a respiratory tract infection, although generalized dissemination may occur. The primary pulmonary form is usually self-limiting and rarely fatal. The rare secondary (progressive, disseminated) form produces abscesses throughout the body and carries a mortality of up to 60%, even with treatment. Such dissemination is more common in dark-skinned men, pregnant women, and patients who are receiving an immunosuppressant. Because of population distribution and an occupational

link (it's common in migrant farm laborers), coccidioidomycosis generally affects Filipino Americans, Mexican Americans, Native Americans, and Blacks.

Causes

■ Inhalation of *C. immitis* spores found in the soil in the southwestern United States or inhalation of spores from dressings or plaster casts of infected persons

Signs and symptoms

■ Chronic pulmonary cavitation, causing hemoptysis with or without chest pain

Primary coccidioidomycosis

■ Acute or subacute respiratory signs and symptoms: dry cough, pleuritic chest pain, and pleural effusion

■ Fever (may last for weeks and can be the sole indication)

■ Sore throat, chills, malaise, and headache

■ Itchy macular rash (primary form)

■ Tender red nodules (erythema nodosum) on the legs, especially the shins, with joint pain in the knees and ankles, occurring from 3 days to several weeks after onset and healing spontaneously within a few weeks

Disseminated coccidioidomycosis

■ Fever

■ Abscesses throughout the body: skeletal, central nervous system (CNS), splenic, hepatic, renal, and subcutaneous tissues

■ Depending on the location of these abscesses, bone pain and meningitis

Diagnostic tests

■ Typical signs and symptoms and skin and serologic studies confirm the diagnosis.

- Positive coccidioidin skin test results occur with the primary and, occasionally, the disseminated form.
- Complement fixation for immunoglobulin G antibodies is diagnostic in the first few weeks.
- Positive serum precipitins (immunoglobulins) confirms diagnosis in the first month.
- Examination of recent immunodiffusion testing of sputum, pus from lesions, and a tissue biopsy may show *C. immitis* spores.
- The presence of antibodies in pleural and joint fluid and a rising serum or body fluid antibody titer indicate dissemination.
- Other abnormal laboratory results include increased white blood cell (WBC) count, increased eosinophil count, and increased erythrocyte sedimentation rate.
- A chest X-ray shows bilaterally diffuse infiltrates.
- In coccidioidal meningitis, cerebrospinal fluid shows the WBC count increased to more than 500/µl (primarily because of mononuclear leukocytes) and increased protein and decreased glucose levels. Ventricular fluid may contain complement fixation antibodies.
- The results of serial skin tests, blood cultures, and serologic testing may document the effectiveness of therapy.

Treatment

- Mild primary coccidioidomycosis requires bed rest and relief of symptoms.
- Severe primary disease and dissemination require long-term I.V. infusion or, with CNS dissemination, intrathecal administration of amphotericin B.
- Excision or drainage of lesions may be necessary.
- Severe pulmonary lesions may require lobectomy.

DRUG CHALLENGE

 Miconazole and ketoconazole suppress *C. immitis* but don't eradicate it. Itraconazole has been used successfully in the treatment of mildly severe cases.

Nursing considerations

- Don't wash off the circle marked on the skin for serial skin tests; this aids in reading test results.
- With mild primary disease, encourage bed rest and adequate fluid intake. Record the amount and color of sputum. Watch for shortness of breath that may point to pleural effusion. In patients with arthralgia, provide an analgesic.
- Coccidioidomycosis requires strict secretion precautions if the patient has draining lesions. No specific isolation precautions are required.
- With CNS dissemination, monitor the patient carefully for a decreased level of consciousness or a change in mood or affect.

DRUG CHALLENGE

 If the patient is to receive I.V. amphotericin B, infuse it slowly; rapid infusion may cause circulatory collapse. During infusion, monitor his vital signs. (His temperature may rise but should return to normal within 1 to 2 hours.) Watch for decreased urine output, and monitor laboratory results for elevated blood urea nitrogen and creatinine levels and hypokalemia. Tell patients to immediately report hearing loss, tinnitus, dizziness, and all signs of toxicity. To ease adverse reactions, give an antihystamine such as diphenhydramine (Benadryl) and an antipyretic.

Cold injuries

Overexposure to cold air or water causes cold injuries. They occur in two major forms: localized injuries (such as frostbite) and systemic injuries (such as hypothermia). Untreated or improperly treated frostbite can lead to gangrene and may necessitate amputation; severe hypothermia can be fatal. The risk of serious cold injuries is increased by youth, lack of insulating body fat, wet or inadequate clothing, old age, drug abuse, cardiac disease, smoking, fatigue, hunger and depletion of caloric reserves, and excessive alcohol intake (which draws blood into the capillaries and away from body organs).

Causes
Frostbite
- Increased capillary permeability due to aggregation of red blood cells and microvascular occlusion
- Localized cold injuries: formulation of ice crystals in the tissues followed by expansion of crystals into extracellular spaces
- Prolonged exposure to freezing temperatures or to cold, wet environments
- Rupture of cell membrane with compression of the tissue cell

Hypothermia
- Cold-water near-drowning and prolonged exposure to cold temperatures
- Slowing of functions of most major organ systems (such as decreased renal blood flow and decreased glomerular filtration)

Signs and symptoms
Frostbite
- Deep frostbite: pain, skin blisters, tissue necrosis, and gangrene, usually extending beyond subcutaneous tissue (most commonly, hands and feet); alteration of skin color from white or yellow to purplish blue (with thawing)
- Superficial frostbite: burning, tingling, numbness, swelling, and a mottled, blue-gray skin color of skin and subcutaneous tissue (face, ears, extremities, and other exposed body areas)

Hypothermia
- Varies with severity:
  – Mild hypothermia with temperature of 89.6° to 95° F (32° to 35° C): severe shivering, slurred speech, and amnesia
  – Moderate hypothermia with temperature of 86° to 89.6° F (30° to 32° C): unresponsiveness or confusion, muscle rigidity, peripheral cyanosis and, with improper rewarming, signs of shock
  – Severe hypothermia with a core temperature of 77° to 86° F (25° to 30° C): loss of deep tendon reflexes, ventricular fibrillation, no palpable pulse or audible heart sounds, dilated pupils, and rigor mortis
  – Temperature drop below 77° F (25° C): cardiopulmonary arrest and death

Diagnostic tests
- Diagnosis is confirmed by the patient's history of severe and prolonged exposure to cold.

Treatment
Frostbite
- Rapidly rewarm the injured part to slightly above ideal body temperature; slow rewarming could increase tissue damage.
- When the affected part begins to rewarm, the patient will feel pain, so administer an analgesic. Check for a pulse. If the injury is on the foot, place cotton

or gauze pads between the toes to prevent maceration. Instruct the patient not to walk.

- After rewarming, the affected part is kept elevated, uncovered, at room temperature. A regimen of whirlpool treatments for 3 or more weeks cleans the skin and debrides sloughing tissue.

Do's & don'ts

 When treating a patient with frostbite, never rub the injured area or rupture blebs because this aggravates tissue damage. Prevent refreezing of thawed tissues because significant tissue damage may occur. Also, it's impossible to assess the depth of frostbite injury in the early stages.

- Give antibiotic and tetanus prophylaxis if the patient has open skin wounds.
- The patient may require surgical intervention or amputation if gangrene develops.

Hypothermia

Action stat!

 If the patient has no pulse or respirations, begin cardiopulmonary resuscitation immediately and continue until he's rewarmed, which may take 2 to 3 hours. Remember, hypothermia helps protect the brain from anoxia, which normally accompanies prolonged cardiopulmonary arrest. Therefore, even after the patient has been unresponsive for a long time, resuscitation may be possible, especially after cold-water near-drownings.

- Move the patient to a warm area, remove wet clothing, and keep him dry. If he's conscious, give warm fluids with high sugar content, such as tea with sugar. If the patient's core temperature is above 89.6° F (32° C), use external

warming techniques. Bathe him in water that's 104° F (40° C), cover him with a heating blanket set at 97.9° to 99.9° F (36.6° to 37.7° C), and cautiously apply hot water bottles at 104° F (40° C) to groin and axillae, guarding against burns.

- If the patient's core temperature is below 89.6° F (32° C), use internal and external warming methods to rewarm his body core and surface 1° to 2° F (0.5° to 1.1° C) per hour concurrently.

Alert

 If you rewarm the surface first, rewarming shock could cause potentially fatal ventricular fibrillation.

- To warm inhalations, provide oxygen heated to 107.6° to 114.8° F (42° to 46° C). Infuse I.V. solutions that have been warmed to 98.6° F (37° C), and perform nasogastric lavage with normal saline solution that has been warmed to the same temperature.
- If indicated, perform peritoneal lavage, using normal saline solution (full or half strength) warmed to 104° to 113° F (40° to 45° C).
- The patient with severe hypothermia may require heart and lung bypass at controlled temperatures and thoracotomy with a direct cardiac warm-saline bath may be required. Avoid using central venous catheters to prevent arrhythmias.

Drug challenge

 Consider giving antibodies if sepsis is the suspected cause of the hypothermia. Consider giving a steroid only if adrenal suppression or insufficiency is the suspected cause.

Nursing considerations

- Before discharging a patient with frostbite, tell him about possible long-term effects: increased sensitivity to cold, burning and tingling, and increased sweating. Warn against smoking; this causes vasoconstriction and slows healing.
- During treatment for hypothermia, monitor arterial blood gas values, intake and output, central venous pressure, temperature, and cardiac and neurologic status every half hour. Monitor laboratory results (complete blood count, blood urea nitrogen and electrolyte levels, and prothrombin and partial thromboplastin times).

ALERT

 If the patient is a child, suspect neglect or abuse; make sure a thorough patient history is performed. If the patient developed a cold injury because of inadequate clothing or housing, refer him to a community social service agency.

- To help prevent future cold injuries, tell the patient to wear mittens (not gloves); windproof, water-resistant, many-layered clothing; two pairs of socks (cotton next to the skin, then wool); and a scarf and a hat that cover the ears (to avoid substantial heat loss through the head).

■ Colorectal cancer

In the United States and Europe, colorectal cancer is the second most common visceral neoplasm. Incidence is equally distributed between men and women. Incidence increases with age, with most patients older than age 55. Higher incidence occurs in patients with a family history of colorectal cancer and in those who have chronic inflammatory bowel disease or polyps. Colorectal malignant tumors are almost always adenocarcinomas. This type of cancer tends to progress slowly and remains localized for a long time; it's curable in 75% of patients if an early diagnosis allows resection before nodal involvement. With early diagnosis, the overall 5-year survival rate is about 50%. (See *Guidelines for detecting colorectal cancer.*)

Causes

- Unknown

Risk factors

- Age (older than age 40)
- Diet (excess animal fat, particularly beef, and low fiber)
- Familial polyposis (cancer almost always develops by age 50)
- History of ulcerative colitis (average interval before onset of cancer is 11 to 17 years)
- Other diseases of the digestive tract

Signs and symptoms

- In the early stages, signs and symptoms are typically vague and depend on the anatomical location and function of the bowel segment containing the tumor. Later, they generally include pallor, cachexia, ascites, hepatomegaly, and lymphangiectasis.

Cancer on the left side

- Intermittent abdominal fullness or cramping, and rectal pressure
- Rectal bleeding (typically ascribed to hemorrhoids)
- Signs and symptoms of an obstruction
- As the disease progresses: constipation, diarrhea, "ribbon" or pencil-shaped stool, pain relief with passage of stool or flatus; obvious signs of bleeding from the colon, such as dark or bright red blood in the stool and mucus in or on the stool

Cancer on the right side

- Abdominal aching, pressure, or dull cramps
- Anemia
- Asymptomatic or black, tarry stool
- Palpable tumor
- As the disease progresses: weakness, fatigue, exertional dyspnea, vertigo, diarrhea, constipation, anorexia, weight loss, vomiting, and other signs and symptoms of intestinal obstruction

Rectal tumor

- Blood or mucus in stool
- Change in bowel habits, usually beginning with an urgent need to defecate on arising ("morning diarrhea") or constipation alternating with diarrhea
- Pain beginning as a feeling of rectal fullness and progressing to a dull ache confined to the rectum or sacral region
- Sense of incomplete evacuation

Diagnostic tests

- Only a tumor biopsy can verify colorectal cancer, but the following tests help detect it:
  - Digital examination may reveal presence of tumor.
  - Hemoccult test (guaiac) may show blood in the stool.
  - Proctoscopy, sigmoidoscopy, or colonoscopy permits visual inspection and allows access for excision and biopsies.
  - Computed tomography scan helps detect areas affected by metastasis.
  - Barium X-ray, using a dual contrast with air, can locate lesions. Barium examination should follow endoscopy or excretory urography because the barium sulfate interferes with these tests.
  - Carcinoembryonic antigen is helpful in monitoring patients before and after treatment to detect metastasis or recurrence.

Guidelines for detecting colorectal cancer

The following recommendations from the American Cancer Society detail screening tests that allow early detection of colorectal cancer. These guidelines apply to men and women age 50 and older.

Screening test	Frequency recommendations
Fecal occult blood test (FOBT)	- Every year
Flexible sigmoidoscopy	- Every 5 years
FOBT plus flexible sigmoidoscopy*	- FOBT every year - Flexible sigmoidoscopy every 5 years
Colonoscopy	- Every 10 years
Double contrast barium enema	- Every 5 years

* Most clinicians prefer the combination of FOBT and flexible sigmoidoscopy over either test alone.

Treatment

- Surgery is needed to remove the malignant tumor and adjacent tissues as well as any lymph nodes that may contain cancer cells. The type of surgery depends on the location of the tumor.
- Chemotherapy is indicated for patients with metastasis, residual disease, or a recurrent inoperable tumor.

DRUG CHALLENGE

 Drugs used in such treatment commonly include fluorouracil combined with levamisole or leucovorin. Patients whose tumor has extended to regional lymph nodes may receive fluorouracil and levamisole for 1 year postoperatively.

■ Radiation therapy induces tumor regression; it may be used before or after surgery or combined with chemotherapy, especially fluorouracil.

Nursing considerations
Before surgery

■ Administer prescribed diets, laxatives, enemas, and antibiotics to clean the bowel and to decrease abdominal and perineal cavity contamination during surgery.
■ If the patient is having a colostomy, teach him and his family about the procedure. Inform the patient that the stoma will be red, moist, and swollen and that postoperative swelling will eventually subside.
■ Show the patient a diagram of the intestine before and after surgery, stressing how much of the bowel will remain intact. Supplement your teaching with instructional aids. Arrange a postsurgical visit from a recovered ostomate.
■ Prepare the patient for postoperative I.V. infusions, a nasogastric tube, and indwelling urinary catheter. Discuss the importance of deep-breathing and coughing exercises.

After surgery

■ Consult with an enterostomal therapist to help set up a regimen for the patient.
■ Encourage the patient to look at the stoma and participate in its care as soon as possible.
■ If appropriate, instruct the patient with a sigmoid colostomy to do his own irrigation as soon as he can after surgery. Advise him to schedule irrigation for the time of day when he normally evacuated before surgery. Many patients find that irrigating every 1 to 3 days is necessary for regularity.
■ If flatus, diarrhea, or constipation occurs, eliminate suspected causative foods from the patient's diet. He may reintroduce them later.
■ After several months, many ostomates establish control with irrigation and no longer need to wear a pouch. A stoma cap or gauze sponge placed over the stoma protects it and absorbs mucoid secretions.
■ Before achieving such control, the patient can resume physical activities, including sports, but he should avoid injury to the stoma or surrounding abdominal muscles.
■ Inform the patient that a structured, gradually progressive exercise program to strengthen abdominal muscles may be instituted under medical supervision. Instruct the patient to avoid heavy lifting because herniation or prolapse may occur.

Common cold

The common cold—an acute, usually afebrile viral infection—causes inflammation of the upper respiratory tract. It accounts for more time lost from school or work than any other cause and is the most common infectious disease. It can also lead to secondary bacterial infections. The common cold is more prevalent in children than in adults, in adolescent boys than in girls, and in women than in men. Transmission occurs through airborne respiratory droplets, contact with contaminated objects, and hand-to-hand transmission. Children acquire new strains from their schoolmates and pass them on to family members.

Causes
- Mycoplasma
- Rhinoviruses, coronaviruses, myxoviruses, adenoviruses, coxsackieviruses, and echoviruses
- Viral infection (90%) of the upper respiratory passages and consequent mucous membrane inflammation

Signs and symptoms
- Burning, watery eyes
- Fever (in children), chills
- Hacking, nonproductive, or nocturnal cough
- Headache
- Myalgia, arthralgia, malaise, and lethargy
- Nasal congestion, rhinitis
- Pharyngitis

Diagnostic tests
- Diagnosis is based on symptoms.
- Despite infection, white blood cell count and differential are within normal limits.

Treatment
- Acetaminophen, ibuprofen, or aspirin eases myalgia and headache.
- For a child with a fever, acetaminophen is the drug of choice.
- Fluids help loosen accumulated respiratory secretions and maintain hydration.
- Rest combats fatigue and weakness.
- Decongestants can relieve congestion.
- Throat lozenges relieve soreness.
- Steam encourages expectoration. In infants, saline nose drops and mucus aspiration with a bulb syringe may be beneficial.
- Pure antitussives relieve severe coughs but are contraindicated with productive

coughs, when cough suppression is harmful.
- Vitamin therapy, interferon administration, and ultraviolet irradiation remain under investigation.

Nursing considerations
- Emphasize to the patient that antibiotics don't cure the common cold.
- Tell the patient to maintain bed rest during the first few days, use a lubricant on his nostrils to decrease irritation, relieve throat irritation with hard candy or cough drops, increase his fluid intake, and eat light meals.
- Inform the patient that warm baths or heating pads can reduce aches and pains, but they don't hasten a cure. Suggest hot or cold steam vaporizers. Commercial expectorants are available, but their effectiveness is questionable.

Drug challenge

 Advise the patient against overuse of nose drops or sprays; they may cause rebound congestion.

- To help prevent colds, warn the patient to minimize contact with people who have colds.
- To avoid spreading colds, teach the patient to wash his hands often, to cover his mouth when he coughs or sneezes, and to avoid sharing towels and drinking glasses.

Common variable immunodeficiency

Also called *acquired hypogammaglobulinemia* and *agammaglobulinemia with immunoglobulin-bearing B cells,* common variable immunodeficiency is characterized by progressive deterioration of B-cell (humoral) immunity. This results in increased susceptibility to infection and usually causes symptoms after infancy and childhood, between ages 25 and 40. It affects men and women equally and usually doesn't interfere with normal life span or with normal pregnancy and off-spring.

Causes
- Unknown; no clear evidence of genetic influence
- Associated with certain cancers (such as leukemia and lymphoma) and autoimmune diseases (such as systemic lupus erythematosus, rheumatoid arthritis, hemolytic anemia, and pernicious anemia)

Signs and symptoms
- Normal circulating B-cell count with defective synthesis or release of immunoglobulins (in most patients)
- Chronic pyogenic bacterial infections (sinopulmonary infections, chronic conjunctivitis)
- Malabsorption (commonly associated with infestation by *Giardia lamblia*)
- Nonseptic inflammatory arthritis or septic arthritis
- Presence of autoimmune diseases (systemic lupus erythematosus, rheumatoid arthritis, hemolytic anemia, and pernicious anemia)

Diagnostic tests
- Decreased serum immunoglobulin (Ig) M, IgA, and IgG detected by immunoelectrophoresis and a normal circulating B-cell count are characteristic diagnostic markers.
- Antigenic stimulation confirms an inability to produce specific antibodies; cell-mediated immunity may be intact or delayed.
- Delayed hypersensitivity skin testing reveals progressive deterioration of T-cell (cell-mediated) immunity.

- X-rays usually show signs of chronic lung disease or sinusitis.

Treatment
- Administer I.V. immune globulin as prescribed (usually weekly to monthly).
- Fresh frozen plasma infusions provide IgA and IgM.
- Antibiotics combat infection.
- Regular X-rays and pulmonary function studies help monitor infection in the lungs.
- Chest physiotherapy clears secretions and deters infection.

Nursing considerations
- To help prevent severe infection, teach the patient and his family how to recognize its early signs. Warn them to avoid crowds and persons who have active infections.
- Stress the importance of good nutrition and regular follow-up care.

Complement deficiencies

A series of circulating enzymatic serum proteins with nine functional components make up complement. When immunoglobulin (Ig) G or IgM reacts with antigens as part of an immune response, they initiate the classic complement pathway, or cascade. Complement then combines with the antigen-antibody complex and undergoes a sequence of reactions that amplify the immune response against the antigen (a complex process called complement fixation). Complement deficiency or dysfunction increases susceptibility to infection due to defective phagocytosis of bacteria; there may also be a relation to certain autoimmune disorders. Primary complement deficiencies are rare. The most common ones are C1, C2, and C4 deficiencies and C5 familial dysfunction.

More common secondary complement abnormalities have been confirmed in select patients with lupus erythematosus, dermatomyositis, scleroderma, gonococcal and meningococcal infections. The prognosis varies with the abnormality and the severity of associated diseases.

Causes
- Primary complement deficiencies: inherited autosomal recessive traits (except the autosomal dominant deficiency of C1 esterase inhibitor)
- Secondary deficiencies: complement-fixing (complement-consuming) immunologic reactions, such as drug-induced serum sickness, acute streptococcal glomerulonephritis, and acute active systemic lupus erythematosus

Signs and symptoms
- C2 and C3 deficiencies and C5 familial dysfunction: increased susceptibility to bacterial infection (which may involve several body systems simultaneously)
- C2 and C4 deficiencies: collagen vascular disease such as lupus erythematosus, and with chronic renal failure
- C5 dysfunction (a familial defect in infants): failure to thrive, diarrhea, and seborrheic dermatitis
- Defects in latter components of the complement cascade (C5 to C9): increased susceptibility to infections with *Neisseria*
- C1 esterase inhibitor deficiency (hereditary angioedema): periodic swelling in the face, hands, abdomen, or throat, with potentially fatal laryngeal edema

Diagnostic tests
- Total serum complement level is low in various complement deficiencies.
- Specific assays are used to confirm deficiencies of specific complement components (for example, detection of complement components and IgG by immunofluorescent examination of glomerular tissues in glomerulonephritis strongly suggests complement deficiency).

Treatment
- Treatment is primarily for associated infection, collagen vascular disease, or renal disease. Controversial adjuncts include:
  – Transfusion of fresh frozen plasma is used to provide temporary replacement of complement components.
  – Bone marrow transplantation may be helpful but can cause a potentially fatal graft-versus-host (GVH) reaction.
  – Anabolic steroids such as danazol, and antifibrinolytic agents, may be used to reduce acute swelling in patients with hereditary angioedema.

Nursing considerations
- Teach the patient or his family the importance of avoiding infection, how to recognize its early signs and symptoms, and the need for prompt treatment if it occurs.
- After bone marrow transplantation, monitor the patient closely for signs of transfusion reaction and GVH reaction.
- Provide meticulous patient care to help speed recovery and prevent complications. A patient with renal infection, for example, will need careful monitoring of intake and output, tests for serum electrolyte levels and acid-base balance, and observation for signs of renal failure.

ACTION STAT!

 When caring for a patient with hereditary angioedema, be prepared for emergency management of laryngeal edema; keep airway equipment on hand. Also, consider giving the patient a medical identification bracelet.

Complex regional pain syndrome

Complex regional pain syndrome (CRPS), also known as *reflex sympathetic dystrophy* (CRPS1) or *causalgia* (CRPS2), is a chronic pain disorder that results from abnormal healing after an major or minor injury to a bone, muscle, or nerve. The development of symptoms is commonly disproportionate to the severity of the injury and seems to result from abnormal functioning of the sympathetic nervous system. One or more extremities and other parts of the body may be affected. CRPS may also be seen in postoperative patients and in patients with diseases that can cause chronic pain, such as cancer and arthritis.

Causes
- Impaired communication between damaged nerves of the sympathetic nervous system and the brain causing interference with signals for sensations, temperature, and blood flow
- Infection
- Injury

Signs and symptoms
- Possible alteration of blood flow to affected area; sensation of warmth or coolness to the touch, with discoloration, sweating, or swelling
- Severe and constant pain
- In time, skin, hair, and nail changes, along with impaired mobility and muscle wasting

Diagnostic tests
- No laboratory test exists for CRPS, so the diagnosis is based on the patient's history and clinical findings.

- Bone X-rays may aid in ruling out other conditions, such as osteomyelitis and stress fractures, which cause similar signs and symptoms.

Treatment
- Drug therapy (such as an anti-inflammatory, antidepressant, vasodilator, and analgesic) is the typical treatment.
- Physical therapy to the injured area (stretching, active and passive exercises, and strengthening exercises) compressive stockings or gloves to control edema, and heat or cold pack applications are helpful for some patients.
- Psychological support may assist with the patient's emotional response to the condition.
- Interrupting the hyperactivity of the sympathetic nervous system through nerve or regional blocks is another treatment.

Nursing considerations
- Monitor effects of prescribed medications.
- Consult a pain care specialist to provide additional options for the patient, and help manage discomfort.
- Offer emotional support to the patient and his family. Teach them about the disease.
- Because chronic pain can be an emotional burden to the patient and his family, provide information on resources, such as counseling, support groups, stress-reduction methods, meditation, relaxation training, and hypnosis.

Concussion

By far the most common head injury, concussion results from an acceleration-deceleration injury or a blow to the head, forceful enough to jostle the brain and make it hit against the skull, (causing temporary neural dysfunction), but not forceful enough to cause a cerebral contusion. Most concussion victims recover completely within 48 hours. Repeated concussions, however, exact a cumulative toll on the brain.

Causes
- Child, spouse, or elder abuse
- Sudden and forceful blow (a fall to the ground, a punch to the head, a motor vehicle accident)

Signs and symptoms
- Anterograde and retrograde amnesia
- Delayed lethargy and somnolence in children
- Dizziness
- Irritability, lethargy, or behavior out of character
- Nausea, vomiting
- Severe headache
- Short-term loss of consciousness

ACTION STAT!

 Although all of the above signs and symptoms occur normally with a concussion, they may also result from more serious head injuries. Medical evaluation is necessary to rule out serious injury to the brain.

- Postconcussion syndrome: headache, dizziness, vertigo, anxiety, and fatigue persisting for several weeks after the injury

Diagnostic tests
- Differentiating between concussion and more serious head injuries requires a thorough history of the trauma and a neurologic examination (level of consciousness [LOC], mental status, cranial nerve and motor function, deep tendon reflexes, and orientation to time, place, and person).
- Computed tomography (CT) scanning and magnetic resonance imaging can

help rule out fractures and more serious injuries.

Treatment
- Treatment is primarily supportive; nonopioid analgesics for headache if there's no serious injury.
- If child abuse is suspected, report to appropriate authorities.
- If the patient has an altered LOC or if a neurologic examination reveals abnormalities, the injury may be more severe than a concussion; in such a case, the patient's practitioner should be consulted immediately.

Nursing considerations
- Monitor vital signs, and check for additional injuries. Palpate the skull for tenderness or hematomas.
- If a neurologic examination reveals no abnormalities, observe the patient in the emergency department. Check his vital signs, LOC, and pupil size and reaction every 15 minutes. The patient whose condition is stable after 4 or more hours of observation can be discharged (with a head injury instruction sheet) under the care of a responsible adult.

Conjunctivitis

Conjunctivitis, or inflammation of the conjunctiva, results from bacterial or viral infection, allergy, or chemical reactions. Bacterial and viral conjunctivitis are highly contagious but self-limiting after 2 weeks. Chronic conjunctivitis may result in degenerative changes to the eyelids. In the Western hemisphere, conjunctivitis is probably the most common eye disorder.

Causes
- Allergic reactions to pollen, grass, topical medications, air pollutants, and smoke

Conjunctival papillae— a sign of vernal conjunctivitis

If you see papillae in the conjunctiva of the upper eyelid, your patient may have vernal (allergic) conjunctivitis. These cobblestone bumps are the telltale sign. They result from swollen lymph tissue within the conjunctival membrane.

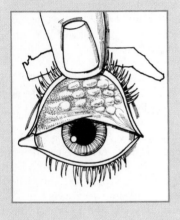

- Bacterial: *Staphylococcus aureus, Streptococcus pneumoniae, Neisseria gonorrhoeae,* and *Neisseria meningitidis*
- Chlamydial: *Chlamydia trachomatis* (inclusion conjunctivitis)
- Idiopathic: accompanies erythema multiforme, chronic follicular conjunctivitis (orphan's conjunctivitis), thyroid disease, and Stevens-Johnson syndrome
- Occupational irritants (acids and alkalies)
- Rickettsial diseases (Rocky Mountain spotted fever); parasitic diseases caused by *Phthirus pubis* and *Schistosoma haematobium;* and, rarely, fungal infections
- Secondary to pneumococcal dacryocystitis or canaliculitis from candidal infection

- Vernal conjunctivitis (seasonal or warm-weather conjunctivitis): allergy to an unidentified allergen (such as grass or pollen) (see *Conjunctival papillae—a sign of vernal conjunctivitis*)
- Viral: adenovirus types 3, 7, and 8; herpes simplex virus type 1

Signs and symptoms
- Hyperemia of the conjunctiva, sometimes accompanied by discharge and tearing
- Onset in one eye with rapid spread to the other by contamination
- Pain and photophobia with corneal involvement
- Vision unaffected without corneal involvement

Acute bacterial form
- Crust of sticky, mucopurulent discharge (if from *N. gonorrhoeae,* profuse, purulent discharge
- Itching, burning, and sensation of a foreign body in the eye

Viral form
- Copious tearing with minimal exudate
- Enlargement of the preauricular lymph node
- Severely disabling in chronic form

Diagnostic tests
- Physical examination reveals injection of the bulbar conjunctival vessels. In children, systemic signs and symptoms may include sore throat and fever.
- Monocytes are predominant in stained smears of conjunctival scrapings if conjunctivitis is caused by a virus.
- Polymorphonuclear cells (neutrophils) predominate if conjunctivitis stems from bacteria.
- Eosinophils predominate if conjunctivitis is related to allergy.

- Culture and sensitivity tests help identify the causative bacterial organism and indicate appropriate antibiotic therapy.

Treatment
- The cause of conjunctivitis dictates the treatment.
- Bacterial conjunctivitis requires topical application of the appropriate antibiotic or sulfonamide.
- If the causative agent is *N. gonorrhoeae,* a single I.M. dose of ceftriaxone is usually given. If the cornea is involved, a 5-day I.M. course is required.
- Although viral conjunctivitis resists treatment, broad-spectrum antibiotic eyedrops may prevent secondary infection.
- Herpes simplex infection treated with vidarabine ointment or oral acyclovir, but the infection may persist for 2 to 3 weeks.
- Treatment of vernal (allergic) conjunctivitis includes administration of corticosteroid drops followed by ketorolac tromethamine (an ophthalmic anti-inflammatory), cold compresses to relieve itching and, occasionally, an oral antihistamine.

DRUG CHALLENGE

 Instillation of a one-time dose of tetracycline or erythromycin ointment into the eyes of neonates prevents gonococcal and chlamydial conjunctivitis.

Nursing considerations
- Teach proper hand-washing technique because some forms of conjunctivitis are highly contagious. Stress the risk of spreading infection by not sharing washcloths, towels, and pillows. Warn against rubbing the infected eye, which can spread the infection to the other eye and to other persons.

DO'S & DON'TS

 Apply warm compresses and therapeutic ointment or drops. Don't irrigate the eye; this will only spread infection. Have the patient wash his hands before he uses the medication and use clean washcloths or towels frequently so he doesn't infect his other eye.

- Teach the patient to correctly instill eyedrops and ointments; stress the important of not allowing the bottle tip to touch the eye or lashes.
- Stress the importance of safety glasses for the patient who works near chemical irritants.
- Notify public health authorities if cultures show *N. gonorrhoeae.*

 # Corneal abrasion

Commonly caused by a foreign body, a corneal abrasion is a scratch on the surface epithelium of the cornea. An abrasion or foreign body in the eye is the most common eye injury. With treatment, the prognosis is usually good. A corneal scratch produced by a fingernail, a piece of paper, or another organic substance may cause a persistent lesion. The epithelium doesn't always heal properly, and a recurrent corneal erosion may develop, with delayed effects more severe than those of the original injury.

Causes
- Falling asleep wearing hard contact lenses
- Foreign body, such as a cinder or a piece of dust, dirt, or grit, embedded under the eyelid

Signs and symptoms
- Pain disproportionate to the size of the injury

- Redness, increased tearing, a sensation of "something in the eye"
- Visual acuity changes, depending on the size and location of the injury

Diagnostic tests

- Staining the cornea with fluorescein stain confirms the diagnosis. The injured area appears green when examined with a Wood's lamp or black light.
- Slit-lamp examination discloses the depth of the abrasion.
- Examining the eye with a flashlight may reveal a foreign body on the cornea; the eyelid must be everted to check for a foreign body embedded under the lid. Before beginning treatment, a test to determine visual acuity provides a medical baseline and a legal safeguard.

Treatment

- If the foreign object is visible, the eye can be irrigated with normal saline solution.
- Removal of a deeply embedded foreign body is done with a foreign-body spud, using a topical anesthetic.
- A rust ring on the cornea must be removed at the slit-lamp examination with an ophthalmic burr, after applying a topical anesthetic. When only partial removal is possible, reepithelialization lifts the ring again to the surface and allows complete removal the next day.
- Cycloplegic eyedrops and broad-spectrum antibiotic eyedrops are instilled in the affected eye every 3 to 4 hours.

Nursing considerations

- Reassure the patient that the corneal epithelium usually heals in 24 to 48 hours.
- Stress the importance of instilling prescribed antibiotic eyedrops because an untreated corneal infection can lead to ulceration and permanent loss of vision.

Teach the patient the proper way to instill eye medications.
- Emphasize the importance of safety glasses and review instructions for wearing and caring for contact lenses.

Corneal ulcers

A major cause of blindness worldwide, corneal ulcers produce corneal scarring or perforation. They occur in the central or marginal areas of the cornea, vary in shape and size, and may be singular or multiple. Marginal ulcers, caused by a sensitivity to *Staphylococcus aureus,* are the most common form. Prompt treatment (within hours of onset) can prevent visual impairment.

Causes

- Allergens
- Bacterial: *Staphylococcus aureus, Pseudomonas aeruginosa, Streptococcus viridans, Streptococcus (Diplococcus) pneumoniae,* and *Moraxella liquefaciens*
- Fungal: *Candida, Fusarium*, and *Cephalosporium*
- Neurotropic ulcers with fifth cranial nerve lesions
- Reactions to bacterial infections
- Trauma, exposure, and toxins
- Tuberculoprotein: classic phlyctenular keratoconjunctivitis
- Viral: herpes simplex type 1 and varicella-zoster viruses
- Xerophthalmia due to vitamin A deficiency

Signs and symptoms

- Pain (aggravated by blinking) and photophobia followed by increased tearing
- Pronounced visual blurring with central corneal ulceration
- Purulent discharge with bacterial ulcer
- Redness of affected eye

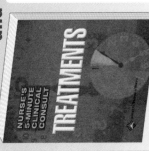

A physicians' favorite expressly for nurses!

Find point-of-care answers on current treatments and the most up-to-date care.

Hallmark, quick-scan page design shows you the full range of disorder treatment details from a nursing point of view, including what the treatment is; its indications and procedural steps; medications, surgeries, and other therapies; care surrounding treatment; potential complications; and nursing interventions. Includes reproducible patient-teaching aids on medications, diet, exercise, daily activities, and more.

☑ **YES! Send *Nurse's 5-Minute Clinical Consult: Treatments* for me to examine FREE.** If I decide to keep it, I'll pay $44.95 plus a small charge for shipping and handling (and sales tax where applicable). Or, I'll return the book within 30 days of receiving it and owe nothing for the book.

Name _____

Address _____ Apt. _____

City _____ State _____ Zip _____

3000000000000H7Z525AD0044955

BRAND NEW

FREE trial!

NURSE'S
5-MINUTE
CLINICAL
CONSULT

TREATMENTS

ISBN: 978-1-58255-512-6
© 2007 Lippincott Williams & Wilkins

Your purchase may qualify as a professional expense for tax purposes in the U.S. Price subject to change. Credit limits may apply. Offer valid in U.S. only.

BUSINESS REPLY MAIL

FIRST-CLASS MAIL   PERMIT NO. 31   HAGERSTOWN, MD

POSTAGE WILL BE PAID BY ADDRESSEE

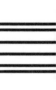

Lippincott Williams & Wilkins

a Wolters Kluwer business

PO BOX 1532
HAGERSTOWN MD 21741-9653

Diagnostic tests

- Flashlight examination reveals an irregular corneal surface, exudate on the cornea, and a hypopyon (accumulation of white cells in the anterior chamber) appearing as a half-moon.
- Fluorescein dye, instilled in the conjunctival sac, shows the outline of the ulcer.
- Culture and sensitivity testing of corneal scrapings identify the causative organism.

Treatment

- Initial treatment consists of administration of a topical broad-spectrum antibiotics until the causative agent is identified.
- *P. aeruginosa* infection is treated with topical ciprofloxacin, gentamicin, or tobramycin.

Do's & don'ts

 A corneal ulcer should never be patched because patching creates the dark, warm, moist environment ideal for bacterial growth. However, it should be protected with a perforated shield.

- Herpes simplex type 1 virus is treated with hourly topical applications of idoxuridine, vidarabine, or trifluridine.
- Fungi are treated with topical instillation of natamycin.
- Cycloplegic eyedrops are given to reduce ciliary body spasms.
- Hypovitaminosis A requires correction of dietary deficiency or GI malabsorption of vitamin A.
- Neurotropic ulcers or exposure keratitis is treated with frequent instillation of artificial tears or lubricating ointments and use of a plastic bubble eye shield or by a tarsorrhaphy (suturing the eyelids together).

Nursing considerations

- Because corneal ulcers are quite painful, give analgesics as needed.
- *P. aeruginosa* infection requires isolation of hospitalized patients.
- Watch for signs of secondary glaucoma (transient vision loss and halos around lights).
- The patient may be more comfortable in a darkened room or when wearing dark glasses.

▍Coronary artery disease

The dominant effect of coronary artery disease (CAD) is the loss of oxygen and nutrients to myocardial tissue because of diminished coronary blood flow. This disease is near epidemic in the Western world. CAD occurs more commonly in men than in women, in whites, and in middle-aged and elderly people. Plaque formation predisposes to thrombosis, which can provoke myocardial infarction (MI).

Causes

- Coronary artery spasms (see *Coronary artery spasm,* page 152)
- Narrowing of the lumen of the coronary arteries due to atherosclerosis, leading to reduced blood flow myocardial ischemia
- Risk factors: family history, hypertension, obesity, smoking, diabetes mellitus, stress, a sedentary lifestyle, and high serum cholesterol and triglyceride levels
- Uncommon causes: dissecting aneurysms, infectious vasculitis, syphilis, and congenital defects in the coronary vascular system

Signs and symptoms

- The classic symptom of CAD: angina—a burning, squeezing, or tight feeling in the substernal or precordial chest,

Coronary artery spasm

A spontaneous, sustained contraction of one or more coronary arteries causes ischemia and dysfunction of the heart muscle in coronary artery spasm. This disorder also causes Prinzmetal's angina and even myocardial infarction in patients with unoccluded coronary arteries.

Cause

Although the cause is unknown, contributing factors include intimal hemorrhage into the medial layer of the blood vessel, hyperventilation, elevated catecholamine levels, fatty buildup in the lumen, and cocaine use.

Signs and symptoms

Severe, prolonged angina pain which occurs spontaneously and may not be related to physical exertion or emotional stress. It may be cyclic, frequently recurring every day at the same time. These ischemic episodes may cause arrhythmias, altered heart rate, lowered blood pressure, and fainting from diminished cardiac output. Spasm in the left coronary artery may result in mitral insufficiency, producing a loud systolic murmur and pulmonary edema, with dyspnea, crackles, hemoptysis, or sudden death.

Diagnosis and treatment

Coronary angiography and electrocardiography facilitate diagnosis. If significant lesions aren't apparent, ergonovine may be given I.V. to precipitate vasospasm. The patient may receive a calcium channel blocker (verapamil, nifedipine, or diltiazem) to reduce coronary artery spasm and vascular resistance as well as a nitrate (nitroglycerin or isosorbide dinitrate) to relieve chest pain.

Nursing considerations

■ When caring for a patient with coronary artery spasm, explain all necessary procedures and teach him how to take his medications safely.
■ For calcium antagonist therapy, monitor blood pressure, pulse rate, and electrocardiogram patterns to detect arrhythmias.
■ For nifedipine and verapamil therapy, monitor digoxin levels and check for signs of digoxin toxicity. Because nifedipine may cause peripheral and periorbital edema, watch for fluid retention.
■ Advise the patient to stop smoking, avoid overeating, use alcohol sparingly, and maintain a balance between exercise and rest.

possibly radiating to the left arm, neck, jaw, or shoulder blade and typically occurring with physical exertion, emotional excitement, exposure to cold, or a large meal
– Stable angina: predictable in frequency and duration; relieved with nitrates and rest
– Unstable angina: increases in frequency and duration; more easily induced
– Prinzmetal's angina: unpredictable coronary artery spasm

ACTION STAT!

 Severe and prolonged anginal pain generally suggests MI, with potentially fatal arrhythmias and mechanical failure. Also, about 50% of women don't have the typical symptoms of angina. These women experience vague symptoms, such as fatigue, shortness of breath, abdominal pain, nausea, or vomiting.

■ Other signs and symptoms:
– Nausea, vomiting
– Fainting

– Sweating
– Cool extremities

Diagnostic tests

- The patient history is crucial in evaluating CAD. Additional diagnostic measures include the following:
- Electrocardiography during angina may show ischemia or be normal; it may also show arrhythmias. The electrocardiogram (ECG) is apt to be normal when the patient is pain-free.
- Treadmill or bicycle exercise test may provoke chest pain and ECG signs of myocardial ischemia (ST-segment depression).
- Coronary angiography reveals narrowing or occlusion of the coronary artery, with possible collateral circulation.
- Myocardial perfusion imaging with thallium-201 or Cardiolite during treadmill exercise detects ischemic areas of the myocardium, visualized as "cold spots."

Treatment

- Reduction of myocardial oxygen demand may be assisted by nitrates, such as nitroglycerin, isosorbide dinitrate, beta-adrenergic blockers (given orally), or calcium channel blockers (given orally).
- Glycoprotein IIb-IIIa inhibitors, such as abciximab, eptifibatide, or tirofiban, may be given to reduce the risk of blood clots.
- Obstructive lesions may necessitate coronary artery bypass grafting (CABG). Keyhole surgery is a minimally invasive coronary artery bypass surgery that may be performed on eligible patients as an alternative to traditional CABG surgery.
- Angioplasty may be performed during cardiac catheterization to compress fatty deposits and relieve occlusion.
- Percutaneous transluminal coronary angioplasty may be done in combination with coronary stenting to provide a framework to hold an artery open.
- Angiogenesis by protein-based therapy with fibroblastic growth factor and vascular endothelial growth factor may be used to increase perfusion in select candidates.

Preventive measures

- Dietary restrictions may include reduced intake of calories (in obesity), dietary fats, and cholesterol.
- Institution of a regular exercise program may be useful.
- Abstention from smoking and reduction of stress are also beneficial.
- Hypertension should be controlled by use of sympathetic blocking agents, such as methyldopa and propranolol, or diuretics such as hydrochlorothiazide.
- Serum cholesterol and triglyceride levels should be controlled by use of antilipemics.
- Administration of aspirin may minimize platelet aggregation and the danger of blood clots.

Nursing considerations

- During anginal episodes, monitor blood pressure and heart rate. Take a 12-lead ECG during anginal episodes and before administering nitroglycerin or other nitrates. Record the duration of pain, amount of medication required to relieve it, and accompanying symptoms.
- Keep nitroglycerin available for immediate use. Instruct the patient to call immediately whenever he feels chest, arm, or neck pain.
- Before cardiac catheterization, explain the procedure to the patient. Make sure he knows why it's necessary, understands the risks, and realizes that it may indicate a need for surgery.
- After catheterization, review the expected course of treatment with the patient and his family. Monitor the catheter

site for bleeding. Also check for distal pulses. To counter the diuretic effect of the dye, make sure the patient drinks plenty of fluids. Maintain bed rest.

■ If the patient is scheduled for surgery, explain the procedure to the patient and his family. Give them a tour of the intensive care unit, and introduce them to the staff.

■ After surgery, monitor blood pressure, intake and output, breath sounds, chest tube drainage, and ECG, watching for signs of ischemia and arrhythmias. Also observe for and treat chest pain and possible dye reactions. Give vigorous chest physiotherapy and guide the patient in coughing and deep-breathing exercises.

■ Before discharge, stress the need to follow the prescribed drug regimen (antihypertensives, nitrates, and antilipemics, for example), exercise program, and diet. Encourage regular, moderate exercise. Refer the patient to a self-help program to stop smoking.

Cor pulmonale

The World Health Organization defines *chronic cor pulmonale* as "hypertrophy of the right ventricle resulting from diseases affecting the function and/or the structure of the lungs, except when these pulmonary alterations are the result of diseases that primarily affect the left side of the heart or of congenital heart disease." It follows a disorder of the lungs, pulmonary vessels, chest wall, or respiratory control center. Because cor pulmonale usually occurs late during the course of chronic obstructive pulmonary disease (COPD) and other irreversible diseases, the prognosis is generally poor. About 85% of patients with cor pulmonale have COPD, and 25% of patients with COPD eventually develop cor pulmonale.

Many patients may live more than 10 to 15 years after diagnosis, but disability slowly increases.

Causes
■ Bronchiectasis and cystic fibrosis
■ COPD
■ Living at high altitudes (chronic mountain sickness)
■ Loss of lung tissue after extensive lung surgery
■ Obesity hypoventilation syndrome (pickwickian syndrome) and upper airway obstruction
■ Pulmonary vascular diseases: recurrent thromboembolism, primary pulmonary hypertension, schistosomiasis, and pulmonary vasculitis
■ Respiratory insufficiency without pulmonary disease: kyphoscoliosis, neuromuscular incompetence resulting from muscular dystrophy or amyotrophic lateral sclerosis, polymyositis, and spinal cord lesions above C6
■ Restrictive lung diseases: pneumoconiosis, interstitial pneumonitis, scleroderma, and sarcoidosis.

Signs and symptoms
■ Chronic productive cough, exertional dyspnea, wheezing respirations, fatigue, and weakness
■ Cor pulmonale and right-sided heart failure: dependent edema, distended neck veins, prominent parasternal or epigastric cardiac impulse, hepatojugular reflux, tachycardia, and enlarged, tender liver
■ Drowsiness and alterations in level of consciousness
■ Progressive disease: dyspnea (even at rest) that worsens on exertion, tachypnea, orthopnea, edema, weakness, and right upper quadrant discomfort
■ Right ventricular early murmur that increases on inspiration
■ Systolic pulmonic ejection click

- Tricuspid insufficiency: pansystolic murmur at the lower left sternal border with increased intensity on inspiration
- Weak pulse and hypotension with decreased cardiac output

Diagnostic tests

- Pulmonary artery pressure (PAP) measurements show increased right ventricular pressure and PAP (systolic pressures will exceed 30 mm Hg; pulmonary artery diastolic pressure will exceed 15 mm Hg).
- Echocardiography or angiography indicates right ventricular enlargement, and echocardiography can estimate PAP.
- Chest X-ray shows large central pulmonary arteries and suggests right ventricular enlargement by rightward enlargement of cardiac silhouette on an anterior chest film.
- Arterial blood gas (ABG) analysis shows decreased partial pressure of arterial oxygen (PaO_2) less than 70 mm Hg.
- Electrocardiography frequently shows arrhythmias, such as premature atrial and ventricular contractions and atrial fibrillation during severe hypoxia; right bundle-branch heart block, right axis deviation, prominent P waves and an inverted T wave in right precordial leads, and right ventricular hypertrophy.
- Pulmonary function tests show results consistent with the underlying pulmonary disease.
- Hematocrit is often greater than 50%.
- Chest examination reveals wheezing, rhonchi, and diminished breath sounds. When secondary to upper airway obstruction or damage to central nervous system respiratory centers, chest findings may be normal except for a right ventricular lift, gallop rhythm, and loud pulmonic component of S_2.

Treatment

- Bed rest

- Treatment may also include administration of:
  - cardiac glycosides (digoxin)
  - antibiotics when respiratory tract infection is present
  - potent pulmonary artery vasodilators (such as diazoxide, nitroprusside, hydralazine, angiotensin-converting enzyme inhibitors, calcium channel blockers, and prostaglandins) in primary pulmonary hypertension
  - oxygen by mask or cannula in concentrations ranging from 24% to 40%, depending on PaO_2, as necessary; in acute cases, therapy may also include mechanical ventilation. Patients with underlying COPD generally shouldn't receive high concentrations of oxygen because of possible subsequent respiratory depression
  - low-sodium diet, restricted fluid intake, and diuretics, such as furosemide, to reduce edema
  - anticoagulation with small doses of heparin to reduce the risk of thromboembolism.
- Lung transplantation may be indicated in end-stage COPD, fibrotic lung disease, or pulmonary hypertension if severe symptoms persist despite maximal medical therapy.
- Tracheotomy may be necessary with upper airway obstruction.
- Steroids may be prescribed for patients with vasculitis autoimmune phenomenon or acute exacerbations of COPD.

Nursing considerations

- The patient will need a diet carefully planned in consultation with the staff dietitian. Because the patient may lack energy and tire easily when eating, provide small, frequent feedings rather than three heavy meals.

DO'S & DON'TS

Living with cor pulmonale

Make sure your patient understands:
■ importance of a low-sodium diet
■ need to weigh himself daily
■ signs and symptoms of edema and the need to report it immediately
■ need for frequent rest periods
■ need to perform breathing exercises daily
■ signs and symptoms of pulmonary infection (increased sputum production, change in sputum color, increased coughing or wheezing, chest pain, fever, tightness in chest) and the need to report it early
■ importance of avoiding crowds and persons with respiratory tract infections, especially during flu season
■ importance of avoiding nonprescribed medications, such as sedatives, which may depress ventilation time.

DRUG CHALLENGE

Monitor serum potassium levels closely if the patient is receiving diuretics. Low serum potassium levels can potentiate the risk of arrhythmias associated with cardiac glycosides.

■ Watch the patient for signs of digoxin toxicity, such as complaints of anorexia, nausea, vomiting, and yellow halos around visual images; monitor for cardiac arrhythmias.
■ Teach the patient to check his radial pulse before taking digoxin or any cardiac glycoside and to report any changes in pulse rate.
■ Reposition the bedridden patient to prevent atelectasis; provide respiratory care (oxygen therapy, pursed-lip breathing exercises).

■ Periodically measure ABG values and watch for signs of respiratory failure, such as a change in pulse rate; deep, labored respirations; and increased fatigue produced by exertion.

Before discharge
■ Provide the patient with information about the disorder. (See *Living with cor pulmonale*.)
■ If the patient needs suctioning or supplemental oxygen therapy at home, refer him to a social service agency that can help him obtain the necessary equipment, and, as necessary, arrange for follow-up examinations.

Creutzfeldt-Jakob disease

Creutzfeldt-Jakob disease (CJD) is a rare, rapidly progressive viral disease that attacks the central nervous system, causing dementia and neurologic signs and symptoms, such as myoclonic jerking, ataxia, aphasia, visual disturbances, and paralysis. It generally affects adults ages 40 to 65 and occurs in more than 50 countries. Males and females are affected equally. CJD is always fatal. A new variant of CJD (vCJD) emerged in Europe in 1996 and is believed to be attributed to *bovine spongiforme encephalopathy,* a fatal disease in cattle also known as *mad cow disease.*

Causes
■ A specific protein called a *prion,* which lacks nucleic acids, resists proteolytic digestion, and spontaneously aggregates in the brain
■ Familial link in 5% to 15% of patients, with an autosomal dominant pattern of inheritance

- Human-to-human transmission with medical procedures, such as corneal and cadaveric dura mater grafts
- Rarely, childhood treatment with human growth hormone and to improperly decontaminated neurosurgical instruments and brain electrodes

Signs and symptoms

- Early, progressive dementia
- Early: slowness in thinking, difficulty concentrating, impaired judgment, and memory loss
- Hallucinations
- With disease progression and mental deterioration: vision disturbances and involuntary movements, such as muscle twitching and trembling

Diagnostic tests

- Neurologic examination is the most effective tool in diagnosing CJD. Difficulty with rapid alternating movements and point-to-point movements are typically evident early in the disease.
- An electroencephalogram may also be performed to assess the patient for typical changes in brain wave activity.
- Computed tomography scan, magnetic resonance imaging of the brain, and lumbar puncture may be useful in ruling out other disorders that cause dementia.
- Definitive diagnosis confirmed by autopsy when brain tissue is examined.

Treatment

- There's no cure for CJD, and its progress can't be slowed. Palliative care is provided to make the patient comfortable and to ease symptoms.

Nursing considerations

- Offer emotional support to the patient and his family. Teach them about the disease, and assist them through the grieving process. Refer the patient and

his family to CJD support groups, and encourage participation.
- Contact social services and hospice, as appropriate, to assist the family with their needs.
- Encourage the family and patient to discuss and complete advance directives.
- To prevent disease transmission, use caution when handling body fluids and other materials from patients suspected of having CJD.

Crohn's disease

Crohn's disease is an inflammation of the alimentary tract characterized by exacerbations and remissions. As the disease progresses, deep ulcers and fissures extend into muscle wall layers, giving rise to characteristic "cobblestone" appearance. Lacteal blockage leads to edema, mucosal inflammation, ulceration, stricturing, and fistula and abscess formation. Absorption is impaired and small bowel obstruction may result. Crohn's disease may lead to intestinal obstruction, fistula formation between the small bowel and the bladder, perianal and perirectal abscesses and fistulas, intra-abdominal abscesses, and perforation.

Crohn's can affect any portion of the tract from the mouth to the anus; 50% of cases involve the colon and small bowel; 33% involve the terminal ileum, and 10% to 20% involve only the colon. The disease can extend through all layers of the intestinal wall and may also involve regional lymph nodes and the mesentery. Crohn's disease occurs equally in both sexes and is more common in people of Jewish ancestry. Onset of the disease is usually before age 30.

Causes

- Allergies
- Genetics
- Immune disorders
- Infection (infecting organism unknown)
- Lymphatic obstruction

Signs and symptoms

Acute disease

- Bleeding (mild or massive)
- Bloody stools
- Diarrhea
- Fever
- Flatulence
- Nausea
- Steady, colicky, pain in the right lower quadrant; cramping; tenderness

Chronic disease

- Abdominal distention and crampy abdominal pain
- Fatigue, weakness
- Fistulas from the colon to small intestine: diarrhea, weight loss, and malnutrition
- Fistulas: asymptomatic or accompanied by fever, chills, tender abdomen, and leukocytosis
- Low-grade fever
- Nonbloody, intermittent diarrhea with right lower quadrant or periumbilical pain
- Weight loss

Diagnostic tests

- Upper GI series with small-bowel follow-through may demonstrate ulcerations, stricture, and fistulas.
- Barium enema showing the string sign (segments of stricture separated by normal bowel) supports the diagnosis.
- Flexible sigmoidoscopy and colonoscopy may show patchy areas of inflammation, ulcers, strictures, and granulomas

- A biopsy is necessary for a definitive diagnosis.
- Laboratory findings usually indicate increased white blood cell count and erythrocyte sedimentation rate, hypokalemia, hypocalcemia, hypomagnesemia, and decreased hemoglobin (Hb) level.

Treatment

- No cure exists for Crohn's disease; treatment is aimed at restoring and maintaining bowel and nutritional status.
- Hyperalimentation may be used to maintain nutrition while resting the bowel.
- Sulfasalazine (an antibacterial) and other 5-ASA (5-amino salicylic acid) agents may be prescribed; metronidazole and ciprofloxacin have proved to be effective in some patients.
- Additional medications may include anti-inflammatory agents, corticosteroids, immunosuppressants (such as azathioprine and mercaptopurine), and an antispasmodic (such as propantheline and dicyclomine) for abdominal cramping.
- Reduced physical activity to help rest the bowel and give it time to heal.
- Dietary changes may include a low-residue diet and, possibly, elimination of dairy products (for lactose intolerance).
- Surgery (colectomy or ileostomy) may be necessary on poor response to medical therapy to correct bowel perforation, massive hemorrhage, intra-abdominal abscess, stricture, fistulas, or acute intestinal obstruction.

Nursing considerations

DRUG CHALLENGE

 If the patient is receiving sulfasalazine, a folic acid supplement should also be given because this medication impairs folate absorption.

- Record fluid intake and output (including the amount of stool), and weigh the patient daily. Watch for dehydration and maintain fluid and electrolyte balance.
- Be alert for signs of intestinal bleeding (bloody stool); check stool daily for occult blood.
- If the patient is receiving a steroid, watch for adverse reactions such as GI bleeding. Remember that steroids can mask signs of infection.
- Check Hb level and hematocrit regularly. Give iron supplements and blood transfusions as needed.
- Observe the patient for fever and pain or pneumaturia, which may signal bladder fistula. Abdominal pain and distention and fever may indicate intestinal obstruction. Watch for stool from the vagina and an enterovaginal fistula.
- Before ileostomy, arrange for a visit by an enterostomal therapist for preoperative education and stoma marking.
- After surgery, frequently check the nasogastric tube for proper functioning. Monitor vital signs and fluid intake and output. Watch for wound infection.
- Provide stoma care, and teach it to the patient and his family.
- Realize that ileostomy changes the patient's body image, so offer reassurance and emotional support.
- Educate the patient regarding stress management techniques; refer to a local support group.

Croup

A severe inflammation and obstruction of the upper airway, croup can occur as acute laryngotracheobronchitis (most common), laryngitis, and acute spasmodic laryngitis. It must always be distinguished from epiglottitis. Croup is a childhood disease affecting boys more commonly than girls (typically between ages 3 months and 3 years) that usually occurs during the winter. Recovery is usually complete.

Causes
- Adenoviruses, respiratory syncytial virus (RSV), influenza and measles viruses
- Bacteria (pertussis and diphtheria)
- Viral infection (parainfluenza viruses in two-thirds of cases)

Signs and symptoms
- Upper respiratory tract infection
- Inspiratory stridor
- Hoarse or muffled vocal sounds
- Laryngeal obstruction and respiratory distress
- Sharp, barklike cough

Laryngotracheobronchitis
- Worsens at night
- Inflammation leading to edema of the bronchi and bronchioles and increasingly difficult expiration
- Fever
- Diffusely decreased breath sounds, expiratory rhonchi, and scattered crackles

Laryngitis
- Usually mild; producing no respiratory distress except in infants
- Sore throat and cough that may progress to hoarseness
- Suprasternal and intercostal retractions
- Inspiratory stridor
- Dyspnea
- Diminished breath sounds
- Restlessness
- In later stages, severe dyspnea and exhaustion

Acute spasmodic laryngitis
- Early: mild to moderate hoarseness and nasal discharge
- Characteristic cough and noisy inspiration (which usually awaken the child at night)
- Labored breathing with retractions
- Rapid pulse and clammy skin
- Anxiety leading to increasing dyspnea and transient cyanosis
- Initially severe symptoms diminishing after several hours but reappearing in a milder form on the next night or two

Diagnostic tests
- Bacterial infection is identified by throat cultures.
- Neck X-rays may show areas of upper airway narrowing and edema in subglottic folds.
- Laryngoscopy may reveal inflammation and obstruction in epiglottal and laryngeal areas.
- Blood cultures can distinguish between bacterial and viral infections.

ACTION STAT!

When evaluating the patient, consider foreign-body obstruction (a common cause of crouplike cough in young children) as well as masses and cysts.

Treatment
- Provide cool humidification during sleep.
- Give antipyretics such as acetaminophen.
- Respiratory distress that interferes with oral hydration requires hospitalization and parenteral fluid replacement to prevent dehydration.
- Antibiotic therapy is necessary for bacterial infection.
- Oxygen therapy may also be required.

- Racemic epinephrine provides temporary relief of stridor; nebulized or parenteral glucocorticoids provide relief in many cases.

Nursing considerations
- Monitor pulse oximetry, and monitor the patient for airway obstruction, which requires endotracheal intubation.

DRUG CHALLENGE

Monitor patient for rebound stridor and respiratory distress, especially if racemic epinephrine is used.

- Carefully monitor cough and breath sounds, hoarseness, severity of retractions, inspiratory stridor, cyanosis, respiratory rate and character (especially prolonged and labored respirations), restlessness, fever, and cardiac rate.
- Keep the child as quiet as possible, but avoid sedation, which can depress respiration.
- If the patient is an infant, position him in an infant seat or prop him up with a pillow; place an older child in high-Fowler's position.
- Isolate patients suspected of having RSV and parainfluenza infections, if possible. Instruct parents and others involved in the care of these children to wash hands thoroughly to prevent spreading the disorder.
- Control fever with sponge baths and an antipyretic. Keep a hypothermia blanket on hand in case the patient's temperatures goes above 102° F (38.9° C). Watch for seizures in infants and young children with high fevers. Give an I.V. antibiotic as necessary.

DO'S & DON'TS

Relieve sore throat with soothing, water-based ices, such as fruit sherbet and ice pops. Avoid thicker, milk-based fluids if the child is producing heavy mucus or has great difficulty swallowing.

- Apply petroleum jelly or another ointment around the nose and lips to soothe irritation from nasal discharge and mouth breathing.
- To relieve croupy spells, tell parents to carry the child into the bathroom, shut the door, and turn on the hot water. Breathing in warm, moist air quickly eases an acute spell of croup. Suggest the use of a cool-mist humidifier (vaporizer).
- Warn parents that complications of croup may include ear infections and pneumonia, which may appear about 5 days after recovery. Stress the importance of reporting earache, productive cough, high fever, or increased shortness of breath immediately.

Cryptococcosis

The airborne fungus *Cryptococcus neoformans* causes cryptococcosis, also called *torulosis* and *European blastomycosis*. Cryptococcosis usually begins as an asymptomatic pulmonary infection but disseminates to extrapulmonary sites, usually to the central nervous system (CNS) but also to the skin, bones, prostate gland, liver, or kidneys. Cryptococcosis is most prevalent in men and is rare in children. It's especially likely to develop in immunocompromised patients, such as those with Hodgkin's disease, sarcoidosis, leukemia, or lymphoma and those who are receiving immunosuppressive agents. Patients with late infection with human immunodeficiency virus are by far the most commonly affected group. With appropriate treatment, the prognosis in pulmonary cryptococcosis is good. CNS infection, however, can be fatal, but treatment dramatically reduces mortality. Complica-tions include optic atrophy, ataxia, hydrocephalus, deafness, paralysis, chronic brain syndrome, and personality changes.

Causes
- Transmission through inhalation of *C. neoformans* in particles of dust contaminated by pigeon stool that harbor the organism

Signs and symptoms
- Bone involvement: painful osseous lesions of the long bones, skull, spine, and joints
- Gradual onset of CNS involvement: progressively severe frontal and temporal headache, diplopia, blurred vision, dizziness, ataxia, aphasia, vomiting, tinnitus, memory changes, inappropriate behavior, irritability, psychotic symptoms, seizures, fever, coma, and death
- Skin involvement: red facial papules and other skin abscesses, with or without ulcerations

Diagnostic tests
- A routine chest X-ray showing a pulmonary lesion may point to pulmonary cryptococcosis.
- Identification of *C. neoformans* is obtained by culture of sputum, urine, prostatic secretions, bone marrow aspirate or biopsy, pleural biopsy, or an India ink preparation of cerebrospinal fluid (CSF) and culture.
- Blood cultures are positive only in severe infection.
- Increased antigen titer in serum and CSF are diagnostic in disseminated infection.
- Increased CSF pressure, protein, and white blood cell count also indicate CNS infection.
- About 50% of patients demonstrate moderately decreased CSF glucose levels.

Treatment

- Disseminated infection is treated with I.V. amphotericin B or fluconazole.
- Patients with acquired immunodeficiency syndrome also need long-term therapy (oral fluconazole).
- Single, intensive course of treatment is given until cultures from the infected site return negative.

Nursing considerations

- Cryptococcosis doesn't require isolation.
- Check the patient's vital functions, and note any changes in mental status, orientation, pupillary response, and motor function.
- Watch for headache, vomiting, and nuchal rigidity.

DRUG CHALLENGE

Before giving I.V. amphotericin B, check for phlebitis. Infuse slowly and dilute—rapid infusion may cause circulatory collapse.

DO'S & DON'TS

Before therapy, draw blood for a serum electrolyte analysis to determine baseline renal status. During drug therapy, watch for decreased urine output, elevated blood urea nitrogen and creatinine levels, and hypokalemia.

- Monitor results of complete blood count, urinalysis, magnesium and potassium levels, and liver function tests. Ask the patient to report hearing loss, tinnitus, or dizziness.
- Provide psychological support to help the patient cope with long-term hospitalization.

Cushing's syndrome

A cluster of clinical abnormalities characterize Cushing's syndrome. These abnormalities result from excessive levels of adrenocortical hormones (particularly cortisol) or related corticosteroids and, to a lesser extent, androgens and aldosterone. Its signs include adiposity of the face (moon face), neck, and trunk and purple striae on the skin. Cushing's syndrome is most common in women. The prognosis depends on the underlying cause; it's poor in untreated persons and in those with untreatable ectopic corticotropin-producing carcinoma. (See *Dealing with lifelong treatment.*)

Causes

- Cortisol-secreting adrenal tumor (about 30% of patients; usually benign)
- Excess production of corticotropin and consequent hyperplasia of the adrenal cortex (about 70% of patients) due to pituitary hypersecretion (Cushing's disease), corticotropin-producing tumor in another organ (particularly bronchogenic or pancreatic carcinoma) or excessive administration of exogenous glucocorticoids
- In infants: adrenal adenoma or carcinoma

Signs and symptoms

- Cardiovascular: hypertension from sodium and water retention, left ventricular hypertrophy, capillary weakness from protein loss leading to bleeding and ecchymosis
- Central nervous system (CNS): irritability and emotional lability (euphoric behavior to depression or psychosis), insomnia
- Endocrine and metabolic: diabetes mellitus, with decreased glucose tolerance, fasting hyperglycemia, and glycosuria

- GI: peptic ulcer from increased gastric secretions and pepsin production, and decreased gastric mucus
- Immunologic: increased susceptibility to infection due to decreased lymphocyte production and suppressed antibody formation, decreased resistance to stress, suppressed inflammatory response
- Musculoskeletal: muscle weakness from hypokalemia, loss of muscle mass from increased catabolism, pathologic fractures from decreased bone mineral, and skeletal growth retardation in children
- Renal and urologic: sodium and secondary fluid retention, increased potassium excretion, inhibited secretion of antidiuretic hormone, ureteral calculi from increased bone demineralization with hypercalciuria
- Reproductive: increased androgen production, with clitoral hypertrophy, mild virilism, and amenorrhea or oligomenorrhea in women; sexual dysfunction
- Skin: acne, purplish striae, little or no scar formation, poor wound healing, hirsutism (in women) and fat pads above the clavicles, over the upper back (buffalo hump), on the face (moon face), and throughout the trunk, with slender arms and legs

Diagnostic tests

- Cortisol levels don't fluctuate and remain consistently elevated; a 24-hour urine sample demonstrates elevated free cortisol levels.
- A low-dose dexamethasone suppression test confirms the diagnosis; high-dose dexamethasone suppression test differentiate pituitary dysfunction (Cushing's disease) from adenoma of the adrenal gland or ectopic corticotropin secretion.
- Stimulation test measure the ability of the pituitary gland and the hypothala-

> ## Dealing with lifelong treatment
>
> The patient who has been treated for Cushing's syndrome with hypophysectomy or adrenalectomy needs careful instruction to help him cope with lifelong steroid replacement. Make sure you teach him to:
> - take replacement steroids with antacids or meals to minimize gastric irritation—two-thirds in the morning and the remaining third in the early afternoon to mimic diurnal adrenal secretion
> - carry a medical identification card
> - immediately report physiologically stressful situations, such as infections, so his steroid dose can be increased
> - watch closely for fatigue, weakness, and dizziness (symptoms of inadequate steroid dose) as well as severe swelling and weight gain (signs of overdose)
> - take his steroids exactly as prescribed; abrupt discontinuation could produce a fatal adrenal crisis.

mus to detect and correct low levels of plasma cortisol by increasing corticotropin production. The patient reacts by secreting an excess of plasma corticotropin as measured by levels of urinary 17-OHCS. If the patient has an adrenal or a nonendocrine corticotropin-secreting tumor, the pituitary gland can't respond normally, so steroid levels remain stable or fall.

- Ultrasonography, a computed tomography (CT) scan, magnetic resonance imaging (MRI), or angiography localizes adrenal tumors; a CT scan and MRI of the head identify pituitary tumors.

Treatment

- Pituitary-dependent Cushing's syndrome with adrenal hyperplasia and severe cushingoid symptoms may require hypophysectomy or pituitary irradiation
- If the patient fails to respond, bilateral adrenalectomy may be performed.
- Nonendocrine corticotropin-producing tumors require excision of the tumor. Drug therapy follows (for example, with mitotane, metyrapone, or aminoglutethimide) to decrease cortisol levels if symptoms persist.
- Aminoglutethimide and ketoconazole decrease cortisol levels.
- Aminoglutethimide alone or with metyrapone is useful in metastatic adrenal carcinoma.

DRUG CHALLENGE

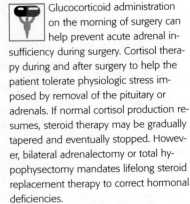 Glucocorticoid administration on the morning of surgery can help prevent acute adrenal insufficiency during surgery. Cortisol therapy during and after surgery to help the patient tolerate physiologic stress imposed by removal of the pituitary or adrenals. If normal cortisol production resumes, steroid therapy may be gradually tapered and eventually stopped. However, bilateral adrenalectomy or total hypophysectomy mandates lifelong steroid replacement therapy to correct hormonal deficiencies.

Nursing considerations

- Frequently monitor vital signs, especially blood pressure. Carefully observe the hypertensive patient who also has cardiac disease.
- Check laboratory reports for hypernatremia, hypokalemia, hyperglycemia, and glycosuria.
- Because the cushingoid patient is likely to retain sodium and water, check for

edema, and monitor daily weight and intake and output carefully.
- To minimize weight gain, edema, and hypertension, ask the dietary department to provide a diet that's high in protein and potassium but low in calories, carbohydrates, and sodium.
- If the patient has osteoporosis and is bedridden, perform passive range-of-motion exercises carefully because of the severe risk for pathologic fractures.

After surgery

- Watch carefully for wound drainage or temperature elevation. Use strict aseptic.
- Monitor urine output and check vital signs carefully, watching for signs of shock (decreased blood pressure, increased pulse rate, pallor, and cold, clammy skin).

DRUG CHALLENGE

 Because mitotane, aminoglutethimide, and metyrapone decrease mental alertness and produce physical weakness, assess neurologic and behavioral status, and warn the patient of adverse CNS effects.

- Watch for severe nausea, vomiting, and diarrhea.
- Check laboratory reports for hypoglycemia from removal of the source of cortisol, a hormone that maintains blood glucose levels.
- Check regularly for signs of adrenal hypofunction—orthostatic hypotension, apathy, weakness, and fatigue—indicators that steroid replacement is inadequate.

ALERT

 In the patient undergoing pituitary surgery, be alert for signs of increased intracranial pressure (confusion, agitation, changes in level of consciousness, nausea, and vomiting). Also, watch for hypopituitarism.

- Teach the patient about the need for continued steroid therapy.

Cystic fibrosis

Sometimes called *mucoviscidosis,* cystic fibrosis, a chronic disease, is a generalized dysfunction of the exocrine glands that affects multiple organ systems. It's the most common fatal genetic disease of White children. Incidence of cystic fibrosis is highest in people of northern European ancestry and lowest in Blacks, Native Americans, and people of Asian ancestry. The immediate causes of symptoms are increased viscosity of bronchial, pancreatic, and other mucous gland secretions and consequent obstruction of glandular ducts. Cystic fibrosis accounts for almost all cases of pancreatic enzyme deficiency in children.

Causes
- Mutation (deletion resulting in absence of phenylalanine) in a gene located on chromosome 7q

Signs and symptoms
- May occur soon after birth or take years to develop
- Sweat gland dysfunction producing increased levels of sodium and chloride in the sweat

Respiratory
- Wheezy respirations
- Dry, nonproductive, paroxysmal cough
- Dyspnea
- Tachypnea
- Thick, tenacious secretions leading to severe atelectasis and emphysema
- Barrel chest, cyanosis, and clubbing of the fingers and toes
- Recurring bronchitis and pneumonia

- Death results from pneumonia, emphysema, or atelectasis

Gastrointestinal
- Meconium ileus in the newborn with symptoms of intestinal obstruction (abdominal distention, vomiting, constipation, dehydration, and electrolyte imbalance)
- Frequent, bulky, foul-smelling, and pale stool with a high fat content
- Poor weight gain, poor growth, ravenous appetite, distended abdomen, thin extremities, and sallow skin with poor turgor from malabsorption
- Deficiency of fat-soluble vitamins (A, D, E, and K), leading to clotting problems, retarded bone growth, and delayed sexual development (congenital bilateral absence of the vas deferens, causing sterility; possible secondary amenorrhea in females
- Rectal prolapse from malnutrition and wasting of perirectal supporting tissues
- Pancreatic insufficiency with insufficient insulin production, abnormal glucose tolerance, and glycosuria
- Biliary obstruction and fibrosis
- Cirrhosis and portal hypertension, possibly leading to esophageal varices, episodes of hematemesis and hepatomegaly, or both

Diagnostic tests
- The Cystic Fibrosis Foundation sets the following standards for a definitive diagnosis:
  - Two sweat tests using a pilocarpine solution (a sweat inducer) are clearly positive; the patient also has either an obstructive pulmonary disease, confirmed pancreatic insufficiency or failure to thrive, or a family history of cystic fibrosis.
  - Chest X-rays indicate early signs of obstructive lung disease.

– Stool specimen analysis indicates the absence of trypsin, suggesting pancreatic insufficiency.
- The following test results may support the diagnosis:
  – Deoxyribonucleic acid testing locates the presence of the Delta F 508 deletion (found in about 70% of patients). This test can also be used for carrier detection and a prenatal diagnosis.
  – Pulmonary function tests reveal decreased vital capacity, elevated residual volume from air entrapments, and decreased forced expiratory volume in 1 second.
  – Liver enzyme test may reveal hepatic insufficiency.
  – Sputum culture reveals organisms chronically colonized (*Staphylococcus* and *Pseudomonas*).
  – Serum albumin levels help assess nutritional status.
  – Electrolyte analysis assesses dehydration and glucose levels.

Treatment

- The aim of treatment is to help the child lead as normal a life as possible. Specific treatment depends on the organ systems involved.
  – To combat sweat electrolyte losses, generous salting of foods and, during hot weather, sodium supplements are given.
  – To offset pancreatic enzyme deficiencies, oral pancreatic enzymes are given with meals and snacks. The diet should be low in fat but high in protein and calories, and include supplements of water-miscible, fat-soluble vitamins (A, D, E, and K).
  – Management of pulmonary dysfunction includes chest physiotherapy, postural drainage, and breathing exercises; a flutter valve may be used in some cases.

DRUG CHALLENGE

Antihistamines are contraindicated; they have a drying effect on mucous membranes, making expectoration of mucus difficult or impossible.

- Aerosol therapy includes intermittent nebulizer treatments before postural drainage to loosen secretions. Dornase alfa, a pulmonary enzyme helps thin airway mucus, improving lung function and reducing the risk of pulmonary infection.
- Broad-spectrum antimicrobials combat infection.
- Oxygen therapy is used as needed.
- Heart-lung transplantation may be necessary to reduce the effects of the disease.
- Aerosol gene therapy shows promise in reducing pulmonary symptoms.

Nursing considerations

- Suggest the use of air conditioners and humidifiers to help decrease vulnerability to respiratory tract infections. Emphasize keeping these units clean to prevent accumulation of organisms that increase the risk of infection.
- Throughout this illness, teach the patient and his family about the disease and its treatment.
- Provide emotional support, and refer the patient and his family for genetic counseling and to the Cystic Fibrosis Foundation.

Cytomegalovirus infection

Also called *generalized salivary gland disease* and *cytomegalic inclusion disease,* cytomegalovirus (CMV) infection is caused by the cytomegalovirus, which is a deoxyribonucleic acid, ether-sensitive virus belonging to the herpes family. The disease occurs worldwide and is transmitted by human contact. About four out of five persons older than age 35 have been infected with CMV, usually during childhood or early adulthood. In most of these people, the disease is so mild that it's overlooked. Immunosuppressed patients, especially those who have received transplanted organs, run a 90% chance of contracting CMV infection. Recipients of blood transfusions from donors with positive CMV antibodies are at some risk. Be aware that CMV infection during pregnancy can be hazardous to the fetus, possibly leading to stillbirth, brain damage, and other birth defects or to severe neonatal illness.

Causes

- Contact with infected secretions (saliva, urine, semen, breast milk, stool, blood, vaginal, cervical)
- Passage through birth canal
- Sexual contact

Signs and symptoms

- Cytomegalovirus mononucleosis with 3 weeks or more of irregular, high fever (in adults)
- Disseminated CMV infection, possibly leading to chorioretinitis (resulting in blindness), colitis, or encephalitis (in patients with acquired immunodeficiency syndrome)
- Infected infants ages 3 to 6 months: usually asymptomatic or, possibly, hepatic dysfunction, hepatosplenomegaly, spider angiomas, pneumonitis, lymphadenopathy, and brain damage
- Mild, nonspecific complaints
- Pneumonia and secondary infections in patients with immunodeficiency and those receiving immunosuppressants

ACTION STAT!

 Occasionally, CMV infection shows up as a rapidly fatal neonatal illness characterized by jaundice, petechial rash, hepatosplenomegaly, thrombocytopenia, hemolytic anemia, microcephaly, psychomotor retardation, mental deficiency, and hearing loss.

Diagnostic tests

- Virus isolation in urine or from saliva, throat, cervix, white blood cell, and biopsy specimens confirm diagnosis.
- Other laboratory tests support the diagnosis, including complement fixation studies, hemagglutination inhibition antibody tests and, for congenital infections, indirect immunofluorescent tests for CMV immunoglobulin M antibody.

Treatment

- Because CMV infection is usually self-limiting, treatment aims to relieve symptoms and prevent complications.
- In the immunosuppressed patient, acyclovir, ganciclovir, valganciclovir, cidofovir, and foscarnet, combined with anti-CMV immune globulin for pneumonitis and possible GI disease.

Nursing considerations

- Provide parents of children with severe congenital CMV infection with counseling to help them cope with the possibility of brain damage or death.
- To help prevent CMV infection, warn immunosuppressed patients and pregnant women to avoid exposure to confirmed or suspected CMV infection. Tell pregnant patients that maternal CMV infection can cause serious fetal abnormalities.

■ Urge patients with CMV infection to wash their hands thoroughly to prevent spreading it.
■ Observe standard precautions when handling body secretions.

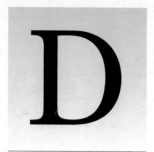

Dermatitis

An inflammation of the skin, dermatitis occurs in several forms: atopic, seborrheic, nummular, contact, chronic, localized neurodermatitis (lichen simplex chronicus), exfoliative, and stasis. (See *Types of dermatitis,* pages 170 to 175.)

Atopic dermatitis (atopic or infantile eczema) is a chronic or recurrent inflammatory response commonly associated with other atopic diseases, such as bronchial asthma and allergic rhinitis. It usually develops in infants and toddlers between ages 1 month to 1 year, commonly in those with strong family histories of atopic disease. These children usually acquire other atopic disorders as they grow older. Typically, this form of dermatitis flares and subsides repeatedly before finally resolving during adolescence. However, it can persist into adulthood. Atopic dermatitis affects about 9 out of every 1,000 persons.

Causes

- Unknown
- Flare-ups: response to sweating, psychological stress, and extremes in temperature and humidity
- Food allergies (eggs, peanuts, milk, and wheat) in about 10% of childhood cases
- Genetic predisposition exacerbated by food allergies, infections, irritating chemicals, temperature and humidity, and emotions
- Secondary cause: irritation that seems to change the epidermal structure, allowing immunoglobulin (Ig) E activity to increase

Signs and symptoms

- Erythematous areas on excessively dry skin; in children, lesions of the forehead, cheeks, and extensor surfaces of the arms and legs; in adults, lesions of flexion points (antecubital fossa, popliteal area, and neck)
- Pruritus and scratching with edema, crusting, and scaling
- Chronic atopic lesions leading to dry, scaly skin, with white dermatographia, blanching, and lichenification
- Secondary conditions: viral, fungal, or bacterial infections and ocular disorders
- Upper eyelid swelling and hyperpigmentation, with a double fold occurring under the lower lid (Morgan's, Dennie's, or Mongolian fold)
- Rarely, atopic cataracts (usually limited to people between ages 20 and 40)
- In patients who are exposed to herpes simplex, Kaposi's varicelliform eruption (eczema herpeticum), a potentially serious widespread cutaneous viral infection

(Text continues on page 174.)

Types of dermatitis

Type	Causes	Signs and symptoms
Contact dermatitis Commonly sharply demarcated inflammation of the skin resulting from contact with an irritating chemical or atopic allergen (a substance producing an allergic reaction in the skin) and irritation of the skin resulting from contact with concentrated substances to which the skin is sensitive, such as perfumes, soaps, or chemicals	■ Mild irritants: chronic exposure to detergents or solvents ■ Strong irritants: damage on contact with acids or alkalis ■ Allergens: sensitization after repeated exposure	■ Mild irritants and allergens: erythema and small vesicles that ooze, scale, and itch ■ Strong irritants: blisters and ulcerations ■ Classic allergic response: clearly defined lesions, with straight lines following points of contact ■ Severe allergic reaction: marked erythema, blistering, and edema of affected areas
Exfoliative dermatitis Severe skin inflammation characterized by redness and widespread erythema and scaling, covering virtually the entire skin surface	■ Preexisting skin lesions progressing to exfoliative stage, such as in contact dermatitis, drug reaction, lymphoma, leukemia, or atopic dermatitis ■ May be idiopathic	■ Generalized dermatitis, with acute loss of stratum corneum, and erythema and scaling ■ Sensation of tight skin ■ Hair loss ■ Possible fever, sensitivity to cold, shivering, gynecomastia, and lymphadenopathy
Hand or foot dermatitis Skin disease characterized by inflammatory eruptions of the hands or feet	■ In many cases, unknown but may result from irritant or allergic contact ■ Excessive skin dryness typically a contributing factor ■ Fifty percent of patients are atopic	■ Redness and scaling of the palms or soles ■ May produce painful fissures ■ Some cases present with blisters (dyshidrotic eczema)

Diagnosis	Treatment and interventions
▪ Patient history, patch testing to identify allergens, and shape and distribution of lesions suggest contact dermatitis.	▪ Elimination of known allergens and decreased exposure to irritants; wearing protective clothing, such as gloves; and washing immediately after contact with irritants or allergens ▪ Topical anti-inflammatory agents (including corticosteroids), systemic corticosteroids for edema and bullae, antihistamines, and local applications of Burow's solution (for blisters) ▪ Same as for atopic dermatitis
▪ Diagnosis requires identification of the underlying cause.	▪ Hospitalization, with protective isolation and hygienic measures to prevent secondary bacterial infection ▪ Open wet dressings, with colloidal baths ▪ Bland lotions over topical corticosteroids ▪ Maintenance of constant environmental temperature to prevent chilling or overheating ▪ Careful monitoring of renal and cardiac status ▪ Systemic antibiotics and steroids ▪ Same as for atopic dermatitis
▪ Patient history and physical findings (distribution of eruption on palms and soles) confirm diagnosis.	▪ Same as for nummular dermatitis ▪ Severe cases may require systemic steroids

(continued)

Types of dermatitis *(continued)*

Type	Causes	Signs and symptoms
Localized neurodermatitis (lichen simplex chronicus, essential pruritus) Superficial inflammation of the skin characterized by itching and papular eruptions that appear on thickened, hyperpigmented skin	▪ Chronic scratching or rubbing of a primary lesion or insect bite, or other skin irritation ▪ May be psychogenic	▪ Intense, sometimes continual scratching ▪ Thick, sharp-bordered, possibly dry, scaly lesions with raised papules and accentuated skin lines (lichenification) ▪ Usually affects easily reached areas, such as ankles, lower legs, anogenital area, back of neck, and ears ▪ One or a few lesions may be present; asymmetric distribution
Nummular dermatitis Subacute form of dermatitis characterized by inflammation in coin-shaped, scaling, or vesicular patches, usually quite pruritic	▪ Possibly precipitated by stress, skin dryness, irritants, or scratching	▪ Round, nummular (coin-shaped), red lesions, usually on arms and legs, with distinct borders of crusts and scales ▪ Possible oozing and severe itching ▪ Summertime remissions common, with wintertime recurrence
Seborrheic dermatitis Subacute skin disease that affects the scalp, face, and occasionally other areas and is characterized by lesions covered with yellow or brownish gray scales	▪ Unknown; stress, immunodeficiency, and neurologic conditions may be predisposing factors; related to the yeast *Pityrosporum ovale* (normal flora)	▪ Eruptions in areas with many sebaceous glands (usually scalp, face, chest, axillae, and groin) and in skin folds ▪ Itching, redness, and inflammation of affected areas; lesions may appear greasy; fissures may occur ▪ Indistinct, occasionally yellowish, scaly patches from excess stratum corneum (Dandruff may be a mild seborrheic dermatitis.)

Diagnosis	Treatment and interventions
■ Physical findings confirm diagnosis.	■ Scratching must stop; then lesions will disappear in about 2 weeks ■ Fixed dressings or Unna's boot to cover affected areas ■ Topical corticosteroids under occlusion or by intralesional injection ■ Antihistamines and open wet dressings ■ Emollients ■ Patient informed about underlying cause
■ Physical findings and patient history confirm nummular dermatitis. ■ Diagnosis must rule out fungal infections, atopic or contact dermatitis, and psoriasis.	■ Elimination of known irritants ■ Measures to relieve dry skin: increased humidification, limited frequency of baths and use of bland soap and bath oils, and application of emollients ■ Application of wet dressings in acute phase ■ Topical corticosteroids (occlusive dressings or intralesional injections) for persistent lesions ■ Tar preparations and antihistamines to control itching ■ Antibiotics for secondary infection ■ Same as for atopic dermatitis
■ Patient history and physical findings, especially distribution of lesions in sebaceous gland areas, confirm seborrheic dermatitis. ■ Diagnosis must rule out psoriasis.	■ Removal of scales with frequent washing and shampooing with selenium sulfide suspension (most effective), zinc pyrithione, or tar and salicylic acid shampoo ■ Application of topical corticosteroids and antifungals to involved area

(continued)

Types of dermatitis *(continued)*

Type	Causes	Signs and symptoms
Stasis dermatitis A condition usually caused by impaired circulation and characterized by eczema of the legs with edema, hyperpigmentation, and persistent inflammation	▪ Secondary to peripheral vascular diseases affecting legs, such as recurrent thrombophlebitis and resultant chronic venous insufficiency	▪ Varicosities and edema common, but obvious vascular insufficiency not always present ▪ Usually affects the lower leg, just above internal malleolus, or sites of trauma or irritation ▪ Early signs: dusky red deposits of hemosiderin in skin, with itching and dimpling of subcutaneous tissue ▪ Later signs: edema, redness, and scaling of large areas of legs ▪ Possible fissures, crusts, and ulcers

Diagnostic tests

▪ A family history of atopic disorders is helpful in diagnosis of atopic dermatitis.
▪ Patch testing and inspecting the distribution of skin lesions help pinpoint the provoking allergen.
▪ Serum IgE levels are commonly elevated but aren't diagnostic.

Treatment

▪ Eliminate allergens.
▪ Avoid irritants (strong soaps, cleansers, and other chemicals), extreme temperature changes, and other precipitating factors.
▪ Application of topical corticosteroid ointment, especially after bathing, usually alleviates inflammation.
▪ Application of a moisturizing cream or petroleum jelly can help the skin retain moisture.
▪ Systemic corticosteroid therapy may be required during extreme exacerbations.
▪ Weak tar preparations and ultraviolet B light therapy are used to increase the thickness of the stratum corneum.
▪ Antibiotics are appropriate for crusted and weeping lesions.

Nursing considerations

▪ Warn the patient that drowsiness is possible with the use of antihistamines to relieve daytime itching. If nocturnal itching interferes with sleep, suggest methods for inducing natural sleep such as drinking a glass of warm milk to prevent overuse of sedatives. Antihistamines may also be useful at bedtime.
▪ Inform the patient about bathing restrictions: use of plain, tepid (96° F [35.6° C]) water and nonfatty, nonperfumed soap; limitation of baths or showers to 5 to 7 minutes; and avoidance of any soap when lesions are acutely inflamed.
▪ For scalp involvement, advise the patient to shampoo frequently and apply corticosteroid solution to the scalp afterward.
▪ Advise him to keep fingernails short to limit excoriation and secondary infections caused by scratching.
▪ Instruct the patient to lubricate the skin after a shower or bath.
▪ To help clear lichenified skin, apply occlusive dressings (such as plastic film) over a corticosteroid cream intermittently as necessary.

Diagnosis	Treatment and interventions
▪ Diagnosis requires positive history of venous insufficiency and physical findings, such as varicosities.	▪ Measures to prevent venous stasis: avoidance of prolonged sitting or standing, use of support stockings, weight reduction in obesity, and leg elevation ▪ Corrective surgery for underlying cause ▪ After ulcer develops, rest periods with legs elevated; open wet dressings; Unna's boot (zinc gelatin dressing provides continuous pressure to affected areas); and antibiotics for secondary infection after wound culture

▪ Inform the patient that irritants, such as detergents and wool, and emotional stress exacerbate atopic dermatitis.

▪ Arrange for counseling, if necessary, to help the patient deal with the condition more effectively.

Dermatophytosis

Also called *tinea* or *ringworm*, dermatophytosis is a disease that can affect the scalp (tinea capitis), body (tinea corporis), nails (tinea unguium), feet (tinea pedis), groin (tinea cruris), and bearded skin (tinea barbae). Tinea infections are quite prevalent in the United States and are usually more common in males than in females. With effective treatment, the cure rate is very high, although about 20% of persons with infected feet or nails develop chronic conditions.

Causes
▪ Contact with animals or soil
▪ Contact with contaminated articles, such as shoes, towels, or shower stalls
▪ Contact with infected lesions
▪ Dermatophytes (noncandidal fungi) of the genera *Trichophyton*, *Microsporum*, and *Epidermophyton* that involve the stratum corneum, nails, or hair

Signs and symptoms
▪ Tinea barbae: uncommon infection of the bearded facial area
▪ Tinea capitis: round erythematous patches on the scalp causing hair loss with scaling; occasional hypersensitivity reaction in children, leading to boggy, inflamed, commonly pus-filled lesions (kerions)
▪ Tinea corporis: flat lesions on the skin at any site except the scalp, bearded skin, groin, palms, or soles; may be dry and scaly or moist and crusty; classic ring-shaped appearance due to growth of edges with central healing
▪ Tinea cruris (jock itch): red, raised, sharply defined, itchy lesions in the groin that may extend to the buttocks, inner thighs, and the external genitalia
▪ Tinea pedis: scaling and blisters between the toes, inflammation, severe itching and pain on walking; and, possibly, dry, squamous inflammation of the entire sole
▪ Tinea unguium (onychomycosis): typically starts at the tip of one or more toe-

nails (fingernail infection is less common) and produces gradual thickening, discoloration, crumbling, and possible destruction of the nail, with accumulation of subungual debris

Diagnostic tests

- Microscopic examination of lesion scrapings prepared in 10% to 20% potassium hydroxide solution usually confirms tinea infection.
- Wood's light examination is useful in only about 5% of cases of tinea capitis.
- Cultures of the affected area may help to identify the infecting organism.

Treatment

- Topical agents (imidazole cream, oral griseofulvin) is especially effective in skin and hair infections.
- Oral terbinafine or itraconazole is helpful in nail infections.

Topical therapy is ineffective for tinea capitis; oral griseofulvin for 1 to 3 months is the treatment of choice. Griseofulvin is contraindicated in the patient with porphyria, and it may necessitate an increase in dosage during anticoagulant (warfarin) therapy.

- Antifungals include naftifine, ciclopirox, terbinafine, and tolnaftate. Topical treatments should continue for 2 weeks after lesions resolve.
- Supportive measures include open wet dressings, removal of scabs and scales, application of keratolytics (such as salicylic acid to soften and remove lesions of the heels or soles).

Nursing considerations

- For all tinea infections except those of the hair and nails, apply topical agents, watch for sensitivity reactions and secondary bacterial infections, and provide patient teaching.
- Monitor liver function of patients on long-term griseofulvin therapy.

DO'S & DON'TS

For tinea capitis, use good hand hygiene, and teach the patient to do the same. To prevent spreading infection to others, advise the patient to wash towels, bedclothes, and combs frequently in hot water and avoid sharing them. Suggest that family members be checked for tinea capitis.

- For tinea corporis, use abdominal pads between skin folds for the patient with excessive abdominal girth; change pads frequently. Check the patient daily for excoriated, newly denuded areas of skin. If the involved area is moist, apply open wet dressings two or three times per day to decrease inflammation and help remove scales.
- For tinea unguium, keep the patient's nails short and straight. Gently remove debris under the nails with an emery board.
- For tinea pedis, encourage the patient to expose feet to air whenever possible and to wear sandals or leather shoes and clean cotton socks. Instruct him to wash the feet twice per day, dry thoroughly, and apply antifungal cream followed by antifungal powder to absorb perspiration and prevent excoriation.
- For tinea cruris, instruct the patient to dry the affected area thoroughly after bathing and to apply a topical antifungal agent followed by antifungal powder. Inform him that warm weather and tight clothing encourage fungus growth. Advise wearing loose-fitting clothing, which should be changed frequently and washed in hot water.

■ For tinea barbae, suggest that the patient let his beard grow. Advise him to trim whiskers with scissors, not a razor. If the patient insists that he must shave, advise him to use an electric razor instead of a blade.

Diabetes insipidus

A disorder of water metabolism, diabetes insipidus results from a deficiency of circulating vasopressin (also called antidiuretic hormone) or from renal resistance to this hormone. Pituitary diabetes insipidus is caused by deficiency of vasopressin, whereas nephrogenic diabetes insipidus is caused by renal tubular resistance to the action of vasopressin. Diabetes insipidus is characterized by excessive fluid intake and hypotonic polyuria. In uncomplicated diabetes insipidus, the prognosis is good with adequate water replacement, and patients usually lead normal lives.

Causes
■ A skull fracture or head trauma that damages the neurohypophyseal structures
■ Granulomatous disease
■ Hypophysectomy or other neurosurgery
■ Idiopathic or, rarely, familial
■ Infection
■ Intracranial neoplastic or metastatic lesions
■ Vascular lesions

Signs and symptoms
■ Abrupt onset of extreme polyuria (usually 4 to 16 L/day of dilute urine, but sometimes as much as 30 L/day), hourly nocturia
■ Extreme thirst
■ Signs and symptoms of dehydration: poor tissue turgor, dry mucous membranes, constipation, muscle weakness, dizziness, and hypotension

Diagnostic tests
■ Urinalysis reveals almost colorless urine of low osmolality (50 to 200 mOsm/kg of water, less than that of plasma) and low specific gravity (less than 1.005).
■ Water deprivation test (dehydration test) is necessary to provide evidence of vasopressin deficiency, resulting in the kidneys' inability to concentrate urine.

Treatment
■ Identify and eliminate cause.
■ Administer vasopressin subcutaneously several times per day.
■ Desmopressin acetate is given orally, nasal spray, subcutaneously or I.V. injection.

Nursing considerations
■ Record fluid intake and output carefully. Maintain fluid intake that's adequate to prevent severe dehydration.
■ Watch for signs of hypovolemic shock, and monitor blood pressure and heart and respiratory rates regularly, especially during the water deprivation test. Check the patient's weight daily.
■ If the patient is dizzy or has muscle weakness, institute safety precautions, including keeping the side rails up. Assist him with walking.
■ Monitor urine specific gravity between doses. Watch for a decrease in specific gravity accompanied by increasing urine output, indicating the recurrence of polyuria and necessitating administration of the next dose of medication or a dosage increase.
■ Teach the patient how to monitor intake and output at home.

■ Advise the patient to wear a medical identification bracelet and to carry his medication with him at all times.
■ Teach the parents of a child with diabetes insipidus about normal growth and development.
■ Refer patients with diabetes insipidus and their families for counseling and psychosocial adjustment or coping and support groups if necessary.

Diabetes mellitus

A chronic disease of relative or absolute insulin deficiency or resistance, diabetes mellitus is characterized by disturbances in carbohydrate, protein, and fat metabolism. The condition occurs in two forms: type 1, characterized by absolute insulin insufficiency, and type 2, characterized by insulin resistance with varying degrees of insulin secretory defects. Onset of type 1 usually occurs before age 30 (although it may occur at any age); the patient is usually thin and requires exogenous insulin and dietary management to achieve control. Conversely, type 2 usually occurs in obese adults after age 40, although it's becoming more common among North American youth. Nearly two-thirds of people with diabetes will die of cardiovascular disease. It's also the leading cause of renal failure and new adult blindness.

Causes
■ Type 1A: autoimmune beta-cell destruction, resulting in insulin deficiency

■ Type 1B: same immunologic markers as type 1A, but results in insulin deficiency and kerosis

Risk factors
■ Antagonizing of insulin effects caused by some medications, including thiazide diuretics, adrenal corticosteroids, and hormonal contraceptives
■ Obesity
■ Physiologic or emotional stress elevating stress hormone levels (cortisol, epinephrine, glucagon, and growth hormone), thereby raising blood glucose levels
■ Pregnancy-related increased levels of estrogen and placental hormones, which antagonize insulin

Signs and symptoms
■ Ketoacidosis or insidious onset in type 1
■ Most commonly, fatigue from energy deficiency and a catabolic state
■ Occasionally, no symptoms (in patients with type 2 diabetes)
■ Osmotic diuresis evident with polyuria, dehydration, polydipsia, dry mucous membranes, and poor skin turgor
■ In ketoacidosis and hyperglycemic hyperosmolar nonketotic state, dehydration potentially leading to hypovolemia and shock.
■ Weight loss and hunger in uncontrolled type 1 diabetes, even if the patient eats voraciously

Long-term effects
■ Retinopathy
■ Nephropathy
■ Atherosclerosis
■ Peripheral neuropathy, usually of the hands and feet
■ Autonomic neuropathy, possibly as gastroparesis (leading to delayed gastric emptying and a feeling of nausea and

fullness after meals), nocturnal diarrhea, impotence, and postural hypotension
- Skin and urinary tract infections and vaginitis

Diagnostic tests

- A diagnosis of diabetes mellitus is confirmed in nonpregnant adults by:
  - at least two occasions of a fasting plasma glucose level greater than or equal to 126 mg/dl
  - typical symptoms of uncontrolled diabetes and a random blood glucose level greater than or equal to 200 mg/dl
  - blood glucose level greater than or equal to 200 mg/dl at 2 hours after ingestion of 75 grams of oral dextrose.
- Two tests are required to confirm the diagnosis; however, it isn't necessary to perform two different tests—the same test may be performed twice. The second test is typically performed at least 24 hours after the first.
  - Ophthalmologic examination may reveal diabetic retinopathy.
  - Urine samples may be assessed for the presence of acetone.
  - Blood samples may reveal glycosylated hemoglobin, which reflects glucose control over the past 2 to 3 months.

Treatment

Effective treatment for both types of diabetes normalizes blood glucose and decreases complications.
- In type 1 diabetes, insulin replacement; human insulin may be rapid-acting (regular), intermediate-acting (NPH or Lente), long-acting (Ultralente, Lantus), or a combination of rapid-acting and intermediate-acting (70/30 or 50/50 of NPH and regular).
- Type 2 diabetes may require oral antidiabetic drugs.

DRUG CHALLENGE

 Studies have shown that treatment with a lipase inhibitor (such as orlistat) combined with a low-calorie diet significantly decreases the weight of overweight patients with type 2 diabetes. Patients following this therapy also displayed mprovements in glycemic control and cardiovascular risk profile; levels of glycosylated hemoglobin, fasting glucose, and postprandial glucose improved significantly.

- Islet cell or pancreas transplantation may be done in Type 1 diabetes; requires chronic immunosuppression.
- Treatment of both types of diabetes requires a diet planned to meet nutritional needs, to control blood glucose levels, and to reach and maintain appropriate body weight.
- Weight reduction may be included in the care plan for an obese patient with type 2 diabetes.
- Treatment of long-term diabetic complications include transplantation or dialysis for renal failure, photocoagulation for retinopathy, and vascular surgery for large-vessel disease. Meticulous blood glucose control is essential.

Nursing considerations

ACTION STAT!

 Watch for acute complications of diabetic therapy, especially hypoglycemia: vagueness, slow cerebration, dizziness, weakness, pallor, tachycardia, diaphoresis, seizures, and coma. Immediately give carbohydrates in the form of fruit juice, hard candy, or honey; if the patient is unconscious, subcutaneous, I.M., or I.V. glucagon or I.V. dextrose may be given.

- Be alert for signs and symptoms of ketoacidosis (acetone breath, dehydration, weak and rapid pulse, Kussmaul's respirations) and hyperosmolar coma (polyuria, thirst, neurologic abnormalities, stupor). These hyperglycemic crises require I.V. fluids, insulin and, usually, potassium replacement.

- Monitor diabetic control by obtaining blood glucose levels.
- Watch for diabetic effects on the cardiovascular system, such as cerebrovascular, coronary artery, and peripheral vascular impairment, and on the peripheral and autonomic nervous systems.
- Treat all injuries, cuts, and blisters (particularly on the legs or feet) meticulously.
- Be alert for signs of urinary tract infection and renal disease.
- Urge regular ophthalmologic examinations to detect diabetic retinopathy.
- Assess for signs of diabetic neuropathy (numbness or pain in the hands and feet, footdrop, neurogenic bladder). Stress the need for personal safety precautions; explain that decreased sensation can mask injuries. Minimize complications by maintaining strict blood glucose control.
- Teach the patient to care for his feet by washing them daily, drying carefully between the toes, and inspecting for corns, calluses, redness, swelling, bruises, and breaks in the skin. Urge him to report any changes. Advise him to wear nonconstricting shoes and to avoid walking barefoot.
- Teach the patient how to manage his diabetes when he has a minor illness such as a cold, flu, or upset stomach.

Disseminated intravascular coagulation

Also called *consumption coagulopathy* and *defibrination syndrome,* disseminated intravascular coagulation (DIC) occurs as a complication of diseases and conditions that accelerate clotting. This accelerated clotting process causes small blood vessel occlusion, organ necrosis, depletion of circulating clotting factors and platelets, and activation of the fibrinolytic system—which, in turn, can provoke severe hemorrhage. (See *Three mechanisms of DIC.*)

DIC is generally an acute condition but may be chronic in cancer patients. The hemorrhage that occurs may largely be the result of the anticoagulant activity of fibrin degradation products as well as depletion of plasma coagulation factors. The prognosis depends on early detection and treatment, the severity of the hemorrhage, and treatment of the underlying disease or condition.

Causes

- Disorders that produce necrosis, such as extensive burns and trauma, brain tissue destruction, transplant rejection, and hepatic necrosis.
- Infection (the most common cause of DIC), including gram-negative or gram-positive septicemia; viral, fungal, or rickettsial infection; and protozoal infection (falciparum malaria)
- Neoplastic disease, including acute leukemia and metastatic carcinoma
- Obstetric complications, such as abruptio placentae, amniotic fluid embolism, and retained dead fetus
- Other causes: heatstroke, shock, poisonous snakebite, cirrhosis, fat embolism, incompatible blood transfusion, cardiac arrest, surgery necessitating cardiopulmonary bypass, giant hemangioma, severe venous thrombosis, and purpura fulminans

Three mechanisms of DIC

However disseminated intravascular coagulation (DIC) begins, accelerated clotting (characteristic of DIC) usually results in excess thrombin, which in turn causes fibrinolysis with excess fibrin formation and fibrin degradation products (FDP), activation of fibrin-stabilizing factor (factor XIII), consumption of platelet and clotting factors and, eventually, hemorrhage.

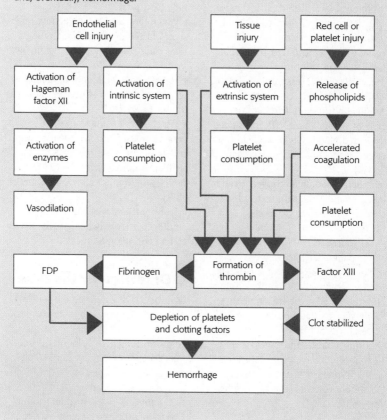

Signs and symptoms

- Abnormal bleeding *without* an accompanying history of a serious hemorrhagic disorder
- Cutaneous oozing
- Petechiae, ecchymoses, hematomas, acrocyanosis
- Bleeding from surgical sites or invasive procedures
- GI tract bleeding
- Oliguria, acute tubular necrosis
- Nausea, vomiting
- Dyspnea
- Seizures, coma
- Shock
- Failure of major organ systems
- Severe muscle, back, and abdominal pain

Diagnostic tests

Initial laboratory findings supporting a tentative diagnosis of DIC include:
- prothrombin time (PT) greater than 15 seconds
- partial thromboplastin time (PTT) greater than 80 seconds
- fibrinogen levels less than 150 mg/dl
- platelet count less than 100,000/µl
- fibrin degradation products commonly greater than 45 mcg/ml or positive at less than 1:100 dilution
- positive D-dimer test specific for DIC; positive at less than 1:8 dilution
- positive fibrin monomers, diminished levels of factors V and VIII, fragmentation of red blood cells (RBCs), and decreased hemoglobin (Hb) (less than 10 g/dl)
- elevated blood urea nitrogen (greater than 25 mg/dl) and serum creatinine (greater than 1.3 mg/dl) levels.

Treatment

- If the patient isn't actively bleeding, supportive care alone may reverse DIC.
- Active bleeding may require administration of blood, fresh frozen plasma, platelets, or packed RBCs to support hemostasis.
- Antithrombin III and gabexate mesylate to inhibit the clotting cascade.
- Heparin therapy is usually mandatory if thrombosis occurs (therapy is otherwise controversial).

Nursing considerations

- To prevent clots from dislodging and causing fresh bleeding, don't scrub bleeding areas. Use pressure, cold compresses, and topical hemostatic agents to control bleeding.
- Protect the patient from injury. Enforce complete bed rest during bleeding episodes. If the patient is agitated, pad the side rails.
- Check all I.V. and venipuncture sites frequently for bleeding. Apply pressure to injection sites for at least 10 minutes. Alert other personnel to the patient's tendency to hemorrhage.
- Monitor intake and output hourly in acute DIC, especially when administering blood products.
- Watch for transfusion reactions and signs of fluid overload. Weigh the patient daily, particularly in renal involvement.
- To measure the amount of blood lost, weigh dressings and linen and record drainage.
- Watch for bleeding from the GI and genitourinary tracts. If you suspect intra-abdominal bleeding, measure the patient's abdominal girth at least every 4 hours, and monitor closely for signs of shock.
- Monitor the results of serial blood studies (particularly hematocrit, Hb level, and coagulation times).

▌Diverticular disease

Diverticular disease is an outpouching of the colon, usually the sigmoid. It develops from the musculature in the colon working against increased intraluminal pressures to move hard stools through. Other typical sites are the duodenum, near the pancreatic border or the ampulla of Vater, and the jejunum. Diverticular disease of the stomach is rare and commonly a precursor of peptic or neoplastic disease. Diverticular disease of the ileum (Meckel's diverticulum) is the most common congenital anomaly of the GI tract. In diverticulosis, diverticula are present but usually the patient is asymptomatic or the symptoms (abdominal pain, fluctuating bowel habits, and constipation) are questionable because they may be related to underlying irritable bowel syndrome. In diverticulitis, diverticula are inflamed and may cause potentially fatal obstruction, infection, or hemorrhage.

Causes
- High intraluminal pressure on areas of weakness in the GI wall, where blood vessels enter; herniation of mucosa occurs through weak areas of the GI tract
- Diet (lack of roughage that reduces fecal residue, narrows the bowel lumen, and leads to higher intra-abdominal pressure)
- Diverticulitis: development of fecalith (hard mass formed from undigested food mixed with bacteria)

Signs and symptoms
Diverticulosis
- Usually causes no symptoms
- Intermittent left lower quadrant pain accompanied by alternating constipation and diarrhea, and relieved by defecation or the passage of flatus
- Possible hemorrhage from colonic diverticula in the right colon (in older patients)

Diverticulitis
- Moderate left lower abdominal pain
- Mild nausea
- Flatus
- Irregular bowel habits (constipation or loose stools)
- Low-grade fever and leukocytosis
- In severe diverticulitis, perforation of the diverticula with abscesses or peritonitis (peritoneal signs of abdominal rigidity and left lower quadrant pain)
- Sepsis and shock (high fever, chills, and hypotension) following peritonitis
- Possibility for microscopic or massive hemorrhage with perforation of diverticulum near a vessel
- Partial obstruction: constipation, thin-caliber stools, intermittent diarrhea, and abdominal distention

- Complete obstruction: abdominal rigidity and pain, diminishing or absent bowel sounds, nausea, and vomiting

Diagnostic tests
- An upper GI series confirms diverticulosis of the esophagus and small bowel.
- Plain X-ray films show evidence of free abdominal air, ileus, or small- or large-bowel obstruction.
- A barium enema confirms diverticulosis of the large bowel and can also identify a stricture or mass. Barium-filled diverticula seen as single, multiple, or clustered like grapes with a wide or narrow mouth.

DO'S & DON'TS

 In patients with acute diverticulitis, a barium enema may rupture the bowel; therefore, this procedure, as well as flexible sigmoidoscopy, shouldn't be performed during the acute stage. A colonoscopic examination can rule out malignancy. A computed tomography scan should be performed 2 to 3 days after initiation of antibiotics to evaluate for abscess.

- A biopsy will confirm cancer; however, colonoscopic biopsy isn't recommended during acute diverticular disease because of the risk of perforation.
- Blood studies show an elevated erythrocyte sedimentation rate in infection.

Treatment
Diverticulosis
- Treatment of diverticulosis includes a liquid or low-residue diet.
- Stool softeners may also be required.
- Occasional doses of mineral oil may be necessary.
- After pain subsides, the patient will require a low-residue diet and bulk medication such as psyllium (1 teaspoon

twice per day) and increased water consumption (8 glasses per day).

Diverticulitis

- Treatment of diverticulitis includes bed rest, a liquid diet, and stool softeners or bulking agents.
- The patient may also need a broad-spectrum antibiotic (such as metronidazole and ciprofloxacin or cotrimoxazole), morphine to control pain and relax smooth muscle, and an antispasmodic such as propantheline to control muscle spasms.
- Diverticulitis that doesn't respond to medical treatment requires surgical resection.
- Perforation, peritonitis, obstruction, or a fistula requires a temporary colostomy for 6 to 8 weeks. The colon can be reconnected after until inflammation or infection subsides.
- Blood replacement and careful monitoring of fluid and electrolyte balance in the patient who develops hemorrhage.
- If bleeding continues, angiography may be necessary to guide catheter placement for infusing vasopressin into the bleeding vessel.

Nursing considerations
Diverticulosis

- Teach the patient about diverticular disease and about how diverticula form.
- Make sure the patient understands the importance of a low-residue diet, harmful effects of constipation and straining. Encourage increased intake of foods high in undigestible fiber, including fresh fruits and vegetables, whole grain bread, and wheat or bran cereals. Warn that a high-fiber diet may temporarily cause flatulence and discomfort.
- Advise the patient to relieve constipation with stool softeners or bulk-forming cathartics. However, caution him against taking bulk-forming cathar-

tics without plenty of water; if swallowed dry, these agents may absorb enough moisture in the mouth and throat to swell and obstruct the esophagus or trachea.
- If the patient is hospitalized, observe stool output for frequency, color, and consistency; and monitor vital signs, including temperature and pulse, because they may signal developing inflammation or complications.

Diverticulitis

- In mild disease, explain diagnostic tests and preparations for such tests, observe stools carefully, and maintain accurate records of temperature, pulse, respirations, and intake and output.
- If the patient requires angiography and catheter placement for vasopressin infusion, inspect the insertion site frequently for bleeding, check pedal pulses often, and keep the patient from flexing his legs at the groin.

After surgery

- Watch for signs of infection and sepsis.
- Provide meticulous wound care; perforation may already have infected the area.
- Check drain sites for signs of infection (purulent drainage, foul odor) or fecal drainage.
- Change dressings as necessary.
- Encourage coughing and deep breathing to prevent atelectasis.
- Watch for signs of bleeding (hypotension, decreased hemoglobin level and hematocrit).
- Record intake and output accurately.
- Provide ostomy care and education.
- Arrange for a visit by an enterostomal therapy nurse.

Down syndrome

Attributed to a chromosomal aberration, Down syndrome (trisomy 21) characteristically produces mental retardation, dysmorphic facial features, and other distinctive physical abnormalities. It's commonly associated with heart defects and other congenital disorders. Life expectancy for patients with Down syndrome has increased significantly because of improved treatment for related complications (heart defects, respiratory and other infections, acute leukemia). Nevertheless, up to 44% of such patients who have associated congenital heart defects die before age 1. Down syndrome occurs in 1 in 800 to 1,000 live births, but the prevalence increases with advanced parental age, especially when the mother is age 34 or older at delivery or the father is older than age 42. At age 20, a woman has about 1 chance in 2,000 of having a child with Down syndrome; by age 49, she has 1 chance in 12.

Causes
- Trisomy 21, a spontaneous chromosomal abnormality in which chromosome 21 has three copies instead of the normal two because of faulty meiosis (nondisjunction) of the ovum or, sometimes, the sperm, resulting in a karyotype of 47 chromosomes instead of the normal 46

Signs and symptoms
- Abnormal fingerprints and footprints
- Clinodactyly (finger that curves inward)
- Craniofacial anomalies: upslanting palpebral fissures, almond-shaped eyes with epicanthic folds, a flat face, a protruding tongue, a small mouth and chin, and a single transverse palmar crease (simian crease)
- Congenital heart disease (septal defects or pulmonary or aortic stenosis)
- Dry, sensitive skin with decreased elasticity
- Duodenal atresia
- Flat bridge across the nose and small ears
- Hypotonic limb muscles impairing reflex development, posture, coordination, and balance
- Megacolon
- Mental retardation (IQ between 30 and 70)
- Pelvic bone abnormalities
- Poorly developed genitalia and delayed puberty; menstruation and fertility possible in females; infertility, low serum testosterone levels and, possibly, undescended testes, in males
- Short extremities, with broad, flat, squarish hands and feet
- Short stature
- Slow dental development, with abnormal or absent teeth
- Small skull and short neck
- Small white spots (Brushfield spots) on the iris, strabismus, and cataracts
- Umbilical hernia
- Wide space between the first and second toes

Diagnostic tests
- Physical findings at birth, especially hypotonia, suggest a diagnosis of Down syndrome.
- A karyotype showing the specific chromosomal abnormality provides a definitive diagnosis.
- Amniocentesis allows prenatal diagnosis and is recommended for pregnant women age 35 or older, or for any pregnant woman if she or the father carries a translocated chromosome.

Treatment

- Surgery may be required to correct heart defects and other related congenital abnormalities.
- Some patients will require antibiotic therapy for recurrent infections.
- Thyroid hormone replacement is given for hypothyroidism.
- Plastic surgery may be indicated to correct the characteristic facial traits, especially a protruding tongue. Benefits include improved speech, reduced susceptibility to dental caries, and fewer orthodontic problems later.
- Special education classes begun as early as possible help the patient with Down syndrome optimize his abilities.

Nursing considerations

- Establish a trusting relationship with the parents, and encourage communication during the difficult period after diagnosis. Recognize signs of grieving.
- Teach parents the importance of a balanced diet. Stress the need for patience while feeding the child, who may have difficulty sucking and may be less demanding and seem less eager to eat than normal babies.
- Encourage the parents to hold and nurture their child.
- Emphasize the importance of adequate exercise and maximal environmental stimulation; refer the parents for infant stimulation classes, which may begin in the early months of life.
- Help the parents set realistic goals for their child. By the time he's age 1, the child's development will clearly lag behind that of other children.
- Refer the parents and older siblings for genetic counseling to help them evaluate future reproductive risks. Discuss options for prenatal testing.
- Inform the parents that their child's level of intellectual function depends greatly on the environment and the amount of early stimulation received in addition to the IQ.
- Encourage the parents to remember the siblings' emotional needs.
- Refer the parents to national or local Down syndrome organizations and support groups.

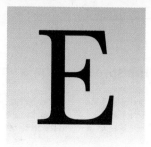

Ebola virus infection

An unclassified ribonucleic acid virus, Ebola virus is morphologically similar to the Marburg virus. Both viruses cause headache, malaise, myalgia, and high fever, progressing to severe diarrhea, vomiting, and internal and external hemorrhage.

The four known strains of the Ebola virus are Ebola Zaire, Ebola Sudan, Ebola–Ivory Coast, and Ebola Reston. The strains are structurally similar but have different antigenic properties. One type, Ebola Reston, affects only monkeys; the other three types affect humans.

The prognosis for Ebola virus disease is extremely poor, with mortality as high as 90%. The incubation period ranges from 2 to 21 days.

Causes
- Direct contact with infected blood, body secretions, or organs

Signs and symptoms
- Flulike signs and symptoms, such as headache, malaise, myalgia, fever, cough, and sore throat (within 3 days of infection)
- Maculopapular eruption (after the fifth day of infection), followed by desquamation
- Bruising
- Melena, hematemesis, epistaxis, and bleeding gums
  If the infection progresses:
- Dehydration
- Hemorrhage
- Liver and kidney dysfunction
  In pregnant women:
- Abortion
- Massive hemorrhage

Diagnostic tests
- Specialized laboratory tests reveal specific antigens or antibodies and may show the isolated virus.
- Blood tests show neutrophil leukocytosis, hypofibrinogenemia, thrombocytopenia, and microangiopathic hemolytic anemia.

Treatment
- No cure exists; treatment consists mainly of intensive supportive care.
- I.V. fluids help offset the effects of severe dehydration.
- Experimental treatments include administration of plasma that contains Ebola virus–specific antibodies.
- Maintain the patient in isolation until diagnostic tests indicate that he's free from the virus, which typically occurs 21 days after onset in the few who survive.

Preventing the spread of Ebola virus

The Centers for Disease Control and Prevention recommends the following guidelines to help prevent the spread of Ebola virus:

Do's
■ Keep the patient in isolation throughout the course of the disease.
■ If possible, place the patient in a negative pressure room at the beginning of hospitalization to avoid the need for transfer as the disease progresses.
■ Restrict nonessential staff members from entering the patient's room.
■ Make sure that anyone who enters the patient's room wears gloves and a gown to prevent contact with any surface in the room that may have been soiled.

■ Use barrier precautions to prevent skin and mucous membrane exposure to blood or other body fluids, secretions, or excretions when caring for the patient.

Don'ts
■ Don't come within 3' (1 m) of the patient without wearing a face shield or a surgical mask and goggles or eyeglasses with side shields.
■ Don't reuse gloves or gowns unless they've been completely disinfected.
■ Make sure a patient who dies of Ebola virus isn't embalmed, but promptly buried or cremated. Precautions to avoid contact with the patient's body fluids and secretions should continue after the patient's death.

Nursing considerations

■ Follow the guidelines for strict isolation precautions formulated by the Centers for Disease Control and Prevention when assessing a patient who may have Ebola virus infection, and take precautions to help prevent the spread of the disease. (See *Preventing the spread of Ebola virus.*)
■ Check the results of complete blood count and coagulation studies for signs of blood loss and coagulopathy.
■ Assess the patient daily for petechiae, ecchymoses, and oozing blood. Note and document the size of ecchymoses at least every 24 hours.
■ Protect all areas of petechiae and ecchymoses from further injury.
■ Test stools, urine, and vomitus for occult blood.
■ Watch for frank bleeding, including GI bleeding and, in women, menorrhagia. Note and document the amount of bleeding at least every 24 hours.

■ Monitor the patient's family and other close contacts for fever and other signs of infection.
■ Watch for any changes in the rate and pattern of respirations.
■ Closely monitor the patient's fluid and electrolyte balance.
■ Provide emotional support for the patient and his family during the course of this devastating disease. Encourage them to ask questions, and discuss any concerns they have about the disease and its treatment.

■ Electric shock

Electric current can cause injury in three ways: true electrical injury as the current passes through the body, arc or flash burns from current that doesn't pass through the body, and thermal surface burns caused by associated heat and flames. Electric shock may cause ventricular fibrillation, respiratory paralysis,

Preventing electric shock

To protect your patient from electric shock:

Do's

■ Check for cut, cracked, or frayed insulation on electric cords, call bells, and electrical devices attached to the bed. Keep these away from hot or wet surfaces and sharp corners. Also check for warm call bells.

■ Report faulty equipment promptly to maintenance personnel. If a machine sparks, smokes, seems unusually hot, or gives you or your patient a slight shock, unplug it immediately if doing so won't endanger the patient's life.

■ Check inspection labels, and report equipment overdue for inspection.

■ Be especially careful when using electrical equipment near patients with pacemakers or direct cardiac lines because a cardiac catheter or pacemaker can create a direct, low-resistance path to the heart. Even a small shock can cause ventricular fibrillation.

■ Remember: Dry, callused, unbroken skin offers more resistance to electric current than mucous membranes, an open wound, or thin, moist skin.

Don'ts

■ Don't use adapters on plugs. Make sure ground connections on electrical equipment are intact. Line cord plugs should have three prongs; the prongs should be straight and firmly fixed. Check that prongs fit wall outlets properly and that outlets aren't loose or broken.

■ Don't apply too much gel to defibrillator paddles. Make sure they're free from dry, caked gel before applying fresh gel because poor electrical contact can cause burns. If the gel runs over the edge of the paddle and touches your hand, you'll receive some of the defibrillator shock, and the patient will lose some of the energy in the discharge.

■ Don't set glasses of water, damp towels, or other wet items on electrical equipment. Wipe up accidental spills before they leak into equipment. Avoid using extension cords because they may circumvent the ground. If they're absolutely necessary, don't place them under carpeting or in areas where they'll be walked on.

---

burns, and death. The prognosis depends on the site and extent of damage, the patient's state of health, and the speed and adequacy of treatment.

The increased use of electrical medical devices in the hospital, many of which are connected directly to the patient, has raised serious concern for electrical safety and has led to the development of electrical safety standards. However, even well-designed equipment with reliable safety features can cause electric shock if it's mishandled. (See *Preventing electric shock*.)

Causes
■ Accidental contact with exposed parts of electrical appliances or wiring
■ Flash of electric arcs from high-voltage power lines or machines
■ Lightning

Signs and symptoms
■ Burns
■ Contusions, fractures, and other injuries resulting from violent muscle contractions or falls during the shock
■ Hyperventilation following muscle contraction (in momentary shock)

- Loss of consciousness; then complaints of muscle pain, fatigue, headaches, and nervous irritability after consciousness is regained
- Muscle contraction
- Myocardial infarction
- Numbness, tingling, or sensorimotor deficits
- Renal shutdown
- Residual hearing impairment
- Respiratory paralysis
- Ventricular fibrillation or another arrhythmia that progresses to fibrillation

Diagnostic tests

- Electrocardiography may be done to assess damage to the heart.
- Arterial blood gas analysis, urine myoglobin test, and X-ray of injured areas are used to evaluate internal damage and guide treatment.

Treatment

ACTION STAT!

 The patient who has undergone an electric shock requires the following emergency measures:

- Separate the victim from the current source by turning it off or unplugging it. If this isn't possible, pull him free with a nonconductive device, such as a loop of dry cloth or rubber, a dry rope, or a leather belt.
- Quickly assess vital functions. If you don't detect a pulse or breathing, start cardiopulmonary resuscitation at once. Continue until vital signs return or emergency help arrives with a defibrillator and other life-support equipment. Then monitor the patient's cardiac rhythm continuously, and obtain a 12-lead electrocardiogram.
- Because internal tissue destruction may be much greater than indicated by skin damage, give a rapid I.V. infusion of 1 to 2 L lactated Ringer's solution, as ordered, to maintain a urine output of 75

to 100 ml/hour. Insert an indwelling urinary catheter, and send the first specimen to the laboratory.

- Measure intake and output hourly, and watch for tea- or port-wine–colored urine, which occurs when coagulation necrosis and tissue ischemia liberate myoglobin and hemoglobin. These proteins can precipitate in the renal tubules, causing tubular necrosis and renal shutdown. To prevent this, give mannitol (Osmitrol) and furosemide (Lasix) as ordered.

Nursing considerations

- Assess the patient's neurologic status frequently.
- Watch for sensorimotor deficits because a spinal cord injury may follow cord ischemia or a compression fracture.
- Check for neurovascular damage in the extremities by assessing peripheral pulses and capillary refill and by asking about numbness, tingling, and pain.
- Elevate injured extremities.
- Apply a temporary sterile dressing. Assist with debridement as needed, and administer topical and systemic antibiotics as prescribed.
- Prepare the patient for grafting or, if his injuries are extreme, amputation.
- Protect patients from electric shock in the hospital.
- Tell patients how to avoid electrical hazards at home and at work.
- Advise parents of young children to put safety guards on all electrical outlets and keep children away from electrical devices.
- Warn patients not to use electrical appliances while showering or wet.
- Warn patients never to touch electrical appliances while touching faucets or cold water pipes in the kitchen because these pipes commonly provide the ground for all circuits in the house.

Encephalitis

A severe inflammation of the brain, encephalitis is usually caused by a mosquito-borne or, in some areas, a tick-borne virus. Viruses transmitted by arthropods are arboviruses (arthropod-borne). Transmission by means other than arthropod bites may occur through ingestion of infected goat's milk and accidental injection or inhalation of the virus. Eastern equine encephalitis may produce permanent neurologic damage and is commonly fatal.

In encephalitis, intense lymphocytic infiltration of brain tissues and the leptomeninges causes cerebral edema, degeneration of the brain's ganglion cells, and diffuse nerve cell destruction.

Causes

- Infection by arboviruses specific to rural areas
- Infection by enteroviruses (coxsackievirus, poliovirus, and echovirus) in urban areas
- Infection by other viruses, including West Nile virus, herpesvirus, mumps virus, human immunodeficiency virus, adenoviruses, and demyelinating diseases after measles, varicella, rubella, or vaccination

Signs and symptoms

- Coma (for days or weeks)
- Fever
- Headache
- Meningeal irritation (stiff neck and back)
- Neuronal damage (drowsiness, paralysis, seizures, ataxia, and organic psychoses)
- Vomiting

Diagnostic tests

- Identification of the virus in cerebrospinal fluid (CSF) or blood confirms the diagnosis.
- Arboviruses and herpesviruses can be isolated by inoculating young mice with specimens taken from patients.
- In herpes encephalitis, serologic studies may show rising titers of complement-fixing antibodies. Virus-specific indirect fluorescent antibody assays have improved diagnosis.
- Lumbar puncture reveals elevated CSF pressure, and despite inflammation, the fluid is clear in many cases.
- White blood cell and protein levels in CSF are slightly elevated, but the glucose level remains normal.
- An EEG study reveals abnormalities.
- Computed tomography scanning or magnetic resonance imaging may rule out cerebral hematoma.

Treatment

- Acyclovir (Zovirax), an antiviral, is prescribed for herpes encephalitis.

Treatment of all other forms of encephalitis is supportive, and includes:
- An anticonvulsant such as phenytoin (Dilantin) is given I.V.
- I.V. mannitol (Osmitrol) and corticosteroids reduce cerebral inflammation and edema.
- Ribavirin (Virazole) and interferon alfa-2b (Intron A) have an effect on West Nile encephalitis.
- Sedatives may be prescribed for restlessness.
- Aspirin or acetaminophen (Tylenol) may be given to relieve headache and reduce fever.
- Ensure adequate fluid and electrolyte intake to prevent dehydration.
- Give antibiotics for an associated infection such as pneumonia.
- Isolation is unnecessary.

Performing a rapid neurologic examination

To assess neurologic function in the patient with encephalitis, include the following:
■ *Orientation:* the patient's knowledge of where he is, the year, season, date, day, and month
■ *Registration and recall:* the patient's ability to recall three objects that you name
■ *Attention and calculation:* the patient's ability to focus on what you're saying
■ *Language:* the patient's ability to name objects, repeat words clearly, read, and follow a written command
■ *Focus on recall of recent events:* the patient's ability to recall your name, what he had for breakfast, and who came to visit.

As you elicit answers, be particularly concerned if the patient is restless or requires greater-than-average stimulation to provide responses.

Nursing considerations

■ Assess neurologic function often. Observe the patient's mental status and cognitive abilities by performing a rapid neurologic examination. (See *Performing a rapid neurologic examination.*) If the tissue within the brain becomes edematous, changes in the patient's mental status and cognitive abilities will occur.
■ Assessment should focus on early changes in level of consciousness. Continued swelling may result in cranial nerve compression, causing changes in pupillary reaction to light, ptosis, eyelid droop, and an eye rotating outward.
■ Monitor for signs of herniation (abnormal posturing movements, such as decerebration, decortication, and flaccidity, to noxious stimuli).

■ Watch for signs of cranial nerve involvement (ptosis, strabismus, diplopia) and for abnormal sleep patterns and behavioral changes.
■ Maintain adequate fluid intake to prevent dehydration, but avoid fluid overload, which may increase cerebral edema. Measure and record intake and output accurately.
■ Give acyclovir (Zovirax) I.V. infusion over at least 1 hour as prescribed to prevent renal tubular damage. Make sure the patient is well hydrated and watch for adverse effects, such as nausea, diarrhea, pruritus, and rash, and adverse effects of other drugs. Check the infusion site often to avoid infiltration and phlebitis.
■ Carefully position the patient to prevent joint stiffness and neck pain, and turn him often. Assist with range-of-motion exercises.
■ Maintain adequate nutrition. It may be necessary to give the patient small, frequent meals or to supplement these meals with nasogastric tube or parenteral feedings.
■ To prevent constipation and minimize the risk of increased intracranial pressure from straining during defecation, give a mild laxative or stool softener as prescribed.
■ Provide good mouth care.
■ Maintain a quiet environment. Darkening the room may decrease photophobia and headache. If the patient naps during the day and is restless at night, plan daytime activities to minimize napping and promote sleep at night.
■ Provide emotional support and reassurance because the patient is apt to be frightened by the illness and frequent diagnostic tests.
■ If the patient is delirious or confused, attempt to reorient him often. Providing a calendar or a clock in the patient's room may be helpful.

- Reassure the patient and his family that behavioral changes caused by encephalitis usually disappear. If a neurologic deficit is severe and appears permanent, refer the patient to a rehabilitation program as soon as the acute phase has passed. Consultation with a speech, occupational, or physical therapist may be indicated.
- Review prevention strategies, such as adequate immunizations and protection against mosquito bites.

Endocarditis

An infection of the endocardium, heart valves, or a cardiac prosthesis, endocarditis results from bacterial or fungal invasion that produces vegetative growths on the heart valves, the endocardial lining of a heart chamber, or the endothelium of a blood vessel. These growths may embolize to the spleen, kidneys, central nervous system, and lungs.

In endocarditis, fibrin and platelets aggregate on the valve tissue and engulf circulating bacteria or fungi that flourish and produce friable verrucous vegetations. Such vegetations may cover the valve surfaces, causing ulceration and necrosis; they may also extend to the chordae tendineae, leading to their upture and subsequent valvular insufficiency.

Untreated endocarditis is commonly fatal, but with proper treatment, about 70% of patients recover. The prognosis is worst when endocarditis causes severe valvular damage, leading to insufficiency and heart failure, or when it involves a prosthetic valve.

Causes
- Gram-negative aerobic organisms, fungi, streptococci, enterococci, or diphtheroids
- Infection by *Staphylococcus aureus* via I.V. drug abuse
- Staphylococcal infection within 60 days of valve insertion
- Streptococci (especially *Streptococcus viridans*), staphylococci, and enterococci (in patients who don't abuse I.V. drugs)

Predisposing factors
- Coarctation of the aorta
- Degenerative heart disease, especially calcific aortic stenosis
- Marfan syndrome
- Pulmonary stenosis
- Subaortic and valvular aortic stenosis
- Tetralogy of Fallot
- Ventricular septal defects

Signs and symptoms
- Anorexia
- Arthralgia
- Chills
- Fatigue
- Intermittent, possibly recurring, fever
- Janeway lesions (purplish macules on the palms or soles)
- Loud, regurgitant murmur (typical of the underlying heart lesion)
- Malaise
- Night sweats
- Osler's nodes (tender, raised subcutaneous lesions on the fingers or toes)
- Petechiae of the skin (especially common on the upper anterior trunk) and the buccal, pharyngeal, or conjunctival mucosa
- Roth's spots (hemorrhagic areas with white centers on the retina)
- Splenomegaly
- Splinter hemorrhages under the nails
- Valvular insufficiency
- Weakness
- Weight loss
- Signs and symptoms of splenic, renal, cerebral, or pulmonary infarction or peripheral vascular occlusion due to em-

bolization from vegetating lesions or diseased valvular tissue:
– Cerebral infarction: hemiparesis, aphasia, or other neurologic deficits
– Peripheral vascular occlusion: numbness and tingling in an arm or a leg, finger, or toe or signs of impending peripheral gangrene
– Pulmonary infarction (most common in right-sided endocarditis, which usually occurs in I.V. drug abusers and after cardiac surgery): cough, pleuritic pain, pleural friction rub, dyspnea, hemoptysis
– Renal infarction: hematuria, pyuria, flank pain, decreased urine output
– Splenic infarction: abdominal rigidity and pain in the left upper quadrant, radiating to the left shoulder

Diagnostic tests

■ Three or more blood cultures in a 24- to 48-hour period identify the causative organism in up to 90% of patients; 10% of patients may have negative blood cultures.
■ Other abnormal but nonspecific laboratory test results may include a normal or elevated white blood cell count, abnormal histiocytes (macrophages), elevated erythrocyte sedimentation rate, positive serum rheumatoid factor (in about 50% of all patients with endocarditis after the disease is present for 6 weeks), and normocytic, normochromic anemia (in 70% to 90% of endocarditis cases).
■ Echocardiography may identify valvular damage.
■ Electrocardiography may show atrial fibrillation and other arrhythmias that accompany valvular disease.

Treatment

■ Antimicrobial therapy is given for 4 to 6 weeks to eradicate the organism. Selection of an anti-infective drug is based on identification of the infecting organism and on sensitivity studies. While awaiting test results or if blood cultures are negative, empiric antimicrobial therapy is based on the likely infecting organism.
■ Place the patient on bed rest and administer aspirin for fever and aches.
■ Valve replacement may be necessary for patients with severe valvular damage or in those requiring replacement of an infected prosthetic valve.

Nursing considerations

■ Obtain the patient's history to determine the presence of allergies before giving antibiotics.
■ Give antibiotics as prescribed to maintain consistent antibiotic blood levels.
■ Observe the venipuncture site for signs of infiltration and inflammation, which are possible complications of long-term I.V. drug administration. To reduce the risk of these complications, rotate venous access sites.
■ Watch for signs of embolization (hematuria, pleuritic chest pain, left upper quadrant pain, and paresis), a common occurrence during the first 3 months of treatment. Tell the patient to watch for and report these signs, which may indicate impending peripheral vascular occlusion or splenic, renal, cerebral, or pulmonary infarction.
■ Monitor the patient's renal status (blood urea nitrogen levels, creatinine clearance, and urine output) to check for signs of renal emboli or evidence of drug toxicity.
■ Observe for signs of heart failure, such as dyspnea, tachypnea, tachycardia, crackles, jugular vein distention, edema, and weight gain.
■ Provide reassurance by teaching the patient and his family about this disease and the need for prolonged treatment. Tell them to watch closely for fever,

anorexia, and other signs of relapse about 2 weeks after treatment stops. Suggest quiet diversionary activities to prevent excessive physical exertion.

■ Make sure a susceptible patient understands the need for prophylactic antibiotics before, during, and after dental work, childbirth, and genitourinary, GI, or gynecologic procedures.

■ Teach the patient how to recognize symptoms of endocarditis, and tell him to notify the practitioner immediately if they occur.

▌Endometriosis

Endometriosis is the formation of endometrial tissue outside the lining of the uterine cavity. Such ectopic tissue is generally confined to the pelvic area, most commonly around the ovaries, uterovesical peritoneum, uterosacral ligaments, and cul-de-sac, but it can appear anywhere in the body.

Ectopic endometrial tissue responds to normal stimulation in the same way the endometrium does. During menstruation, the ectopic tissue bleeds, causing the surrounding tissues to become inflamed. This inflammation causes fibrosis, leading to adhesions that produce pain and cause infertility.

Active endometriosis usually occurs between ages 30 and 40, especially in women who postpone childbearing; it may be seen less commonly before age 20. Severe symptoms of endometriosis may have an abrupt onset or develop over many years. The disorder usually becomes progressively severe during the menstrual years; after menopause, it tends to subside. The primary complication of endometriosis is infertility.

Causes
■ Unknown

■ Familial susceptibility or recent hysterotomy may be predisposing factors

Signs and symptoms
■ Cyclic pain in the lower abdomen, vagina, posterior pelvis, and back beginning 5 to 7 days before menses, reaching its peak on days of bleeding, and lasting for 2 to 3 days

■ Other signs and symptoms depending on the location of the ectopic tissue:
 – bladder: suprapubic pain, dysuria, hematuria
 – cervix, vagina, and perineum: bleeding from endometrial deposits in these areas during menses
 – ovaries and oviducts: infertility and profuse menses
 – ovaries or cul-de-sac: deep thrust dyspareunia
 – rectovaginal septum and colon: painful defecation, rectal bleeding with menses, pain in the coccyx or sacrum
 – small bowel and appendix: abdominal cramps, nausea and vomiting, which worsen before menses

Diagnostic tests
■ Laparoscopy is used to confirm the diagnosis and determine the stage of the disease before treatment is started.

Treatment
■ Androgens such as danazol are prescribed in stages I and II (mild forms with superficial endometria and filmy adhesions) for young women who want to have children.

■ Progestins and hormonal contraceptives also relieve symptoms.

■ Gonadotropin-releasing hormone agonists suppress estrogen production, which causes atrophic changes in the ectopic endometrial tissue and allows healing.

■ Laparoscopy permits laser vaporization of implants (followed by hormonal therapy) or may be used therapeutically to lyse adhesions, remove small implants, and cauterize implants.

- Surgery may be required to rule out cancer (when ovarian masses are present).
- Severe endometriosis may require a total abdominal hysterectomy and, possibly, bilateral salpingo-oophorectomy.

Nursing considerations

- Because infertility is a possible complication, advise the patient who wants children not to postpone childbearing.
- Recommend to all patients that they have an annual pelvic examination and Papanicolaou test.
- Provide emotional support.

Epicondylitis

Also known as *tennis elbow* and *epitrochlear bursitis,* epicondylitis is inflammation of the forearm extensor supinator tendon fibers at their common attachment to the lateral humeral epicondyle. This inflammation produces acute or subacute pain. If it isn't treated, epicondylitis may become disabling.

Causes

- Activity requiring a forceful grasp, wrist extension against resistance, or frequent rotation of the forearm (such as playing tennis)

Signs and symptoms

- Elbow pain that gradually worsens and commonly radiates to the forearm and back of the hand whenever the patient grasps an object or twists his elbow
- Local heat, swelling, and restricted range of motion (ROM) (in rare instances)
- Tenderness over the involved lateral or medial epicondyle or over the head of the radius

Diagnostic tests

- X-rays are almost always negative.
- Neuromuscular test results may reveal a weak grasp.

Treatment

- Treatment may include systemic anti-inflammatory therapy or local injection of a corticosteroid and a local anesthetic.
- Immobilizing the arm with a splint from the distal forearm to the elbow may provide relief.
- Heat therapy (such as warm compresses, short-wave diathermy, and ultrasound) may be useful, alone or in combination with diathermy.
- Physical therapy, consisting of manipulation and massage to detach the tendon from the chronically inflamed periosteum, may be indicated.
- A "tennis elbow strap" has helped many patients. This strap, which is wrapped snugly around the forearm about 1" (2.5 cm) below the epicondyle, helps relieve the strain on affected forearm muscles and tendons.
- Surgical release of the tendon at the epicondyle may be necessary if other measures fail to relieve pain.

Nursing considerations

- Assess the patient's level of pain, ROM, and sensory function.
- Monitor heat therapy to prevent burns.
- Instruct the patient to rest the elbow until inflammation subsides.
- Remove the support daily, and gently move the arm to prevent stiffness and contracture.
- Instruct the patient to follow the prescribed exercise program. For example, he may stretch his arm and flex his wrist to the maximum, then press the back of his hand against a wall until he can feel a pull in his forearm, and hold this position for 1 minute.

- Advise the patient to warm up for 15 to 20 minutes before beginning any sports activity.
- Urge the patient to wear an elastic support or splint during any activity that stresses the forearm or elbow.

Epididymitis

This infection of the epididymis, the testicle's cordlike excretory duct, is one of the most common infections of the male reproductive tract. It usually affects adults and is rare before puberty. Epididymitis may spread to the testicle itself, causing orchitis; bilateral epididymitis may cause sterility.

Causes

- Chemical irritation by extravasation of urine through the vas deferens
- Complication of prostatectomy
- Infection by organisms such as *Chlamydia trachomatis* or *Neisseria gonorrhoeae* in sexually active men younger than age 35 and from urinary pathogens in older men
- Trauma (may reactivate a dormant infection or initiate a new one), gonorrhea, syphilis, or chlamydial infection
- Urinary tract infection or prostatitis

Signs and symptoms

- Acute hydrocele (as a reaction to the inflammatory process)
- Characteristic waddle (an attempt to protect the groin and scrotum during walking)
- Extreme tenderness, pain, and swelling in the groin and scrotum
- Heavy feeling in scrotum
- High fever
- Malaise

Diagnostic tests

- Urinalysis showing an increased white blood cell count confirms infection.
- Urine culture and sensitivity tests may identify the causative organism.
- A serum WBC count of more than 10,000/µl indicates infection.
- Scrotal ultrasonography may help differentiate acute epididymitis from conditions such as testicular torsion, which is a surgical emergency.

Treatment

- Place the patient on bed rest.
- Provide scrotal elevation with towel rolls or adhesive strapping.
- Give broad-spectrum antibiotics as prescribed.
- Give analgesics as prescribed for associated pain.
- An ice bag applied to the area may reduce swelling and relieve pain. (Heat is contraindicated because it may damage germinal cells, which are viable only at or below normal body temperature.)
- When pain and swelling subside and the patient is allowed to walk, wearing an athletic supporter may prevent resumption of pain.
- Epididymectomy under local anesthetic may be necessary if epididymitis is refractory to antibiotic therapy.

Nursing considerations

- Watch closely for abscess formation (a localized hot, red, tender area) and extension of the infection into the testes. Closely monitor temperature, and ensure adequate fluid intake.
- Because the patient is usually uncomfortable, give analgesics as necessary. During bed rest, check often for proper scrotum elevation.
- Before discharge, emphasize the importance of completing the prescribed antibiotic therapy, even after symptoms subside. Infected sexual partners may also need treatment.

■ If the patient faces the possibility of sterility, suggest supportive counseling as needed.

Epiglottiditis

Acute epiglottiditis is an inflammation of the epiglottis that tends to cause airway obstruction. It typically strikes children ages 2 to 8. A critical emergency, epiglottiditis can prove fatal in 8% to 12% of victims unless it's recognized and treated promptly.

Causes
■ *Haemophilus influenzae* type B (Hib) infection
■ Pneumococci and group A streptococci (occasionally) infection

Signs and symptoms
■ Breathing difficulties as indicated by hyperextension of the neck, sitting upright but in a forward-leaning position, with mouth open, tongue protruding, and nostrils flaring
■ Complete upper airway obstruction within 2 to 5 hours of onset
■ Drooling
■ Dysphagia
■ High fever
■ Inspiratory retractions and rhonchi
■ Irritability and restlessness
■ Laryngeal obstruction from inflammation and edema of the epiglottis
■ Sore throat
■ Stridor

Diagnostic tests
■ In acute epiglottiditis, throat examination reveals a large, edematous, bright red epiglottis. Such examination should follow lateral neck X-rays and, generally, shouldn't be performed if the suspected obstruction is large or if immediate intubation isn't possible.

ACTION STAT!

 Special equipment (a laryngoscope and endotracheal [ET] tubes) should be available because a tongue blade can cause sudden, complete airway obstruction. An anesthesiologist or other trained personnel should be on hand during throat examination to secure an emergency airway.

Treatment
■ A child with acute epiglottiditis and airway obstruction may need emergency ET intubation or a tracheotomy and should be monitored in an intensive care unit.
■ Parenteral fluid administration is necessary to prevent dehydration.
■ A 10-day course of parenteral antibiotics is indicated (usually ampicillin; if the child is allergic to penicillin, chloramphenicol or another antibiotic may be substituted).
■ Corticosteroids may be prescribed to reduce edema during early treatment.
■ Oxygen therapy and arterial blood gas (ABG) level monitoring may be desirable.
■ The Hib vaccine is recommended as a preventive measure by the American Academy of Pediatrics, beginning at age 2 months and continuing for 3 or 4 doses (depending on the manufacturer).

Nursing considerations
■ Keep the following equipment available in case of sudden, complete airway obstruction: a tracheotomy tray, ET tubes, a handheld resuscitation bag, oxygen equipment, and a laryngoscope with blades of various sizes.
■ Monitor ABG levels for hypoxia and hypercapnia.
■ Keep the child calm; agitation can worsen symptoms.

- Don't examine the child's throat; doing so may cause laryngospasm.

 Watch for increasing restlessness, rising heart rate, fever, dyspnea, and retractions, which may indicate the need for an emergency tracheotomy.

- Maintain fluid hydration with I.V. therapy as prescribed, or give oral clear liquid or ice pops as tolerated.
- After tracheotomy, anticipate the patient's needs because he won't be able to cry or call out, and provide emotional support. Reassure the patient and his family that the tracheotomy is a short-term intervention (usually from 4 to 7 days).
- Monitor the patient for rising temperature and pulse rate and for hypotension, which are signs of secondary infection.

Epilepsy

Seizure disorder, or epilepsy, is a condition of the brain characterized by a susceptibility to recurrent seizures (paroxysmal events associated with abnormal electrical discharges of neurons in the brain). Epilepsy is believed to affect 1% to 2% of the population. The prognosis is good if the patient adheres strictly to the prescribed treatment. Recurring seizures are classified as partial, generalized, status epilepticus, or unclassified. Some patients may be affected by more than one type of seizure.

Causes

- Unknown (in about one-half of all patients)
- Anoxia
- Birth trauma (inadequate oxygen supply to the brain, blood incompatibility, or hemorrhage)
- Brain tumors
- Perinatal infection
- Head injury or trauma
- Infectious diseases (meningitis, encephalitis, or brain abscess)
- Ingestion of toxins (mercury, lead, or carbon monoxide)
- Inherited disorders or degenerative disease, such as phenylketonuria or tuberous sclerosis
- Metabolic disorders, such as hypocalcemia, hypoglycemia, and hypoparathyroidism
- Stroke (hemorrhage, thrombosis, or embolism)

Status epilepticus
- Abrupt withdrawal of anticonvulsant medications
- Acute head trauma
- Hypoxic encephalopathy
- Metabolic encephalopathy
- Septicemia resulting from encephalitis or meningitis

Signs and symptoms
Partial seizures
- Focal symptoms arising from a localized area of the brain and classified by their effect on consciousness; may be simple or complex
- Complex partial seizure: 1 to 3 minutes in duration, impaired consciousness, amnesia related to events during and immediately after the seizure (differentiating characteristic) and, possibly, some ability to follow simple commands during course of seizure
- Simple partial seizure: brief duration (typically a few seconds), no preceding or provoking events, localized, typically no alteration in consciousness, sensory symptoms (lights flashing, smells, hearing hallucinations), autonomic symptoms (sweating, flushing, pupil dilation), and psychic symptoms (dream states, anger, fear)

Generalized seizures

- Absence seizure: most common in children, 1 to 10 seconds duration, brief change in level of consciousness (LOC) with blinking or rolling of the eyes, a blank stare, and slight mouth movements (at onset); uninterrupted maintenance of posture and preseizure activity; commonly recurrent up to 100 times per day; generally nonconvulsive but, possibly, progressing to generalized tonic-clonic seizure
- Myoclonic seizure: brief, involuntary muscular jerks of the body or extremities, possibly occurring in a rhythmic manner, no alteration in LOC
- Generalized tonic-clonic seizure: 2 to 5 minutes' duration, loud cry at onset (due to air rushing from the lungs through the vocal cords), loss of consciousness, falling and stiffening of the patient's body (tonic phase) with alternating episodes of muscle spasm and relaxation (clonic phase); possibly, tongue biting, incontinence, labored breathing, apnea, and subsequent cyanosis; and postseizure signs and symptoms of confusion, speech difficulties, drowsiness, fatigue, headache, muscle soreness, arm or leg weakness and, possibly, deep sleep
- Atonic seizure: occurs in young children, general loss of postural tone and temporary loss of consciousness

Status epilepticus

- Abnormally prolonged seizure (lasting longer than 5 minutes) or inability to fully regain consciousness between seizures
- Respiratory distress

Diagnostic tests

- Computed tomography scanning or magnetic resonance imaging offer densi-

ty readings of the brain and may indicate abnormalities in internal structures.
- Paroxysmal abnormalities on the EEG confirm the diagnosis by providing evidence of the continuing tendency to have seizures. A negative EEG doesn't rule out epilepsy because the paroxysmal abnormalities occur intermittently.
- Other tests include serum glucose and calcium studies, skull X-rays, lumbar puncture, brain scan, and cerebral angiography.

Treatment

- Treatment focuses on identifying and correcting the underlying disorder or condition causing the seizures.
- Drug therapy is specific to the type of seizure. The most commonly prescribed drugs include phenytoin (Dilantin), carbamazepine (Tegretol), phenobarbital, valproic acid (Depakene), and primidone (Mysoline) given individually for generalized tonic-clonic seizures and complex partial seizures.

DRUG CHALLENGE

 I.V. fosphenytoin (Cerebyx) is an alternative to phenytoin that's just as effective, with a long half-life and minimal central nervous system depression. In addition, it can be given rapidly without the adverse cardiovascular effects that occur with phenytoin.

- Valproic acid, clonazepam (Klonopin), and ethosuximide (Zarontin) are commonly prescribed for absence seizures. A patient taking an anticonvulsant requires monitoring for signs of toxicity, such as nystagmus, ataxia, lethargy, dizziness, drowsiness, slurred speech, irritability, nausea, and vomiting.
- If drug therapy fails, a vagus nerve stimulator implant may help reduce the

Guidelines for seizures

Generalized tonic-clonic seizures may necessitate basic interventions. Use this checklist when teaching the patient's family what to do in the event of a seizure.

Do's

- To support the airway, turn the patient's head to the side.
- After the seizure subsides, reassure the patient that he's all right, orient him to time and place, and inform him that he has had a seizure.

Don'ts

- Don't restrain the patient during a seizure. Instead, help him to a supine position, loosen any tight clothing, and place something flat and soft, such as a pillow, jacket, or hand, under his head. Clear the area of hard objects.
- Never put anything in the mouth of a patient having a seizure.
- If the patient is having a complex partial seizure, don't restrain him. Protect him from injury by gently calling his name and directing him away from the source of danger.

incidence of focal seizure. Transcranial magnetic stimulators are also under study and have been shown to help some patients.

- A demonstrated focal lesion may be surgically removed in an attempt to stop seizures.
- A ketogenic diet rich in fats and low in carbohydrates may be beneficial to some patients. A dietitian should be consulted if this is prescribed.

Action stat!

Emergency treatment of status epilepticus usually consists of I.V. administration of diazepam or lorazepam, phenytoin, or phenobarbital; dextrose 50% (when seizures are secondary to hypoglycemia); and thiamine (in chronic alcoholism or withdrawal).

Nursing considerations

- When the patient has a seizure, describe the seizure in detail instead of classifying it. List precipitating events, how the seizure began and progressed, its duration, all movements and activities, LOC, and postseizure activity.
- Encourage the patient and his family to express their feelings about the patient's condition. Answer their questions, and help them cope by dispelling some of the myths about epilepsy—that it's contagious, for example. Assure them that epilepsy is controllable for most patients who follow a prescribed medication regimen and that most patients maintain a normal lifestyle.
- Teach the family how to give the patient first aid when a seizure occurs. (See *Guidelines for seizures*.)
- Because drug therapy is the treatment of choice for most patients with epilepsy, information about the medications is invaluable.
- Stress the need for compliance with the prescribed drug schedule. Assure the patient that anticonvulsant drugs are safe when taken as prescribed.
- Reinforce dosage instructions, and find methods to help the patient remember to take medications. Caution him to

monitor the amount of medication left so he doesn't run out of it.

- Warn against possible adverse effects, such as drowsiness, lethargy, hyperactivity, confusion, and vision and sleep disturbances, which indicate the need for dosage adjustment. Phenytoin therapy may lead to hyperplasia of the gums, which may be relieved by conscientious oral hygiene. Instruct the patient to report adverse effects immediately.
- Warn the patient against drinking alcoholic beverages.
- Emphasize the importance of having anticonvulsant blood levels checked at regular intervals as well as during periods of stress or illness, even if the seizures are under control.
- Know which social agencies in your community can help patients with epilepsy. Refer the patient to the Epilepsy Foundation of America for general information and to the state motor vehicle department for information about a driver's license.

Epistaxis

Nosebleed, or epistaxis, may be a primary disorder, or it may occur because of another underlying condition. Nosebleeds in children usually originate in the anterior nasal septum and tend to be mild. In adults, such bleeding is most likely to originate in the posterior septum and can be severe. Epistaxis is twice as common in children as in adults.

Causes

- Acute or chronic infections, such as sinusitis or rhinitis, that cause congestion and eventual bleeding from capillary blood vessels
- Inhalation of chemicals that irritate the nasal mucosa
- Polyps
- Sudden mechanical decompression (caisson disease) and violent exercise
- Trauma from external or internal causes: a blow to the nose, nose picking, or insertion of a foreign body

Predisposing factors

- Anticoagulant therapy
- Aspirin use on a chronic basis
- Blood dyscrasias (hemophilia, purpura, leukemia, and anemias)
- Hemorrhagic telangiectasia
- Hodgkin's disease
- Hypertension
- Neoplastic disorders
- Rheumatic fever
- Sclerotic vessel disease
- Scurvy
- Vitamin K deficiency

Signs and symptoms

- Bright red blood oozing from the nostrils originating in the anterior nose
- Dark or bright red blood from the back of the throat originating in the posterior nose (commonly mistaken for hemoptysis because of expectoration)
- Moderate epistaxis: light-headedness, dizziness, and slight respiratory difficulty
- Severe epistaxis: seepage behind the nasal septum, in the middle ear, and in the corners of the eyes
- Severe hemorrhage (persisting longer than 10 minutes after application of pressure): hypotension, rapid and bounding pulse, dyspnea, and pallor; potential for blood loss up to 1 L/hour in adults

Diagnostic tests

- Inspection with a bright light and nasal speculum locates the site of bleeding.
- Blood studies showing gradual reduction in hemoglobin levels and hemat-

Insertion of an anterior-posterior nasal pack

The first step in the insertion of an anterior-posterior nasal pack is the insertion of catheters in the nostrils. After drawing the catheters through the mouth, a suture from the pack is tied to each catheter, which positions the pack in place as the catheters are drawn back through the nostrils.

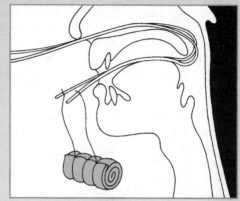

While the sutures are held tightly, packing is inserted into the anterior nose.

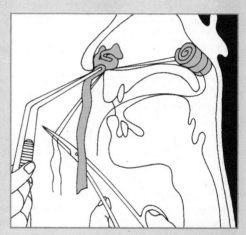

The sutures are then secured around a dental roll; the middle suture extends from the mouth and is tied to the cheek.

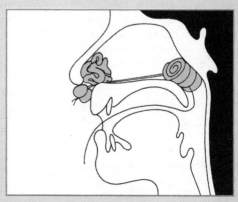

ocrit are commonly inaccurate immediately after epistaxis because of hemoconcentration.

- The patient with blood dyscrasia may have a decreased platelet count.
- Prothrombin time and partial thromboplastin time show a coagulation time two times the control because of a bleeding disorder or anticoagulant therapy.
- Diagnosis must rule out underlying systemic causes of epistaxis, especially disseminated intravascular coagulation and rheumatic fever. Bruises or simultaneous bleeding elsewhere probably indicates a hematologic disorder. Recurrent epistaxis may indicate a nasopharyngeal angiofibroma.

Treatment

- The bleeding is stopped by applying a cotton ball saturated with epinephrine to the bleeding site, external pressure, and cauterization with electrocautery or a silver nitrate stick (anterior bleeding). If these measures don't control the bleeding, petroleum gauze nasal packing may be needed. (See *Insertion of an anterior-posterior nasal pack,* page 203.)
- Methods to control posterior bleeding include inserting a nasal balloon catheter, gauze packing (inserted through the nose), or postnasal packing (inserted through the mouth), depending on the bleeding site. (Gauze packing generally remains in place for 24 to 48 hours; postnasal packing remains in place for 3 to 5 days.)
- Antibiotics may be appropriate if the packing must remain in place for longer than 24 hours.
- Supplemental vitamin K is given for severe bleeding.
- Blood transfusions and surgical ligation or embolization of a bleeding artery may be necessary if local measures fail to control bleeding.

Nursing considerations

- Compress the soft portion of the nostrils against the septum continuously for 5 to 10 minutes. Apply an ice collar or cold, wet compresses to the nose. Bleeding should stop after 10 minutes.
- Give oxygen as prescribed and needed.
- Monitor vital signs and skin color; record blood loss.
- Tell the patient to breathe through his mouth and not to swallow blood, talk, or blow his nose.
- Monitor oxygen saturation levels.
- Keep vasoconstrictors, such as phenylephrine (Sinex), handy.
- Reassure the patient and his family that epistaxis usually looks worse than it is.

To prevent a recurrence

- Instruct the patient not to pick his nose or insert foreign objects into it and to avoid bending and lifting. Emphasize the need for follow-up examinations and periodic blood studies after an episode of epistaxis. Advise the patient to get prompt treatment for nasal infection or irritation.
- Suggest a humidifier for patients who live in dry climates or at high elevations or whose homes are heated with circulating hot air.
- Instruct the patient to sneeze with his mouth open.
- Caution the patient against inserting cotton or tissues into the nose on his own because these objects are difficult to remove and may further irritate the nasal mucosa.

Escherichia coli and other Enterobacteriaceae infections

Enterobacteriaceae—a group of mostly aerobic gram-negative bacilli—cause local and systemic infections, including an invasive diarrhea that resembles shigella and, more commonly, a noninvasive toxin-mediated diarrhea that resembles cholera.

Escherichia coli and other Enterobacteriaceae cause most nosocomial infections. Noninvasive, enterotoxin-producing *E. coli* infections may be a major cause of diarrheal illness in children in the United States.

The incidence of *E. coli* infection is highest among travelers returning from other countries, particularly Mexico, and those in Southeast Asia and South America. *E. coli* infection also induces other diseases, especially in people whose resistance is low. One strain, *E. coli* O157:H7, associated with undercooked ground beef, produces hemorrhagic colitis and hemolytic uremic syndrome in children—a principal cause of acute kidney failure in children. This strain of *E. coli* may also be transmitted by swimming in or drinking sewage-contaminated water; consuming infected spinach, lettuce, sprouts, or unpasteurized milk or juice; and by encountering contaminated railings, feed bins, soil, or fur of animals in petting zoos.

The prognosis in mild to moderate infection is good. Severe infection requires immediate fluid and electrolyte replacement to avoid fatal dehydration, especially among children, in whom mortality may be quite high.

Causes
- Infection with certain nonindigenous strains of *E. coli*

Signs and symptoms
- Abrupt onset of watery diarrhea with cramping abdominal pain
- In *E. coli* O157:H7 infection: bloody diarrhea
- In infants: vomiting, listlessness, irritability, and anorexia followed by diarrhea with loose, watery stools that change from yellow to green and contain little mucus or blood; possibility of fever, severe dehydration, acidosis, and shock
- In invasive infection: chills, abdominal cramps, and diarrhea that contains blood and pus
- In severe illness: metabolic acidosis

Diagnostic tests
- Diagnosis depends on clinical observation alone.
- Diagnosis must rule out salmonellosis, shigellosis, and other common infections that produce similar signs and symptoms.

Treatment
- Treatment focuses on isolating the causative organism and correcting fluid and electrolyte imbalances.
- Antibiotics haven't been shown to improve the course of the disease and may precipitate kidney complications.
- For cramping and diarrhea, bismuth subsalicylate may be given; antidiarrheals, such as loperamide (Imodium), should be avoided.

Nursing considerations
- Keep accurate intake and output records. Measure stool volume, and note the presence of blood and pus. Replace fluids and electrolytes as prescribed, monitoring for decreased serum sodium

and chloride levels and signs of gram-negative septic shock. Watch for signs of dehydration, such as poor skin turgor and dry mouth.

To prevent the spread of this infection:
- Screen all hospital personnel and visitors for diarrhea, and prevent them from making direct patient contact during epidemics.
- Report cases to the local public health authorities.
- Use standard precautions: private room, gown and gloves while handling feces, and hand washing before entering and after leaving the patient's room.
- To prevent the accumulation of these water-loving organisms, discard suction bottles, irrigating fluid, and open bottles of saline solution every 24 hours according to facility policy.
- Change I.V. tubing according to facility policy, and empty the ventilator water reservoirs before refilling them with sterile water.
- Advise travelers to foreign countries to consume only bottled water and to avoid uncooked vegetables.
- Instruct the patient to thoroughly cook ground beef (to 160° F [71.1° C] on a food thermometer), avoid unpasteurized milk, and wash hands thoroughly.

Esophageal cancer

Nearly always fatal, esophageal cancer usually develops in men older than age 60. This disease occurs worldwide, but incidence varies geographically. It's most common in Japan, Russia, China, the Middle East, and the Transkei region of South Africa.

Esophageal tumors are usually fungating and infiltrating. Most arise in squamous cell epithelium, a few are adenocarcinomas, and fewer still are melanomas and sarcomas.

Esophageal cancer has a 5-year survival rate below 5%, and regional metastasis occurs early by way of submucosal lymphatics. Metastasis produces such serious complications as tracheoesophageal fistulas, mediastinitis, and aortic perforation. Common sites of distant metastasis include the liver and lungs.

Causes
- Unknown

Predisposing factors
- Chronic irritation caused by heavy smoking and excessive use of alcohol
- Nutritional deficiency
- Previous head and neck tumors
- Stasis-induced inflammation

Signs and symptoms
- Initially causes no symptoms
- Dysphagia (mild and intermittent initially; constant in later stages) and weight loss
- Pain, hoarseness, coughing, and esophageal obstruction
- Cachexia

Diagnostic tests
- X-rays of the esophagus with barium swallow and motility studies reveal structural and filling defects and reduced peristalsis.
- Endoscopic examination of the esophagus, punch and brush biopsies, and an exfoliative cytologic test confirm the diagnosis.

Treatment
- The patient with esophageal cancer requires palliative therapy with treatment to keep the esophagus open, including dilation of the esophagus.
- Gastrostomy or jejunostomy can help provide adequate nutrition.

- The patient may be given laser or radiation therapy.
- Chemotherapy and radiation therapy can slow the growth of the tumor.
- The patient may require insertion of prosthetic tubes (such as the Celestin tube) to bridge the tumor and alleviate dysphagia.
- Radical surgery can excise the tumor and resect either the esophagus alone or the esophagus and the stomach.
- Analgesics are given as prescribed for pain.

Nursing considerations

- Before surgery, answer the patient's questions and let him know what to expect after surgery, such as gastrostomy tubes, closed chest drainage, and nasogastric suctioning.
- After surgery, monitor vital signs, maintain sequential compression device, encourage incentive spirometry use, and watch for unexpected changes.
- Promote adequate nutrition, and assess the patient's nutritional and hydration status to determine the need for supplementary parenteral feedings.
- Expect to start oral intake on the sixth day, with sips of water every 15 to 30 minutes.
- As diet advances, prevent aspiration of food by placing the patient in Fowler's position for meals and allowing plenty of time to eat. Provide high-calorie, high-protein, pureed food as needed.
- Because the patient will probably regurgitate some food, clean his mouth carefully after each meal. Keep mouthwash handy.
- If the patient has a gastrostomy tube, give food slowly, using gravity to adjust the flow rate. The prescribed amount usually ranges from 200 to 500 ml. Offer him something to chew before each feeding to promote gastric secretions and a semblance of normal eating.

- Instruct the family in gastrostomy tube care (checking tube patency before each feeding, providing skin care around the tube, and keeping the patient upright during and after feedings).
- Provide emotional support for the patient and his family; refer them to appropriate organizations such as the American Cancer Society.

Esophageal diverticula

An esophageal diverticulum is an epithelial-lined mucosal pouch that protrudes from the esophageal lumen. Esophageal diverticula are classified according to their location: just above the upper esophageal sphincter (Zenker's, or pulsion, diverticulum, the most common type), near the midpoint of the esophagus (traction diverticulum), and just above the lower esophageal sphincter (epiphrenic diverticulum).

Generally, esophageal diverticula occur later in life, although they can affect infants and children. They're three times more common in men than in women. Zenker's diverticula occur in patients ages 30 to 50.

Causes

- Primary muscle abnormalities that may be congenital or inflammatory processes adjacent to the esophagus

Zenker's diverticulum

- Increased intraesophageal pressure caused by developmental muscle weakness of the posterior pharynx above the border of the cricopharyngeal muscle
- Pressure of swallowing or contraction of the pharynx before relaxation of the sphincter

Traction diverticulum
- Pressure from adjacent inflamed tissue or lymph nodes
- Tuberculosis

Epiphrenic diverticulum
- Abnormally elevated pressure within the lumen of the esophagus

Signs and symptoms
- In early stages, regurgitation soon after eating; in later stages, delayed regurgitation (possibly during sleep) leading to food aspiration and pulmonary infection
- Noise when liquids are swallowed, chronic cough, hoarseness, a bad taste in the mouth, and halitosis
- Traction diverticulum: commonly no symptoms
- Traction and epiphrenic diverticula with an associated motor disturbance (achalasia or spasm): dysphagia, heartburn, and regurgitation from associated esophageal conditions, such as hiatal hernia, diffuse esophageal spasm, achalasia, reflux esophagitis, and cancer
- Zenker's diverticulum: initially, throat irritation; later, dysphagia and near-complete obstruction

Diagnostic tests
- A barium esophagogram usually confirms the diagnosis by showing characteristic outpouching.
- Esophagoscopy isn't performed because the scope may be passed into the diverticulum and can cause a rupture.
- Traction diverticulum is diagnosed as an incidental finding on a barium esophagogram.

Treatment
- For a small, asymptomatic Zenker's diverticulum, treatment includes a bland diet, thorough chewing, and drinking water after eating to flush out the sac. Symptomatic patients may require surgery to remove the sac or to facilitate drainage. An esophagomyotomy to prevent recurrence is required in most cases.
- A traction diverticulum seldom requires therapy except when esophagitis aggravates the risk of rupture. Then, treatment includes antacids and an antireflux regimen: keeping the head elevated, maintaining an upright position for 2 hours after eating, eating small meals, controlling chronic coughing, and avoiding constrictive clothing.
- Epiphrenic diverticulum requires treatment of accompanying motor disorders, such as achalasia, by repeated dilatations of the esophagus, of acute spasm by anticholinergic administration and diverticulum excision, and of dysphagia or severe pain by surgical excision; if there's an associated hiatal hernia or incompetent lower esophageal sphincter, an antireflux operation is performed. Calcium channel blockers may be used to relax smooth muscles, decrease esophageal pressure, and improve swallowing.
- Depending on the patient's nutritional status, treatment may also include insertion of a nasogastric tube (passed carefully to prevent perforation) and tube feedings to prepare for the stress of surgery.

Nursing considerations
- Carefully observe and document symptoms.
- Assess nutritional status (weight, caloric intake, and appearance).
- If the patient has dysphagia, record well-tolerated foods and what circumstances ease swallowing. Provide a pureed diet with vitamin or protein supplements, and encourage thorough chewing.
- If the patient regurgitates food and mucus, protect against aspiration by

placing him in high Fowler's position to elevate his head.

- To prevent aspiration, tell the patient to empty any visible outpouching in the neck by massage or postural drainage before retiring.

- Teach the patient about this disorder. Explain the proposed treatment and diagnostic procedures.

Esophagitis, corrosive

Inflammation and damage to the esophagus after ingestion of a caustic chemical is called corrosive or caustic esophagitis. Similar to a burn, this injury may be temporary or lead to permanent stricture (narrowing or stenosis) of the esophagus that requires corrective surgery.

Severe injury can quickly lead to esophageal perforation, mediastinitis, and death from infection, shock, and massive hemorrhage (due to aortic perforation). The type and amount of chemical ingested determine the severity and location of the damage.

In children, household chemical ingestion is accidental; in adults, it's usually a suicide attempt or gesture. (See *Advice for corrosive esophagitis.*) The chemical may damage only the mucosa or submucosa, or it may damage all layers of the esophagus.

Esophageal tissue damage occurs in three phases: in the acute phase, edema and inflammation; in the latent phase, ulceration, exudation, and tissue sloughing; and in the chronic phase, diffuse scarring.

Causes
- Ingestion of lye or other strong alkalies
- Ingestion of strong acids (less common)

Advice for corrosive esophagitis

- The adult who has ingested a corrosive agent has usually done so with suicidal intent. Encourage and assist the patient and his family to seek psychological counseling.
- Provide emotional support for parents whose child has ingested a chemical. They'll be distraught and may feel guilty about the accident.
- After the emergency and without emphasizing blame, teach appropriate preventive measures, such as locking accessible cabinets and keeping all corrosive agents out of a child's reach.

Signs and symptoms
- Acute phase lasting 3 to 4 days
- Bloody vomitus that contains pieces of esophageal tissue (with severe damage)
- Dysphagia with development of stricture (usually within weeks)
- Esophageal perforation and mediastinitis, especially crepitation (destruction of the entire esophagus)
- Fever (if secondary infection)
- Inability to speak (if laryngeal damage)
- Inability to swallow
- Marked salivation
- No pain to intense pain in the mouth and anterior chest
- Tachypnea

Diagnostic tests
- Endoscopy (in the first 24 hours after ingestion) delineates the extent and location of the esophageal injury and assesses the depth of the burn. This procedure may also be performed a week after ingestion to assess stricture development.
- Barium swallow also assesses esophageal damage; it's performed 1 week after

chemical ingestion and every 3 weeks thereafter, as ordered, to identify segmental spasm or fistula.

Treatment

- Conservative treatment includes monitoring the patient's condition and administering medications as ordered, including opioids, corticosteroids, and broad-spectrum antibiotics.
- Bougienage involves passing a slender, flexible, cylindrical instrument called a *bougie* into the esophagus to dilate it and minimize stricture. Some practitioners begin bougienage immediately and continue it regularly to maintain a patent lumen and prevent stricture; others delay it for a week to avoid the risk of esophageal perforation.
- Immediate surgery may be necessary for esophageal perforation; it may also be performed later to correct stricture that isn't treatable with bougienage.
- Corrective surgery may involve transplanting a piece of the colon to the damaged esophagus. Even after surgery, stricture may recur at the site of the anastomosis.
- I.V. therapy is started to replace fluids.
- Total parenteral nutrition is given while the patient can't swallow, after which the patient may gradually progress to clear liquids and a soft diet.

Nursing considerations

ACTION STAT!

 If you're the first health care professional to see the patient who has ingested a corrosive chemical, the quality of your emergency care is critical. Follow these important guidelines.

- Don't induce vomiting or lavage because this exposes the esophagus and oropharynx to injury a second time.
- Don't perform gastric lavage because the corrosive chemical may further damage the mucous membrane of the GI lining.
- Provide vigorous support of vital functions as needed, such as oxygen therapy, mechanical ventilation, I.V. fluids, and treatment for shock, depending on the severity of the injury.
- Carefully observe and record intake and output.
- Before X-rays and endoscopy, explain the procedure to the patient to lessen anxiety during the tests and to enhance his cooperation.

- Teach patients and families how to prevent future incidents of chemical ingestion, and make referrals for psychological counseling as appropriate.

Extraocular motor nerve palsies

Dysfunctions of the third, fourth, and sixth cranial nerves are called extraocular motor nerve palsies. Each of these nerves innervates specific muscles.

- The oculomotor (third cranial) nerve innervates the inferior, medial, and superior rectus muscles; the inferior oblique extraocular muscles; the pupilloconstrictor muscles; and the levator palpebrae muscles.
- The trochlear (fourth cranial) nerve innervates the superior oblique muscles.
- The abducens (sixth cranial) nerve innervates the lateral rectus muscles.

The superior oblique muscles control downward rotation, intorsion, and abduction of the eye. Complete dysfunction of the third cranial nerve is called total oculomotor ophthalmoplegia and may be associated with other central nervous system abnormalities. Myasthenia and dysthyroid disease should be examined as differential diagnoses.

Causes

- Diabetic neuropathy
- Pressure from an aneurysm or brain tumor
- Third-nerve (oculomotor) palsy (acute ophthalmoplegia, congenital or acquired: aneurysm (particularly in the posterior communicating artery), tumor, trauma, or microvascular disease, such as diabetes or hypertension; rarely, uncal herniation, cavernous sinus mass lesion, orbital disease, herpes zoster, leukemia and, in children, ophthalmic migraine
- Fourth-nerve (trochlear) palsy: closed head trauma (blowout fracture) or sinus surgery
- Sixth-nerve (abducens) palsy: increased intracranial pressure, trauma, idiopathic thyroid disease, and vasculopathic entities, such as diabetes, hypertension, and atherosclerosis; less commonly, giant cell arteritis, cavernous sinus mass (meningiomas, aneurysms, or metastasis), multiple sclerosis, and stroke

Signs and symptoms

- Diplopia of recent onset
- Third-nerve palsy: ptosis, exotropia (in which the eye looks outward), pupil dilation, unresponsiveness to light, immobility of the eye
- Fourth-nerve palsy: diplopia, inability to rotate the eye downward or upward, tilting of the head
- Sixth-nerve palsy: turning of one eye, inability of the eye to abduct beyond the midline, tilting of head to unaffected side

Diagnostic tests

- Magnetic resonance imaging, computed tomography scanning, or skull X-rays rule out tumors, and cerebral angiography evaluates possible vascular abnormalities such as aneurysms.
- Laboratory studies assess for diabetes.

- An erythrocyte sedimentation rate rules out giant cell arteritis.
- Culture and sensitivity tests may be used to identify the causative organism and determine therapy for sixth-nerve palsy.

Treatment

- Treatment focuses on correcting the underlying cause of the condition.
- Neurosurgery is necessary if the patient has an intracranial tumor or aneurysm.
- High-dose corticosteroids are given I.V. (for giant cell arteritis).
- Massive doses of an I.V. antibiotic may be given for infection.

Nursing considerations

- Give medications as prescribed and monitor for adverse effects.
- Assess the patient's neurologic status.
- Obtain blood samples for laboratory testing as ordered.
- Prepare the patient for surgery if indicated.
- Provide postoperative craniotomy care if indicated.
- Maintain patient safety.

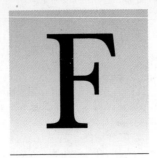

Fatty liver

Steatosis, or fatty liver, is the accumulation of triglycerides and other fats in liver cells. In severe fatty liver, fat constitutes as much as 40% of the liver's weight (as opposed to 5% in a normal liver); the liver's weight may increase from 3.3 lb (1.5 kg) to as much as 11 lb (5 kg).

Minimal fatty changes are temporary and produce no symptoms; severe or persistent changes may cause liver dysfunction. Fatty liver is usually reversible by simply eliminating the cause. (See *Reversing fatty liver.*) This disorder may result in recurrent infection or sudden death from fat emboli in the lungs. Whatever the cause, fatty infiltration of the liver probably results from mobilization of fatty acids from adipose tissues or from altered fat metabolism.

Causes
- Acquired immunodeficiency syndrome
- Carbon tetrachloride intoxication
- Chronic alcoholism (most common cause; severity of liver disease directly related to the amount of alcohol consumed)
- Cushing's syndrome
- DDT poisoning
- Diabetes mellitus
- Drug toxicity
- Jejunoileal bypass surgery
- Malnutrition (especially protein deficiency)
- Obesity
- Pregnancy
- Prolonged total parenteral nutrition (TPN)
- Reye's syndrome

Signs and symptoms
- Ascites
- Edema
- Fever
- Jaundice
- Large, tender liver (hepatomegaly)
- Nausea, vomiting, and anorexia (less common)
- Right upper quadrant pain (with massive or rapid infiltration)
- Spider angiomas, varices, transient gynecomastia, and menstrual disorders (rare)
- Splenomegaly (with cirrhosis)

Diagnostic tests
- A liver biopsy confirms excessive fat in the liver.
- The following findings on liver function tests support this diagnosis:
  - albumin—low
  - globulin—usually elevated
  - cholesterol—usually elevated
  - total bilirubin—elevated
  - alkaline phosphatase—elevated

Reversing fatty liver

■ Suggest counseling for patients with alcoholism, and provide emotional support for their families.

■ Teach patients with diabetes and their families about proper care, such as the purpose of insulin injections or oral diabetic agents, diet, and exercise. Refer patients to diabetes care classes to promote compliance with the treatment plan. Emphasize the need for long-term medical supervision, and urge diabetic patients to report changes in their health immediately.

■ Instruct patients who are obese and their families about proper diet. Warn against fad diets because they may be nutritionally inadequate.

■ Recommend medical supervision for patients who are more than 20% overweight.

■ Encourage the patient to attend a group diet and exercise program and, if necessary, suggest a behavior modification program to correct eating habits.

■ Advise patients who are receiving hepatotoxins and those at risk for occupational exposure to DDT to watch for and immediately report signs of toxicity.

■ Inform all patients that fatty liver is reversible only if they strictly follow the therapeutic program; otherwise, they risk permanent liver damage.

– aminotransferase—usually low
– prothrombin time—possibly prolonged.
■ Other laboratory tests look for anemia, leukocytosis, albuminuria, hyperglycemia or hypoglycemia, and deficiencies of iron, folic acid, and vitamin B_{12}.

Treatment
■ Treatment focuses on correcting the underlying condition or eliminating its cause.
■ Fatty liver that results from I.V. TPN may be corrected by decreasing the rate of carbohydrate infusion.
■ In alcoholic fatty liver, abstinence from alcohol and a proper diet can begin to correct liver changes within 4 to 8 weeks. This requires comprehensive patient teaching.
■ Depending on the degree of severity, the patient may need to undergo liver transplantation.

Nursing considerations
■ Assess for malnutrition, especially protein deficiency, in those with chronic illness. Instruct the patient about what constitutes an adequate diet.
■ Monitor an obese patient's progress in losing weight. Provide positive reinforcement for any weight loss.
■ Perform comprehensive patient teaching, especially for obese, alcoholic, and diabetic patients.

Fibromyalgia syndrome

A diffuse pain syndrome, fibromyalgia syndrome (FMS, previously called *fibrositis*) is one of the most common causes of chronic musculoskeletal pain; it's observed in up to 15% of patients seen in a general rheumatology practice and 5% of general medicine clinic patients. Women are affected more commonly than men, and although FMS can affect all age-groups, its peak incidence is between ages 20 and 60. It may occur as a primary disorder or in association with an underlying disease, such as systemic lupus erythematosus, rheumatoid arthritis, osteoarthritis, and sleep apnea

Tender points of fibromyalgia

The patient with fibromyalgia syndrome may report specific areas of tenderness, which are indicated in these illustrations.

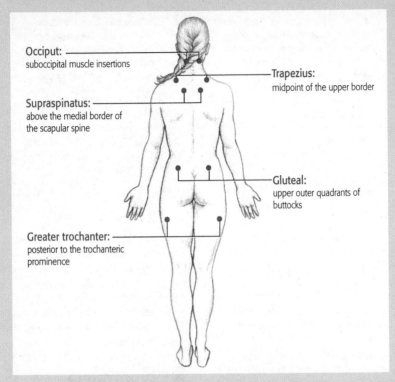

Occiput:
suboccipital muscle insertions

Trapezius:
midpoint of the upper border

Supraspinatus:
above the medial border of
the scapular spine

Gluteal:
upper outer quadrants of
buttocks

Greater trochanter:
posterior to the trochanteric
prominence

syndromes. FMS has also been reported in children, who tend to have more diffuse pain and sleep disturbances than adult patients. Children may have fewer tender points, and many improve over 2 to 3 years.

Causes

- Unknown (in primary form)
- Systemic lupus erythematosus, rheumatoid arthritis, osteoarthritis, and sleep apnea syndromes (in secondary form)

Signs and symptoms

- Chronic musculoskeletal pain and stiffness: diffuse, dull, typically concentrated across the neck, shoulders, lower back, and proximal limbs, possibly involving all four body quadrants; typically lessening as the day progresses; varying from day to day; aggravating factors including stress, lack of sleep, weather changes, and inactivity
- Cognitive impairment
- Dizziness
- Dry eyes and mouth
- Irritable bowel syndrome

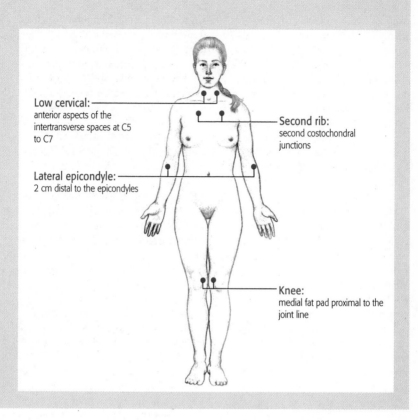

Low cervical:
anterior aspects of the
intertransverse spaces at C5
to C7

Second rib:
second costochondral
junctions

Lateral epicondyle:
2 cm distal to the epicondyles

Knee:
medial fat pad proximal to the
joint line

- Multiple tender points in specific areas on examination
- Paresthesia
- Sensation of hand swelling ("puffy hands"), especially in the morning
- Sensitivities to odors, loud noises, bright lights, and prescribed medications
- Skin sensitivities
- Sleep disturbances: light sleep, frequent awakening, fragmented sleep in some patients (possibly due to pain in those patients who have underlying illnesses, such as osteoarthritis and rheumatoid arthritis); in others, inability to feel rested after a night's sleep leading to fatigue occurring 30 minutes to several hours after awakening and remaining throughout the day
- Tension headaches

Diagnostic tests

- Tenderness can be elicited by applying a moderate amount of pressure to specific locations. (See *Tender points of fibromyalgia.*) Although this examination can be fairly subjective, many FMS patients with true tender points wince or withdraw when pressure is applied to a tender point. Pressure can also be applied to nontender control points, such as the midforehead, distal forearm, and midanterior thigh, to assess for conversion reactions (psychogenic rheumatism), in which patients hurt everywhere, or for other psychosomatic illnesses.

▪ Diagnostic testing for FMS that isn't associated with an underlying disease doesn't usually reveal significant abnormalities. For example, an examination of joints doesn't reveal synovitis or significant swelling; a neurologic examination is normal; and no laboratory or radiologic abnormalities are common to FMS patients.

Treatment

▪ Treatment includes informing the patient that although FMS pain can be severe and is commonly chronic, it's common and doesn't lead to deforming or life-threatening complications.

▪ A regular, low-impact aerobic exercise program can help improve muscle conditioning, energy levels, and an overall sense of well-being. The FMS patient should stretch before and after exercising to minimize injury. Any exercise program, such as walking, bicycling, and swimming, should be started at a low intensity with a slow, gradual increase as tolerated.

▪ Pain control measures may include physical therapy, massage therapy, or injection of tender points.

▪ Ultrasound treatments may be beneficial for particularly problematic areas.

▪ Acupuncture, phototherapy, and mind-body exercises, such as yoga and tai chi, may be beneficial.

▪ Tricyclic antidepressants, such as amitriptyline, nortriptyline, or cyclobenzaprine, given at bedtime may improve sleep, but these agents produce anticholinergic adverse effects and daytime drowsiness.

▪ Nonsteroidal anti-inflammatory drugs may be used for coexisting tendinitis or arthritis but are typically ineffective against FMS pain.

▪ A serotonin reuptake inhibitor such as fluoxetine (Prozac) taken during the day may also be useful in combination with a tricyclic antidepressant at bedtime.

▪ Opioids should be used only with extreme caution to control pain, preferably under the guidance of a pain clinic.

Nursing considerations

▪ Reassure the patient that FMS is common and, although chronic, can be treated.

▪ Explain to the patient that he may experience increased muscle pain when starting a new exercise program. If this occurs, suggest that he decrease the duration or intensity of the exercise. Encourage the patient not to stop exercising altogether, unless otherwise indicated, because even a limited amount of exercise each day may be beneficial.

▪ Advise the patient whose drug regimen includes a tricyclic antidepressant to take the dose 1 to 2 hours before bedtime, which may improve its benefits for sleep and reduce morning drowsiness.

▪ FMS shouldn't be confused with chronic myofascial pain, which is characterized by unilateral and commonly focal or regional pain (as opposed to FMS, in which the pain is bilateral and diffuse), minimal fatigue or stiffness, and few focal tender points (usually distinguished as trigger points) that may produce a radiating pain along a muscle group or tendon (unlike in FMS, where tender points aren't usually associated with radiating pain). Myofascial pain is treated with local measures, such as stretching, physical therapy, heat, and trigger point injections; the symptoms are usually temporary, but may recur.

Folic acid deficiency anemia

A common, slowly progressive megaloblastic anemia, folic acid deficiency anemia is most prevalent in infants, adolescents, pregnant and lactating women, alcoholics, elderly people, and people with malignant or intestinal diseases.

Causes

- Decreased level or lack of folate, a vitamin that's essential for red blood cell production and maturation, that occurs in the following:
  - Alcohol abuse (may suppress metabolic effects of folate)
  - Bacteria competing for available folic acid
  - Impaired absorption (due to intestinal dysfunction from such disorders as celiac disease, tropical sprue, and regional jejunitis and from bowel resection)
  - Inadequate diet (common in alcoholics, elderly people who live alone, and infants, especially those with infections or diarrhea)
  - Increased folic acid requirement during pregnancy, during rapid growth in infancy, during childhood and adolescence, and in patients with neoplastic diseases and some skin diseases (chronic exfoliative dermatitis)
  - Limited storage capacity in infants
  - Overcooking, which can destroy a high percentage of folic acids in foods
  - Prolonged drug therapy (with anticonvulsants, hormonal contraceptives, sulfa antibiotics, and estrogens)

Signs and symptoms

- Dyspnea
- Glossitis
- Headache, fainting, irritability, and forgetfulness
- Nausea and anorexia
- Pallor and slight jaundice
- Palpitations
- Paranoid behavior
- Progressive fatigue
- Weakness

Diagnostic tests

- Schilling test and a therapeutic trial of vitamin B_{12} injections help distinguish between folic acid deficiency anemia and pernicious anemia.
- Blood tests show macrocytosis, a decreased reticulocyte count, increased mean corpuscular volume, low platelet count, and a serum folate level less than 4 mg/ml.

Treatment

- Folic acid supplements are given orally (usually 1 to 5 mg/day) or parenterally (to patients who are severely ill, have malabsorption, or can't take oral medication).
- Provide a well-balanced diet.
- Folic acid replenishment alone may aggravate neurologic dysfunction if the patient has combined vitamin B_{12} and folate deficiencies.

Nursing considerations

- Encourage the patient to meet daily folic acid requirements by including a food from each food group in every meal.
- If the patient has a severe deficiency, explain that diet only reinforces folic acid supplementation but isn't therapeutic by itself.
- Urge compliance with the prescribed course of therapy. Advise the patient not to stop taking the supplements when he begins to feel better.
- Emphasize the importance of good oral hygiene for the patient with glossitis. Suggest regular use of mild or diluted mouthwash and a soft toothbrush. Oral anesthetics may reduce discomfort.

■ Monitor fluid and electrolyte balance, particularly in the patient who has severe diarrhea and is receiving parenteral fluid replacement therapy.

■ Because anemia causes severe fatigue, schedule regular rest periods until the patient can resume normal activity.

■ To prevent folic acid deficiency anemia, emphasize the importance of a well-balanced diet high in folic acid (dark green, leafy vegetables, organ meats, eggs, milk, oranges, bananas, dry beans, and whole grains). Identify alcoholics with poor dietary habits, and try to arrange for appropriate counseling.

■ Tell mothers who aren't breast-feeding to use commercially prepared formulas.

Folliculitis, furunculosis, and carbunculosis

A bacterial infection of the hair follicle, folliculitis causes the formation of a pustule of the hair follicle opening. The infection can be superficial (follicular impetigo or Bockhart's impetigo) or deep (sycosis barbae).

Furuncles, commonly known as *boils*, are another form of deep folliculitis. Carbuncles are a group of interconnected furuncles. The prognosis depends on the severity of the infection and the patient's physical condition and ability to resist infection.

Causes
■ *Staphylococcus aureus* (most common)

Predisposing factors
■ Chemical exposure (cutting oils)
■ Debilitation
■ Diabetes mellitus
■ Friction
■ Immunosuppressive therapy
■ Incorrect shaving technique
■ Infected wound

■ Moisture
■ Obesity
■ Occlusive cosmetics
■ Poor hygiene
■ Skin disease
■ Tight clothes

Signs and symptoms
■ Folliculitis: a primary lesion in a small pustule located over a sebaceous orifice; may be perforated by a hair
■ Furuncles: hard, painful nodules on the neck, face, breasts, perineum, thighs, axillae, and buttocks; rupturing after several days' growth, discharging pus and necrotic material; pain relieved after rupture but persistent erythema and edema (days or weeks)
■ Carbuncles: multiple pustules or deep abscesses that drain through multiple openings onto the skin surface, usually around several hair follicles; possibly accompanied by fever and malaise

Diagnostic tests
■ Wound culture usually shows *S. aureus*.
■ A complete blood count may show an elevated white blood cell count (leukocytosis).

Treatment
■ Folliculitis is treated by cleaning the infected area thoroughly with antibacterial soap (such as Hibiclens) and water; applying warm, wet compresses to promote vasodilation and drainage from the lesions; applying topical antibiotics, such as mupirocin (Bactroban) ointment, clindamycin or erythromycin solution; and, in extensive infection, administering systemic antibiotics (a cephalosporin or dicloxacillin) after culture and sensitivity results return.
■ Furuncles may require incision and drainage of ripe lesions after application of warm, wet compresses and systemic

antibiotics, as indicated by culture results, after drainage.
■ Carbuncles require systemic antibiotic
therapy as well as incision and drainage.

Nursing considerations
■ Clean the infected area with an antibacterial.

<u>**DO'S & DON'TS**</u>

 Teach your patient the following:
Do's
■ Observe scrupulous personal and family hygiene measures to prevent spreading the infection.
■ Wash items such as bedsheets, towels,
and linens in hot water before they're
reused.
■ Change dressings frequently, and discard them promptly in paper bags.
■ Change clothes and bedsheets daily.
■ Have a physical examination if furuncles are recurrent because they may indicate an underlying disease such as diabetes.
Don'ts
■ Never squeeze a boil because this may
cause it to rupture into the surrounding
area.
■ Don't share towels and washcloths.

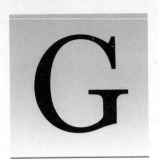

Gallbladder and bile duct cancers

Cancer of the gallbladder is rare, constituting less than 1% of all cancer cases. It's usually found coincidentally in patients with cholecystitis. This disease is most prevalent in women over age 60. It's rapidly progressive and usually fatal; patients seldom live 1 year after diagnosis. The poor prognosis is because of late diagnosis; gallbladder cancer usually isn't diagnosed until after cholecystectomy, when it's typically in an advanced, metastatic stage.

Extrahepatic bile duct cancer is the cause of about 3% of all cancer deaths in the United States. It occurs in both men and women between ages 60 and 70 (incidence is slightly higher in men). The usual site is at the bifurcation in the common duct.

Cancer at the distal end of the common duct is commonly confused with pancreatic cancer. Characteristically, metastasis occurs in local lymph nodes and in the liver, lungs, and peritoneum. Lymph node metastasis is present in up to 70% of patients at diagnosis. Direct extension to the liver is common (affecting up to 90% of patients); direct extension to the cystic and the common bile ducts as well as the stomach, colon, duodenum, and jejunum produces ob-structions. Metastasis also occurs through the portal or hepatic veins to the peritoneum, ovaries, and lower lung lobes.

Causes
- Adenocarcinoma (85% to 95% of cases)
- Extrahepatic bile duct cancer (unknown)
- Gallstones
- Mixed-tissue types (rare)
- Squamous cell carcinoma (5% to 15% of cases)

Signs and symptoms
Gallbladder cancer
- Signs and symptoms identical to those of cholecystitis
- Abdominal distention
- Anorexia, nausea, and vomiting
- Hepatosplenomegaly (in some patients)
- Jaundice
- Pain in the epigastrium or right upper quadrant (chronic, progressively severe pain with cancer; sporadic pain with gallstones)
- Palpable gallbladder (in the right upper quadrant) with obstructive jaundice
- Weight loss

Bile duct cancer
- Black, tarry stools

- Chills and fever (with acute cholecystitis)
- Chronic pain in the epigastrium or right upper quadrant, radiating to the back
- Progressive, profound jaundice (first sign of obstruction)
- Pruritus and skin excoriations

Diagnostic tests
Gallbladder cancer

- Liver function tests typically reveal elevated serum bilirubin, urine bile and bilirubin, and urobilinogen levels in more than 50% of patients with gallbladder cancer. These patients also have consistently elevated serum alkaline phosphatase levels.
- A liver-spleen scan detects abnormalities.
- Cholecystography may demonstrate stones or calcification ("porcelain" gallbladder).
- Magnetic resonance imaging may show areas of tumor growth.
- Cholangiography may outline a common bile duct obstruction.

Bile duct cancer

- Liver function test results showing elevated levels of bilirubin (5 to 30 mg/dl), alkaline phosphatase, and blood cholesterol along with prolonged prothrombin time confirm biliary obstruction.
- Endoscopic retrograde pancreatography identifies the tumor site and allows access for obtaining a biopsy specimen.

Treatment

- Palliative surgery may include cholecystectomy, common bile duct exploration, T-tube drainage, and wedge excision of hepatic tissue.
- Surgery to relieve the obstruction and jaundice that result from extrahepatic bile duct cancer may include cholecystoduodenostomy and T-tube drainage of

the common duct, depending on the site of the cancer.
- Other palliative measures for both kinds of cancer include radiation therapy, radiation implants (used mostly for local and incisional recurrences), and chemotherapy (infrequently used).

Nursing considerations
After biliary resection

- Monitor vital signs.
- Use strict sterile technique when caring for the incision and the surrounding area.
- Place the patient in low Fowler's position.
- Prevent respiratory problems by encouraging deep breathing, coughing, and incentive spirometry use. The high incision makes the patient want to take shallow breaths; taking analgesics and splinting his abdomen with a pillow or an abdominal binder may make breathing easier.
- Monitor bowel sounds and bowel movements. Observe the patient's tolerance of his diet.
- Provide pain-control measures.
- Check intake and output carefully. Watch for electrolyte imbalance; monitor I.V. solutions to avoid overloading the cardiovascular system.
- Monitor the nasogastric tube, which will be in place for 24 to 72 hours postoperatively to relieve distention, and the T tube. Record the amount and color of drainage each shift. Secure the T tube to minimize tension on it and to prevent it from being pulled out.
- Help the patient and his family cope with their initial fears and reactions to the diagnosis by offering information and support.
- Before discharge, teach the patient how to manage the biliary catheter.
- Advise the patient of the adverse effects of both chemotherapy and radia-

tion therapy, and monitor him for these effects.

Gastric cancer

Common throughout the world, gastric cancer affects all races. However, unexplained geographic and cultural differences in incidence occur; for example, mortality is high in Japan, Iceland, Chile, and Austria. In the United States, incidence has decreased 50% during the past 25 years. The decrease in gastric cancer incidence in the United States has been attributed to a decreased consumption of salty, smoked, and cured foods, refrigeration, which reduces the number of nitrate-producing bacteria in food, and a high vitamin C intake.

Incidence is highest in men over age 40. The prognosis depends on the stage of the disease at the time of diagnosis; overall, the 5-year survival rate is about 15%.

According to gross appearance, gastric cancer can be classified as polypoid, ulcerating, ulcerating and infiltrating, or diffuse. The parts of the stomach affected by gastric cancer, listed in order of decreasing frequency, are the pylorus and antrum (50%), the lesser curvature (25%), the cardia (10%), the body of the stomach (10%), and the greater curvature (2% to 3%).

Gastric cancer metastasizes rapidly to the regional lymph nodes, omentum, liver, and lungs by the following routes: walls of the stomach, duodenum, and esophagus; lymphatic system; adjacent organs; bloodstream; and peritoneal cavity.

Causes
- Unknown
- Commonly associated with gastritis, chronic inflammation of the stomach, gastric ulcers, *Helicobacter pylori* bacteria, and gastric atrophy

Predisposing factors
- Dietary factors: some methods of food preparation and preservation (especially smoking, pickling, and salting) and physical properties of some foods
- Environmental influences, such as smoking and high alcohol intake
- Genetics
- Having type A blood (increases risk by 10%)

Signs and symptoms
- Abdominal distention
- Chronic dyspepsia
- Chronic epigastric discomfort
- Early symptoms: dysphagia (with cancer of the cardia), blood in stools
- Later symptoms: vomiting, weight loss, anorexia, a feeling of fullness after eating, anemia, and fatigue

Diagnostic tests
- Barium X-rays of the GI tract, with fluoroscopy, showing a tumor or filling defect in the outline of the stomach, loss of flexibility and distensibility, and abnormal gastric mucosa with or without ulceration.
- Gastroscopy with fiber-optic endoscopy helps rule out other diffuse gastric mucosal abnormalities by allowing direct visualization and gastroscopic biopsy to evaluate gastric mucosal lesions.
- Endoscopy for biopsy and cytologic washings and photography with fiber-optic endoscopy provides a permanent record of gastric lesions that can later be used to determine the progress of the disease and the effect of treatment.
- A gastric acid stimulation test discloses whether the stomach secretes acid properly.
- The following studies may rule out metastasis to specific organs: computed

tomography scans, chest X-rays, liver and bone scans, and a liver biopsy.

Treatment

- Surgery is commonly the treatment of choice. Excision of the lesion with appropriate margins is possible in more than one-third of patients. Even in patients whose disease isn't considered surgically curable, resection offers palliation and improves potential benefits from chemotherapy and radiation therapy. Common surgical procedures include subtotal gastrectomy and total gastrectomy.
- When cancer involves the pylorus and antrum, gastrectomy removes the lower stomach and duodenum (gastrojejunostomy or Billroth II). If metastasis has occurred, the omentum and spleen may also have to be removed.
- If gastric cancer has spread to the liver, peritoneum, or lymph glands, palliative surgery may include gastrostomy, jejunostomy, or a total or subtotal gastrectomy. Such surgery may temporarily relieve vomiting, nausea, pain, and dysphagia while allowing enteral nutrition to continue.
- Chemotherapy for GI cancers may help to control symptoms and prolong survival. Adenocarcinoma of the stomach has responded to several agents, including fluorouracil, carmustine (BiCNU), doxorubicin (Rubex), and mitomycin (Mutamycin).
- Antiemetics can control nausea, which increases as the cancer advances. In the more advanced stages, sedatives and tranquilizers may be necessary to control overwhelming anxiety. Opioids are necessary in many cases to relieve severe and unremitting pain.
- Radiation therapy has been particularly useful when combined with chemotherapy in patients who have unre-

sectable or partially resectable disease. It should be given on an empty stomach and shouldn't be used preoperatively because it may damage viscera and impede healing.
- Antispasmodics and antacids may help relieve GI distress.

Nursing considerations

- Prepare the patient for surgery and for procedures such as insertion of a nasogastric (NG) tube for drainage and I.V. lines as indicated.
- Reassure the patient who's having a subtotal gastrectomy that he may eventually be able to eat normally.
- Prepare the patient who's having a total gastrectomy for slow recovery and only partial return to a normal diet.
- After any type of gastrectomy, pulmonary complications may result, and oxygen may be needed. Regularly assist the patient with coughing and deep breathing. Turn the patient hourly, and give opioid analgesics to help prevent pulmonary problems. Incentive spirometry may also be needed for complete lung expansion. Proper positioning is important as well: Semi-Fowler's position facilitates breathing and drainage.
- After gastrectomy, little (if any) drainage comes from the NG tube because no secretions form after stomach removal. Without a stomach for storage, many patients experience dumping syndrome. Intrinsic factor is absent from gastric secretions, leading to malabsorption of vitamin B_{12}.
- After gastric surgery, don't irrigate or check placement of the NG tube because this may cause pressure at the incision site and possible rupture.
- Instruct the patient about the importance of taking a replacement vitamin for the rest of his life to prevent vitamin B_{12} deficiency.

■ During radiation therapy, encourage the patient to eat high-calorie, well-balanced meals. Offer fluids, such as ginger ale, to minimize such adverse effects as nausea and vomiting.

■ Patients who experience poor digestion and absorption after gastrectomy need a special diet: frequent feedings of small amounts of clear liquids, increasing to small, frequent feedings of bland food.

■ Inform the patient that after total gastrectomy, he must eat small, frequent meals for the rest of his life.

■ Instruct the patient to take pancreatin (Kutrase) and sodium bicarbonate (Neut) after meals to prevent or control steatorrhea and dyspepsia if prescribed.

■ Observe the wound regularly for redness, swelling, failure to heal, and warmth. Parenteral administration of vitamin C may improve wound healing.

■ Give ascorbic acid, thiamine, riboflavin, nicotinic acid, and vitamin K supplements as prescribed.

■ Anabolic agents may induce nitrogen retention. Steroids, antidepressants, wine, and brandy may boost the appetite.

■ Keep the patient comfortable and free from pain, and provide as much psychological support as possible when treatment fails.

■ Discuss continuing care needs with the caregiver or refer the patient to an appropriate home health care agency if the patient is going home.

Gastritis

An inflammation of the gastric mucosa, gastritis may be acute or chronic. *Acute gastritis* produces mucosal reddening, edema, hemorrhage, and erosion. *Chronic gastritis* is common among elderly people and those with pernicious anemia. It's commonly present as chronic atrophic gastritis, in which all stomach mucosal layers are inflamed, with reduced numbers of chief and parietal cells.

Causes
Acute gastritis

■ Chronic ingestion of irritating foods such as hot peppers

■ Drugs (aspirin, nonsteroidal anti-inflammatory drugs, alcohol, caffeine, corticosteroids

■ Endotoxins released from infecting bacteria (staphylococci, *Escherichia coli*, and salmonella)

■ Infection with *Helicobacter pylori* or with other acute infecting organisms

■ Ingested poisons

Chronic atrophic gastritis

■ Autoimmune factors; found predominantly in the body of the stomach (type A)

■ Chronic reflux of pancreatic secretions, bile, and bile acids from the duodenum into the stomach (for example, with peptic ulcer disease or gastrostomy)

■ *H. pylori;* found predominantly in the antral part of the stomach (type B)

■ Recurrent exposure to irritating substances (drugs, alcohol, cigarette smoke)

Signs and symptoms
Acute gastritis

■ Anorexia
■ Cramping
■ Epigastric discomfort
■ Indigestion
■ Nausea, vomiting, and hematemesis

Chronic gastritis

■ Similar to those of acute gastritis or mild epigastric pain

Erosive gastritis

■ None (commonly)

- Anorexia
- Epigastric pain
- Melena
- Nausea and vomiting (possibly coffee-ground emesis)

Diagnostic tests

- Fecal occult blood test detects occult blood in vomitus and stools of the patient with gastric bleeding.
- Hemoglobin level and hematocrit are low if significant bleeding has occurred.
- Upper GI endoscopy with biopsy confirms the diagnosis when performed within 24 hours of bleeding. Biopsy reveals the inflammatory process. An upper GI series may also be performed to exclude serious lesions. Upper endoscopy is contraindicated after ingestion of a corrosive agent.

Treatment

- Antibiotics are prescribed to treat *H. pylori* infection if the patient is immunocompromised.
- Histamine-2 receptor antagonists such as cimetidine (Tagamet), ranitidine (Zantac), or famotidine (Pepcid) may block gastric secretions.
- Antacids may be used as buffers.
- Analgesics may be given for associated pain.
- Initiate fluid and electrolyte replacement as needed.
- The patient experiencing major bleeding may require blood replacement, nasogastric lavage, angiography with vasopressin (Pitressin) infused in normal saline solution and, possibly, surgery.
- Vagotomy and pyloroplasty have achieved limited success when conservative treatments have failed.
- Partial or total gastrectomy may be required (rarely).
- Vitamin B_{12} may be given parenterally (if pernicious anemia is the cause).

Nursing considerations

- For vomiting, give antiemetics and I.V. fluids as prescribed.
- Monitor fluid intake and output and electrolyte levels.
- Monitor the patient for recurrent symptoms as food is reintroduced; provide a bland diet.
- Offer smaller, more frequent meals to reduce irritating gastric secretions. Eliminate foods that cause gastric upset.
- If the patient smokes, refer him to a smoking-cessation program.
- Urge the patient to seek immediate attention for recurring symptoms, such as hematemesis, nausea, and vomiting.
- Urge the patient to take prophylactic medications as prescribed.

DRUG CHALLENGE

 If pain or nausea interferes with the patient's appetite, give analgesics or antiemetics 1 hour before meals.

- Advise the patient to take steroids with milk, food, or antacids to reduce gastric irritation.
- Instruct the patient to take antacids between meals and at bedtime and to avoid aspirin-containing compounds.

Gastroenteritis

Also called *intestinal flu, traveler's diarrhea, viral enteritis,* and *food poisoning,* gastroenteritis is a self-limiting disorder characterized by diarrhea, nausea, vomiting, and abdominal cramping. It occurs in all age-groups and is a major cause of morbidity and mortality in underdeveloped nations.

It can also be life-threatening in children, elderly people, and debilitated people, due to their inability to tolerate electrolyte and fluid losses.

Causes

- Amebas: especially *Entamoeba histolytica*
- Bacteria (responsible for acute food poisoning): *Staphylococcus aureus, Salmonella, Shigella, Clostridium botulinum, Escherichia coli, Clostridium perfringens*
- Drug reactions: antibiotics
- Enzyme deficiencies
- Food allergens
- Ingestion of toxins: plants or toadstools (mushrooms)
- Parasites: *Ascaris, Enterobius, Trichinella spiralis*
- Viruses (may be responsible for traveler's diarrhea): adenovirus, echovirus, rotovirus, calcivirus, astrovirus, norovirus, or coxsackievirus

Signs and symptoms

- Abdominal discomfort (ranging from cramping to pain)
- Borborygmi
- Bowel hypermotility
- Diarrhea
- Fever
- Intracellular fluid depletion
- Malaise
- Nausea and vomiting

Diagnostic tests

- Laboratory studies, such as Gram stain, blood culture, and stool sample, identify the causative bacteria, parasites, or amebas.

Treatment

- Provide nutritional support, and increase the patient's fluid intake.
- Fluid and electrolyte replacement is necessary for severe symptoms that last for more than 3 or 4 days in a young child or an elderly or debilitated person.
- Antibiotics treat the causative infection.
- Antiemetics are used to control nausea and vomiting.

Nursing considerations

- Give medications as prescribed; correlate dosages, routes, and times appropriately with the patient's meals and activities—for example, give antiemetics 30 to 60 minutes before meals.
- Encourage the patient to replace lost fluids and electrolytes with clear liquids and sports-type drinks.
- Vary the patient's diet to make it more enjoyable, and allow some choice of foods.
- Instruct the patient to avoid milk and milk products, which may exacerbate the condition.
- Record strict intake and output. Watch for signs of dehydration, such as dry skin and mucous membranes, fever, and sunken eyes.
- Wash your hands thoroughly after giving care to avoid spread of infection.
- Instruct the patient to take warm sitz baths three times per day to relieve anal irritation.
- Contact public health authorities to interview patients and food handlers, and take samples of the suspected contaminated food if food poisoning is suspected.
- Instruct patients to thoroughly cook foods, especially pork; to refrigerate perishable foods, such as milk, mayonnaise, potato salad, and cream-filled pastry; and to always wash their hands with warm water and soap before handling food, especially after using the bathroom.
- Teach patients to clean utensils thoroughly, to avoid drinking water or eating raw fruit or vegetables when visiting a foreign country, and to eliminate flies and roaches in their homes.

Gastroesophageal reflux

The backflow or reflux of gastric and duodenal contents into the esophagus and past the lower esophageal sphincter (LES), without associated belching or vomiting, is called *gastroesophageal reflux*. Reflux may not cause symptoms or pathologic changes. Persistent reflux may cause reflux esophagitis (inflammation of the esophageal mucosa). The prognosis varies with the underlying cause.

Causes

- Abnormal esophageal clearance
- Deficient LES pressure or pressure within the stomach exceeding LES pressure
- Delayed gastric emptying resulting from partial gastric outlet obstruction or gastroparesis

Predisposing factors

- Any agent that lowers LES pressure, such as food, alcohol, cigarettes, anticholinergics (atropine, belladonna, and propantheline), and other drugs (morphine, diazepam [Valium], and meperidine [Demerol])
- Any condition or position that increases intraabdominal pressure
- Hiatal hernia (especially in children)
- Long-term nasogastric (NG) intubation (more than 5 days)
- Pyloric surgery (alteration or removal of the pylorus)

Signs and symptoms

- Asymptomatic (in some cases)
- Bleeding (bright red or dark brown)
- Chronic pain, possibly radiating to the neck, jaws, and arms
- Chronic pulmonary disease or nocturnal wheezing, bronchitis, asthma, morning hoarseness, and cough (due to reflux of gastric contents into the throat and subsequent aspiration)
- Dysphagia
- Failure to thrive and forceful vomiting from esophageal irritation (in children)
- Indigestion and heartburn (possibly increasing in severity 1 to 2 hours after meals, on reclining, and with vigorous exercise, bending, or lying down)
- Nocturnal regurgitation
- Odynophagia and, possibly, a dull substernal ache

Diagnostic tests

- Barium swallow fluoroscopy, esophageal pH probe, endoscopy, and esophagoscopy all confirm the diagnosis.
- The esophageal acidity test is the most sensitive and accurate measure of gastroesophageal reflux. Degree of reflux may be determined with 12- to 36-hour esophageal pH monitoring.
- In children, barium esophagography under fluoroscopic control can show reflux. Recurrent reflux after age 6 weeks is abnormal.
- Esophagoscopy and a biopsy allow visualization and confirmation of pathologic changes in the mucosa.

Treatment

- Place the patient in the reverse Trendelenburg position (with the head of the bed elevated) for sleeping.
- Positional therapy is especially useful in infants and children. The patient is also encouraged to reduce his weight to help reduce symptoms.
- Over-the-counter antisecretory agents may be helpful in mild cases.
- Histamine-2 receptor blocking agents (cimetidine [Tagamet], ranitidine [Zantac], famotidine [Pepcid], nizatidine [Axid]) for 6 to 12 weeks provide symptom relief in moderate cases.

Coping with reflux

■ Teach the patient what causes reflux, how to avoid reflux with an antireflux regimen (medication, diet, and positional therapy), and what symptoms to watch for and report.
■ Instruct the patient to avoid any circumstance that increases intra-abdominal pressure (such as bending, coughing, vigorous exercise, tight clothing, constipation, and obesity) or any substance that reduces sphincter control (such as cigarettes, alcohol, fatty foods, and certain drugs).
■ Advise the patient to sit upright, particularly after meals, and to eat small, frequent meals. Tell him to avoid highly seasoned food, acidic juices, alcoholic drinks, bedtime snacks, and foods high in fat or carbohydrates, which reduce lower esophageal sphincter pressure. Advise him to avoid lying down for 3 hours after eating a meal.
■ Tell the patient to take antacids as ordered (usually 1 hour and 3 hours after meals and at bedtime).

■ Proton pump inhibitors, such as omeprazole (Prilosec), lansoprazole (Prevacid), pantoprazole (Protonix), or rabeprazole (Aciphex) are necessary for erosive esophagitis.
■ Surgical intervention may be necessary to control severe and refractory symptoms, such as pulmonary aspiration, hemorrhage, obstruction, severe pain, perforation, incompetent LES, and associated hiatal hernia. Surgical procedures include antireflux surgery, in which the fundus is wrapped around the esophagus (fundoplication). Also, vagotomy or pyloroplasty may be combined with an antireflux regimen to modify gastric contents.

Nursing considerations
■ Give medications as prescribed.
■ Explain the preparations required for diagnostic testing. For example, instruct the patient not to eat for 6 to 8 hours before having a barium X-ray or endoscopy.
■ After surgery using a thoracic approach, carefully watch and record chest tube drainage and respiratory status. If needed, give chest physiotherapy and oxygen. Encourage incentive spirometry use. Place the patient with an NG tube in semi-Fowler's position to help prevent reflux. Offer reassurance and emotional support.
■ Teach the patient how to avoid and treat reflux. (See *Coping with reflux*.)

Glaucoma

Glaucoma is a group of disorders characterized by intraocular pressure (IOP) high enough to damage the optic nerve. If untreated, it leads to gradual peripheral vision loss and, ultimately, blindness.

Glaucoma occurs in several forms: primary open-angle (chronic), acute angle-closure (narrow-angle), low tension (normal IOP that's too high for a particular person), and congenital (inherited as an autosomal recessive trait) glaucomas; and glaucoma that results from an underlying condition.

Glaucoma is one of the leading causes of blindness in the United States. About 2% of Americans between ages 40 and 50 and 8% of Americans older than age 70 are afflicted with the disease. Its incidence is highest among blacks, and it's the single most common cause of blindness in that population. In the United States, the visual prognosis is good with early treatment.

Causes

Primary open-angle glaucoma

- Obstructed outflow of aqueous humor through the trabecular meshwork or the canal of Schlemm (commonly runs in families; affects 90% of all patients with glaucoma)
- Overproduction of aqueous humor

Acute angle-closure glaucoma

- Adhesions in the angle between the anterior iris and the posterior corneal surface (referred to as peripheral anterior synechiae)
- Neovascularization in the angle due to vein occlusion or diabetes
- Obstructed outflow of aqueous humor caused by anatomically narrow angles between the anterior iris and the posterior corneal surface, shallow anterior chambers, a thickened iris that causes angle closure on pupil dilation, or a bulging iris that presses on the trabeculae, closing the angle

Secondary glaucoma

- Diabetes
- Drugs such as corticosteroids
- Trauma
- Uveitis
- Venous occlusion

Signs and symptoms

Bilateral, primary open-angle glaucoma

- Loss of peripheral vision
- Mild aching in the eyes
- Reduced visual acuity (especially at night) that's uncorrectable with glasses
- Seeing halos around lights

Acute angle-closure glaucoma

- Blurring and decreased visual acuity
- Cloudy cornea

- Moderate pupil dilation that's nonreactive to light
- Nausea and vomiting
- Photophobia
- Pressure over the eye
- Seeing halos around lights
- Unilateral eye inflammation and pain

Diagnostic tests

- Tonometry (using an applanation, Schiøtz or pneumatic tonometer) measures IOP and provides a baseline for reference. Normal IOP ranges between 8 and 21 mm Hg, but some patients who fall in the normal range develop signs and symptoms of glaucoma. On the other hand, some patients who have abnormally high pressure have no clinical effects. Fingertip tension is another way to measure IOP. On gentle palpation of closed eyelids, one eye feels harder than the other in acute angle-closure glaucoma.
- Slit-lamp examination provides a look at the anterior structures of the eye, including the cornea, iris, and lens.
- Gonioscopy, by determining the angle of the anterior chamber of the eye, allows differentiation between primary open-angle glaucoma and acute angle-closure glaucoma. The angle is normal in primary open-angle glaucoma. In older patients, partial closure of the angle may also occur, so two forms of glaucoma may coexist.
- Ophthalmoscopy provides a look at the fundus, where cupping of the optic disk is visible in chronic open-angle glaucoma. This change appears later in chronic angle-closure glaucoma if the disease isn't brought under control. A pale disk appears in acute angle-closure glaucoma.
- Perimetry or visual field tests help evaluate the extent of primary open-angle deterioration by determining peripheral vision loss.

- Fundus photography can monitor the disk for any changes.

Treatment
For primary open-angle glaucoma

- Beta-adrenergic blockers, such as timolol (Betimol) (contraindicated for patients with asthma or bradycardia) and betaxolol (Betoptic) (a beta$_1$-receptor antagonist), reduce pressure by decreasing aqueous humor production.
- Alpha agonists such as brimonidine (Alphagan P) lower IOP.
- Topical carbonic anhydrase inhibitors such as dorzolamide (Trusopt) reduce pressure by decreasing aqueous humor production.
- Miotic eyedrops, such as pilocarpine, facilitate the outflow of aqueous humor.
- Trabeculectomy, a surgical filtering procedure that creates an opening for aqueous outflow, may be necessary if the condition doesn't respond to medical treatment.
- Tube shunt or valve may be required to decrease IOP in end-stage disease.
- Argon laser trabeculoplasty, in which an argon laser beam is focused on the trabecular meshwork of an open angle, produces a thermal burn that changes the surface of the meshwork and increases the outflow of aqueous humor.

For acute angle-closure glaucoma

- Immediate treatment is necessary to lower the high IOP. If the pressure doesn't decrease with drug therapy, laser iridotomy or surgical peripheral iridectomy must be performed promptly to save the patient's vision.
- Iridectomy relieves pressure by excising part of the iris to reestablish aqueous humor outflow. A prophylactic iridectomy is performed a few days later on the

patient's other eye to prevent an acute episode of glaucoma in that eye.
- I.V. mannitol (Osmitrol) and steroid drops are given preoperatively to lower and quell the inflammation. Acetazolamide (Diamox) is used as well as pilocarpine (which constricts the pupil, forcing the iris away from the trabeculae and allowing fluid to escape) or oral glycerin (50%) to force fluid from the eye by making the blood hypertonic.
- Timolol (Betimol) is used to decrease IOP.
- Opioid analgesics are given to relieve severe pain.

Nursing considerations

- Stress the importance of meticulous compliance with prescribed drug therapy to prevent disk changes, loss of vision, and an increase in IOP.
- Give the patient with acute angle-closure glaucoma medications, and prepare him physically and psychologically for laser iridotomy or surgical peripheral iridectomy.

DRUG CHALLENGE

 Postoperative care after laser peripheral iridectomy includes cycloplegic eyedrops (apraclonidine [Iopidine]) to relax the ciliary muscle and decrease inflammation, thus preventing adhesions. Cycloplegics must be used only in the affected eye. The use of these drops in the normal eye may precipitate an attack of acute angle-closure glaucoma in this eye, threatening the patient's residual vision.

- Encourage ambulation immediately after surgery.
- After surgical filtering, postoperative care includes cycloplegic dilation and topical antibiotic steroids to quell the inflammatory response to surgery.

- Stress the importance of glaucoma screening for early detection and prevention. All people over age 35, especially those with a family history of glaucoma, should have an annual tonometric examination.

Glomerulonephritis, acute poststreptococcal

Also called *acute glomerulonephritis*, acute poststreptococcal glomerulonephritis (APSGN) is a relatively common bilateral inflammation of the glomeruli. It follows a streptococcal infection of the respiratory tract or, less commonly, a skin infection such as impetigo. The damaged and inflamed glomerulus loses the ability to be selectively permeable and allows red blood cells (RBCs) and proteins to filter through as the glomerular filtration rate (GFR) falls. Uremic poisoning may result.

APSGN is most common in boys ages 3 to 7 but can occur at any age. Up to 95% of children and up to 70% of adults with APSGN recover fully; the remainder of patients may progress to chronic renal failure within months.

Causes
- Entrapment and collection of antigen-antibody complexes (produced as an immunologic mechanism in response to streptococci) in the glomerular capillary membranes, inducing inflammatory damage and impeding glomerular function
- Untreated pharyngitis

Signs and symptoms
- Fatigue
- Mild to moderate edema
- Mild to severe hypertension
- Pulmonary edema (in heart failure due to hypervolemia)
- Oliguria (less than 400 ml/24 hours), proteinuria, azotemia, and hematuria

Diagnostic tests
- Urinalysis typically reveals proteinuria and hematuria. The presence of RBCs, white blood cells, protein, and mixed cell casts in urine indicate renal failure.
- Blood tests show elevated serum creatinine levels, low creatinine clearance, and impaired glomerular filtration.
- Elevated antistreptolysin-O titers (in 80% of patients), elevated streptozyme and anti-DNase B titers, and low serum complement levels verify recent streptococcal infection.
- Throat culture may also show group A beta-hemolytic streptococci.
- Renal ultrasonography may show a normal or slightly enlarged kidney.
- Renal biopsy may confirm the diagnosis in a patient with APSGN or may be used to assess renal tissue status.

Treatment
- Supportive care includes bed rest, fluid and dietary sodium restrictions, and correction of electrolyte imbalances (possibly with dialysis, although this is seldom necessary).
- Diuretics, such as metolazone (Zaroxolyn) and furosemide (Lasix), reduce extracellular fluid overload; vasodilators, such as hydralazine (Apresoline), may also be prescribed to lower blood pressure.
- Antibiotics are given to eliminate streptococcal infection.

Nursing considerations
- APSGN usually resolves within 2 weeks, so patient care is primarily supportive.
- Give medications as prescribed.
- Check vital signs and electrolyte values. Monitor intake and output and daily weight. Assess renal function daily

through serum creatinine and blood urea nitrogen levels and urine creatinine clearance. Watch for signs of acute renal failure (oliguria, azotemia, and acidosis).

■ Consult the dietitian to provide a diet high in calories and low in protein, sodium, potassium, and fluids.

■ Protect the debilitated patient against secondary infection by providing good nutrition, using good hygienic technique, and preventing contact with infected people.

■ Bed rest is necessary during the acute phase. Encourage the patient to gradually resume normal activities as symptoms subside.

■ Provide emotional support for the patient and his family. If the patient is on dialysis, explain the procedure fully.

■ Advise the patient with a history of chronic upper respiratory tract infections to report signs of infection (fever, sore throat) immediately.

■ Tell the patient that follow-up examinations are necessary to detect chronic renal failure. Stress the need for regular blood pressure, urine protein, and renal function assessments during the convalescent months to detect recurrence. After APSGN, gross hematuria may recur during nonspecific viral infections; abnormal urinary findings may persist for years.

■ Encourage pregnant women with a history of APSGN to have frequent medical evaluations because pregnancy further stresses the kidneys and increases the risk of chronic renal failure.

Glomerulonephritis, chronic

A slowly progressive disease, chronic glomerulonephritis is characterized by inflammation of the glomeruli, which results in sclerosis, scarring and, eventually, renal failure.

This condition usually remains subclinical until the progressive phase begins, marked by proteinuria, cylindruria (presence of granular tube casts), and hematuria. By the time it produces symptoms, chronic glomerulonephritis is usually irreversible.

Causes
■ Diabetes mellitus
■ Focal glomerulosclerosis
■ Goodpasture's syndrome
■ Lupus erythematosus
■ Membranoproliferative glomerulonephritis
■ Membranous glomerulopathy
■ Poststreptococcal glomerulonephritis
■ Rapidly progressive glomerulonephritis

Signs and symptoms
■ Asymptomatic initially, possibly for many years
■ Hematuria
■ Hypertension
■ Nephrotic syndrome
■ Proteinuria

In late stages
■ Advanced renal failure (accelerated in patients with concurrent severe hypertension) eventually necessitating dialysis or kidney transplantation
■ Azotemia
■ Nausea and vomiting
■ Pruritus
■ Dyspnea
■ Malaise and fatigue
■ Mild to severe edema and anemia
■ Severe hypertension causing cardiac hypertrophy leading to heart failure

Diagnostic tests
■ Urinalysis reveals proteinuria, hematuria, cylindruria, and red blood cell casts.

- Rising blood urea nitrogen and serum creatinine levels indicate advanced renal insufficiency.
- X-ray or ultrasonography shows smaller kidneys.
- Kidney biopsy identifies underlying disease and provides data needed to guide therapy.

Treatment

- Antihypertensives and a sodium-restricted diet are prescribed to lower blood pressure.
- Correction of fluid and electrolyte imbalances is achieved through restrictions and replacement.
- Diuretics, such as furosemide (Lasix), are used to reduce edema and prevent heart failure.
- Antibiotics are used to treat symptomatic urinary tract infections.
- Dialysis or kidney transplant may be used to control symptoms of kidney failure or to keep the patient alive.

Nursing considerations

- Monitor the patient closely and provide supportive care.
- Accurately monitor vital signs, intake and output, and daily weight to evaluate fluid retention.
- Observe for signs of fluid, electrolyte, and acidbase imbalances.
- Ask the dietitian to plan low-sodium, highcalorie meals with adequate protein.
- Administer medications, as prescribed, and provide good skin care (because of pruritus and edema) and oral hygiene.
- Instruct the patient to continue taking prescribed antihypertensives as scheduled, even if he's feeling better, and to report any adverse effects.
- Advise the patient to take diuretics in the morning so he won't need to disrupt his sleep to void, and teach him how to assess ankle edema.

- Warn the patient to report signs of infection, particularly urinary tract infection, and to avoid contact with people who have infections. Urge follow-up examinations to assess renal function.

Glycogen storage disease

Consisting of at least eight distinct errors of metabolism—all inherited—glycogen storage disease alters the synthesis or degradation of glycogen, the form in which glucose is stored in the body.

Normally, muscle and liver cells store glycogen. Muscle glycogen is used in muscle contraction; liver glycogen can be converted into free glucose, which can then diffuse out of the liver cells to increase blood glucose levels.

Glycogen storage disease manifests as a dysfunction of the liver, heart, or musculoskeletal system. Symptoms vary from mild and easily controlled hypoglycemia to severe organ involvement that may lead to cardiac and respiratory failure.

The most common type of glycogen storage disease is type I, glucose-6-phosphatase deficiency, or von Gierke's disease, which results from a deficiency of the liver enzyme glucose-6-phosphatase. This enzyme converts glucose-6-phosphate into free glucose and is necessary for the release of stored glycogen and glucose into the bloodstream to relieve hypoglycemia.

Infants may die of acidosis before age 2; if they survive past this age, with proper treatment, they may grow normally and live to adulthood with only minimal hepatomegaly.

Types of glycogen storage disease

Type	Deficiency	Inheritance pattern
I (von Gierke's)	Glucose-6-phosphatase	Autosomal recessive
II (Pompe's)	Alpha 1,4-glucosidase (acid maltase)	Probably autosomal recessive in most patients (late onset may be autosomal dominant)
III (Cori's)	Debranching enzyme (amylo-1,6-glucosidase)	Autosomal recessive
IV (Andersen's)	Branching enzyme (amylo-1,4-1,6-tansglucosidase)	Autosomal recessive
V (McArdle)	Muscle phosphorylase	Autosomal recessive
VI (Hers')	Possible hepatic phosphorylase	Probably autosomal recessive
VII	Muscle phosphofructokinase	Probably autosomal recessive (rare)
VIII	Hepatic phosphorylase kinase	X-linked and autosomal recessive forms

Causes

- Types I through V and type VII: transmitted as autosomal recessive traits (see *Types of glycogen storage disease*)
- Type VI: transmission mode unknown
- Type VIII: may be an X-linked trait

Signs and symptoms

- Type I:
  - Infants: acidosis, hyperlipidemia, GI bleeding, coma
  - Children: low resistance to infection and, without proper treatment, short stature
  - Adolescents: gouty arthritis and nephropathy, chronic tophaceous gout, bleeding (especially epistaxis), small superficial vessels visible in skin because of impaired platelet function, and fat deposits in cheeks, buttocks, and subcutaneous tissues
- Hepatomegaly and rapid onset of hypoglycemia and acidosis when food is withheld (types I, III, IV, VI, and VIII)
- Muscle glycogen storage disease (types II, V, and VII): poor muscle tone; risk of death from heart failure in type II
- Poor muscle tone, enlarged kidneys, xanthomas over extensor surfaces of the arms and legs, steatorrhea, osteoporosis (probably secondary to a negative calcium balance), and multiple, bilateral, yellow lesions in fundi

Diagnostic tests

- Liver biopsy is the key diagnostic tool because it shows normal glycogen synthetase and phosphorylase enzyme activities but reduced or absent glucose-6-

phosphatase activity. Glycogen structure is normal, but levels are elevated.

■ Laboratory studies of plasma demonstrate low glucose levels but high levels of free fatty acids, triglycerides, cholesterol, and uric acid. Serum analysis reveals high pyruvic acid and lactic acid levels. Diagnosis can be made prenatally for types II, III, and IV.

■ Injection of glucagon or epinephrine increases pyruvic and lactic acid levels but doesn't increase blood glucose levels. The glucose tolerance test curve typically shows depletional hypoglycemia and reduced insulin output. An intrauterine diagnosis is possible.

Treatment

■ For type I, the aims of treatment are to maintain glucose homeostasis and prevent secondary consequences of hypoglycemia through frequent feedings and a constant nocturnal nasogastric (NG) drip with an enteral nutrition formula or dextrose. Uncooked cornstarch is given and acts as a slow-release form of glucose. Treatment includes a low-fat diet with normal amounts of protein and calories; carbohydrates should contain glucose or glucose polymers only.

■ No effective treatment exists for type II.

■ Therapy for type III includes frequent feedings and a highprotein diet.

■ Type IV requires a high-protein, high-calorie diet; bed rest; diuretics; sodium restriction; and paracentesis, if necessary, to relieve ascites.

■ Types V and VII require no treatment except avoidance of strenuous exercise.

■ No treatment is necessary for types VI and VIII.

Nursing considerations
Managing type I disease

■ Consult with a registered dietitian to help educate the family regarding dietary restrictions and adjustments.

■ Before discharge, teach the patient or a family member how to insert an NG tube, use a pump with alarm capacity, monitor blood glucose levels, and recognize symptoms of hypoglycemia (including fatigue, headache, hunger, malaise, and a rapid heart rate).

■ Watch for signs of infection (fever, chills, myalgia) and hepatic encephalopathy (mental confusion, stupor, asterixis, coma) due to increased blood ammonia levels.

Managing other types

■ Type II: Explain test procedures, such as electromyography and EEG, thoroughly.

■ Type III: Instruct the patient to eat a high-protein diet (eggs, nuts, fish, meat, poultry, and cheese). If hypoglycemia is present, high-carbohydrate meals with cornstarch supplements may be provided.

■ Type IV: Watch for signs of hepatic failure (nausea, vomiting, irregular bowel function, clay-colored stools, right upper quadrant pain, jaundice, dehydration, electrolyte imbalance, edema, and changes in mental status progressing to coma).

■ When caring for patients with type II, III, or IV glycogen storage disease, offer the parents reassurance and emotional support. Recommend and arrange for genetic counseling if appropriate.

■ Types V through VIII: Care for these patients is minimal. Explain the disorder to the patient and his family, and help them accept the limitations imposed by his particular type of glycogen storage disease.

Goiter

Nontoxic or simple goiter—thyroid gland enlargement not caused by inflammation or a neoplasm—is commonly classified as endemic or sporadic. It occurs when the thyroid gland can't produce and secrete enough hormones to meet metabolic requirements. As a result, the level of thyroid-stimulating hormone (TSH) increases, which causes the thyroid gland to enlarge to compensate for inadequate hormone synthesis. Such compensation usually overcomes mild to moderate hormonal impairment.

Endemic goiter affects females more than males, especially during adolescence and pregnancy, when the demand on the body for thyroid hormone increases. Sporadic goiter affects no particular population segment. With appropriate treatment, the prognosis is good for either type.

Patient instructions in goiter

- To maintain constant hormone levels, instruct the patient to take prescribed thyroid hormone preparations at the same time each day on an empty stomach.
- Instruct the patient and family members to identify and immediately report signs and symptoms of thyrotoxicosis. Such signs include increased pulse rate, palpitations, diarrhea, sweating, tremors, agitation, and shortness of breath.
- Instruct the patient with endemic goiter to use iodized salt to supply the daily 150 to 300 mcg of iodine necessary to prevent goiter.

Causes

- Both types of goiter: inherited defects possibly leading to insufficient T_4 synthesis or impaired iodine metabolism
- Endemic goiter: inadequate dietary intake of iodine, leading to inadequate production and secretion of thyroid hormone
- Sporadic goiter: ingestion of large amounts of goitrogenic foods or the use of goitrogenic drugs
  - Goitrogenic drugs: propylthiouracil (PTU), methimazole (Tapazole), iodides, and lithium (Lithobid) (may affect fetus if taken during pregnancy)
  - Goitrogenic foods: rutabagas, cabbage, soybeans, peanuts, peaches, peas, strawberries, spinach, and radishes

Signs and symptoms

- Mildly enlarged gland to massive, multinodular goiter
- Respiratory distress and dysphagia from compression of the trachea and esophagus and from swelling and distention of the neck
- Large goiter: obstructed venous return producing venous engorgement and, in rare cases, development of collateral venous circulation in the chest, possibly with dizziness or syncope (if patient raises his arms above his head)

Diagnostic tests

- Ultrasound of the thyroid reveals thyroid mass.
- Biopsy reveals the type of lesion.
- TSH levels may be high or normal.
- Serum T_4 concentration is low normal or normal.
- Iodine 131 uptake is normal or increased (50% of the dose at 24 hours).

Treatment

- Exogenous thyroid hormone replacement with levothyroxine (Synthroid) is

the treatment of choice; it decreases TSH secretion and allows the gland to rest. (See *Patient instructions in goiter*.)
■ Small doses of iodine (Lugol's or potassium iodide solution) commonly relieve goiter caused by iodine deficiency. Sporadic goiter requires avoidance of known goitrogenic drugs and foods.
■ A large goiter that's unresponsive to treatment may require subtotal thyroidectomy.

Nursing considerations
■ Measure the patient's neck circumference to check for progressive thyroid gland enlargement. Also check for the development of hard nodules in the gland, which may indicate carcinoma.
■ Monitor the patient taking goitrogenic drugs for signs of sporadic goiter.
■ Teach the patient about iodized salt, medications, and the symptoms of thyrotoxicosis.

Gonorrhea

A common sexually transmitted disease, gonorrhea is an infection of the genitourinary tract (especially the urethra and cervix) and, occasionally, the rectum, pharynx, and eyes. Untreated gonorrhea can spread through the blood to the joints, tendons, meninges, and endocardium; in females, it can also lead to chronic pelvic inflammatory disease (PID) and sterility.

After adequate treatment, the prognosis in both males and females is excellent, although reinfection is common. Gonorrhea is especially prevalent among young people and people with multiple partners.

Causes
■ Infection with *Neisseria gonorrhoeae*, the organism that causes gonorrhea

■ Exposure during passage through the birth canal (gonococcal ophthalmia neonatorum)
■ Gonococcal conjunctivitis: touching eyes with contaminated hands
■ Sexual contact with an infected person

Signs and symptoms
■ Engorged, red, swollen vagina with profuse purulent discharge
■ Fever
■ Friable cervix and a greenish, yellow discharge
■ Ocular infection
■ Pain and a cracking noise when moving an involved joint
■ Papillary skin lesions on the hands and feet
■ Perihepatitis
■ Pharyngeal infection
■ PID
■ Purulent discharge from urethral meatus
■ Rectal infection
■ Red, swollen female urethral meatus

Diagnostic tests
■ A culture from the site of infection (urethra, cervix, rectum, or pharynx), grown on a Thayer-Martin medium, usually establishes the diagnosis by isolating the organism.
■ A Gram stain showing gram-negative diplococci supports the diagnosis and may be sufficient to confirm gonorrhea in males.
■ Confirmation of gonococcal arthritis requires identification of gram-negative diplococci on smears made from joint fluid and skin lesions. Complement fixation and immunofluorescent assays of serum reveal antibody titers four times the normal rate.
■ Culture of conjunctival scrapings confirms gonococcal conjunctivitis.

Treatment

■ For adults and adolescents with uncomplicated gonorrhea caused by susceptible non-penicillinase-producing *N. gonorrhoeae*, a single dose of ceftriaxone (Rocephin) I.M. is indicated.

■ For presumptive treatment of concurrent *Chlamydia trachomatis* infection, doxycycline (Vibramycin) is given orally two times per day for 7 days.

■ A single dose of ceftriaxone and erythromycin for 7 days is recommended for pregnant patients and those allergic to penicillin.

■ The recommended initial regimen for disseminated gonococcal infection in adults and adolescents is 1 g ceftriaxone I.M. or I.V. every 24 hours.

■ All regimens should be continued for 24 to 48 hours after improvement begins; then therapy may be switched to oral cefixime (Suprax) two times per day, to complete 1 full week of antimicrobial therapy. Ciprofloxacin is no longer recommended by the Centers for Disease Control and Prevention (CDC) for the treatment of gonorrhea in California, Hawaii, Asia, and the Pacific because of the high incidence of fluoroquinolone-resistant *N. gonorrhoeae* cases in those areas. It's also contraindicated in children, adolescents, and pregnant or lactating women.

■ Gonorrhea may also be treated with a single 1-g dose of azithromycin (Zithromax) per CDC guidelines.

■ Treatment of gonococcal conjunctivitis requires a single 1 g dose of ceftriaxone I.M. and lavage of the infected eye with normal saline solution once.

■ Routine instillation of 1% silver nitrate or erythromycin drops into neonates' eyes has greatly reduced the incidence of gonococcal ophthalmia neonatorum.

Nursing considerations

■ Before treatment, establish whether the patient has any drug sensitivities, and watch closely for adverse effects during therapy.

■ Warn the patient that until cultures prove negative, he's still infectious and can transmit gonococcal infection.

■ Practice standard precautions.

■ In the patient with gonococcal arthritis, apply moist heat to ease pain in affected joints.

■ Urge the patient to inform sexual contacts of his infection so that they can seek treatment, even if cultures are negative. Advise them to avoid sexual intercourse until treatment is complete.

■ Report all cases of gonorrhea to local public health authorities for follow-up on sexual contacts. Examine and test all people exposed to gonorrhea as well as neonates of infected mothers.

■ Routinely instill two drops of 1% silver nitrate or erythromycin in the eyes of all neonates immediately after birth. Check neonates of infected mothers for signs of infection. Take specimens for culture from the infant's eyes, pharynx, and rectum.

■ To prevent gonorrhea, tell patients to avoid anyone even *suspected* of being infected, to use condoms during intercourse, to wash their genitalia with soap and water before and after intercourse, and to avoid sharing washcloths or douche equipment.

■ Report all cases of gonorrhea in children to child abuse authorities.

Gout

Also known as *gouty arthritis*, gout is a metabolic disease marked by urate deposits in the joints, which cause painfully arthritic joints. It can strike any joint but favors those in the feet and legs. Primary gout usually occurs in men older than age 30 and in postmenopausal women. Secondary gout occurs in older people.

Gout follows an intermittent course and commonly leaves patients free from symptoms for years between attacks. Gout can lead to chronic disability or incapacitation and, rarely, severe hypertension and progressive renal disease. The prognosis is good with treatment.

Causes
- Unknown
- Genetic defect in purine metabolism
- Pseudogout: calcium pyrophosphate crystals in the periarticular joint structures (see *Pseudogout*)
- Secondary gout: associated with obesity, diabetes mellitus, hypertension, sickle cell anemia, renal disease, and drug therapy (especially hydrochlorothiazide or pyrazinamide)

Signs and symptoms
Asymptomatic gout
- Serum urate levels elevated (no symptoms)

Acute stage
- Acute attack of swift, sudden onset and rapid peaking, attacking only one or a few joints with extreme pain; hot, tender, inflamed, dusky red, or cyanotic joints
- Hypertension or nephrolithiasis with severe back pain
- Initial inflammation of the metatarsophalangeal joint of the great toe (podagra), followed by the instep, ankle, heel, knee, or wrist joints
- Low-grade fever (occasionally)
- Mild acute attacks of quick resolution and irregular recurrence
- Severe attacks of days' or weeks' duration

Pseudogout

Also called *calcium pyrophosphate disease*, pseudogout results when calcium pyrophosphate crystals collect in periarticular joint structures. Without treatment, it leads to permanent joint damage in about one-half of the patients it affects, most of whom are elderly.

Signs and symptoms
Like gout, pseudogout causes abrupt joint pain and swelling, most commonly in the knee, wrist, ankle, and other peripheral joints. These recurrent, self-limiting attacks may be triggered by stress, trauma, surgery, severe dieting, thiazide therapy, and alcohol abuse. Associated symptoms are similar to those of rheumatoid arthritis.

Diagnosis and treatment
In pseudogout, the diagnosis depends on joint aspirations and a synovial biopsy to detect calcium pyrophosphate crystals. X-rays reveal calcific densities in the fibrocartilage and linear markings along bone ends. Blood tests may detect an underlying endocrine or metabolic disorder.

Effective treatment of pseudogout includes joint aspiration to relieve fluid pressure; instillation of steroids; administration of analgesics, salicylates, or other nonsteroidal anti-inflammatory drugs; and, if appropriate, treatment of the underlying endocrine or metabolic disorder.

Intercritical stage
- Migratory attacks sequentially striking various joints and the Achilles tendon; associated with either subdeltoid or olecranon bursitis
- Polyarticular attacks affecting joints in the feet and legs; accompanied by fever

- Second attack: longer lasting, more severe; commonly occurring within 6 months to 2 years, but occasionally 5 to 10 years (in untreated cases)
- Symptom-free intervals between gout attacks

Chronic stage
- Chronic inflammation and tophaceous deposits precipitating secondary joint degeneration, with eventual erosions, deformity, and disability
- Hypertension and albuminuria (in some patients)
- Kidney involvement with associated tubular damage leading to chronic renal dysfunction
- Persistent painful polyarthritis with large, subcutaneous tophi in cartilage, synovial membranes, tendons, and soft tissue
- Tophi formulation in the fingers, hands, knees, feet, ulnar sides of the forearms, helix of the ear, Achilles tendons and, rarely, internal organs, such as the kidneys and myocardium
- Ulceration of skin over the tophus with release of chalky, white exudate or pus
- Urolithiasis (common)

Diagnostic tests
- Monosodium urate monohydrate crystals in synovial fluid from an inflamed joint or a tophus establishes the diagnosis.
- Aspiration of synovial fluid (arthrocentesis) or tophaceous material reveals needlelike intracellular crystals of sodium urate.
- Although hyperuricemia isn't specifically diagnostic of gout, the serum uric acid level is above normal. The urine uric acid level is usually higher in secondary gout than in primary gout.
- Initially, X-ray examinations are normal. However, in chronic gout, X-rays

show damage of the articular cartilage and subchondral bone. Outward displacement of the overhanging margin from the bone contour characterizes gout.

Treatment
Acute gout
- Primary treatment includes bed rest, local application of heat or cold, and immobilization and protection of the inflamed, painful joints.
- Analgesics, such as acetaminophen (Tylenol), relieve the pain associated with mild attacks, but acute inflammation requires nonsteroidal anti-inflammatory drugs or intramuscular corticotropin.
- Oral corticosteroids or intra-articular corticosteroid injections are occasionally needed to treat acute attacks.

Chronic gout
- A continuing maintenance dosage of allopurinol (Zyloprim) is given in many cases to suppress uric acid formation or control uric acid levels, preventing further attacks. This powerful drug should be used cautiously in patients with renal failure.
- Uricosuric agents promote uric acid excretion and inhibit its accumulation.
- Dietary restrictions include avoidance of alcohol and purine-rich foods. Obese patients should try to begin a weight-loss program because obesity puts additional stress on painful joints.
- Surgery may be necessary to improve joint function or correct deformities.
- Surgical excision and drainage is necessary for infected or ulcerated tophi.

Nursing considerations
- Encourage bed rest, but use a bed cradle to keep bedcovers off extremely sensitive, inflamed joints.

- Give pain medication as needed, especially during acute attacks. Apply hot or cold packs to inflamed joints. Administer anti-inflammatory medication and other drugs, and watch for adverse effects. Be alert for GI disturbances with colchicine.
- Urge the patient to drink plenty of fluids (up to 2 qt [2 L]/day) to prevent formation of renal calculi.
- When forcing fluids, record intake and output accurately. Be sure to monitor serum uric acid levels regularly. Alkalinize urine with sodium bicarbonate or another agent as needed.
- Watch for acute gout attacks 24 to 96 hours after surgery. Even minor surgery can precipitate an attack. Before and after surgery, administer colchicine to help prevent gout attacks as needed.
- Make sure the patient understands the importance of having serum uric acid levels checked periodically. Tell him to avoid high-purine foods, such as anchovies, liver, sardines, kidneys, sweetbreads, lentils, and alcoholic beverages (especially beer and wine), all of which raise the urate level.
- Explain the principles of a gradual weight reduction diet to obese patients. Such a diet features foods that contain moderate amounts of protein and little fat.

DRUG CHALLENGE

Advise the patient who's receiving allopurinol, probenecid, or other drugs to immediately report adverse effects, such as drowsiness, dizziness, nausea, vomiting, urinary frequency, and dermatitis.

- Warn the patient taking probenecid or sulfinpyrazone to avoid aspirin and other salicylates. Their combined effect causes urate retention.

- Inform the patient that long-term colchicine therapy is essential during the first 3 to 6 months of treatment with uricosuric drugs or allopurinol.

Graft rejection syndromes

As the clinical practice of solid organ transplantation evolves in sophistication and frequency, the focus on the mechanisms and subsequent treatment of graft rejection grows. Tissues commonly transplanted include the kidney, liver, heart, lung, and cornea. Bone marrow transplantation is unique in that the host's immune system is markedly suppressed and an immune-mediated response can occur when cells in the transplanted bone marrow react against host antigens (called *graft versus host disease*). The incidence of graft rejection has declined significantly with the improvement in compatibility screening techniques and immunosuppressive regimens.

Graft rejection syndromes can be divided into three subtypes, based on timing of onset and mechanisms involved.

Fifty percent of transplant patients experience acute rejection (with only 10% progressing to graft loss), which may occur several hours to days (even weeks) after transplantation. The incidence of acute rejection has decreased significantly with the successful use of immunosuppressants, such as cyclosporine (Sandimmune) and azathioprine (Imuran). The incidence of graft loss has been reduced by newer antirejection therapies.

Chronic rejection occurs in 50% of transplant patients within 10 years after transplantation. This form of rejection is characterized by the development of blood vessel luminal occlusion from progressive thickening of the intimal layers of medium and large arterial walls.

Hyperacute rejection occurs within minutes to days after graft transplantation. This type of rejection has become rare, affecting less than 1% of transplant recipients because of improved pretransplant screenings.

Causes
- Immune response to a graft

Signs and symptoms
- Vary markedly, depending on type of rejection, underlying illness, and type of organ transplanted
- Edema in the heart
- Heart failure
- Hypotension
- Rapid or gradual progression of organ dysfunction, such as oliguria and rising serum blood urea nitrogen and creatinine levels in the kidney

Diagnostic tests
- Biopsy of the transplanted tissue:
  – Tissue in acute rejection displays focal regions of perivascular infiltration of leukocytes, which become more widespread as the process progresses. Eventually, tissue distortion, cellular necrosis, and debris are seen.
  – In chronic rejection, graft vessels display markedly thickened walls that may be occluded, and diffuse interstitial fibrosis is prominent. Leukocyte infiltration is usually mild or absent.
  – Graft tissue undergoing hyperacute rejection is characterized by large numbers of polymorphonuclear leukocytes within the graft blood vessels, widespread microthrombi, platelet accumulation, and interstitial hemorrhage. There's little or no interstitial inflammation.
- Transaminase levels become elevated.
- Albumin levels become decreased.

Treatment
- Management of transplant patients involves postoperative care after transplantation, close monitoring of the function of the grafted organ, immunosuppressive therapy for prevention and control of acute rejection, and surveillance with prophylactic measures against opportunistic infections.
- The primary method for managing hyperacute rejection is prevention. Avoidance of high-risk donor-recipient combinations and the use of thorough pretransplant screening for cross-reactive antibodies are important. When a hyperacute rejection reaction is initiated, no pharmacologic agents can halt it. Management becomes supportive until another donor organ can be found.
- In acute rejection, immunosuppressants, usually given in combination regimens, can be effective. Commonly used agents include corticosteroids, cyclosporine, tacrolimus (FK506, Prograf), and azathioprine. Newer antirejection therapies such as muromonab-CD3 (Orthoclone OKT3), an immunosuppressive monoclonal antibody directed at the CD3 molecule on T cells, are promising.
- There's no accepted therapeutic strategy for treating chronic rejection. Preventive strategies to minimize peritransplant ischemia and reperfusion injury are under investigation and include such measures as the use of pulsatile graft perfusion devices during transport and peritransplant graft treatments to minimize release of mediators in response to vascular trauma.
- Because graft rejection can be compounded by coexisting opportunistic infections, prophylaxis and early antibiotic or antiviral interventions are commonly indicated.

Nursing considerations

- Provide emotional and social support to the patient and his family.
- Teach the patient how to recognize signs and symptoms of organ dysfunction. Instruct him to report fever, chills, or symptoms of infection immediately.
- Stress the importance of complying with immunosuppressive treatment. Explain to the patient that this compliance may be long term, if not lifelong.

▌Granulocytopenia and lymphocytopenia

In *granulocytopenia*, a marked reduction in the number of circulating granulocytes occurs. Although this implies that all the granulocytes (neutrophils, basophils, and eosinophils) are reduced, granulocytopenia usually refers only to decreased neutrophils.

This disorder, which can occur at any age, is associated with infections and ulcerative lesions of the throat, GI tract, other mucous membranes, and skin. Its most severe form is known as *agranulocytosis*.

Lymphocytopenia (lymphopenia), a rare disorder, is a deficiency of circulating lymphocytes (leukocytes produced mainly in lymph nodes).

In granulocytopenia and lymphocytopenia, the total white blood cell (WBC) count may reach dangerously low levels, leaving the body unprotected against infection. The prognosis in both disorders depends on the underlying cause and whether it can be treated. Untreated, severe granulocytopenia can be fatal in 3 to 6 days.

Causes
Granulocytopenia

- Radiation or drug therapy
- Splenic sequestration
- Viral and bacterial infections

Lymphocytopenia

- Aplastic anemia
- Chemotherapy (with alkylating agents)
- Elevated plasma corticoid levels (due to stress, corticotropin or steroid treatment, and heart failure)
- Genetic or thymic abnormality
- Hodgkin's disease
- Immunodeficiency disorders, such as ataxiatelangiectasia and thymic dysplasia
- Impaired intestinal lymphatic drainage (as in Whipple's disease)
- Intestinal lymphangiectasia
- Leukemia
- Lupus erythematosus
- Myasthenia gravis
- Protein-calorie malnutrition
- Radiation therapy
- Renal failure
- Sarcoidosis
- Severe combined immunodeficiency disease (in infants)
- Terminal cancer
- Thoracic duct drainage
- Tuberculosis

Signs and symptoms
Granulocytopenia

- Pharyngeal ulceration, possibly with associated necrosis
- Pneumonia
- Septicemia, possibly leading to septic shock and death
- Slowly progressive fatigue and weakness (not present if caused by an idiosyncratic drug reaction)
- Sudden onset of signs of overwhelming infection (fever, chills, tachycardia, anxiety, headache, and extreme prostration)
- Ulcers in the mouth or colon

Lymphocytopenia

- Enlarged lymph nodes, spleen, and tonsils
- Signs of an associated disease

Diagnostic tests

- Complete blood count (CBC) reveals a marked reduction in neutrophils (less than 500/μl leads to severe bacterial infections) and a WBC count lower than 2,000/μl with few observable granulocytes.
- Examination of bone marrow generally shows a scarcity of granulocytic precursor cells beyond the most immature forms, but this finding may vary, depending on the cause.
- Lymphocyte count less than 1,500/μl in adults or less than 3,000/μl in children indicates lymphocytopenia. Identifying the cause by evaluation of the patient's clinical status, bone marrow and lymph node biopsies, and other appropriate diagnostic tests helps establish the diagnosis.

Treatment
Granulocytopenia

- Treatment focuses on eliminating the underlying cause and controlling infection until the bone marrow can generate more leukocytes. Drug or radiation therapy must be stopped and antibiotic treatment begun immediately, even while awaiting test results.
- Antifungals may be added to the treatment regimen if fever is unresponsive in 4 to 5 days (or if it recurs) with broad-spectrum antibiotics.
- Colony-stimulating factor, such as filgrastim (G-CSF; Neupogen) or sargramostim (GM-CSF; Leukine), stimulates bone marrow production of neutrophils. Spontaneous restoration of leukocyte production in bone marrow generally occurs within 1 to 3 weeks.

Lymphocytopenia

- Treatment focuses on eliminating the cause and managing any underlying disorders.

- Bone marrow transplantation may be necessary for infants with severe combined immunodeficiency disease.

Nursing considerations

- Monitor vital signs frequently.
- Obtain cultures from blood, throat, urine, and sputum.
- Administer antibiotics as prescribed.
- Explain the necessity for protective isolation (preferably with laminar air flow) to the patient and his family.
- Teach proper hand hygiene and how to correctly use gowns and masks. Prevent patient contact with staff members or visitors with respiratory tract infections.
- Maintain adequate nutrition and hydration because malnutrition aggravates immunosuppression. Make sure the patient with mouth ulcers receives a high-calorie, liquid diet—for example, high-protein milk shakes. Offer a straw to make drinking less painful.
- Provide warm saline water gargles and rinses, analgesics, and anesthetic lozenges because good oral hygiene promotes patient comfort and facilitates the healing process.
- Ensure adequate rest, which is essential to the mobilization of the body's defenses against infection. Provide good skin and perineal care.
- Monitor CBC and differential, blood culture results, serum electrolyte levels, intake and output, and daily weight.
- Advise the patient with known or suspected sensitivity to a drug that may lead to granulocytopenia or lymphocytopenia to alert medical personnel to this sensitivity in the future.

▌Guillain-Barré syndrome

Also known as *infectious polyneuritis, Landry-Guillain-Barré syndrome,* and *acute idiopathic polyneuritis,* Guillain-Barré syndrome is an acute, rapidly progressive, and potentially fatal form of polyneuritis that causes muscle weakness and mild distal sensory loss.

This syndrome can occur at any age but is most common between ages 30 and 50; it occurs equally in both sexes. It affects about 2 of every 100,000 people.

The clinical course of Guillain-Barré syndrome is divided into three phases:
- The initial phase begins when the first definitive symptom develops; it ends 1 to 3 weeks later, when no further deterioration is noted.
- The plateau phase lasts from several days to 2 weeks.
- The recovery phase is believed to coincide with remyelination and axonal process regrowth. This phase extends over 4 to 6 months; patients with severe disease may take up to 2 years to recover, and recovery may not be complete.

Significant complications of Guillain-Barré syndrome include mechanical ventilatory failure, aspiration pneumonia, sepsis, joint contractures, and deep vein thrombosis. Unexplained autonomic nervous system involvement may cause sinus tachycardia or bradycardia, hypertension, postural hypotension, and loss of bladder and bowel sphincter control.

Causes
- Unknown; possibly a cell-mediated immune response with an attack on peripheral nerves in response to a virus leading to segmental demyelination of the peripheral nerves

Predisposing factors
- Hodgkin's or some other malignant disease
- Rabies or swine influenza vaccination
- Recent history of minor febrile illness, usually an upper respiratory tract infection or, less commonly, gastroenteritis
- Surgery
- Systemic lupus erythematosus
- Viral illness

Signs and symptoms
- Areflexia
- Dysphagia or dysarthria and, less commonly, weakness of the muscles supplied by cranial nerve XI (spinal accessory nerve)
- Facial diplegia, possibly with ophthalmoplegia (ocular paralysis)
- Hypotonia
- Muscle weakness possibly limited to the cranial nerves (in mild type)
- Muscle weakness, initially in legs with (ascending type) and spreading to the arms and facial nerves within 24 to 72 hours; initially in arms (descending type)
- Paresthesia preceding muscle weakness and vanishing quickly (occasionally)
- Simultaneous loss of sensory and motor function
- Stiffness and pain in the form of a severe "charley horse" (common)

Diagnostic tests
- Several days after onset of signs and symptoms, the cerebrospinal fluid (CSF) protein level begins to rise, peaking in 4 to 6 weeks, probably as a result of widespread inflammatory disease of the nerve roots.
- CSF white blood cell count remains normal, but in severe disease, CSF pressure may rise above normal.
- Complete blood count shows leukocytosis with the presence of immature forms early in the illness, but blood study results soon return to normal.

- Electromyography may show repeated firing of the same motor unit, instead of widespread sectional stimulation.
- Electrophysiologic testing may reveal marked slowing of nerve conduction velocities.

Treatment

- Endotracheal (ET) intubation or tracheotomy is necessary for the patient who has difficulty clearing secretions.
- Mechanical ventilation is necessary if the patient has respiratory difficulties.
- A trial dose of prednisone may be given if the course of the disease is relentlessly progressive. If prednisone produces no noticeable improvement after 7 days, the drug is discontinued.
- Plasmapheresis is useful during the initial phase but offers no benefit if begun 2 weeks after onset.
- High doses of immunoglobulins may be administered I.V. to decrease the autoimmune response but must be started as soon as possible to have an effect.
- Continuous electrocardiogram monitoring is needed to identify cardiac arrhythmias. Propranolol (Indural) is prescribed to treat tachycardia and hypotension; atropine (Sal-Tropine) to treat bradycardia; and volume replacement to treat hypotension.

Nursing considerations

- Watch for ascending sensory loss, which precedes motor loss. Also, monitor vital signs and level of consciousness.
- Assess and treat respiratory dysfunction. If respiratory muscles are weak, take serial vital capacity recordings. Use a respirometer with a mouthpiece or a face mask for bedside testing. Some patients require ventilatory assistance.
- Obtain arterial blood gas measurements as ordered. Because neuromuscular disease results in primary hypoventilation with hypoxemia and hypercapnia, watch for a partial pressure of oxygen (PaO_2) below 70 mm Hg, which signals respiratory failure. Be alert for signs of a rising partial pressure of carbon dioxide (confusion, tachypnea).
- Auscultate for breath sounds, turn and reposition the patient regularly, and encourage coughing and deep breathing.
- Begin respiratory support at the first sign of dyspnea (in adults, a vital capacity less than 800 ml; in children, less than 12 ml/kg of body weight) or a decreasing PaO_2.
- Establish an emergency airway and prepare for ET intubation if respiratory failure appears imminent.
- Give meticulous skin care to prevent skin breakdown and contractures.
- Establish a strict turning schedule; inspect the skin (especially the sacrum, heels, and ankles) for breakdown, and reposition the patient every 2 hours.
- Use foam, gel, or alternating-pressure pads at points of contact to prevent skin breakdown.
- Perform passive range-of-motion exercises within the patient's pain limits. Remember that the proximal muscle groups of the thighs, shoulders, and trunk will be the most tender and cause the most pain on passive movement and turning.
- When the patient's condition stabilizes, change to gentle stretching and active assistance exercises.
- Assess the patient for signs of dysphagia (coughing, choking, "wet-sounding" voice, increased presence of rhonchi after feeding, drooling, delayed swallowing, regurgitation of food, and weakness in cranial nerves V, VII, IX, X, XI, or XII).
- Take measures to minimize aspiration: elevate the head of the bed, position the patient upright and leaning forward

when eating, feed semi-solid food, and check the mouth for food pockets.

■ Encourage the patient to eat slowly and remain upright for 15 to 20 minutes after eating.

■ A speech pathologist and modified video fluoroscopy can assist in identifying the best feeding strategies.

■ If aspiration can't be minimized by diet and position modification, nasogastric feeding is recommended.

■ As the patient regains strength and can tolerate a vertical position, be alert for orthostatic hypotension. Monitor blood pressure and pulse rate during tilting periods and, if necessary, apply toe-to-groin elastic bandages or an abdominal binder to prevent orthostatic hypotension.

■ Inspect the patient's legs regularly for signs of thrombophlebitis (localized pain, tenderness, erythema, edema, positive Homans' sign), a common complication of Guillain-Barré syndrome.

■ To prevent thrombophlebitis, apply antiembolism stockings and sequential compression devices, and give prophylactic anticoagulants as prescribed.

■ If the patient has facial paralysis, give eye and mouth care every 4 hours.

■ Protect the corneas with isotonic eyedrops and conical eye shields.

■ Encourage adequate fluid intake (2 qt [2 L]/day), unless contraindicated.

■ Watch for urine retention. Measure and record intake and output every 8 hours, and offer the bedpan every 3 to 4 hours.

■ If urine retention develops, begin intermittent catheterization as needed. Because the abdominal muscles are weak, the patient may need manual pressure on the bladder (Credé's method) before he can urinate.

■ To prevent and relieve constipation, offer prune juice and a high-bulk diet. If necessary, give daily or alternate-day

suppositories (glycerin or bisacodyl) or enemas as ordered.

■ Before discharge, prepare a home care plan. Teach the patient how to transfer from bed to wheelchair and from wheelchair to toilet or tub and how to walk short distances with a walker or cane.

■ Teach the family how to help the patient eat, compensating for facial weakness, and how to help him avoid skin breakdown. Stress the need for a regular bowel and bladder routine.

■ Refer the patient for physical therapy, occupational therapy, and speech therapy as needed.

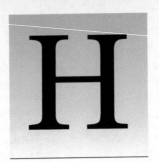

Haemophilus influenzae infection

Haemophilus influenzae is a common cause of laryngotracheobronchitis, epiglottiditis, pneumonia, bronchiolitis, otitis media, and meningitis. Less commonly, it causes bacterial endocarditis, conjunctivitis, facial cellulitis, septic arthritis, and osteomyelitis.

H. influenzae type B (Hib) infection predominantly affects children, at a rate of 3% to 5%. This incidence was higher before vaccinations were widely used. The vaccine is given at age 2, 4, 6, and 15 months. The incidence of meningitis in black children is higher because of Hib infection.

Causes
- *H. influenzae*

Signs and symptoms
- Acute suppurative inflammation
- Bronchopneumonia
- Epiglottitis, generally affecting both the laryngeal and the pharyngeal surfaces
- High fever
- Malaise
- Mucosal edema and thick exudate when *H. influenzae* infects the larynx, trachea, and bronchial tree
- Reddened pharyngeal mucosa, possibly with a soft yellow exudate

Diagnostic tests
- Isolation of the organism, usually with a blood culture, confirms *H. influenzae* infection.
- Polymorphonuclear leukocytosis (15,000 to 30,000/µl) also confirms the diagnosis.
- Hib meningitis is detectable in cerebrospinal fluid cultures.
- A positive nasopharyngeal culture result isn't diagnostic because this may be a normal finding in healthy people.

Treatment
- A 2-week course of ampicillin is standard, but about 30% to 50% of *H influenzae* strains are resistant.
- Ceftriaxone (Rocephin), cefotaxime (Claforan), or chloramphenicol may be used concurrently until sensitivities are identified.

Nursing considerations
- Maintain adequate respiratory function through proper positioning, humidification in children and, possibly, suctioning.
- Monitor the rate and type of respirations.

- Watch for signs of cyanosis and dyspnea, which necessitate intubation or a tracheotomy.
- For home treatment, suggest using a room humidifier or breathing moist air from a shower or bath, as necessary.
- Check the patient's history for drug allergies before giving antibiotics.
- Monitor the complete blood count for signs of bone marrow depression when therapy includes chloramphenicol.
- Monitor intake (including I.V. infusions) and output. Watch for signs of dehydration, such as decreased skin turgor, parched lips, concentrated urine, decreased urine output, and increased pulse rate.
- Take preventive measures, such as encouraging parents to have their young children receive the *H. influenzae* vaccine to prevent these infections, maintaining respiratory isolation, using proper hand-washing technique, properly disposing of respiratory secretions, placing soiled tissues in a plastic bag, and decontaminating all equipment.

▌Hantavirus pulmonary syndrome

Mainly occurring in the southwestern United States, hantavirus pulmonary syndrome was first reported in May 1993. The syndrome, which rapidly progresses from flulike symptoms to respiratory failure, is known for its high mortality.

The hantavirus strain that causes disease in Asia and Europe—mainly hemorrhagic fever and kidney disease—is distinctly different from the strain described in North America.

Despite efforts to identify clinical and laboratory features that distinguish hantavirus pulmonary syndrome from other infections with similar features, diagnosis is based on clinical suspicion along with a process of elimination developed by the Centers for Disease Control and Prevention with the Council of State and Territorial Epidemiologists. (See *Screening for hantavirus pulmonary syndrome*, page 250.)

Causes

- Hantavirus (typically following exposure to infected rodents, the primary reservoir for this virus)

Signs and symptoms

- Noncardiogenic pulmonary edema (distinguishing feature)
- Fever, myalgia (within 1 to 5 weeks of exposure)
- Coughing and shortness of breath (ventilation necessary within 24 hours)
- Headache
- Nausea and vomiting
- Hypoxia
- Serious hypotension (in some patients)
- Increased respiratory rate (28 breaths/minute or more)
- Increased heart rate (greater than 120 beats/minute)

Diagnostic tests

- Laboratory tests usually reveal elevated hematocrit, decreased platelet count, prolonged partial thromboplastin time, a normal fibrinogen level, and an elevated white blood cell count with a predominance of neutrophils, myeloid precursors, and atypical lymphocytes.
- Laboratory findings commonly demonstrate only minimal abnormalities in renal function, with serum creatinine levels no higher than 2.5 mg/dl.
- Chest X-rays eventually show bilateral diffuse infiltrates in almost all patients (findings consistent with acute respiratory distress syndrome).

Screening for hantavirus pulmonary syndrome

The Centers for Disease Control and Prevention (CDC) has developed a screening procedure to track cases of hantavirus pulmonary syndrome. The screening criteria identify potential and actual cases.

Potential cases

For a diagnosis of possible hantavirus pulmonary syndrome, a patient must have one of the following:

■ a febrile illness (temperature equal to or above 101° F [38.3° C]) occurring in a previously healthy person and characterized by unexplained acute respiratory distress syndrome

■ bilateral interstitial pulmonary infiltrates that develop within 1 week of hospitalization with respiratory compromise that requires supplemental oxygen

■ an unexplained respiratory illness resulting in death and autopsy findings demonstrating noncardiogenic pulmonary edema without an identifiable specific cause of death.

Exclusions

Of the patients who meet the criteria for potential hantavirus pulmonary syndrome, the CDC excludes those who have any of the following:

■ a predisposing underlying medical condition; for example, severe underlying pulmonary disease, solid tumors or hematologic cancers, congenital or acquired immunodeficiency disorders, and medical conditions, such as rheumatoid arthritis and organ transplantation, that require immunosuppressive therapy, such as steroids and cytotoxic chemotherapy

■ an acute illness that provides a likely explanation for the respiratory illness (for example, recent seizure disorder, major trauma, burn, or surgery; a history of aspiration, bacterial sepsis; or another respiratory disorder such as respiratory syncytial virus in young children, influenza, and legionella pneumonia).

Confirmed cases

Cases of confirmed hantavirus pulmonary syndrome must include the following:

■ at least one serum sample or tissue specimen available for laboratory testing for evidence of hantavirus infection

■ in a patient with a compatible clinical illness, serologic evidence (presence of hantavirus-specific immunoglobulin [Ig] M or rising titers of IgG), polymerase chain reaction for hantavirus ribonucleic acid, or positive immunohistochemistry for the hantavirus antigen.

Treatment

■ Intubation and aggressive respiratory management within the first few hours are critical. Supportive care includes maintaining adequate oxygenation, monitoring vital signs, and intervening to stabilize the patient's heart rate and blood pressure.

■ Vasopressors, such as dopamine or epinephrine, may be administered for hypotension.

■ Fluid volume replacement may be necessary; take precautions against overhydrating the patient.

■ Ribavirin (Virazole) in aerosol form has been used for children, but its efficacy for adults hasn't been proven.

Nursing considerations

■ Assess the patient's respiratory status and arterial blood gas values frequently.

- Maintain a patent airway by suctioning. Ensure adequate humidification, and check ventilator settings frequently.
- Assess neurologic status frequently, along with heart rate and blood pressure in the patient with hypoxemia.
- Administer drug therapy as prescribed, and monitor the patient's response.
- Monitor the patient's serum electrolyte levels, and administer electrolyte replacements as prescribed.
- Administer I.V. fluid therapy as prescribed and in accordance with the results of hemodynamic monitoring.
- Provide emotional support for the patient and his family.
- Report cases of hantavirus pulmonary syndrome to the state health department.
- Provide prevention guidelines to the patient and his family. (Until more is known about hantavirus pulmonary syndrome, preventive measures focus on rodent control.)

Headache

The most common patient complaint, headache usually occurs as a symptom of an underlying disorder. Ninety percent of all headaches result from vascular causes, muscle contraction, or a combination of the two; 10% are due to underlying intracranial, systemic, or psychological disorders.

Migraine headaches, probably the most intensively studied, are throbbing, vascular headaches that usually begin to appear in childhood or adolescence and recur throughout adulthood. Affecting up to 10% of people in the United States, they're more common in females and have a strong familial incidence.

Causes
Migraine headache
- Unknown
- Constriction and dilation of intracranial and extracranial arteries
- Genetic

Muscle contraction headache
- Abscess
- Aneurysm
- Diseases of the scalp, teeth, extracranial arteries, or external or middle ear
- Glaucoma
- Head trauma and tumor
- Hypertension
- Hypoxia
- Inflammation of the eyes or mucosa of the nasal or paranasal sinuses
- Intracranial bleeding
- Muscle contraction due to emotional stress, fatigue, menstruation, or environmental stimuli (such as noise, crowds, and bright lights)
- Muscle spasms of the face, neck, or shoulders
- Systemic disease
- Vasodilators (such as nitrates, alcohol, and histamines)

Signs and symptoms
Migraine headache
- Scintillating scotoma, hemianopsia, unilateral paresthesia, or speech disorders (preceding onset)
- Unilateral, pulsating pain at onset, later becoming more generalized
- Irritability, anorexia, nausea, vomiting, and photophobia (see *Clinical features of headaches,* page 252)

Muscle contraction headache
- Dull, persistent ache
- Feeling of tightness around the head, with a characteristic "hatband" distribution

Clinical features of headaches

The International Headache Society classifies migraines as occurring with or without an aura. The differentiating characteristics of each type are listed below.

Migraines without an aura

Formerly called *common migraines* or *hemicrania simplex,* migraine headaches without an aura are diagnosed when the patient has five attacks that include the following symptoms:

■ untreated or unsuccessfully treated headache lasting 4 to 72 hours
■ two of the following: pain that's unilateral, pulsating, moderate or severe in intensity, or aggravated by activity
■ nausea, vomiting, photophobia, or phonophobia.

Migraines with an aura

Previously called classic, classical, ophthalmic, hemiplegic, or aphasic migraines, migraine headaches with an aura are diagnosed when the patient has at least two attacks with three of the following characteristics:

■ one or more reversible aura symptoms (indicates focal cerebral cortical or brain stem dysfunction)
■ one or more aura symptoms that develop over more than 4 minutes or two or more symptoms that occur in succession
■ an aura symptom that lasts less than 60 minutes (per symptom)
■ headache begins before, occurs with, or follows an aura with a free interval of less than 60 minutes.

Migraines with an aura also must have one of the following to be classified as a typical aura:

■ homonymous vision disturbance
■ unilateral paresthesia or numbness, or both
■ unilateral weakness
■ aphasia or other speech difficulty.

Migraines also have one of the following characteristics:
■ history and physical and neurologic examinations are negative for a disorder
■ examinations suggest a disorder that's ruled out by appropriate investigation
■ a disorder is present but migraines don't occur for the first time in relation to the disorder.

Tension-type headaches

In contrast to migraines, episodic tension-type headaches are diagnosed when the headache occurs on fewer than 180 days per year or the patient has fewer than 15 headaches per month and the following characteristics are present:

■ headache lasting from 30 minutes to 7 days
■ pain that's pressing or tightening in quality, mild to moderate, bilateral, and not aggravated by activity
■ photophobia or phonophobia occurring sometimes but usually not nausea or vomiting.

Cluster headaches

Cluster headaches are a treatable type of vascular headache syndrome. Characteristics include:

■ episodic type (more common)—one to three short-lived attacks of periorbital pain per day over a 4- to 8-week period followed by a pain-free interval averaging 1 year
■ chronic type—recurrences of established episodic pattern
■ unilateral pain occurring without warning, reaching a crescendo within 5 minutes, and described as excruciating and deep
■ attacks lasting from 30 minutes to 2 hours
■ associated symptoms including tearing, reddening of the eye, nasal stuffiness, lid ptosis, and nausea.

- Neurologic deficits, such as paresthesia and muscle weakness (if intracranial hemorrhage)
- Severe, unrelenting pain (with tumor, most severe when patient awakens)
- Tender spots on the head and neck

Diagnostic tests

- Magnetic resonance imaging, computed tomography scans, lumbar puncture, and serology may be beneficial in diagnosing the condition.
- Aneurysm, neurologic deficits (such as stroke or brain tumors), and metabolic processes (such as thyroid disease or diabetes) must be ruled out if the patient describes the headache as so intensely painful that it's "the worst" he's ever experienced.

Treatment

- Depending on the type of headache, treatment may include pharmacologic agents, relaxation techniques, massage, and biofeedback.
- Antidepressants, beta-adrenergic blockers, and calcium channel blockers may be prescribed for migraine headaches.
- Prevention focuses on identifying and eliminating causative factors, stressors, or stimuli that might trigger an attack such as in the migraine-type headache. Diet history and examination of lifestyle patterns may help identify causative agents.
- Analgesics, ranging from aspirin to codeine or meperidine, may provide symptomatic relief.
- For migraine headaches, ergotamine alone or with caffeine may be effective.

Nursing considerations

- Obtain a complete patient history, including duration and location of the headache, time of day it usually begins, nature of the pain, the concurrence of headache with other symptoms such as blurred vision, and precipitating factors, such as tension, menstruation, loud noises, menopause, alcohol use, prolonged fasting, and use of such medications as hormonal contraceptives.
- Instruct the patient to keep a journal describing the events surrounding the headache. The journal can be used as a guide to aid the patient in avoiding precipitating factors.
- Advise the patient to lie down in a dark, quiet room during an attack and to place ice packs on his forehead or a cold cloth over his eyes.
- Instruct the patient to take the prescribed medication at the onset of migraine symptoms, to prevent dehydration by drinking plenty of fluids after nausea and vomiting subside, and to use other headache-relief measures.

Hearing loss

Loss of hearing results from a mechanical or nervous impediment to the transmission of sound waves. Hearing loss is classified into three major forms:

- Conductive loss is the interrupted passage of sound from the external ear to the junction of the stapes and oval window.
- Sensorineural loss is impaired cochlear or acoustic (eighth cranial) nerve dysfunction, causing failure of transmission of sound impulses within the inner ear or brain.
- Mixed loss is a combination of conductive and sensorineural hearing loss.

Hearing loss may be partial or complete and is calculated using the American Medical Association formula: Hearing is 1.5% impaired for every decibel (dB) that the pure tone average exceeds 25 dB.

Causes
Conductive hearing loss
- Blockage of the external ear
- Cerumen impaction
- Otitis media, otitis externa
- Otosclerosis
- Serous otitis
- Thickening, retraction, scarring, or perforation of the tympanic membrane

Sensorineural hearing loss
- Acoustic neuroma
- Arteriosclerosis
- Brief exposure to very loud noise (greater than 90 dB)
- Drug toxicity
- Head or ear trauma
- Impairment of the cochlea or the acoustic (eighth cranial) nerve
- Infectious diseases
- Loss of hair cells and nerve fibers in the cochlea
- Otospongiosis
- Organ of Corti degeneration
- Perilymphatic fistula
- Prolonged exposure to loud noise (85 to 90 dB)
- Vascular occlusion of the anterior cerebellar artery

Congenital hearing loss
- Dominant, autosomal dominant, autosomal recessive, or sex-linked recessive trait

Hearing loss in neonates
- Congenital abnormalities of the ears, nose, or throat
- Drug toxicity
- Maternal infection during pregnancy or delivery
- Maternal exposure to rubella or syphilis during pregnancy
- Prolonged fetal anoxia during delivery
- Trauma during delivery
- Use of ototoxic drugs during pregnancy

Sudden hearing loss
- Acoustic neuroma
- Bacterial and viral infections
- Blood dyscrasias
- Ménière's disease
- Occlusion of internal auditory artery by spasm or thrombosis
- Ototoxic drugs
- Subclinical mumps

Signs and symptoms
- Deficient response to auditory stimuli within 2 to 3 days after birth (neonatal hearing loss)
- Impaired speech development
- Obvious hearing difficulty

Diagnostic tests
- Weber's and Rinne tests and other specialized audiologic tests differentiate between conductive and sensorineural hearing loss.
- Auditory brain response is used to measure activity in the auditory nerve and brain stem.
- A computed tomography (CT) scan helps to evaluate vestibular and auditory pathways, and pure tone audiometry assesses the presence and degree of hearing loss.
- CT scanning and magnetic resonance imaging are performed to determine soft-tissue involvement and the presence and location of tumors.
- Otoscopic or microscopic examination can be used to diagnose middle ear disorders or remove debris of infection.

Treatment
- The patient may require a hearing aid or other aids to communication.
- Cochlear implant may be required.
- Surgery may be performed to correct tympanic membrane perforation.
- Antibiotics are prescribed when infection is the causative mechanism.

- Cerumenolytics are prescribed to dissolve cerumen.
- Decongestants clear congestion, thereby improving hearing.
- Analgesics may be given to promote comfort.

Nursing considerations

- Approach the patient within his visual range, and elicit his attention by raising your arm or waving; touching him may be unnecessarily startling. Face the patient when speaking, and enunciate words clearly, slowly, and in a normal tone.
- Don't smile, chew gum, or cover your mouth when talking. It makes lip reading more difficult.
- Make other staff members and hospital personnel aware of the patient's disability and his established method of communication.
- Carefully explain all diagnostic tests and hospital procedures in a way the patient understands.
- Write out important statements or information for the patient. He may be embarrassed to tell you he didn't hear everything you said.
- Make sure the patient with a hearing loss is in an area in which he can observe unit activities and people approaching because such a patient depends totally on visual clues.
- Provide emotional support and encouragement to the patient who's learning to use a hearing aid. Teach him how the aid works and how to maintain it.
- To help prevent hearing loss, watch for signs of hearing impairment in patients receiving ototoxic drugs. Emphasize the danger of excessive exposure to noise; stress the danger of exposure to drugs, chemicals, and infection (especially rubella) to pregnant women; and encourage the use of protective devices in a noisy environment.

Heart failure

A syndrome characterized by myocardial dysfunction, heart failure leads to impaired pump performance (reduced cardiac output) or to frank heart failure and abnormal circulatory congestion. Congestion of systemic venous circulation may result in peripheral edema or hepatomegaly; congestion of pulmonary circulation may cause pulmonary edema, an acute, life-threatening emergency.

Pump failure usually occurs in a damaged left ventricle (left-sided heart failure) but may occur in the right ventricle (right-sided heart failure) either as a primary disorder or secondary to left-sided heart failure. Left- and right-sided heart failure usually develop simultaneously.

Although heart failure may be acute (as a direct result of myocardial infarction [MI]), it's usually a chronic disorder associated with sodium and water retention by the kidneys. Advances in diagnostic and therapeutic techniques have greatly improved the outlook for patients with heart failure, but the prognosis still depends on the underlying cause and its response to treatment.

Causes

- Anemia
- Arrhythmias
- Atherosclerosis with MI
- Constrictive pericarditis
- Emotional stress
- Hypertension
- Increased salt or water intake
- Infections
- Mitral or aortic insufficiency
- Mitral stenosis secondary to rheumatic heart disease, constrictive pericarditis, or atrial fibrillation
- Myocarditis
- Pregnancy

Pulmonary edema: How to intervene

Obtain the patient history, assist with diagnostic tests, and assess respiratory, mental, and cardiovascular status.

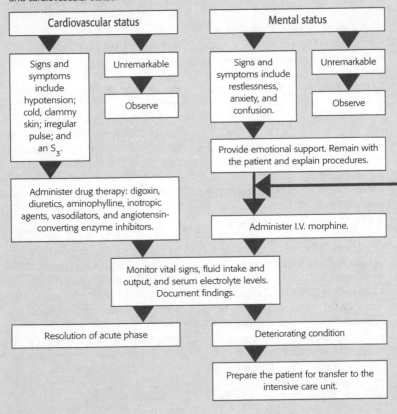

- Pulmonary embolism
- Thyrotoxicosis
- Ventricular and atrial septal defects

Signs and symptoms

Heart failure is usually classified by the site of failure (left-sided, right-sided, or both). It may also be classified as systolic or diastolic. These classifications represent different clinical aspects of

heart failure, not distinct diseases. (See *Pulmonary edema: How to intervene*.)

Left-sided heart failure
- Arrhythmias
- Cough
- Crackles may be accompanied by wheezing
- Cyanosis or pallor
- Dyspnea
- Elevated blood pressure

- Dependent peripheral edema
- Dizziness
- Fatigue
- Hepatojugular reflex
- Hepatomegaly
- Jugular vein distention
- Nausea and vomiting
- Slow weight gain
- Splenomegaly
- Syncope
- Weakness

Diastolic heart failure
- Elevated blood pressure
- Normal or near normal ejection fraction
- S_4 heart sound

Systolic heart failure
- Ejection fraction of less than 40%
- Normal or low blood pressure
- S_3 gallop

Diagnostic tests
- Electrocardiography reflects heart strain, enlargement, and ischemia. It may also reveal atrial enlargement, tachycardia, and extrasystole.
- Chest X-ray shows increased pulmonary vascular markings, interstitial edema, pleural effusion, and cardiomegaly.
- Pulmonary artery monitoring typically demonstrates elevated pulmonary artery and pulmonary artery wedge pressures, elevated left ventricular end-diastolic pressure in left-sided heart failure, and elevated right atrial pressure or central venous pressure in right-sided heart failure.
- Echocardiography demonstrates left ventricular dysfunction with a reduced ejection fraction.
- Brain natriuretic peptide (BNP) assay detects abnormal hormone levels produced by failing ventricles.

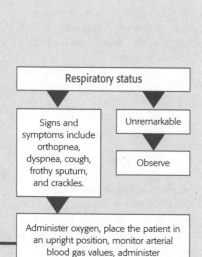

- Hypoxia
- Orthopnea
- Palpitations
- Pulsus alternans
- Respiratory acidosis

Right-sided heart failure
- Abdominal distention
- Anorexia
- Arrhythmias
- Ascites

■ Cardiopulmonary exercise testing determines oxygen consumption and severity of heart failure.

Treatment
■ Diuretics, such as furosemide (Lasix) or spironolactone (Aldactone), a potassium-sparing diuretic, are administered to reduce total blood volume and circulatory congestion.
■ Nesiritide (Natrecor), a recombinant form of human BNP, is given to increase diuresis and to decrease ventricular outflow (afterload).
■ Vasodilators and angiotensin-converting enzyme inhibitors increase cardiac output by reducing the impedance to afterload.
■ Digoxin (Lanoxin) strengthens myocardial contractility.
■ Carvedilol (Coreg), a nonselective beta-adrenergic blocker, reduces mortality and improves quality of life.
■ Institute dietary restrictions, such as restricting sodium and limiting fluid intake to 2 qt (2 L)/day.
■ A biventricular pacemaker controls ventricular dyssynchrony.
■ Antiembolism stockings prevent venostasis and thromboembolus.

Nursing considerations
During the acute phase
■ Monitor the patient closely for signs of pulmonary edema.
■ Place the patient in high Fowler's position and give him supplemental oxygen to help him breathe more easily.
■ Weigh the patient daily, and check for peripheral edema. Carefully monitor his I.V. intake and urine output, vital signs, and mental status. Auscultate the heart for abnormal sounds (S_3 gallop) and the lungs for crackles or rhonchi.
■ Frequently monitor levels of blood urea nitrogen and serum creatinine, potassium, sodium, chloride, and magnesium.
■ The patient should have continuous cardiac monitoring during acute and advanced stages to identify and treat arrhythmias promptly.
■ To prevent deep vein thrombosis due to vascular congestion, assist the patient with range-of-motion exercises. Enforce bed rest and apply antiembolism stockings. Check regularly for calf pain and tenderness.
■ Allow adequate rest periods.

Before discharge
■ Advise the patient to avoid foods high in sodium, such as canned or commercially prepared foods and dairy products, to curb fluid overload.
■ Explain to the patient that the potassium he loses through diuretic therapy must be replaced by taking a prescribed potassium supplement and eating potassium-rich foods, such as bananas, apricots, and orange juice.
■ Stress the need for regular checkups.
■ Emphasize the importance of taking digoxin exactly as prescribed. Tell the patient to watch for and immediately report signs of toxicity, such as anorexia, vomiting, and yellow vision.
■ Tell the patient to promptly report any pulse irregularities. He should also report dizziness, blurred vision, shortness of breath, persistent dry cough, palpitations, increased fatigue, paroxysmal nocturnal dyspnea, swollen ankles, decreased urine output, and rapid weight gain (3 to 5 lb [1.5 to 2.5 kg] in a week).

Heat syndrome
Resulting from environmental or internal conditions that increase heat production or impair heat dissipation, heat syndrome falls into three categories:

Recognizing and managing heat syndrome

Type and predisposing factors	Signs and symptoms	Management
Heat cramps ■ Commonly affect young adults ■ Strenuous activity without training or acclimatization ■ Normal to high temperature or high humidity	■ Muscle twitching and spasms, weakness, severe muscle cramps ■ Nausea ■ Normal temperature or slight fever ■ Normal central nervous system findings ■ Diaphoresis	■ Hospitalization is usually unnecessary. ■ To replace fluid and electrolytes, give a balanced electrolyte drink. ■ Loosen patient's clothing, and have him lie down in a cool place. If muscle cramps are severe, start an I.V. infusion with normal saline solution.
Heat exhaustion ■ Commonly affects young adults ■ Physical activity without acclimatization ■ Decreased heat dissipation ■ High temperature and humidity	■ Muscle cramps (infrequent) ■ Nausea and vomiting ■ Decreased blood pressure ■ Thready, rapid pulse ■ Cool, pallid skin ■ Headache, mental confusion, syncope, giddiness ■ Oliguria, thirst ■ No fever ■ Sweating	■ Hospitalization is usually unnecessary but patient may need emergency evaluation. ■ Immediately give patient a balanced electrolyte drink. ■ Loosen patient's clothing, and put him in a shock position in a cool place. Massage his muscles. If cramps are severe, start an I.V. infusion. ■ If needed, give oxygen.
Heatstroke ■ Exertional: commonly affecting young, healthy adults involved in strenuous activity ■ Classic: commonly affecting elderly, inactive people who have cardiovascular disease or who take drugs that influence temperature regulation ■ High temperature and humidity without any wind	■ Hypertension followed by hypotension ■ Atrial or ventricular tachycardia ■ Hot, dry, red skin, which later turns gray; no diaphoresis ■ Confusion, progressing to seizures and loss of consciousness ■ Temperature higher than 104° F (40° C) ■ Dilated pupils ■ Slow, deep respirations followed by Cheyne-Stokes respirations	■ Initiate airway, breathing, and circulation measures. ■ To lower patient's body temperature, cool rapidly with ice packs on arterial pressure points and hypothermia blankets. ■ To replace fluids and electrolytes, start an I.V. infusion. ■ Hospitalization is needed. ■ Insert nasogastric tube to prevent aspiration. ■ Give a benzodiazepine to control seizures or I.V. chlorpromazine to reduce shivering. ■ Monitor temperature, intake and output, and cardiac status. Give dobutamine to correct cardiogenic shock. (Vasoconstrictors are contraindicated.)

heat cramps, heat exhaustion, and heat-stroke.

Causes
- Dehydration
- Drugs, such as phenothiazines, anticholinergics, and amphetamines
- Endocrine disorders
- Excessive clothing
- Excessive physical activity
- Heart disease
- Hot environment without ventilation
- Illness
- Inadequate fluid intake
- Infection
- Neurologic disorder
- Sudden discontinuation of Parkinson's disease medications

Signs and symptoms
- See *Recognizing and managing heat syndrome,* page 259.

Nursing considerations
- Advise patients to avoid heat syndrome by taking the following precautions in hot weather: rest frequently, avoid hot places, drink adequate fluids, and wear loose-fitting, lightweight clothing.
- Advise patients who are obese, elderly, or taking drugs that impair heat regulation to avoid overheating.
- Tell patients who have had heat cramps or heat exhaustion to increase their salt and water intake. They should also refrain from exercising until symptoms resolve, then resume exercises gradually with plenty of electrolyte-containing fluids and precautions to prevent overheating.
- Warn patients with heatstroke that residual hypersensitivity to high temperatures may persist for several months.

- Parents should be aware that young children and infants are at risk for overheating in hot weather.
- Monitor the patient's vital signs frequently.
- Assess the patient's cardiovascular, respiratory, renal, and neurologic status.
- Cool the patient with ice packs and a hypothermia blanket.
- Administer replacement I.V. fluids.

■ Hemophilia

A hereditary bleeding disorder, hemophilia results from the deficiency of specific clotting factors. *Hemophilia A* (classic hemophilia), which affects more than 80% of all people with hemophilia, results from a deficiency of factor VIII; *hemophilia B* (Christmas disease), which affects 15% of people with hemophilia, results from a deficiency of factor IX. After a person with hemophilia forms a platelet plug at a bleeding site, clotting factor deficiency impairs the capacity to form a stable fibrin clot.

The severity and prognosis of bleeding disorders vary with the degree of deficiency and the site of bleeding. The overall prognosis is best in mild hemophilia, which doesn't cause spontaneous bleeding and joint deformities.

Advances in treatment have greatly improved the prognosis, and many people with hemophilia live normal life spans. Surgical procedures can be done safely at special treatment centers for hemophiliacs under the guidance of a hematologist.

Causes
- Deficiency of genetically transmitted clotting factors (see *X factor*)

Signs and symptoms
- Abnormal bleeding tendency

- Limited joint range of motion (ROM)
- Painful and swollen joints

Diagnostic tests

- Specific coagulation factor assays can diagnose the type and severity of hemophilia. For example, those characteristic of hemophilia A include:
  - factor VIII assay 0% to 25% of normal
  - prolonged partial thromboplastin time (PTT)
  - normal platelet count and function, bleeding time, and prothrombin time.
- Characteristics of hemophilia B include:
  - deficient factor IX assay
  - baseline coagulation results similar to those in hemophilia A, with normal factor VIII.
- In hemophilia A or hemophilia B, the *degree* of factor deficiency determines severity.
  - Mild hemophilia—factor levels 5% to 25% of normal
  - Moderate hemophilia—factor levels 1% to 5% of normal
  - Severe hemophilia—factor levels less than 1% of normal

Treatment

- During a bleeding episode, correct treatment quickly stops bleeding by increasing plasma levels of deficient clotting factors.
- Gene therapy has shown promise as a treatment for both types of hemophilia.

Hemophilia A

- Cryoprecipitated antihemophilic factor (AHF), lyophilized AHF, or both, may be given in doses large enough to raise clotting factor levels above 25% of normal.
- Desmopressin (Stimate) may be given to stimulate the release of stored factor VIII, raising the level in the blood.

X factor

Hemophilia A and hemophilia B are inherited as X-linked recessive traits. Female carriers, therefore, have a 50% chance of transmitting the gene to each daughter, who would also be a carrier, and a 50% chance of transmitting the gene to each son, who would be born with hemophilia.

Hemophilia B

- Factor IX concentrate is administered during bleeding episodes.
- Administer aminocaproic acid for oral bleeding.
- Preventive treatment teaches the patient how to avoid trauma, manage minor bleeding, and recognize bleeding that requires immediate medical intervention. (See *Managing hemophilia,* page 262.)

Nursing considerations
During bleeding episodes

- Administer deficient clotting factor or plasma as prescribed. The body uses up AHF in 48 to 72 hours, so administer repeat infusions, as needed, until bleeding stops.
- Apply cold compresses or ice bags, and raise the injured part.
- Restrict activity for 48 hours after bleeding is under control.
- Control pain with an analgesic, such as acetaminophen (Tylenol), propoxyphene, codeine, or morphine as ordered.
- Avoid I.M. injections because of possible hematoma formation at the injection site.
- Explain the importance of avoiding aspirin and aspirin-containing medications because they decrease platelet adherence and may increase the bleeding.

Managing hemophilia

Include the information below when teaching parents how to care for a child with hemophilia.

Risk of injury and bleeding

■ Instruct parents to notify the practitioner immediately after even a minor injury but especially after an injury to the head, neck, or abdomen. Such injuries may require special blood factor replacement. Also, they should check with the practitioner before allowing dental extractions or any other surgery.

■ Stress the importance of regular, careful toothbrushing to prevent the need for dental surgery. The child should use a soft toothbrush.

■ Teach parents to be alert for signs of internal bleeding, such as severe pain or swelling in a joint or muscle, stiffness, decreased joint movement, severe abdominal pain, severe headache, blood in the urine, and black, tarry stools.

Risk of other disorders

■ Because the child receives blood components, he's at risk for hepatitis. Early signs—headache, fever, decreased appetite, nausea, vomiting, abdominal tenderness, and pain over the liver—may appear 3 weeks to 6 months after treatment with blood components.

■ Discuss the increased risk of human immunodeficiency virus (HIV) infection if the child received a blood product before routine screening of blood products for HIV began. Tell his parents to ask the practitioner about periodic testing for HIV.

Precautions and treatment

■ Urge parents to make sure their child wears a medical identification bracelet at all times.

■ Warn parents never to give the child aspirin, which can increase the tendency to bleed. Advise them to give acetaminophen (Tylenol) instead.

■ Instruct parents to protect the child from injury but to avoid unnecessary restrictions that impair his development. For example, they can sew padded patches into the knees and elbows of a toddler's clothing to protect these joints during falls. They must forbid an older child to play contact sports such as football but can encourage swimming or golf.

■ Teach parents to apply cold compresses or ice bags to an injured area and to elevate or apply light pressure to a bleeding site. To prevent recurrence of bleeding, advise parents to restrict their child's activity for 48 hours after his bleeding is under control.

■ If parents have been trained to give blood factor components at home to avoid hospitalization, make sure they know how to perform venipuncture and infusion techniques and don't delay treatment during bleeding episodes.

■ Instruct parents to keep blood factor concentrate and infusion equipment on hand at all times, including during vacations.

■ Emphasize the importance of having the child keep routine appointments at the local hemophilia center.

Importance of genetic screening

■ Hemophilia A and B are inherited as X-linked recessive traits.

■ Female children should have genetic screening and testing to determine whether they are hemophilia carriers. Affected males should have counseling as well. Female carriers have a 50% chance of transmitting the gene to each daughter, who would then be a carrier, and a 50% chance of transmitting the gene to each son, who would then be born with hemophilia.

■ Refer the parents to the National Hemophilia Foundation for additional information.

If the patient has bled into a joint
- Immediately elevate the joint.
- Begin ROM exercises at least 48 hours after the bleeding is controlled to improve joint mobility.
- Tell the patient to avoid weight bearing until the bleeding stops and swelling subsides.

After bleeding episodes and surgery
- Watch closely for signs of further bleeding, such as increased pain and swelling, fever, and shock.
- Closely monitor PTT.
- Teach parents special precautions to prevent bleeding episodes, signs of internal bleeding, and how to administer emergency first aid.
- Refer new patients to a hemophilia treatment center for evaluation. The center will devise a treatment plan for the patient's primary physician and serve as a resource for everyone involved in the patient's care.
- Referral to a local or national acquired immunodeficiency syndrome support group may be helpful for patients who test positive for human immunodeficiency virus.
- Refer the patient and family for genetic counseling to understand how the disease is inherited, and discuss prenatal testing.

Hemorrhoids

Hemorrhoidal varices are part of the normal anatomy. Dilation and enlargement of the superior plexus of the superior hemorrhoidal veins located above the dentate line produce internal hemorrhoids. Enlargement of the plexus of the inferior hemorrhoidal veins located below the dentate line produces external hemorrhoids. External hemorrhoids may protrude from the rectum. Hemorrhoids occur in both sexes. Incidence is generally highest between ages 20 and 50.

Causes
- Activities that increase intravenous pressure in the hemorrhoidal plexus
- Alcoholism
- Anorectal infections
- Hepatic disease, such as cirrhosis, amebic abscesses, or hepatitis

Predisposing factors
- Constipation
- Low-fiber diet
- Obesity
- Pregnancy
- Prolonged sitting or standing
- Straining at defecation

Signs and symptoms
Internal hemorrhoids
- May cause no symptoms
- Painless, intermittent bleeding during defecation

External hemorrhoids
- Constant discomfort and prolapse with any increase in intra-abdominal pressure
- Sudden rectal pain and a large, firm, subcutaneous lump (with external hemorrhoid thrombosis)

Diagnostic tests
- Anoscopy and flexible sigmoidoscopy are used to confirm internal hemorrhoids and rule out other possible causes of symptoms, such as rectal polyps and anal fistulas.

Treatment
- Institute a high-fiber diet and increase fluid intake to eight to ten 8-oz glasses of water per day. Fiber may be added to the diet by using bulking agents such as psyllium.

- Local anesthetic agents (lotions, creams, or suppositories) or astringents help control pain.
- Hydrocortisone can relieve itching or inflammation.
- Cold compresses followed by warm sitz baths may alleviate discomfort.
- Injection sclerotherapy and rubber band ligation are outpatient procedures that may be used to treat hemorrhoids.
- Infrared photocoagulation bipolar diathermy may be used to affix the mucosa to the underlying muscle.
- Hemorrhoidectomy may be required for severe bleeding, intolerable pain, pruritus, and large prolapsed hemorrhoids.

Nursing considerations
- Prepare the patient for outpatient hemorrhoidectomy by telling him that he may require an enema the night before and morning of surgery.
- Postoperatively, check for signs of prolonged rectal bleeding, administer adequate analgesics, and provide sitz baths.
- Before discharge, tell the patient that he can resume his regular diet.
- Instruct the patient to take a bulking agent, such as psyllium, about 1 hour after the evening meal to help ensure a daily bowel movement. Advise him to maintain regular bowel habits and avoid straining.
- Instruct the patient to avoid vigorous wiping and harsh soaps.

Hemothorax

In hemothorax, blood from damaged intercostal, pleural, mediastinal and, rarely, lung parenchymal vessels enters the pleural cavity. Depending on the amount of bleeding and the underlying cause, hemothorax may be associated with varying degrees of lung collapse and mediastinal shift. Pneumothorax—air in the pleural cavity—commonly accompanies hemothorax.

Causes
- Anticoagulant therapy
- Blunt or penetrating chest trauma (in about 25% of trauma cases)
- Dissecting thoracic aneurysm
- Neoplasm
- Pulmonary infarction
- Thoracic surgery

Signs and symptoms
- Anxiety
- Chest pain
- Cyanosis
- Expansion and stiffening of the affected side of the chest; rising and falling of the unaffected side during respiration
- Hypotension and shock (if marked blood loss)
- Mild to severe dyspnea
- Restlessness
- Tachypnea

Diagnostic tests
- Percussion reveals dullness and, on auscultation, decreased to absent breath sounds over the affected side.
- Thoracentesis yields blood or serosanguineous fluid.
- Chest X-rays show pleural fluid with or without mediastinal shift.
- Arterial blood gas (ABG) analysis may document respiratory failure.
- Hemoglobin level may be decreased, depending on blood loss.

Treatment
- Mild hemothorax usually clears rapidly in 10 to 14 days, requiring only observation for further bleeding.
- Thoracentesis is used to remove blood and other fluids from the pleural cavity.
- The patient with breathing difficulty may benefit from supplemental oxygen therapy.

- Analgesics may be given to control pain.
- I.V. therapy may be used to restore fluid volume.
- Autotransfusion is necessary with significant blood loss (exceeding 1 L).
- Some patients may require insertion of a chest tube.
- Thoracotomy is necessary if the chest tube doesn't improve the patient's condition, to evacuate blood and clots and to control bleeding.

Nursing considerations
- Give supplemental oxygen, I.V. fluids, and blood transfusions as prescribed.
- Monitor pulse oximetry, ABG results, and hemoglobin levels.
- Explain all procedures to the patient to allay his fears.
- Assist with chest tube insertion if indicated.
- Observe chest tube drainage carefully, and record the volume drained at least every hour. Keep the chest tube open and free from clots.
- Assist with thoracentesis as needed. Warn the patient not to cough during this procedure.
- Watch the patient closely for pallor and gasping respirations. Monitor his vital signs diligently. Falling blood pressure and rising pulse and respiratory rates may indicate shock or massive bleeding.

Hepatic encephalopathy

Also known as *hepatic coma*, hepatic encephalopathy is a neurologic syndrome that results from the liver's failure to detoxify noxious agents that arise from the GI tract. Most common in patients with cirrhosis, this syndrome is caused primarily by ammonia intoxication of the brain. It may be acute and self-limiting or chronic and progressive.

In advanced stages, the prognosis is extremely poor, despite vigorous treatment.

Causes
- Unknown
- Ammonia intoxication of the brain

Signs and symptoms
Grade or stage I (prodromal stage)
- Forgetfulness
- Mood fluctuation
- Sleep-wake reversal
- Slight tremor

Grade or stage II (impending stage)
- Aberrant behavior
- Apraxia
- Confusion
- Disorientation
- Incontinence
- Lethargy
- Tremor progressing to asterixis (quick, irregular extensions and flexions of the wrists and fingers when the wrists are held out straight and the hands flexed upward)

Grade or stage III (stuporous stage)
- Hyperventilation
- Stuporous to noisy and abusive when aroused

Grade or stage IV (comatose stage)
- Coma
- Fetor hepaticus (musty, sweet breath odor)
- Hyperactive reflexes
- Positive Babinski's sign

Diagnostic tests

- Elevated serum ammonia levels in venous and arterial samples, along with characteristic signs and symptoms, strongly suggest hepatic encephalopathy.
- An EEG shows slowing waves as the disease progresses.
- Computed tomography scanning or magnetic resonance imaging may be needed to rule out structural disease.

Treatment

- Lactulose traps ammonia in the bowel and promotes its excretion.
- Sorbitol produces osmotic diarrhea, which eliminates ammonia from the GI tract.
- Neomycin 3 to 4 g per day orally or by retention enema may be used as a second-line treatment to suppress bacterial flora and prevent the conversion of amino acids into ammonia.
- Potassium supplements correct alkalosis.
- Salt-poor albumin may be used to maintain fluid and electrolyte balance, replace depleted albumin levels, and restore plasma.

Nursing considerations

- Frequently assess and record the patient's vital signs and neurologic status. Continually orient him to place and time.
- Monitor intake and output and fluid and electrolyte balance. Check daily weight and measure abdominal girth. Immediately report signs of anemia (decreased hemoglobin levels), infection, alkalosis (increased serum bicarbonate levels), and GI bleeding (melena, hematemesis).
- Give prescribed drugs, and monitor the patient for adverse effects.
- Consult with the dietitian to provide the specified low-protein diet, with carbohydrates supplying most of the calories.
- Provide good mouth care.
- Promote rest, comfort, and a quiet atmosphere. Discourage strenuous exercise.
- Protect the comatose patient's eyes from corneal injury by using artificial tears or eye patches.
- Provide emotional support for the family of the patient with end-stage liver disease.

Hepatitis, nonviral

Classified as toxic or drug-induced (idiosyncratic) hepatitis, nonviral hepatitis is an inflammation of the liver. Most patients recover from this illness, although a few develop fulminating hepatitis or cirrhosis.

Causes

- Alcohol overuse: follows heavy alcohol consumption
- Cholestatic reactions: lack of bile excretion, direct hepatotoxicity from hormonal contraceptives or anabolic steroids, and hypersensitivity to phenothiazine derivatives, such as chlorpromazine, antibiotics, thyroid medications, antidiabetic drugs, and cytotoxic drugs
- Direct hepatotoxicity: hepatocellular damage and necrosis due to toxins; dose-dependent and occurring primarily in connection with acetaminophen (Tylenol) overdose
- Idiosyncratic hepatotoxicity: initial sensitization period of several weeks; host hypersensitivity to medications (isoniazid [Nydrazid], methyldopa, mercaptopurine [Purinethol], lovastatin [Mevacor], pravastatin [Pravachol], dipyridamole [Persantine], and halothane)
- Infectious agents: systemic viruses, such as cytomegalovirus, mononucleosis

or Epstein-Barr virus, measles virus, varicella zoster, adenovirus, herpes simplex virus, coxsackievirus, and human immunodeficiency virus; and spirochetes such as those that cause syphilis and leptospirosis
- Metabolic and autoimmune disorders: acute exacerbations of subclinical liver disease, such as autoimmune hepatitis and Wilson's disease

Signs and symptoms
All types
- Abdominal pain (with acute onset and massive necrosis)
- Anorexia
- Clay-colored stools
- Dark urine
- Hepatomegaly
- Jaundice
- Nausea and vomiting
- Pruritus

Carbon tetrachloride poisoning
In addition to the common signs and symptoms:
- Dizziness
- Drowsiness
- Headache
- Vasomotor collapse

Halothane-related hepatitis
In addition to the common signs and symptoms:
- Eosinophilia
- Fever
- Moderate leukocytosis

Chlorpromazine-related hepatitis
In addition to the common signs and symptoms:
- Abrupt fever
- Arthralgia
- Epigastric or right upper quadrant pain

- Lymphadenopathy
- Rash

Diagnostic tests
- Confirm diagnosis by studies showing elevation in serum aspartate aminotransferase, alanine aminotransferase, both total and direct bilirubin (with cholestasis), and alkaline phosphatase levels; white blood cell (WBC) count; and eosinophil count (possible in the drug-induced type).
- Liver biopsy may help identify the underlying condition, especially infiltration with WBCs and eosinophils.
- Liver function tests have limited value in distinguishing between nonviral and viral hepatitis.

Treatment
- Lavage, catharsis, or hyperventilation may be used to eliminate the causative agent, depending on the route of exposure.
- Acetylcysteine (Mucomyst) may serve as an antidote for toxic hepatitis caused by acetaminophen poisoning but doesn't prevent drug-induced hepatitis caused by other substances.
- Corticosteroids may be prescribed for patients with drug-induced hepatitis.

Nursing considerations
- Assess the patient's vital signs, GI status, and neurologic status.
- Administer medications as prescribed and note their effectiveness.
- Provide emotional support to the patient and his family.
- Teach the patient the proper use of drugs and the proper handling of cleaning agents and solvents.
- Explain the disorder and treatment regimen. If alcohol abuse was the cause, explain the importance of alcohol cessation.

Hepatitis, viral

A fairly common systemic disease, viral hepatitis is marked by hepatocellular destruction, necrosis, and autolysis, leading to anorexia, jaundice, and hepatomegaly. In most patients, hepatic cells eventually regenerate with little or no residual damage. Advanced age and serious underlying disorders make complications more likely. The prognosis is poor if edema and hepatic encephalopathy develop.

The six types of hepatitis are:

■ Type A (infectious or short-incubation hepatitis) is rising among homosexuals and in people with immunosuppression related to human immunodeficiency virus (HIV) infection. It's usually self-limiting and without a chronic form. About 40% of cases in the United States result from hepatitis A virus.

■ Type B (serum or long-incubation hepatitis) is also increasing among HIV-positive individuals. Hepatitis B is considered a sexually transmitted disease because of its high incidence and rate of transmission by this route.

Routine screening of donor blood for the hepatitis B surface antigen (HBsAg) has decreased the incidence of post-transfusion cases, but transmission by needles shared by drug abusers remains a major problem. Acute signs and symptoms usually begin insidiously and last for 1 to 4 weeks. Urticaria or arthralgia that's experienced before any signs of jaundice is highly suggestive of hepatitis B infection. A chronic, potentially infectious state develops in about 10% of infected adults and in 70% to 90% of infected infants. This chronic state is associated with progressive liver disease in some individuals. Fulminant hepatitis can ensue, and there's an increased risk of primary hepatocellular carcinoma.

■ Type C accounts for about 20% of all viral hepatitis cases and is primarily transmitted through blood and body fluids or obtained during tattooing.

■ Type D (delta hepatitis) is responsible for about 50% of all cases of fulminant hepatitis, which has a high mortality. Developing in 1% of patients, fulminant hepatitis causes unremitting liver failure with encephalopathy. It progresses to coma and commonly leads to death within 2 weeks.

In the United States, type D hepatitis is confined to people who are frequently exposed to blood and blood products, such as I.V. drug users and hemophiliacs. It's transmitted parenterally and, less commonly, sexually.

■ Type E (formerly grouped with type C under the name non-A, non-B hepatitis) occurs primarily in people who have recently returned from an endemic area (such as India, Africa, Asia, or Central America); it's more common in young adults and more severe in pregnant women.

■ Type G is a newly discovered form of hepatitis. Transmission is blood-borne, and it occurs most commonly in those who receive blood transfusions.

Causes
Hepatitis A

■ Fecal-oral or parenteral transmission
■ Ingestion of contaminated food, milk, or water
■ Ingestion of seafood from polluted water

Hepatitis B

■ Contact with contaminated human blood, secretions, or stool
■ Intimate sexual contact
■ Perinatal transmission

Hepatitis C
- Transfused blood from asymptomatic donors, sharing of needles by I.V. drug users, and receiving tattoos

Hepatitis D
- Limited to patients with an acute or chronic episode of hepatitis B

Hepatitis E
- Oral-fecal transmission
- Water-borne

Hepatitis G
- Blood-borne

Signs and symptoms
Prodromal stage
- Anorexia (possibly with mild weight loss)
- Arthralgia
- Dark-colored urine and clay-colored stools (usually appearing 1 to 5 days before the onset of the clinical jaundice stage)
- Depression
- Easy fatigue
- Generalized malaise
- Headache
- Myalgia
- Nausea and vomiting
- Photophobia
- Taste and smell changes
- Temperature of 100° to 102° F (37.8° to 38.9° C)
- Weakness

Clinical jaundice stage
- Abdominal pain or tenderness especially in the right upper quadrant
- Anorexia (in early stages)
- Enlarged and tender liver
- Indigestion
- Jaundice
- Pruritus

- Rashes, erythematous patches, and urticaria of the skin, especially if the patient has hepatitis B or C
- Splenomegaly and cervical adenopathy (in some cases)

Recovery stage
- Commonly lasts 2 to 12 weeks, or longer with hepatitis B, C, or E
- Decrease or resolution of most symptoms
- Decrease in liver enlargement

Diagnostic tests
- A hepatitis profile identifies antibodies specific to the causative virus, establishing the type of hepatitis as follows:
  - Type A: Detection of an antibody to hepatitis A confirms the diagnosis.
  - Type B: The presence of HBsAg and hepatitis B antibodies confirms the diagnosis.
  - Type C: The diagnosis depends on serologic testing for the specific antibody 1 or more months after the onset of acute hepatitis. Until then, the diagnosis is established primarily by obtaining negative test results for hepatitis A, B, and D.
  - Type D: Detection of intrahepatic delta antigens or immunoglobulin (Ig) M antidelta antigens in acute disease (or IgM and IgG in chronic disease) establishes the diagnosis.
  - Type E: Detection of hepatitis E antigens supports the diagnosis; the diagnosis may also be determined by ruling out hepatitis C.
  - Type G: Detection of hepatitis G ribonucleic acid supports the diagnosis; serologic assays are being developed.
- Additional findings from liver function studies support the diagnosis:
  - Serum aspartate aminotransferase and serum alanine aminotransferase levels are increased in the prodromal stage of acute viral hepatitis.

Preventing a recurrence of hepatitis

Provide the following information before discharging the patient with hepatitis:
- Emphasize the importance of having regular medical checkups for at least 1 year. The patient will have an increased risk of developing hepatocellular carcinoma.
- Warn the patient against using alcohol or nonprescription drugs for 1 year.
- Teach the patient to recognize the signs of recurrence.
- Encourage appropriate vaccinations.
- Discuss the use of medications.
- Teach the patient how to protect himself against other viruses.
- Stress the need for personal safety.

– Serum alkaline phosphatase levels are slightly increased.
– Serum bilirubin levels are elevated. Levels may continue to be high late in the disease, especially if the patient has severe disease.
- Prothrombin time more than 3 seconds longer than normal indicates severe liver damage.
- White blood cell counts commonly reveal transient neutropenia and lymphopenia followed by lymphocytosis.
- Liver biopsy is performed if chronic hepatitis is suspected. (It's performed for acute hepatitis only if the diagnosis is questionable.)

Treatment
- Hepatitis B immunoglobulin and hepatitis B vaccine are given to individuals exposed to blood or body secretions of infected individuals. The hepatitis B vaccine is given also as part of the routine childhood immunization schedule.
- No vaccine exists for hepatitis C, but it's usually treated somewhat successfully with interferon alfa-2b and peginterferon alfa-2a, more recently approved by the Food and Drug Administration.
- Rest is advised in the early stages of the illness.
- Combat anorexia by eating small, high-protein meals. The largest meal should be eaten in the morning because nausea tends to intensify as the day progresses.
- A low-protein diet should be followed if signs of precoma (lethargy, confusion, mental changes) develop.
- Parenteral nutrition may be required if the patient experiences persistent vomiting and can't maintain oral intake.
- Antiemetics (trimethobenzamide [Tigan]) may be given 30 minutes before meals to relieve nausea and prevent vomiting; phenothiazines have a cholestatic effect and should be avoided.
- Resin cholestyramine (Questran) may relieve severe pruritus.

Nursing considerations
- Before the patient is discharged, discuss restrictions and how to prevent a recurrence of hepatitis. (See *Preventing a recurrence of hepatitis*.)
- Enteric precautions are used when caring for patients with type A or E hepatitis. Practice standard precautions for all patients.
- Stress the importance of thorough hand washing.
- Inform visitors about isolation precautions.
- Provide rest periods throughout the day. Schedule treatments and tests so the patient can rest between bouts of activity.
- Because inactivity may make the patient anxious, include diversional activi-

ties as part of his care. Gradually add activities as the patient begins to recover.

- Encourage the patient to eat. Provide small, frequent meals. Minimize medications.
- Encourage fluids (at least 1 gal [4 L]/ day). Encourage the anorexic patient to drink fruit juices. Also offer ice chips and effervescent soft drinks to maintain hydration without inducing vomiting.
- Give supplemental vitamins and commercial feedings. If symptoms are severe and the patient can't tolerate oral intake, provide parenteral nutrition and hydration.
- Monitor the patient's weight daily, and record intake and output. Observe stools for color, consistency, and amount, and record the frequency of bowel movements.
- Watch for signs of fluid shift, such as weight gain and orthostasis.
- Watch for signs of hepatic coma, dehydration, pneumonia, vascular problems, and pressure ulcers.
- In fulminant hepatitis, maintain electrolyte balance and a patent airway, prevent infections, and control bleeding. Correct hypoglycemia and any other complications while awaiting liver regeneration and repair.

▌Herniated disk

Also called a *ruptured* or *slipped disk* or a *herniated nucleus pulposus,* a herniated disk occurs when all or part of the nucleus pulposus—the soft, gelatinous, central portion of an intervertebral disk—is forced through the disk's weakened or torn outer ring (anulus fibrosus).

When this happens, the extruded disk may impinge on spinal nerve roots as they exit from the spinal canal or on the spinal cord itself, resulting in back pain and other signs of nerve root irritation. Herniated disks usually occur in adults (mostly men) younger than age 45.

About 90% of herniated disks occur in the lumbar and lumbosacral regions, 8% occur in the cervical area, and 1% to 2% occur in the thoracic area.

Patients with a congenitally small lumbar spinal canal or with osteophyte formation along the vertebrae may be more susceptible to nerve root compression with a herniated disk and more likely to have neurologic symptoms.

Causes
- Intervertebral joint degeneration
- Minor trauma in older patients whose disks have begun to degenerate
- Severe trauma or strain

Signs and symptoms
- Muscle spasms
- Pain (sudden onset, initially brief duration followed by recurrences at shorter intervals and with increasingly progressive intensity (in trauma-related herniated disk)
- Sciatic pain: begins as a dull pain in the buttocks; intensified by Valsalva's maneuver, coughing, sneezing, and bending
- Sensory and motor loss in the area innervated by the compressed spinal nerve root
- Severe lower back pain radiating to the buttocks, legs, and feet, usually unilaterally
- Weakness and atrophy of leg muscles (in later stages)

Diagnostic tests
- The straight-leg-raising test and its variants are perhaps the best tests for diagnosing a herniated disk. For this test, the patient lies in a supine position while the examiner places one hand on the patient's ilium, to stabilize the pelvis,

and the other hand under the ankle and then slowly raises the patient's leg. The test is positive only if the patient complains of posterior leg (sciatic) pain, not back pain.

- In Lasègue's test, the patient lies flat while the thigh and knee are flexed to a 90-degree angle. Resistance and pain as well as loss of ankle or knee-jerk reflex indicate spinal root compression.
- X-rays of the spine are essential to show degenerative changes and to rule out other abnormalities but may not diagnose a herniated disk because a marked disk prolapse can be present despite a normal X-ray.
- Peripheral vascular status check, including posterior tibial and dorsalis pedis pulses and the skin temperature of extremities, helps rule out ischemic disease, another cause of leg pain or numbness.
- Myelography pinpoints the level of the herniation.
- Computed tomography scanning shows bone and soft-tissue abnormalities and can also show spinal canal compression that results from herniation.
- Magnetic resonance imaging (MRI) defines tissues in areas usually obscured by bone on other imaging tests such as those done with X-rays. MRI is the method of choice to confirm the diagnosis and determine the exact level of herniation.

Treatment

- Treatment for symptoms includes bed rest (possibly with pelvic traction), heat or ice applications, and an exercise program.
- Nonsteroidal anti-inflammatory drugs reduce inflammation and edema at the site of injury.
- Epidural corticosteroids, short-term oral corticosteroids, nerve root blocks, or physical therapy may be prescribed.

- Muscle relaxants may also be beneficial.
- Laminectomy (excision of a portion of the lamina and removal of the protruding disk) may be necessary if conservative treatment fails.
- Spinal fusion may be necessary to overcome segmental instability.
- Laminectomy and spinal fusion are sometimes performed concurrently to stabilize the spine.
- Chemonucleolysis—injection of the enzyme chymopapain into the herniated disk to dissolve the nucleus pulposus—is a possible alternative to laminectomy.
- Percutaneous automated diskectomy or microdiskectomy can also be used to remove fragments of the nucleus pulposus.

Nursing considerations

- Provide supportive care, careful patient teaching, and strong emotional support to help the patient cope with the discomfort and frustration of chronic lower back pain.
- Reinforce the need for myelography and tell the patient to expect some pain. Assure him that he'll receive a sedative before the test, if needed, to keep him as calm and comfortable as possible.
- Before myelography, question the patient carefully about allergies to iodides, iodine-containing substances, or seafood because such allergies may indicate sensitivity to the test's radiopaque dye.
- After myelography, urge the patient to remain in bed with his head elevated and to drink plenty of fluids. Monitor intake and output. Watch for seizures and an allergic reaction.
- During conservative treatment, watch for any deterioration in neurologic status (especially during the first 24 hours after admission), which may indicate an urgent need for surgery.

- Apply antiembolism stockings and sequential compression devices as prescribed, and encourage the patient to move his legs as allowed. Provide high-topped sneakers to prevent footdrop. Work closely with the physical therapy department to ensure a consistent regimen of leg- and back-strengthening exercises.
- Remind the patient to cough, deep-breathe, and use an incentive spirometer to prevent pulmonary complications.
- Use a fracture bedpan for the patient on complete bed rest.
- After laminectomy, microdiskectomy, or spinal fusion, enforce bed rest. If a blood drainage system (such as Hemovac) is in use, check the tubing frequently for kinks and a secure vacuum. Empty the blood drainage system at the end of each shift, and record the amount and color of drainage.
- Report colorless moisture on dressings (possibly cerebrospinal fluid leakage) or excessive drainage immediately. Observe the neurovascular status of the legs (color, motion, temperature, and sensation).
- Monitor vital signs, and check for bowel sounds and abdominal distention. Use the logrolling technique to turn the patient.
- Give analgesics, especially 30 minutes before initial attempts at sitting or walking. Help the patient during his first attempt to walk. Provide a straight-backed chair for limited sitting.
- Teach the patient who has undergone spinal fusion how to wear a brace. Assist with straight-leg-raising and toe-pointing exercises, as necessary.
- Before discharge, teach proper body mechanics—bending at the knees and hips (never at the waist), standing straight, and carrying objects close to the body.
- Advise the patient to lie down when tired and to sleep on his side (never on his abdomen) on an extra-firm mattress or a bed board. Urge him to maintain proper weight to prevent lordosis caused by obesity.
- Before chemonucleolysis, ask the patient about allergies to meat tenderizers (chymopapain is a similar substance). Such an allergy contraindicates the use of this enzyme, which can produce severe anaphylaxis in a sensitive patient. Enforce bed rest. Give analgesics and apply heat as needed. Assist with special exercises, and tell the patient to continue these exercises after discharge.
- Tell the patient who must receive a muscle relaxant of possible adverse effects, especially drowsiness. Warn him to avoid activities that require alertness until he has built up a tolerance to the drug's sedative effects.

▌ Herpes simplex viral infection

A recurrent viral infection, herpes simplex virus (HSV) produces no symptoms in about 85% of cases. The other cases produce localized lesions and systemic reactions. After the first infection, a patient is a carrier susceptible to recurrent infections, which may be provoked by fever, menses, stress, heat, and cold. In recurrent infections, the patient usually has no constitutional signs and symptoms.

Herpesvirus hominis, a widespread infectious agent, causes two serologically distinct HSV types. Type 1 (HSV-1) is transmitted primarily by contact with oral secretions and is the leading cause of gingivostomatitis in children ages 1 to 3. It causes the most common nonepidemic encephalitis and is the second most common viral infection in pregnant women. It can pass to the fetus transplacentally and, in early pregnancy, may cause spontaneous abortion or pre-

Treating and preventing herpes simplex

■ Teach the patient with genital herpes to use warm compresses or take sitz baths several times per day. Tell him to use a drying agent, such as povidone-iodine solution, to increase his fluid intake, and to avoid all sexual contact during the active stage.

■ Advise the pregnant woman with *Herpesvirus hominis* infection to have weekly viral cultures of the cervix and external genitalia starting at 32 weeks' gestation.

■ Instruct patients with herpetic whitlow not to share towels or utensils with uninfected people. Educate staff members and other susceptible people about the risk of contracting the disease.

■ Tell patients with cold sores not to kiss infants or people with eczema. (Those with genital herpes pose no risk to infants if their hygiene is meticulous.)

Type 2 herpes
■ Cross-infection (in orogenital contact)
■ Sexual contact

Signs and symptoms
Primary perioral HSV
■ Increased salivation
■ Severe mouth pain, halitosis
■ Small vesicles on an erythematous base
■ Sore throat, fever, anorexia, adenopathy

Diagnostic tests
■ Confirmation requires isolation of the virus from local lesions and a histologic biopsy.
■ A rise in antibodies and moderate leukocytosis may support the diagnosis.

Treatment
■ Analgesics and antipyretics relieve pain and reduce fever.
■ Anesthetic mouthwashes such as viscous lidocaine help reduce the pain of gingivostomatitis.
■ Drying agents, such as calamine lotion, reduce pain of labial lesions.
■ Acyclovir (Zovirax) may bring relief to patients with genital herpes or to immunosuppressed patients with severe and frequent recurrences. The drug is available in topical, oral, and I.V. form (usually reserved for severe infections). (See *Treating and preventing herpes simplex*.)

Nursing considerations
■ Abstain from direct patient care if you have active oral or cutaneous infections.
■ Patients with central nervous system infection alone need no isolation.
■ Teach patients how to apply medications, using sterile technique, and how to avoid infecting others.

mature birth. Primary infection in childhood may be generalized or localized. Type 2 (HSV-2) is transmitted primarily by contact with genital structures.

Herpes is equally common in males and females. It occurs worldwide and is most prevalent among children in lower socioeconomic groups who live in crowded environments. Saliva, stool, urine, skin lesions, and purulent eye exudate are potential sources of infection.

Causes
■ The infectious agent *H. hominis*

Type 1 herpes
■ Oral and respiratory secretions

Herpes zoster

Also called *shingles,* herpes zoster is an acute unilateral and segmental inflammation of the dorsal root ganglia caused by infection with the herpesvirus varicella-zoster, which also causes chickenpox. This infection usually occurs in adults. It produces localized vesicular skin lesions confined to a dermatome and severe neuralgic pain in peripheral areas innervated by the nerves arising in the inflamed root ganglia. A positive diagnosis of herpes zoster usually isn't possible until the characteristic skin lesions develop. Before then, the pain may mimic that of appendicitis, pleurisy, or other conditions.

The prognosis is good unless the infection spreads to the brain. Eventually, most patients recover completely, except for possible scarring and, in corneal damage, vision impairment. Occasionally, neuralgia may persist for months or years.

Herpes zoster is found primarily in adults, especially those older than age 50. It seldom recurs.

Causes
- Reactivation of dormant varicella virus

Signs and symptoms
Onset of disease
- Fever and malaise
- Severe deep pain, pruritus, and paresthesia or hyperesthesia, usually on the trunk and occasionally on the arms and legs in a dermatomal distribution (onset within 2 to 4 days; duration 1 to 4 weeks)

Skin lesions
- Up to 2 weeks after the first symptoms: possible eruption of small, red, nodular skin lesions on the painful areas, with unilateral spreading around

Skin lesions in herpes zoster

Characteristic skin lesions in herpes zoster are fluid-filled vesicles that dry and form scabs after about 10 days.

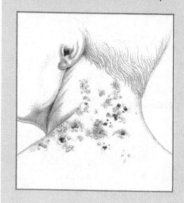

the thorax or vertical spreading over the arms or legs followed by progression to fluid or pus-filled vesicles
- About 10 days after appearance: drying and scabbing of vesicles (see *Skin lesions in herpes zoster*)
- When lesions rupture: possibility of infected lesions leading to enlargement of regional lymph nodes and, possibly, development of gangrene

Cranial nerve involvement
- Oculomotor involvement: conjunctivitis, extraocular weakness, ptosis, and paralytic mydriasis
- Trigeminal ganglion involvement: eye pain and, possibly, corneal and scleral damage and impaired vision
- Vesicle formation in the external auditory canal, ipsilateral facial palsy, hearing loss, dizziness, and loss of taste

Diagnostic tests

■ Examination of vesicular fluid and infected tissue shows eosinophilic intranuclear inclusions and varicella virus.
■ Lumbar puncture shows increased cerebrospinal fluid (CSF) pressure; examination of CSF shows increased protein levels and, possibly, pleocytosis.
■ Staining antibodies from vesicular fluid and identification under fluorescent light differentiate herpes zoster from localized herpes simplex.

Treatment

■ Calamine lotion or another antipruritic relieve itching.
■ Neuralgic pain is relieved with analgesics (such as aspirin, acetaminophen [Tylenol] or, possibly, codeine).
■ Systemic antibiotics are necessary for bacterial infection of ruptured vesicles.
■ Idoxuridine ointment or another antiviral agent may be necessary for trigeminal zoster with corneal involvement.
■ Systemic corticosteroids such as cortisone or corticotropin help relieve the intractable pain of postherpetic neuralgia. Tricyclic antidepressants may also be beneficial to help relieve neuritic pain.
■ Oral acyclovir (Zovirax) therapy accelerates healing of lesions and resolution of zoster-associated pain.
■ I.V. acyclovir may be administered to immunocompromised patients (children and adults).

Nursing considerations

■ Keep the patient comfortable, maintain meticulous hygiene, and prevent infection. During the acute phase, encourage him to get adequate rest and give supportive care to promote proper healing of lesions.
■ Apply calamine lotion liberally to the lesions. If lesions are severe and widespread, apply a wet dressing.
■ Instruct the patient to avoid scratching the lesions.
■ Apply a cold compress if vesicles rupture.
■ Tell the patient to use a soft toothbrush, eat a soft diet, and use saline mouthwash to decrease the pain of oral lesions.
■ Never withhold or delay administration of analgesics. Give them exactly on schedule because the pain of herpes zoster can be severe. In postherpetic neuralgia, avoid opioid analgesics because of the danger of addiction.
■ Repeatedly reassure the patient that herpetic pain will eventually subside. Provide the patient with diversionary activity to take his mind off the pain and pruritus.

Hiatal hernia

Hiatal hernia is a defect in the diaphragm that permits a portion of the stomach to pass through the diaphragmatic opening into the chest. Three types of hiatal hernia can occur: *sliding hernia, paraesophageal (rolling) hernia,* and *mixed hernia,* which includes features of both. (See *Types of hiatal hernia.*)

In a sliding hernia, both the stomach and the gastroesophageal junction slip up into the chest, so that the gastroesophageal junction is above the diaphragmatic hiatus. In paraesophageal hernia, a part of the greater curvature of the stomach rolls through the diaphragmatic defect. Treatment can prevent such complications as strangulation of the herniated intrathoracic portion of the stomach. A mixed hernia is one that includes features of sliding and rolling hernias.

The incidence of hiatal hernia is higher in women than in men (especially the paraesophageal type), and incidence increases with age. By age 60, about 60% of people have hiatal hernias; however, most have no symptoms.

Causes

- Diaphragmatic malformations causing congenital weakness
- Increased intra-abdominal pressure due to ascites, pregnancy, obesity, constrictive clothing, bending, straining, coughing, Valsalva's maneuver, or extreme physical exertion
- Loosening of the muscular collar around the esophageal and diaphragmatic junction allowing the lower portion of the esophagus and the stomach to rise into the chest
- Muscle weakening due to aging, esophageal cancer, kyphoscoliosis, trauma, and certain surgical procedures

Signs and symptoms

Paraesophageal hernia

- Possibly no symptoms
- Feeling of fullness in the chest or pain that resembles angina pectoris

Sliding hernia

- Without incompetent lower esophageal sphincter (LES): No symptoms
- With incompetent LES: Pyrosis (heartburn), onset 1 to 4 hours after eating, aggravated by reclining, belching, and increased intra-abdominal pressure, possibly accompanied by regurgitation or vomiting; retrosternal or substernal chest pain due to reflux of gastric contents, distention of the stomach, and spasm or altered motor activity, common after meals or at bedtime and aggravated by reclining, belching, and increased intra-abdominal pressure
- Symptoms reflecting possible complications
  - Bleeding: mild or massive, frank or occult, caused by esophagitis or erosions of the gastric pouch

Types of hiatal hernia

Normal stomach

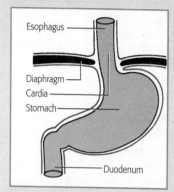

Sliding hiatal hernia

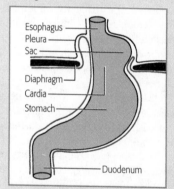

Paraesophageal or rolling hernia

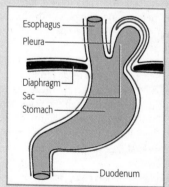

– Dysphagia due to esophagitis, esophageal ulceration, or stricture, especially with ingestion of very hot or cold foods, alcoholic beverages, or a large amount of food
– Severe pain and shock due to incarceration, possibly leading to perforation of a gastric ulcer as well as strangulation and gangrene of the herniated portion of the stomach

Diagnostic tests

▪ Chest X-ray occasionally shows an air shadow behind the heart with a large hernia and infiltrates in the lower lobes if the patient has aspirated.
▪ Barium swallow with fluoroscopy is the most specific test for detecting a hiatal hernia. The hernia may appear as an outpouching that contains barium at the lower end of the esophagus. (Small hernias are difficult to recognize.) This study also shows diaphragmatic abnormalities.
▪ Endoscopy and biopsy differentiate between hiatal hernia, varices, and other small gastroesophageal lesions; identify the mucosal junction and the edge of the diaphragm indenting the esophagus; and can rule out malignant tumors that otherwise might be difficult to detect.
▪ Esophageal motility studies assess the presence of esophageal motor abnormalities before surgical repair of the hernia.
▪ pH studies assess for reflux of gastric contents.
▪ Acid perfusion (Bernstein) test indicates that heartburn results from esophageal reflux when perfusion of hydrogen chloride through the nasogastric (NG) tube provokes this symptom.

The following laboratory tests may indicate GI bleeding as a complication of hiatal hernia:
▪ Complete blood count may show hypochromic microcytic anemia when bleeding from esophageal ulceration occurs.
▪ Stool guaiac test may be positive.
▪ Analysis of gastric contents may reveal blood.

Treatment

▪ Medical therapy attempts to modify or reduce reflux by changing the quantity or quality of refluxed gastric contents, strengthening the LES muscle pharmacologically, or decreasing the amount of reflux through gravity.
▪ Restrict any activity that increases intra-abdominal pressure (coughing, straining, bending).
▪ Institute a smoking cessation program because smoking stimulates gastric acid production.
▪ Start the following dietary modifications: eating small, frequent meals at least 2 hours before lying down (no bedtime snacks); eating slowly; and avoiding irritating foods, alcoholic beverages, and coffee.
▪ Antacids modify the fluid refluxed into the esophagus and are probably the best treatment for intermittent reflux.
▪ To reduce the amount of reflux, the overweight patient should lose weight to decrease intra-abdominal pressure. Elevating the head of the bed about 6″ to 12″ (15.2 to 30 cm) reduces gastric reflux by gravity.
▪ Drug therapy to strengthen cardiac sphincter tone may include a cholinergic agent such as bethanechol (Duvoid).
▪ Metoclopramide (Reglan) has also been used to stimulate smooth-muscle contraction, increase LES tone, and decrease reflux after eating.

Surgery

▪ Antireflux surgical repair is necessary when attempts to control symptoms medically fail or complications such as stricture, bleeding, pulmonary aspiration, strangulation, or incarceration occur.

- Surgery creates an artificial closing mechanism at the gastroesophageal junction to strengthen the LES's barrier function.
- A transabdominal fundoplication is performed by wrapping the fundus of the stomach around the lower esophagus to prevent reflux of stomach contents. An abdominal or a thoracic approach may be used.
- Laparoscopic surgery to repair the hernia is now commonplace.
- A newer treatment involves thoracoscopic surgery, with the hernia repaired microscopically.
- Even if it produces no symptoms, paraesophageal hernia needs surgical treatment because of the high risk of strangulation.

Nursing considerations

- To enhance compliance with treatment, instruct the patient about the causes of this disorder. Explain proposed treatments, diagnostic tests, and significant symptoms.
- Prepare the patient for diagnostic tests as needed. After endoscopy, watch for signs of perforation (falling blood pressure, rapid pulse, shock, and sudden pain).
- Before surgery, reinforce patient teaching about the procedure and any preoperative and postoperative considerations.
- Postoperatively, monitor intake and output, including NG tube drainage.
- Never manipulate an NG tube in a patient with hiatal hernia surgical repair.
- If a thoracic approach was used, the patient will have chest tubes in place. Carefully observe chest tube drainage and respiratory status, and perform pulmonary physiotherapy.
- Monitor NG tube patency and security to prevent distention of the stomach during the healing period. Distention can cause a breakdown of the repair.

- Instruct the patient that a barium swallow will be performed on the sixth or seventh postoperative day to look for the unobstructed passage of barium into the stomach before starting solid foods.
- Inform the patient that slight dysphagia may be experienced in the first few weeks after surgery. This will gradually disappear.
- Instruct the patient to eat small, frequent meals.
- Counsel the patient that increased flatus and mild gastric distention (gas bloat syndrome) may occur due to trapping of air in the stomach from air swallowing. Air swallowing should be consciously avoided.
- Instruct the patient to take all medications in liquid or crushed form for at least 6 months to avoid a drug-induced esophageal injury.
- Instruct the patient to avoid wearing constrictive clothing.

Hodgkin's disease

A neoplastic disease, Hodgkin's disease is characterized by painless, progressive enlargement of lymph nodes, spleen, and other lymphoid tissue resulting from proliferation of lymphocytes, histiocytes, eosinophils, and Reed-Sternberg giant cells. The latter cells are its special histologic feature.

Untreated, Hodgkin's disease follows a variable but relentlessly progressive and ultimately fatal course. Advances in therapy have made Hodgkin's disease potentially curable, even in advanced stages, and appropriate treatment yields a 5-year survival rate of about 90%.

This disease is most common in young adults and occurs more commonly in men than in women. It occurs in all races but is slightly more common in whites. Incidence peaks in two age-groups: ages 15 to 38 and after age 50,

Staging Hodgkin's disease

Treatment of Hodgkin's disease depends on the stage it has reached—that is, the number, location, and degree of involved lymph nodes. The Ann Arbor Classification System, adopted in 1971, divides Hodgkin's disease into four stages, which are then subdivided into categories.

Stage I

Hodgkin's disease appears in a single lymph node region (I) or a single extralymphatic organ (IE).

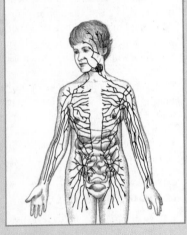

Stage II

The disease appears in two or more nodes on the same side of the diaphragm (II) and in an extralymphatic organ (IIE).

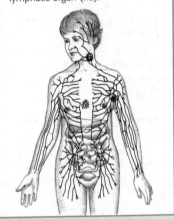

except in Japan, where it occurs exclusively among people older than age 50.

Causes
- Unknown

Predisposing factors
- Environmental
- Genetic
- Viral

Signs and symptoms
Early signs
- Enlargement of lymph nodes: rapid onset with pain and obstruction or slow (months or years) painless onset; or, possibly, "waxing and waning" of lymph note enlargement (without a return to normal size)
- Painless swelling of one of the cervical lymph nodes (or, occasionally, the axillary, mediastinal, or inguinal lymph nodes)
- Persistent fever, night sweats, fatigue, weight loss, and malaise (in older patients)
- Pruritus (initially mild, becoming acute as the disease progresses)
- Respiratory symptoms (with involvement of mediastinum)

Late signs
- Edema of the face and neck
- Increased susceptibility to infection
- Nerve pain
- Possibly jaundice

Category A includes patients with undefined signs and symptoms, and category B includes patients who experience such defined signs as recent unexplained weight loss, fever, and night sweats.

Stage III

Hodgkin's disease spreads to both sides of the diaphragm (III) and perhaps to an extralymphatic organ (IIIE).

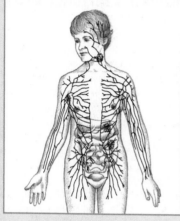

Stage IV

The disease disseminates, involving one or more extralymphatic organs or tissues, with or without associated lymph node involvement.

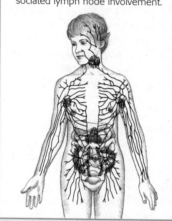

- Progressive anemia
- Systemic manifestations: enlargement of retroperitoneal nodes and nodular infiltrations of the spleen, liver, and bones

Diagnostic tests

- Lymph node biopsy shows abnormal histiocyte proliferation of Reed-Sternberg cells (a giant atypical tumor cell) and nodular fibrosis and necrosis.
- Bone marrow, liver, mediastinal, lymph node, and spleen biopsies, chest X-ray, abdominal computed tomography scan, lung scan, bone scan, and lymphangiography may be used to detect lymph node or organ involvement.
- Laparoscopy and a lymph node biopsy are performed to complete staging.

- Hematologic tests show mild to severe normocytic anemia, normochromic anemia (in 50% of patients), and an elevated, normal, or reduced white blood cell count and differential showing any combination of neutrophilia, lymphocytopenia, monocytosis, and eosinophilia.
- An elevated serum alkaline phosphatase level indicates liver or bone involvement.
- A staging laparotomy is necessary for patients younger than age 55 and those without obvious stage III or stage IV disease, lymphocyte predominance subtype histology, or medical contraindications. (See *Staging Hodgkin's disease*.)

Treatment

- Radiation therapy is used alone for stage I and stage II and in combination with chemotherapy for stage III.
- Chemotherapy, usually with a combination of agents, is used for stage IV, sometimes inducing a complete remission.
- Antiemetics, sedatives, or antidiarrheals to combat GI adverse effects of radiation and chemotherapy.
- High-dose chemotherapeutic agents may be used in conjunction with autologous bone marrow transplantation.
- Autologous peripheral blood sternal transfusions or autologous bone marrow transplantation are other treatments.
- Biotherapy alone hasn't proven effective.

Nursing considerations

- Watch for and promptly report adverse effects of radiation therapy and chemotherapy (particularly anorexia, nausea, vomiting, diarrhea, fever, and bleeding).
- Minimize adverse effects of radiation therapy by maintaining good nutrition (aided by eating small, frequent meals of favorite foods), drinking plenty of fluids, pacing activities to counteract therapy-induced fatigue, and keeping the skin in radiated areas dry.
- Control pain and bleeding of stomatitis by using a soft toothbrush, cotton swab, or anesthetic mouthwash such as viscous lidocaine; by applying petroleum jelly to the patient's lips; and by avoiding astringent mouthwashes.
- If a female patient is of childbearing age, advise her to delay pregnancy until prolonged remission because radiation therapy and chemotherapy can cause genetic mutations and spontaneous abortions.
- Because the patient with Hodgkin's disease has usually been healthy until this point, he's likely to be especially distressed. Provide emotional support and offer appropriate reassurance. Ease the patient's anxiety by sharing your optimism about his prognosis.
- Make sure the patient and his family know that the local chapter of the American Cancer Society is available for information, financial assistance, and supportive counseling.

Human immunodeficiency virus infection

One of the most widely publicized diseases, acquired immunodeficiency syndrome (AIDS), caused by human immunodeficiency virus (HIV), is marked by progressive failure of the immune system. Although it's characterized by gradual destruction of cell-mediated (T-cell) immunity, it also affects humoral immunity and autoimmunity because of the central role of the CD4+ T lymphocyte in immune reactions. The resultant immunodeficiency makes the patient susceptible to opportunistic infections, unusual cancers, and other abnormalities that characterize AIDS.

This syndrome was first described by the Centers for Disease Control and Prevention (CDC) in 1981. Since then, the CDC has declared a case surveillance definition for AIDS and has modified it several times, most recently in 1993.

Two major strains of the retrovirus exist: HIV-1 (the primary causative agent, closely related to the primate retrovirus, simian immunodeficiency virus) and HIV-2 (associated with immunodeficiency but less pathogenic than HIV-1). The disease is transmitted through contact with infected blood or body fluids and is associated with identifiable high-risk behaviors. It's therefore disproportionately represented in homosexual and bisexual men, I.V. drug users, neonates of HIV-infected women, recipients of contaminated blood or blood products (dramatically decreased since mid-1985), and heterosexual partners of people in the former groups. Because of similar routes of transmission, AIDS shares epidemiologic patterns with hepatitis B and sexually transmitted diseases (STDs).

The natural history of AIDS infection begins with infection by the HIV retrovirus, which is detectable only by laboratory tests, and ends with the severely immunocompromised, terminal stage of this disease. The infection process takes three forms:

- autoimmunity (lymphoid interstitial pneumonia, arthritis, hypergammaglobulinemia, and production of autoimmune antibodies)
- immunodeficiency (opportunistic infections and unusual cancers)
- neurologic dysfunction (AIDS dementia complex, HIV encephalopathy, and peripheral neuropathies)

Patients develop antibodies to the virus within 6 to 8 weeks of exposure, with an average of 8 to 10 years between exposure and diagnosis. Depending on individual variations and the presence of cofactors that influence progression, the time elapsed from acute HIV infection to the appearance of symptoms (mild to severe) to the diagnosis and, eventually, to death varies greatly. Current combination antiretroviral therapy (for example, with zidovudine [Retrovir], ritonavir [Norvir], and others) and treatment and prevention of common opportunistic infections can delay the natural progression of HIV disease and prolong survival.

Causes
- Exposure to HIV-1, through direct inoculation during intimate sexual contact, especially associated with the mucosal trauma of receptive rectal intercourse; transfusion of contaminated blood or blood products (a risk diminished by routine testing of all blood products); sharing of contaminated needles; or transplacental or postpartum transmission from an infected mother to the fetus (by cervical or blood contact at delivery and in breast milk)

Signs and symptoms
- Initially: mononucleosis-like syndrome, possibly followed by an asymptomatic period lasting for years
- Neurologic symptoms resulting from HIV encephalopathy
- Nonspecific symptoms (weight loss, fatigue, night sweats, fevers)
- Opportunistic infection or cancer
- Persistent generalized adenopathy

In children
- Mean incubation period of 17 months; signs and symptoms resembling those in adults, except for those related to STDs
- Opportunistic infections also observed in adult patients, but higher incidence of bacterial infections, such as otitis media, sepsis, chronic salivary gland enlargement, *Mycobacterium avium* complex function, and pneumonias, including *Pneumocystis carinii* and lymphoid interstitial pneumonias

Diagnostic tests
- The CDC's current AIDS surveillance case definition requires laboratory confirmation of HIV infection in people who have a CD4+ T-cell count of 200 cells/ml or who have an associated clinical condition or disease.
- Antibody tests indicate HIV infection indirectly by revealing HIV antibodies. The recommended protocol requires initial screening of individuals and blood products with an enzyme-linked im-

munosorbent assay (ELISA). A positive ELISA should be repeated and then confirmed by an alternate method, usually the Western blot or an immunofluorescence assay.

- Antibody testing isn't always reliable. Because the body takes a variable amount of time to produce a detectable level of antibodies, a "window" varying from a few weeks to as long as 35 months in one documented case allows an HIV-infected person to test negative for HIV antibodies.
- Antibody tests are also unreliable in neonates because transferred maternal antibodies persist for 6 to 10 months.
- Direct tests include antigen tests (p24 antigen), HIV cultures, nucleic acid probes of peripheral blood lymphocytes with determination of HIV-1 ribonucleic acid levels, and the polymerase chain reaction.
- Additional tests to support the diagnosis and help evaluate the severity of immunosuppression include CD4$^+$ and CD8$^+$ T-lymphocyte subset counts, erythrocyte sedimentation rate, complete blood count, serum beta$_2$-microglobulin, p24 antigen, neopterin levels, and anergy testing.
- Because many opportunistic infections in patients are reactivations of previous infections, patients are also tested for syphilis, hepatitis B, tuberculosis, toxoplasmosis and, in some areas, histoplasmosis.

Treatment

- No cure has yet been found for the disorder; however, primary therapy for HIV infection includes three different types of antiretrovirals. Used in various combinations, they're designed to inhibit HIV viral replication:
  - protease inhibitors (PIs), such as ritonavir, indinavir (Crixivan), nelfinavir (Viracept), and saquinavir (Invirase)
  - nucleoside reverse transcriptase inhibitors (NRTIs), such as zidovudine, didanosine (Videx), zalcitabine (Hivid), lamivudine (Epivir), and stavudine (Zerit)
  - nonnucleoside reverse transcriptase inhibitors, such as nevirapine (Viramune) and delavirdine (Rescriptor).
- Immunomodulatory agents strengthen the weakened immune system.
- Anti-infectives and antineoplastics combat opportunistic infections and associated cancers; some are used prophylactically to help patients resist opportunistic infections.
- Current treatment protocols combine three agents in an effort to gain the maximum benefit with the fewest adverse reactions. Such regimens include one PI and are considered the most effective treatment. Many variations and drug interactions are under study. Combination therapy helps inhibit the production of resistant, mutant strains.
- Supportive treatments help maintain nutritional status and relieve pain and other distressing physical and psychological symptoms.
- Many pathogens respond to anti-infectives but tend to recur after treatment ends. Therefore, most patients need continuous anti-infective treatment, presumably for life or until the drug is no longer tolerated or effective.
- Zidovudine has proven effective in slowing the progression of HIV infection, decreasing opportunistic infections, and prolonging survival. However, it commonly produces serious adverse reactions and toxicities. The drug is typically combined with other agents (such as lamivudine) but has also been used as a single agent for pregnant HIV-positive women. Other NRTIs, such as didanosine and zalcitabine, may also be used in combination regimens for patients who

can't tolerate or no longer respond to zidovudine.

Nursing considerations

- Health care workers and the public are advised to use precautions in all situations that risk exposure to blood, body fluids, and secretions. Diligently practicing standard precautions can prevent the inadvertent transmission of HIV, hepatitis B, and other infectious diseases that are transmitted by similar routes.
- Combination antiretroviral therapy aims to maximally suppress HIV replication, thereby improving survival odds. However, poor drug compliance may lead to resistance and treatment failure. Patients must understand that medication regimens must be followed closely and may be required for many years, if not throughout life.
- Recognize that a diagnosis is profoundly distressing because of the disease's social impact and the discouraging prognosis. The patient may lose his job and financial security as well as the support of family and friends. Coping with an altered body image, the emotional burden of serious illness, and the threat of death may overwhelm the patient.

Huntington's disease

Also called *Huntington's chorea, hereditary chorea, chronic progressive chorea,* and *adult chorea,* Huntington's disease is a hereditary disease in which degeneration in the cerebral cortex and basal ganglia causes chronic progressive chorea (dancelike movements) and cognitive deterioration, ending in dementia.

Huntington's disease usually strikes people between ages 25 and 55 (the average age is 35); however, 2% of cases occur in children, and 5%, as late as age 60. Males and females are equally affected. Death usually results 10 to 15 years after onset from suicide, heart failure, or pneumonia.

Because of hereditary transmission, Huntington's disease is prevalent in areas in which affected families have lived for several generations. Genetic testing is offered to those with a known family history of the disease.

The diagnosis is based on a characteristic clinical history: progressive chorea and dementia, onset of the disorder early in middle age (ages 35 to 40), and confirmation of a genetic link.

Causes

- Autosomal dominant trait transmitted and inherited by both sexes, with a 50% risk for each child of a parent who has the disease

Signs and symptoms
Neurologic manifestations

- Bradykinesia (slow movements) accompanied by rigidity but without loss of muscle strength
- Choreic movements: rapid, usually violent, purposeless; initially, unilateral with greater involvement of the face and arms than the legs; progressing from mild fidgeting to grimacing, tongue smacking, dysarthria (indistinct speech), athetoid movements (slow, twisting muscle contractions, especially of the hands) related to emotional state, and torticollis (neck muscle contractions)
- Combination of chorea, bradykinesia, and normal muscle strength resulting in impairment of both voluntary and involuntary movement
- Dysarthria (early onset); possibly complicated by perseveration (persistent repetition of a reply), oral apraxia (difficulty coordinating movement of the mouth), and aprosody (inability to accurately reproduce or interpret the tone of language)

- Dysphagia (common in advanced stages)

Cognitive manifestations

- Deficits of executive function (planning, organizing, regulating, and programming)
- Dementia (early onset, subcortical in origin)
- Impairment of impulse control

Psychiatric manifestations

- Depression (possibly with manic component)
- Irritability, lability, impulsiveness, and aggressive behavior
- Psychosis and obsessive-compulsive behavior (rare)

Diagnostic tests

- Huntington's disease can be detected by positron emission tomography and deoxyribonucleic acid analysis.
- A computed tomography scan shows brain atrophy and magnetic resonance imaging demonstrates characteristic butterfly-shaped dilation of the brain's lateral ventricles.
- Molecular genetics may detect the gene for Huntington's disease in people at risk while they're still asymptomatic.

Treatment

- Dopamine blockers, such as haloperidol (Haldol), help control choreic movements and reduce abnormal behaviors.
- Amantadine (Symmetrel) may be used to control extra movements.
- Some evidence suggests the coenzyme Q10 may minimally decrease progression of the disease.
- Psychotherapy to decrease anxiety and stress may also be helpful.
- Institutionalization is usually necessary because of mental deterioration.

Nursing considerations

- Provide physical support by attending to the patient's basic needs, such as hygiene, skin care, bowel and bladder care, and nutrition. Increase this support as mental and physical deterioration make him increasingly immobile.
- Assist in designing a behavioral plan that deals with the disruptive and aggressive behavior and impulse control problems. Reinforce positive behaviors, and maintain consistency with all caregiving.
- Offer emotional support to the patient and his family. Teach them about the disease, and listen to their concerns and special problems. Keep in mind the patient's dysarthria, and allow him extra time to express himself, thereby decreasing frustration. Teach the family to participate in the patient's care.
- Stay alert for possible suicide attempts. Control the patient's environment to protect him from suicide or other self-inflicted injury. Pad the side rails of the bed but avoid restraints, which may cause the patient to injure himself with violent, uncontrolled movements.
- If the patient has difficulty walking, provide a walker to help him maintain his balance.
- If the patient has dysphagia, minimize the potential for aspiration, infection, malnutrition, and pneumonitis.
- Make sure affected families receive genetic counseling. All affected family members should realize that each of their offspring has a 50% chance of inheriting this disease.
- Refer people at risk who desire genetic testing to specialized centers where psychosocial support is available.
- Refer the patient and his family to appropriate community organizations.
- For more information about this degenerative disease, refer the patient and

his family to the Huntington's Disease Association.

Hydrocephalus

An excessive accumulation of cerebrospinal fluid (CSF) within the ventricular spaces of the brain, hydrocephalus occurs most commonly in neonates. It can also occur in adults as a result of injury or disease. In infants, hydrocephalus enlarges the head, and in both infants and adults, the resulting compression can damage brain tissue.

With early detection and surgical intervention, the prognosis improves but remains guarded. Even after surgery, such complications as developmental delay, impaired motor function, and vision loss can persist. Without surgery, the prognosis is poor: Mortality may result from increased intracranial pressure (ICP) in people of all ages; infants may also die prematurely of infection and malnutrition.

Causes
- Faulty absorption of CSF (communicating hydrocephalus)
- Obstruction in CSF flow (noncommunicating hydrocephalus)

Noncommunicating hydrocephalus
- Faulty fetal development, infection (syphilis, granulomatous diseases, meningitis), a tumor, a cerebral aneurysm, or a blood clot
- Obstruction between the third and fourth ventricles, at the aqueduct of Sylvius, at the outlets of the fourth ventricle (foramina of Luschka and Magendie) or, rarely, at the foramen of Monro

Characteristics of hydrocephalus

In infants, changes characteristic of hydrocephalus include marked enlargement of the head, distended scalp veins, underdeveloped neck muscles, and thin, shiny, and fragile-looking scalp skin.

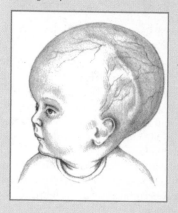

Communicating hydrocephalus
- Faulty absorption of CSF due to surgical repair of a myelomeningocele, adhesions between meninges at the base of the brain, or meningeal hemorrhage
- Tumor in the choroid plexus causing overproduction of CSF (rare)

Signs and symptoms
In infants
- Distended scalp veins; thin, shiny, fragile-looking scalp skin; and underdeveloped neck muscles (see *Characteristics of hydrocephalus*)
- Enlargement of the head clearly disproportionate to the infant's growth
- Truly tense fontanels present in the sitting position
- In severe hydrocephalus: depression of roof of the orbit, downward displace-

ment of the eyes, prominent sclerae, abnormal muscle tone in the legs, irritability, anorexia, projectile vomiting, and high-pitched, shrill cry

In adults and older children
■ Decreased level of consciousness (LOC), headache, nausea, vomiting, and other symptoms of increased ICP
■ Possibly: ataxia, incontinence, and impaired intellect

Diagnostic tests
■ In infants, skull X-rays show thinning of the skull with separation of sutures and widening of the fontanels.
■ Angiography, computed tomography scans, and magnetic resonance imaging can differentiate between hydrocephalus and intracranial lesions and can also demonstrate the Arnold-Chiari deformity (a type of neural tube defect), which may occur in an infant with hydrocephalus.

Treatment
■ Surgical correction consists of insertion of a ventriculoperitoneal shunt, which transports excess fluid from the lateral ventricle into the peritoneal cavity.
■ A less common procedure, used if a concurrent abdominal problem exists, is insertion of a ventriculoatrial shunt, which drains fluid from the brain's lateral ventricle into the right atrium of the heart, where the fluid makes its way into the venous circulation.
■ Endoscopic third ventriculostomy involves creating a passage between the third ventricle and the basal cisterns. This procedure is used for noncommunicating hydrocephalus in patients older than age 2.

Nursing considerations
■ Obtain a complete history from the patient or the family. Note the patient's general behavior, especially irritability, apathy, and decreased LOC.
■ Perform a neurologic assessment. Examine the eyes: pupils should be equal and reactive to light. In adults and older children, evaluate movements and motor strength in the extremities. (Watch especially for ataxia.)
■ Irritability, restlessness, and change in cognitive function are all indicators of increased ICP in adults and children. A change in eating, sleeping, and pitch of cry are strong indicators of increased ICP in infants.

Before surgery to insert a shunt
■ Encourage maternal-neonatal bonding when possible. When caring for the neonate yourself, hold him on your lap for feeding, stroke and cuddle him, and speak soothingly.
■ Check the fontanels for tension or fullness, and measure and record head circumference.
■ To appropriately assess fontanels, lay the infant down, and then raise him to a sitting position. Truly tense fontanels will be present in the sitting position. Remember that if the infant is crying, fontanel pressure will increase. This wouldn't be indicative of hydrocephalus.
■ On the patient's chart, draw a picture showing where to measure the head so that other staff members measure it in the same place, or mark the forehead with ink.
■ To prevent postfeeding aspiration and hypostatic pneumonia, place the infant on his side and reposition him every 2 hours, or prop him up in an infant seat.
■ To prevent skin breakdown, make sure the infant's earlobe is flat, and place a

sheepskin or rubber foam under his head.

■ When turning the infant, move his head, neck, and shoulders with his body to reduce strain on his neck.

■ Feed the infant slowly. To lessen the strain from the weight of the infant's head on your arm while holding him during feeding, place his head, neck, and shoulders on a pillow.

After surgery

■ Place the infant on the side opposite the operative site, with his head level with his body.

■ Check temperature, pulse rate, blood pressure, and LOC. Also check the fontanelles daily for fullness. Watch for irritability, which may be an early sign of increased ICP and shunt malfunction.

■ Watch for signs of infection, especially meningitis: fever, stiff neck, irritability, or tense fontanelles. Also watch for redness, swelling, and other signs of local infection over the shunt tract. Check the dressing often for drainage.

■ Listen for bowel sounds after ventriculoperitoneal shunt.

■ Check the infant's growth and development periodically, and help the parents set goals consistent with the infant's ability and potential.

■ Help the parents focus on their child's strengths, not his weaknesses. Discuss special education programs, and emphasize the infant's need for sensory stimulation appropriate for his age.

■ Teach the parents to watch for signs of shunt malfunction, infection, and paralytic ileus. Tell them that shunt insertion requires periodic surgery to lengthen the shunt as the child grows older, to correct malfunctioning, or to treat infection.

▌ Hydronephrosis

An abnormal dilation of the renal pelvis and the calyces of one or both kidneys, hydronephrosis is caused by an obstruction of urine flow in the genitourinary tract. Although partial obstruction and hydronephrosis may not produce symptoms initially, the pressure built up behind the area of obstruction eventually results in symptomatic renal dysfunction.

The most common complication of an obstructed kidney is infection (pyelonephritis) due to urinary stasis that worsens renal damage and may create a life-threatening crisis. Paralytic ileus commonly accompanies acute obstructive uropathy.

Causes

■ Benign prostatic hyperplasia (BPH), urethral strictures, and calculi

■ Less commonly: strictures or stenosis of the ureter or bladder outlet, congenital abnormalities, abdominal tumors, blood clots, neurogenic bladder, and tumors of the ureter and bladder

■ Obstruction of a ureter (usually unilateral)

■ Obstruction of the urethra or bladder (usually bilateral)

■ Total obstruction of urine flow with dilation of the collecting system leading to complete cortical atrophy and cessation of glomerular filtration

Signs and symptoms

■ None, initially

■ Decreased urine flow

■ Hematuria, pyuria, dysuria, alternating oliguria and polyuria, and complete anuria

■ Mild pain

■ Nausea, vomiting, abdominal fullness, pain on urination, dribbling, and hesitancy

■ Severe, colicky renal pain or dull flank pain that may radiate to the groin
■ Unilateral pain (commonly in the flank area) with unilateral obstruction

Diagnostic tests
■ Excretory urography, retrograde pyelography, renal ultrasonography, and renal function study results are positive for hydronephrosis.

Treatment
■ Treatment preserves renal function and prevents infection through surgical removal of the obstruction, such as dilation for stricture of the urethra and prostatectomy for BPH.
■ If renal function has been affected, therapy may include a diet low in protein, sodium, and potassium. This diet is designed to stop the progression of renal failure before surgery.
■ Inoperable obstructions may require decompression and drainage of the kidney, using a nephrostomy tube placed temporarily or permanently in the renal pelvis.
■ Concurrent infection requires appropriate antibiotic therapy.

Nursing considerations
■ Explain hydronephrosis as well as the purpose of excretory urography and other diagnostic procedures. Find out whether the patient is allergic to the dye used in excretory urography.
■ Give prescribed pain medication as needed.
■ Postoperatively, closely monitor intake and output, vital signs, and fluid and electrolyte status. Watch for a rising pulse rate and cold, clammy skin, which indicate possible impending hemorrhage and shock. Monitor renal function studies daily.
■ If a nephrostomy tube has been inserted, check it frequently for bleeding and

patency. Irrigate the tube but don't clamp it.
■ If the patient will be discharged with a nephrostomy tube in place, teach him how to care for it properly.
■ To prevent progression of hydronephrosis to irreversible renal disease, urge older men (especially those with family histories of BPH or prostatitis) to have routine medical checkups. Teach them to recognize and report symptoms of hydronephrosis (colicky pain and hematuria) or urinary tract infection.

Hyperaldosteronism

In hyperaldosteronism (also called *aldosteronism*), hypersecretion of the mineralocorticoid aldosterone by the adrenal cortex causes excessive reabsorption of sodium and water and excessive renal excretion of potassium.

The incidence of primary hyperaldosteronism is three times higher in women than in men and is highest between ages 30 and 50.

If hypokalemia develops in a hypertensive patient shortly after starting treatment with potassium-wasting diuretics (such as thiazides), and if it persists after the diuretic has been discontinued and potassium replacement therapy has been instituted, evaluation for hyperaldosteronism is necessary.

Causes
Primary hyperaldosteronism
■ Benign aldosterone-producing adrenal adenomas (common)
■ Bilateral adrenal hyperplasia (less common)
■ Adrenal carcinoma (rare)
■ Excessive ingestion of English black licorice or a similar substance; produces a similar syndrome because of the mineralocorticoid action of glycyrrhizic acid

Secondary hyperaldosteronism

- Extra-adrenal abnormality leading to stimulation of the adrenal gland, resulting in increased aldosterone production
- Nephrotic syndrome, hepatic cirrhosis with ascites, and heart failure (commonly induce edema); Bartter's syndrome and salt-losing nephritis (don't induce edema)
- Wilms' tumor, hormonal contraceptives, and pregnancy (conditions that induce hypertension through increased renin production)

Signs and symptoms

- Azotemia
- Fatigue
- Headaches
- Hypertension
- Hypokalemia
- Intermittent, flaccid paralysis
- Muscle weakness
- Neuromuscular irritability
- Paresthesia
- Polydipsia
- Polyuria
- Worsening of glucose control in diabetic patients

Diagnostic tests

- Persistently low serum potassium levels in a nonedematous patient who isn't taking diuretics, doesn't have obvious GI losses (from vomiting or diarrhea), and has a normal sodium intake suggest hyperaldosteronism.
- A low plasma renin level that fails to increase appropriately during volume depletion (upright posture, sodium depletion) and a high plasma aldosterone level during volume expansion by salt loading confirm primary hyperaldosteronism in a hypertensive patient without edema.
- The serum bicarbonate level is commonly elevated, with ensuing alkalosis

due to hydrogen and potassium ion loss in the distal renal tubules.
- Markedly increased urine aldosterone levels and increased plasma aldosterone levels are seen.
- In secondary hyperaldosteronism, plasma renin levels are increased.
- A suppression test is useful to differentiate between primary and secondary hyperaldosteronism. During this test, the patient receives oral desoxycorticosterone acetate for 3 days while plasma aldosterone levels and urine metabolites are continuously measured. These levels decrease in secondary hyperaldosteronism but remain the same in primary hyperaldosteronism. Simultaneously, renin levels are low in primary hyperaldosteronism and high in secondary hyperaldosteronism.
- Electrocardiogram shows signs of hypokalemia (ST-segment depression and flattened U waves).
- Chest X-ray shows left ventricular hypertrophy from chronic hypertension.
- Localization of the tumor by adrenal angiography, computed tomography scans, or magnetic resonance imaging.

Treatment

- Unilateral adrenalectomy is required for an aldosterone-producing adenoma.
- Potassium-sparing diuretics (spironolactone [Aldactone]) control hyperaldosteronism.
- Treatment should also correct underlying cause (secondary hyperaldosteronism).

Nursing considerations

- Monitor and record urine output, blood pressure, weight, and serum potassium levels.
- Watch for hypokalemia-induced cardiac arrhythmias, paresthesia, and weakness. Give potassium replacement as ordered.

- Ask the dietitian to provide a low-sodium, high-potassium diet.
- Watch for weakness, hyponatremia, rising serum potassium levels, and signs of adrenal hypofunction, especially hypotension after the patient undergoes adrenalectomy.
- Advise the patient taking spironolactone or amiloride to watch for signs of hyperkalemia. Tell him that impotence and gynecomastia may follow long-term use of spironolactone.
- Tell the patient who must take steroid hormone replacement to wear a medical identification bracelet.

▌Hyperhidrosis

The excessive secretion of sweat from the eccrine glands, hyperhidrosis usually occurs in the axillae (typically after puberty) and on the palms and soles (commonly starting during infancy or childhood).

Causes

- Certain drugs, such as antipyretics, emetics, meperidine (Demerol), and anticholinesterase
- Exercise and a hot climate
- Genetic factors

Predisposing conditions

- Cardiovascular disorders, such as shock and heart failure
- Central nervous system disturbances (most commonly lesions of the hypothalamus)
- Diabetes during a hypoglycemic crisis
- Graves' disease
- Infections and chronic diseases, such as tuberculosis, malaria, and lymphoma
- Menopause
- Pheochromocytomas
- Withdrawal from drugs or alcohol

Signs and symptoms

- Contact dermatitis from clothing dyes
- Extreme axillary sweating
- Extreme sweating of the soles
- Profuse sweating of the palms

Diagnostic tests

- None

Treatment

- Aluminum chloride 20% in absolute ethanol decreases excessive perspiration. (Most antiperspirants contain a 5% solution.)
- Formaldehyde may also be used but may lead to allergic contact sensitization.
- Glutaraldehyde produces less contact sensitivity than formaldehyde but stains the skin; it's used more commonly on the feet than on the hands as a soak or applied directly several times per week and then weekly as needed.
- Anticholinergics, except in patients with glaucoma or benign prostatic hyperplasia.
- Local axillary removal of sweat glands or, as a last resort, a cervicothoracic or lumbar sympathectomy may be required for severe hyperhidrosis unresponsive to conservative therapy.
- Iontophoresis of water into involved areas of skin can be achieved with a device that may be purchased by the patient.

Nursing considerations

- Provide support and reassurance because hyperhidrosis may be socially embarrassing.
- Tell the patient to apply aluminum chloride in absolute ethanol nightly to dry axillae, soles, or palms, as prescribed. The area should be covered with plastic wrap for 6 to 8 hours, preferably overnight, and then washed with soap and water. Repeat this proce-

dure for several nights until profuse daytime sweating subsides. Frequency of treatments can then be reduced.

- Advise the patient with hyperhidrosis of the soles to wear leather sandals and white or colorfast cotton socks.

Hyperlipoproteinemia

Hyperlipoproteinemia is an inherited disorder marked by increased plasma concentrations of one or more lipoproteins. Hyperlipoproteinemia may also occur secondary to other conditions, such as diabetes, pancreatitis, hypothyroidism, and renal disease.

This disorder affects lipid transport in serum and produces varied clinical changes, from relatively mild symptoms that can be corrected by dietary management to potentially fatal pancreatitis.

Hyperlipoproteinemia occurs as five distinct metabolic disorders. Types I and III are transmitted as autosomal recessive traits; types II, IV, and V are transmitted as autosomal dominant traits.

Causes

See *Types of hyperlipoproteinemia,* pages 294 and 295.

Signs and symptoms
Type I hyperlipoproteinemia

- Abdominal spasm, rigidity, or rebound tenderness
- Anorexia
- Fever
- Hepatosplenomegaly with liver or spleen tenderness
- Lipemia retinalis (reddish white retinal vessels)
- Malaise
- Papular or eruptive xanthomas (pinkish yellow cutaneous deposits of fat) over pressure points and extensor surfaces

- Recurrent attacks of severe abdominal pain similar to pancreatitis, usually preceded by fat intake

Type II hyperlipoproteinemia

- Accelerated atherosclerosis and premature coronary artery disease (CAD)
- Juvenile corneal arcus (opaque ring surrounding the corneal periphery)
- Recurrent polyarthritis
- Tendinous xanthomas (firm masses) on the Achilles tendons and tendons of the hands and feet
- Tenosynovitis
- Tuberous xanthomas
- Xanthelasma

Type III hyperlipoproteinemia

- Palmar xanthomas on the hands, particularly fingertips
- Peripheral vascular disease manifested by claudication or tuberoeruptive xanthomas (soft, inflamed, pedunculated lesions) over the elbows and knees
- Premature atherosclerosis

Type IV hyperlipoproteinemia

- Diabetes
- Hypertension
- Obesity
- Predisposition to atherosclerosis and early CAD

Type V hyperlipoproteinemia

- Abdominal pain (most common)
- Eruptive xanthomas on extensor surfaces of the arms and legs
- Hepatosplenomegaly
- Lipemia retinalis
- Pancreatitis
- Peripheral neuropathy

Diagnostic tests

Diagnostic findings vary among the five types of hyperlipoproteinemia. (See *Types of hyperlipoproteinemia,* pages 294 and 295.)

Types of hyperlipoproteinemia

Type	Causes and incidence	Diagnostic findings
I (Frederickson's hyperlipoproteinemia, fat-induced hyperlipemia, idiopathic familial)	■ Deficient or abnormal lipoprotein lipase, resulting in decreased or absent postheparin lipolytic activity ■ Relatively rare ■ Present at birth	■ Chylomicrons (very-low-density lipoprotein [VLDL], low-density lipoprotein [LDL], and high-density lipoprotein) in plasma 14 hours or more after last meal ■ Highly elevated serum chylomicron and triglyceride levels; slightly elevated serum cholesterol levels ■ Lower serum lipoprotein lipase levels ■ Leukocytosis
II (Familial hyperbetalipoproteinemia, essential familial hypercholesterolemia)	■ Deficient cell surface receptor that regulates LDL degradation and cholesterol synthesis, resulting in increased levels of plasma LDL over joints and pressure points ■ Onset between ages 10 and 30	■ Increased plasma concentrations of LDL ■ Increased serum LDL and cholesterol levels ■ Increased LDL levels in amniotic fluid
III (Familial broad-beta disease, xanthoma tuberosum)	■ Unknown underlying defect resulting in deficient conversion of triglyceride-rich VLDL to LDL ■ Uncommon; usually occurring after age 20 (or earlier in men)	■ Abnormal serum beta-lipoprotein levels ■ Elevated cholesterol and triglyceride levels ■ Slightly elevated glucose tolerance ■ Hyperuricemia
IV (Endogenous hypertriglyceridemia hyperbetalipoproteinemia)	■ Primary defect unknown; secondary to obesity, diabetes, and hypertension ■ Relatively common, especially in middle-age men	■ Elevated VLDL levels ■ Moderately increased plasma triglyceride levels ■ Normal or slightly elevated serum cholesterol levels ■ Mildly abnormal glucose tolerance ■ Family history ■ Early coronary artery disease ■ Chylomicrons in plasma

Types of hyperlipoproteinemia (continued)

Type	Causes and incidence	Diagnostic findings
V (Mixed hypertriglyceridemia, mixed hyperlipidemia)	■ Defective triglyceride clearance causing pancreatitis; usually secondary to another disorder, such as obesity or nephrosis ■ Uncommon; onset usually occurring late in adolescence or early in adulthood	■ Elevated plasma VLDL levels ■ Elevated serum cholesterol and triglyceride levels

Treatment

■ Treat any underlying problem such as diabetes.

■ Patients with types II, III, and IV without underlying problems respond to dietary management.

■ Drug therapy (cholestyramine [Questran], clofibrate, gemfibrozil [Lopid], lovastatin [Mevacor], pravastatin [Pravachol], simvastatin [Zocor], or pharmaceutical nonflush niacin) may also be used to lower the plasma triglyceride or cholesterol level when diet alone is ineffective.

Type I

■ Initiate long-term weight reduction, with fat intake restricted to less than 20 g/day. A 20- to 40-g/day medium-chain triglyceride diet may be ordered to supplement caloric intake.

■ Avoid alcoholic beverages to decrease plasma triglycerides.

Type II

■ Dietary management restores normal lipid levels and decreases the risk of atherosclerosis. Restrict cholesterol intake to less than 300 mg/day for adults and less than 150 mg/day for children; triglyceride levels must be restricted to less than 100 mg/day for children and adults.

■ Diet should be high in polyunsaturated fats.

■ Atorvastatin (Lipitor) and fenofibrate (Tricor) may help lower levels when they're combined with diet therapy.

Type III

■ Dietary management includes restriction of cholesterol intake to less than 300 mg/day; carbohydrates must also be restricted, and polyunsaturated fats are increased.

■ Clofibrate, atorvastatin, and niacin are used to help lower blood lipid levels.

■ Weight reduction is helpful.

Type IV

■ Weight reduction may normalize blood lipid levels without additional treatment.

■ Long-term dietary management includes restricted cholesterol intake, increased polyunsaturated fats, and avoidance of alcoholic beverages.

■ Clofibrate, atorvastatin, fenofibrate, and niacin may lower plasma lipid levels.

Type V

■ Weight reduction and long-term maintenance of a low-fat diet constitute treatment.

- Alcoholic beverages must be avoided.
- Niacin, clofibrate, gemfibrozil, and a 20- to 40-g/day medium-chain triglyceride diet may prove helpful.

Nursing considerations
- Monitor the patient for adverse reactions to drugs.
- Teach the importance of long-term dietary management.
- Give cholestyramine before meals or before bedtime as prescribed. This drug must not be given with other medications. Watch for adverse reactions, such as nausea, vomiting, constipation, steatorrhea, rashes, and hyperchloremic acidosis. Also watch for malabsorption of other medications and fat-soluble vitamins.
- Give clofibrate as prescribed. Watch for adverse reactions, such as cholelithiasis, cardiac arrhythmias, intermittent claudication, thromboembolism, nausea, weight gain (from fluid retention), and myositis.

DRUG CHALLENGE

Don't give niacin to patients with active peptic ulcers or liver disease. Use with caution in patients with diabetes. In other patients, watch for adverse reactions, such as flushing, pruritus, hyperpigmentation, and worsening of inactive peptic ulcers.

- Urge the patient to adhere to his diet (usually 1,000 to 1,500 calories/day), to avoid excess sugar and alcoholic beverages, to minimize intake of saturated fats (higher in meats, coconut oil), and to increase intake of polyunsaturated fats (vegetable oils).
- Instruct the patient, for the 2 weeks preceding serum cholesterol and serum triglyceride tests, to maintain a steady weight and to adhere strictly to the pre-

scribed diet. He should also fast for 12 hours before the test.
- Instruct women with elevated serum lipid levels to avoid hormonal contraceptives or drugs that contain estrogen.

Hyperparathyroidism

Characterized by overactivity of one or more of the four parathyroid glands, hyperparathyroidism results from excessive secretion of parathyroid hormone (PTH). Such hypersecretion of PTH promotes bone resorption and leads to hypercalcemia and hypophosphatemia. The signs and symptoms of primary hyperparathyroidism result from hypercalcemia and are typically present in several body systems. (See *Bone resorption in primary hyperparathyroidism.*) Increased renal and GI absorption of calcium occurs.

Primary hyperparathyroidism is commonly diagnosed by elevated calcium levels found on laboratory profiles in asymptomatic patients. It affects women two to three times more commonly than men.

Causes
- Adenoma
- Chronic renal failure
- Decreased intestinal absorption of vitamin D or calcium
- Dietary vitamin D or calcium deficiency
- Genetic disorders
- Idiopathic
- Ingestion of drugs such as phenytoin
- Laxative ingestion
- Multiple endocrine neoplasia
- Osteomalacia

Signs and symptoms
- Central nervous system: psychomotor and personality disturbances, depres-

Bone resorption in primary hyperparathyroidism

In primary hyper-
parathyroidism,
bone X-rays show
demineralization
and erosion.

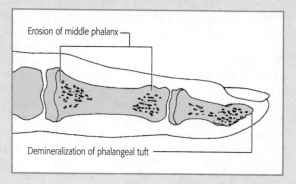

Erosion of middle phalanx

Demineralization of phalangeal tuft

sion, overt psychosis, stupor and, possibly, coma
- GI: pancreatitis causing constant, severe epigastric pain that radiates to the
back; peptic ulcers causing abdominal
pain, anorexia, nausea, and vomiting
- Neuromuscular: muscle weakness and
atrophy, particularly in the legs
- Renal (most common): polyuria,
nephrocalcinosis due to elevated levels
of calcium and, possibly, recurring
nephrolithiasis, possibly leading to renal
insufficiency
- Skeletal and articular: chronic lower
back pain and easy fracturing due to
bone degeneration; bone tenderness;
chondrocalcinosis; osteopenia and osteoporosis, especially on the vertebrae;
erosions of the juxta-articular surface;
subchondral fractures; traumatic synovitis; and pseudogout
- Other: skin necrosis, cataracts, calcium
microthrombi to lungs and pancreas,
polyuria, anemia, and subcutaneous calcification

Diagnostic tests
Primary disease
- High concentration of serum PTH on
radioimmunoassay with accompanying
hypercalcemia confirms the diagnosis.
- X-rays show diffuse demineralization
of bones, bone cysts, outer cortical bone
absorption, and subperiosteal erosion of
the phalanges and distal clavicles.
- Microscopic examination of the bone
with such tests as X-ray spectrophotom-
etry typically demonstrates increased
bone turnover.
- Laboratory tests reveal elevated urine
and serum calcium and chloride levels
and decreased serum phosphorus levels.
- Hyperparathyroidism may increase
uric acid and creatinine levels, as well as
basal acid secretion and the serum im-
munoreactive gastrin level.
- Increased serum amylase levels may
indicate acute pancreatitis.

Secondary disease
- In patients with secondary hyperparathyroidism, laboratory test results
show normal or slightly decreased
serum calcium level and a variable
serum phosphorus level, especially

when hyperparathyroidism is due to rickets, osteomalacia, or kidney disease.
- Other laboratory values and physical examination findings identify the cause of secondary hyperparathyroidism.

Treatment
Primary disease
- Surgery removes the adenoma or, depending on the extent of hyperplasia, all but one-half of one gland (the remaining part of the gland is necessary to maintain normal PTH levels).
- Increase fluid intake.
- Restrict dietary intake of calcium.
- Initiate I.V. infusion of normal saline solution (up to 6 L in life-threatening circumstances).
- Furosemide or ethacrynic acid promotes sodium and calcium excretion (thereby decreasing calcium levels) through forced diuresis.
- Oral sodium or potassium phosphate, calcitonin, or plicamycin are also used to promote sodium and calcium excretion.
- I.V. administration of magnesium and phosphate or sodium phosphate solution given by mouth or retention enema may be given for potential postoperative magnesium and phosphate deficiencies.
- Supplemental calcium is given during the first 4 to 5 days after surgery, when serum calcium falls to low-normal levels.
- Vitamin D or calcitriol may also be used to raise the serum calcium level.

Secondary disease
- Correct the underlying cause of parathyroid hypertrophy with vitamin D therapy or, in the patient with kidney disease, give an oral calcium preparation for hyperphosphatemia.
- Dialysis is necessary in the patient with renal failure to lower the calcium level.

Nursing considerations
- Obtain pretreatment baseline serum potassium, calcium, phosphate, and magnesium levels because these values may change abruptly during treatment.
- During hydration to reduce the serum calcium level, record intake and output accurately. Strain the urine to check for calculi. Provide at least 3 qt (3 L) of fluid per day, including cranberry or prune juice to increase urine acidity and help prevent calculus formation.
- Obtain blood samples and urine specimens to measure sodium, potassium, and magnesium levels, especially for the patient taking furosemide.
- Auscultate for breath sounds often. Listen for signs of pulmonary edema in the patient receiving large amounts of saline solution I.V., especially if he has lung or heart disease.
- Monitor the patient receiving cardiac glycosides carefully because elevated calcium levels can rapidly produce toxic effects.
- Because the patient is predisposed to pathologic fractures, take safety precautions to minimize the risk of injury. Assist him with walking, keep the bed at its lowest position, and raise the side rails. Lift the immobilized patient carefully to minimize bone stress.
- Schedule care to allow the patient with muscle weakness as much rest as possible.
- Watch for signs of peptic ulcer, and administer antacids as appropriate.

After parathyroidectomy
- Check frequently for respiratory distress, and keep a tracheotomy tray at the bedside. Watch for postoperative complications, such as laryngeal nerve damage and, rarely, hemorrhage. Monitor intake and output carefully.
- Check for swelling at the operative site. Place the patient in semi-Fowler's

position, and support his head and neck with sandbags to decrease edema, which may cause pressure on the trachea.

■ Watch for signs of mild tetany such as complaints of tingling in the hands and around the mouth. These symptoms should subside quickly but may be prodromal signs of tetany, so keep calcium gluconate I.V. available for emergency administration. Watch for increased neuromuscular irritability and other signs of severe tetany.

■ Ambulate the patient as soon as possible postoperatively, even though he may find this uncomfortable, because pressure on bones speeds up bone recalcification.

■ Check laboratory results for low serum calcium and magnesium levels.

■ Monitor the patient's mental status, and watch for listlessness. In the patient with persistent hypercalcemia, check for muscle weakness and psychiatric symptoms.

■ Before discharge, advise the patient of the possible adverse effects of drug therapy. Emphasize the need for periodic follow-up through laboratory blood tests. If hyperparathyroidism wasn't corrected surgically, warn the patient to avoid calcium-containing antacids and thiazide diuretics.

Hypertension

An intermittent or sustained elevation in diastolic or systolic blood pressure, hypertension occurs as two major types: essential (also called *primary* or *idiopathic*) hypertension, the most common, and secondary hypertension, which results from kidney disease or another identifiable cause. Malignant hypertension is a severe, fulminant form of hypertension common to both types.

Hypertension is a major cause of stroke, heart disease, and renal failure.

Incidence of hypertension

Gender and age play a role in who develops hypertension.

■ Before age 55, men are more likely than women to have high blood pressure.

■ Between ages 55 and 74, women are *slightly* more likely than men to have high blood pressure, but after age 74, the incidence of high blood pressure in women becomes *significantly* higher than in men.

■ Women taking hormonal contraceptives (especially women who are overweight or obese) are two to three times more likely to have high blood pressure than women not taking contraceptives.

The prognosis is good if this disorder is detected early and if treatment begins before complications develop. Severely elevated blood pressure (hypertensive crisis) may be fatal.

Blacks are twice as likely as Whites to be affected. If untreated, hypertension carries a high mortality. In many cases, however, treatment with stepped care offers patients an improved prognosis. (See *Incidence of hypertension*.)

Systolic hypertension poses a risk equal to or greater than diastolic elevations. It's commonly seen in elderly people and presents a risk of stroke or myocardial infarction (MI).

Hypertension usually doesn't produce clinical effects until vascular changes in the heart, brain, or kidneys occur. Highly elevated blood pressure damages the intima of small vessels, resulting in fibrin accumulation in the vessels, development of local edema and, possibly, intravascular clotting.

Causes
Essential hypertension
- Unknown

Predisposing factors
- Aging
- Family history
- High intake of saturated fats or sodium
- Insulin resistance
- Obesity
- Race (most common in blacks)
- Sedentary lifestyle
- Stress
- Tobacco use

Secondary hypertension
- Coarctation of the aorta
- Cushing's syndrome
- Drugs, such as cocaine, epoetin alfa, and cyclosporine
- Hormonal contraceptive use
- Neurologic disorders
- Pheochromocytoma
- Pregnancy
- Primary hyperaldosteronism
- Thyroid, pituitary, or parathyroid dysfunction

Signs and symptoms
Symptoms produced by this process depend on the location of the damaged vessels.
- Brain: stroke
- Retina: blindness
- Heart: increases the heart's workload, causing left ventricular hypertrophy and, later, left- and right-sided heart failure, MI, and pulmonary edema
- Kidneys: proteinuria, edema and, eventually, renal failure

Diagnostic tests
- Serial blood pressure measurements that are greater than 120/80 mm Hg but less than 140/90 mm Hg indicate prehypertension; measurements greater than 140/90 mm Hg confirm hypertension.

Stage 1 hypertension is defined as a systolic blood pressure greater than 139 but less than 160 mm Hg or a diastolic blood pressure greater than 89 but less than 100 mm Hg. Stage 2 hypertension is defined as a systolic blood pressure greater than or equal to 159 mm Hg or diastolic blood pressure greater than or equal to 99 mm Hg.
- Auscultation reveals bruits over the abdominal aorta and the carotid, renal, and femoral arteries.
- Ophthalmoscopy reveals arteriovenous nicking and, in hypertensive encephalopathy, papilledema.

The following tests may show predisposing factors and help identify an underlying cause:
- Urinalysis: The presence of protein, red blood cells, and white blood cells may indicate glomerulonephritis.
- Excretory urography: Renal atrophy indicates chronic kidney disease; one kidney that's more than 1.5 cm shorter than the other suggests unilateral kidney disease.
- Serum potassium: Levels less than 3.5 mEq/L may indicate adrenal dysfunction (primary hyperaldosteronism).
- Blood urea nitrogen (BUN) and serum creatinine levels: A BUN level that's normal or elevated to more than 20 mg/dl and a serum creatinine level that's normal or elevated to more than 1.5 mg/dl suggest kidney disease.
- Electrocardiography may show left ventricular hypertrophy or ischemia.
- Chest X-ray may show cardiomegaly.
- Echocardiography may show left ventricular hypertrophy.
- Oral captopril challenge tests for renovascular hypertension. This functional diagnostic test depends on the abrupt inhibition of circulating angiotensin II by angiotensin-converting enzyme inhibitors (ACEIs), removing the major support for perfusion through a stenotic

kidney. The acutely ischemic kidney immediately releases more renin and undergoes a marked decrease in glomerular filtration rate and renal blood flow.
- Renal arteriography may show renal artery stenosis.

Treatment

- Secondary hypertension treatment focuses on correcting the underlying cause and controlling hypertensive effects. The National Institutes of Health recommends the following approach for treating primary hypertension:
  - First, help the patient initiate necessary lifestyle modifications, including weight reduction, moderation of alcohol intake, regular physical exercise, reduction of sodium intake, and smoking cessation.
  - If the patient fails to achieve the desired blood pressure or make significant progress, continue lifestyle modifications and begin drug therapy.
  - For stage 1 hypertension in the absence of compelling indications (heart failure, post-MI, high coronary disease risk, diabetes, chronic kidney disease, or recurrent stroke prevention), give most patients thiazide-type diuretics. Consider using an ACEI, angiotensin receptor blocker (ARB), beta-adrenergic blocker (BB), calcium channel blocker (CCB), or a combination.
  - For stage 2 hypertension in the absence of compelling indications, give most patients a two-drug combination (usually a thiazide-type diuretic and an ACEI, ARB, BB, or CCB).
- If the patient has one or more compelling indications, base drug treatment on benefits from outcome studies or existing clinical guidelines. Treatment may include the following, depending on indication:
  - Heart failure: diuretic, BB, ACEI, ARB, or aldosterone antagonist
  - Post-myocardial failure: BB, ACEI, or aldosterone antagonist
  - High coronary disease risk: diuretic, BB, ACEI, or CCB
  - Diabetes: diuretic, BB, ACEI, ARB, or CCB
  - Chronic kidney disease: ACEI or ARB
  - Recurrent stroke prevention: diuretic or ACEI
  - Other antihypertensive drugs as needed
- If the patient fails to achieve the desired blood pressure, continue lifestyle modifications and optimize drug dosages or add additional drugs until the goal blood pressure is achieved. Also, consider consultation with a hypertension specialist.
- Studies have shown that omega-3 fatty acids used in the treatment of hypertension significantly reduce total cholesterol, low-density lipoprotein cholesterol, and triglyceride levels and lower systolic and diastolic blood pressure.
- The treatment for renal artery stenosis includes the use of ACEIs and renal artery stents.

ACTION STAT!

 Hypertensive emergencies include hypertensive encephalopathy, intracranial hemorrhage, acute left-sided heart failure with pulmonary edema, and dissecting aortic aneurysm. Hypertensive emergencies are also associated with eclampsia and severe gestational hypertension, unstable angina, and acute MI.

Typically, hypertensive emergencies require parenteral administration of a vasodilator or an adrenergic inhibitor or oral administration of a selected drug, such as nifedipine (Procardia), captopril (Capoten), clonidine (Catapres), or labetalol (Trandate), to rapidly reduce blood pressure.

Nursing considerations

■ Instruct the patient to establish a daily routine for taking his medication. Warn him that uncontrolled hypertension may cause stroke and MI.
■ Tell the patient to report adverse reactions to drugs.
■ Advise the patient to avoid high-sodium antacids and over-the-counter cold and sinus medications, which contain harmful vasoconstrictors.
■ Encourage the patient to change his dietary habits if indicated. Help the obese patient plan a weight-reduction diet; tell him to avoid high-sodium foods (pickles, potato chips, canned soups, and cold cuts) and table salt.
■ Help the patient examine and modify his lifestyle, for example, by reducing stress and exercising regularly.

For a hospitalized patient with hypertension

■ Monitor the patient's vital signs, cardiovascular and neurologic status.
■ Find out if he was taking his prescribed medication. If he wasn't, ask why. If the patient can't afford the medication, consult social services.
■ Tell the patient and his family to keep a record of drugs used in the past, noting especially which ones were and weren't effective. Suggest recording this information on a card so that the patient can show it to his physician.
■ Tell the patient who has a renal artery stent to expect an increase in urine output the first few days after the procedure.

When routine blood pressure screening shows elevated pressure

■ Make sure the cuff size is appropriate for the patient's upper arm circumference.
■ Measure the pressure in both arms in lying, sitting, and standing positions.
■ Ask the patient if he smoked, drank a beverage containing caffeine, or was emotionally upset before the measurement.
■ Advise the patient to return for blood pressure testing at frequent and regular intervals.

To help identify hypertension and prevent untreated hypertension

■ Participate in public education programs dealing with hypertension and ways to reduce risk factors.
■ Encourage public participation in blood pressure screening programs. Routinely screen all patients, especially those at risk (blacks and people with family histories of hypertension, stroke, or MI).

Hypoglycemia

An abnormally low glucose level in the bloodstream, hypoglycemia occurs when glucose burns up too rapidly, when the glucose release rate falls behind tissue demands, or when excessive insulin enters the bloodstream.

Hypoglycemia is classified as reactive or fasting. Reactive hypoglycemia results from the reaction to the disposition of meals or the administration of excessive insulin. Fasting hypoglycemia causes discomfort during long periods of abstinence from food, for example, in the early morning hours before breakfast.

Although hypoglycemia is a specific endocrine imbalance, its symptoms are commonly vague and depend on how quickly the patient's glucose levels drop. If not corrected, severe hypoglycemia may result in coma, irreversible brain damage, and death.

Causes
Reactive hypoglycemia
- Administration of too much insulin
- Administration of too much oral antidiabetic medication
- Delayed and excessive insulin production after carbohydrate ingestion
- Gastric dumping syndrome
- Idiopathic
- Impaired glucose tolerance
- Sharp increase in insulin output after a meal (postprandial hypoglycemia)

Fasting hypoglycemia
- Excess of insulin or insulin-like substance or decrease in counterregulatory hormones
- External factors such as alcohol or drug ingestion
- Tumors

Hypoglycemia in infants and children
- Maternal disorders that can produce hypoglycemia in infants within 24 hours after birth, such as diabetes mellitus, pregnancy-induced hypertension, erythroblastosis, and glycogen storage disease
- Nesidioblastosis, a benign condition of the insulin-producing islet cells

Signs and symptoms
Reactive hypoglycemia
- Cold sweats
- Fatigue
- Headache
- Hunger
- Irritability
- Malaise
- Nervousness
- Rapid heart rate
- Trembling

Fasting hypoglycemia
- Blurred or double vision
- Coma
- Confusion
- Hemiplegia
- Motor weakness
- Same signs and symptoms as reactive hypoglycemia
- Seizures

Hypoglycemia in infants and children
- Coma
- Limpness
- Refusal to eat
- Seizures
- Sweating
- Tremors
- Twitching
- Weak or high-pitched cry

Diagnostic tests
- Glucometer readings provide quick screening methods for determining blood glucose levels.
- Laboratory testing confirms the diagnosis by showing decreased blood glucose values. The following values indicate hypoglycemia:
  - Full-term neonates: less than 50 mg/dl before or after a feeding
  - Preterm neonates: less than 50 mg/dl before or after a feeding
  - Children and adults: less than 40 mg/dl before a meal; less than 50 mg/dl after a meal.
- A 5-hour glucose tolerance test may be administered to provoke reactive hypoglycemia. After a 12-hour fast, laboratory testing to detect plasma insulin and plasma glucose levels may identify fasting hypoglycemia.

Treatment

 Urgent treatment may be provided by glucose tablets, candy, or fluids if the patient is alert. Dextrose 50% solution is given for emergency treatment, followed by a constant infusion in children and adults.

Reactive hypoglycemia

■ Dietary modification to help delay glucose absorption and gastric emptying includes small, frequent meals; ingestion of complex carbohydrates, fiber, and fat; and avoidance of simple sugars, alcohol, and fruit drinks.
■ Anticholinergic drugs slow gastric emptying and intestinal motility and inhibit vagal stimulation of insulin release.

Fasting hypoglycemia

■ Surgery and drug therapy may be required.
■ Removal of the tumor is the treatment of choice for an insuloma.
■ Drug therapy may include nondiuretic thiazides, such as diazoxide (Hyperstat), to inhibit insulin secretion, streptozocin (Zanosar), and hormones, such as glucocorticoids and long-acting glycogen.

Hypoglycemia in infants and children

■ Hypertonic solution of dextrose 10% in water, calculated at 5 to 10 ml/kg of body weight administered I.V. over 10 minutes and followed by 4 to 8 mg/kg/minute for severe hypoglycemia in neonates.
■ Administer feedings of either breast milk or a commercially prepared infant formula as soon after birth as possible to reduce the chance of hypoglycemia in high-risk neonates.

Nursing considerations

■ Watch for signs of hypoglycemia (such as poor feeding) in high-risk neonates.
■ Monitor diabetic patients for hypoglycemia; administer a carbohydrate immediately if hypoglycemia is detected.
■ Monitor the patient's glucose levels as needed.
■ Monitor infusion of hypertonic glucose in the neonate to avoid hyperglycemia, circulatory overload, and cellular dehydration. Terminate glucose solutions gradually to prevent hypoglycemia caused by hyperinsulinemia.
■ Monitor the effects of drug therapy, and watch for the development of adverse effects.
■ Teach the patient which foods to include in his diet (complex carbohydrates, fiber, and fat) and which foods to avoid (simple sugars and alcohol). Refer the patient and his family for dietary counseling as appropriate.

Hypoparathyroidism

A deficiency of parathyroid hormone (PTH), hypoparathyroidism is caused by disease, injury, surgical removal, or congenital malfunction of the parathyroid glands. Because the parathyroid glands primarily regulate calcium balance, hypoparathyroidism causes hypocalcemia, producing neuromuscular symptoms ranging from paresthesia to tetany.

The clinical effects of hypoparathyroidism are usually correctable with replacement therapy. Some complications of long-term hypocalcemia, such as cataracts and basal ganglion calcifications, are irreversible.

Hypoparathyroidism may be acute or chronic and is classified as idiopathic or acquired.

The incidence of the idiopathic and reversible forms is highest in children; incidence of the irreversible acquired form is highest in older patients who have undergone surgery for hyperthyroidism or other head and neck conditions.

Causes
- Abnormalities of the calcium-sensor receptor
- Accidental removal of or injury to one or more of the parathyroid glands during surgery
- Amyloidosis
- Autoimmune genetic disorder
- Congenital absence or malformation of the parathyroid gland
- Delayed maturation of parathyroid function
- Hemochromatosis
- Hypomagnesemia-induced impairment of hormone secretion
- Ischemia or infarction of the parathyroid glands during surgery
- Massive thyroid irradiation
- Neoplasms
- Sarcoidosis
- Suppression of normal gland function due to hypercalcemia
- Trauma
- Tuberculosis

Signs and symptoms
Acute hypoparathyroidism
- Abdominal pain
- Brittle fingernails that develop ridges or fall out
- Cataracts
- Cyanosis
- Dry, lusterless hair
- Dry, scaly skin
- Hypocalcemia (may induce cardiac arrhythmias and eventually lead to heart failure)
- Laryngospasm
- Pain that varies with the degree of muscle tension
- Seizures
- Spontaneous hair loss

- Stridor
- Tetany
- Weakened tooth enamel, causing teeth to stain, crack, and decay easily

Chronic hypoparathyroidism
- Chvostek's sign (hyperirritability of the facial nerve, producing a characteristic spasm when it's tapped)
- Dysphagia
- Increased deep tendon reflexes
- Mental deficiency in children
- Neuromuscular irritability
- Organic brain syndrome
- Psychosis
- Tetany (may cause difficulty in walking and a tendency to fall; may lead to laryngospasm, stridor and, eventually, cyanosis and seizures)

Diagnostic tests
- Radioimmunoassay for PTH reveals decreased PTH concentration.
- Serum and urine calcium levels are decreased, serum phosphate levels are increased, and urine creatinine levels are decreased.
- Electrocardiography (ECG) reveals prolonged QT and ST intervals due to hypocalcemia.
- Inflating a blood pressure cuff on the upper arm to between diastolic and systolic blood pressure and maintaining this inflation for 3 minutes elicits Trousseau's sign (carpal spasm).

Treatment
- Administration of vitamin D and calcium supplements is usually lifelong, except for the reversible form of the disease.
- Calcitriol (Rocaltrol) may be used if the patient can't tolerate vitamin D.
- Immediate I.V. administration of 10% calcium gluconate, 10% calcium gluceptate, or 10% calcium chloride raises serum calcium levels if acute, life-threat-

Discharge instructions in hypoparathyroidism

■ Advise the patient to follow a high-calcium, low-phosphorus diet, and tell him which foods are permitted.

■ For the patient on drug therapy, emphasize the importance of checking serum calcium levels at least three times per year. Instruct him to watch for signs of hypercalcemia and to keep medications away from light and heat.

■ Instruct the patient with scaly skin to use creams to soften his skin.

■ Tell the patient to keep his nails trimmed to prevent them from splitting.

ening tetany occurs. The patient who's awake and able to cooperate can help raise serum calcium levels by breathing into a paper bag and then inhaling his own carbon dioxide; this produces hypoventilation and mild respiratory acidosis.

■ Sedatives and anticonvulsants may control spasms until calcium levels rise.

■ Maintenance therapy for the patient with chronic tetany consists of oral calcium and vitamin D supplements.

Nursing considerations

■ Maintain a patent I.V. line and keep I.V. calcium gluconate and calcium chloride available.

■ Maintain seizure precautions.

■ Keep a tracheotomy tray and endotracheal (ET) tube at bedside because laryngospasm may result from hypocalcemia.

■ Administer 10% calcium gluconate slow I.V. (1 mg/minute) as prescribed, and maintain a patent airway if the patient suffers acute tetany. Assist with ET intubation if needed.

■ Administer I.V. lorazepam for sedation, and monitor vital signs frequently after administration.

■ When caring for the patient with chronic hypoparathyroidism, particularly a child, stay alert for minor muscle twitching (especially in the hands) and for signs of laryngospasm (respiratory stridor or dysphagia) because these effects may signal onset of tetany.

■ Monitor the patient's ECG for heart block and signs of decreasing cardiac output because the patient with chronic disease has prolonged QT intervals.

■ Closely monitor the patient receiving both digoxin and calcium gluconate because calcium potentiates the effect of digoxin. Stay alert for signs of digoxin toxicity (arrhythmias, nausea, fatigue and vision changes).

■ Perform careful patient teaching. (See *Discharge instructions in hypoparathyroidism.*)

▌Hypopituitarism

Hypopituitarism, also known as *panhypopituitarism,* is a complex syndrome marked by metabolic dysfunction, sexual immaturity, and growth retardation (when it occurs in childhood), resulting from a deficiency of the hormones secreted by the anterior pituitary gland. Panhypopituitarism refers to a generalized condition caused by partial or total failure of all six of this gland's vital hormones—corticotropin, thyroid-stimulating hormone (TSH), luteinizing hormone, follicle-stimulating hormone (FSH), human growth hormone (hGH), and prolactin. Partial hypopituitarism and complete hypopituitarism occur in adults and children; in children, these diseases may cause dwarfism and delayed puberty. The prognosis may be good with adequate replacement therapy and correction of the underlying causes.

Causes

- Congenital defects
- Deficiency of hypothalamus releasing hormones
- Granulomatous disease
- Idiopathic
- Infection
- Partial or total hypophysectomy by surgery, irradiation, or chemical agents
- Pituitary infarction
- Trauma
- Tumor

Signs and symptoms
Gonadotropin deficiency in women

- Amenorrhea
- Dyspareunia
- Infertility
- Reduced libido

Gonadotropin deficiency in men

- Impotence
- Reduced libido

TSH deficiency

- Cold intolerance
- Constipation
- Lethargy
- Menstrual irregularity
- Severe growth retardation in children despite treatment

Corticotropin deficiency

- Fatigue
- Nausea, vomiting, and anorexia
- Weight loss

Prolactin deficiency

- Absent postpartum lactation
- Amenorrhea

Diagnostic tests

- Low serum levels of thyroxine (T_4) indicate diminished thyroid gland function, but further tests are necessary to identify the source of dysfunction.
- Radioimmunoassay showing decreased plasma levels of some or all pituitary hormones, accompanied by end-organ hypofunction, including low levels of T_4, estrogen, and testosterone, suggests pituitary failure and eliminates target gland disease.
- Failure of thyrotropin-releasing hormone administration to increase TSH or prolactin concentrations rules out hypothalamic dysfunction as the cause of hormonal deficiency.
- Provocative tests are helpful in pinpointing the source of low cortisol levels. Oral metyrapone blocks cortisol synthesis, which should stimulate pituitary secretion of corticotropin and the adrenal precursors of cortisol, measured in urine as hydroxycorticosteroids. Insulin-induced hypoglycemia also stimulates corticotropin secretion. Persistently low levels of corticotropin indicate pituitary or hypothalamic failure. These tests require careful medical supervision because they may precipitate an adrenal crisis.
- Measurement of hGH levels in the blood after administration of regular insulin (inducing hypoglycemia) or levodopa show low levels of hGH. These drugs should provoke increased secretion of hGH. Persistently low hGH levels, despite provocative testing, confirm hGH deficiency.
- Computed tomography scan, magnetic resonance imaging, or cerebral angiography confirms the presence of intrasellar or extrasellar tumors.

Treatment

- Hormone replacement therapy includes cortisol, thyroxine, and androgen

or cyclic estrogen. The patient of reproductive age may benefit from cyclic administration of FSH and human chorionic gonadotropin to induce ovulation.
■ Somatrem, identical to GH but the product of recombinant DNA technology, and other agents have replaced growth hormones derived from human sources.
■ Children may require adrenal and thyroid hormone replacement and, as they approach puberty, sex hormones.

Nursing considerations

■ Provide emotional support.
■ Monitor the results of all laboratory tests for hormonal deficiencies, and know what they mean. Until hormone replacement therapy is complete, check for signs of thyroid deficiency (increasing lethargy), adrenal deficiency (weakness, orthostatic hypotension, hypoglycemia, fatigue, and weight loss), and gonadotropin deficiency (decreased libido, lethargy, and apathy).
■ Watch for anorexia in the patient with panhypopituitarism. Help plan a menu that contains his favorite foods—ideally, high-calorie foods. Monitor for weight loss or gain.
■ Record temperature, blood pressure, and heart rate every 4 to 8 hours. Check eyelids, nail beds, and skin for pallor, which indicates anemia.
■ Prevent infection by giving meticulous skin care. Because the patient's skin is probably dry, use oil or lotion instead of soap. If the patient's body temperature is low, provide additional clothing and covers, as needed, to keep him warm.
■ Darken the room if the patient has a tumor that's causing headaches and vision disturbances. Help with any activity that requires good vision such as reading the menu. The patient with bilateral hemianopsia has impaired peripheral vision, so be sure to stand where he can

see you, and advise his family to do the same.
■ During insulin testing, monitor closely for signs of hypoglycemia (initially, slow cerebration, tachycardia, diaphoresis, and nervousness, progressing to seizures). Keep dextrose 50% in water available for I.V. administration to correct hypoglycemia rapidly.
■ To prevent orthostatic hypotension, be sure to keep the patient in a supine position during levodopa testing.
■ Instruct the patient to wear a medical identification bracelet. Teach him and his family how to administer steroids parenterally in case of an emergency.
■ Refer the family of a child with dwarfism to appropriate community resources for psychological counseling because the emotional stress caused by this disorder increases as the child becomes more aware of his condition.

Hypothyroidism in adults

Hypothyroidism, a state of low serum thyroid hormone, results from hypothalamic, pituitary, or thyroid insufficiency. The disorder can progress to life-threatening myxedema coma. Hypothyroidism is more prevalent in women than in men; in the United States, incidence is rising significantly in people ages 40 to 50.

Causes

■ Amyloidosis
■ Antithyroid drugs
■ Autoimmune thyroiditis
■ Congenital defects
■ Drugs, such as iodides and lithium
■ Endemic iodine deficiency
■ External radiation of the neck
■ Idiopathic
■ Inflammatory conditions

- Pituitary failure to produce thyroid-stimulating hormone (TSH)
- Pituitary tumor
- Radioactive iodine therapy
- Sarcoidosis
- Thyroid gland surgery

Signs and symptoms
Early stages
- Constipation
- Fatigue
- Forgetfulness
- Sensitivity to cold
- Unexplained weight gain

Later stages
- Anorexia and abdominal distention
- Ataxia
- Cardiovascular involvement leading to decreased cardiac output, slow pulse rate, signs of poor peripheral circulation and, occasionally, an enlarged heart
- Decreased libido
- Decreasing mental stability
- Delayed relaxation time in reflexes (especially in the Achilles tendon)
- Dry, flaky, inelastic skin
- Dry, sparse hair
- Hoarseness
- Infertility
- Menorrhagia
- Nystagmus
- Periorbital edema
- Progression to myxedema coma (usually gradual but can be abrupt when stress aggravates severe or prolonged hypothyroidism)
- Puffy face, hands, and feet
- Thick, brittle nails
- Upper eyelid droop

Diagnostic tests
- Radioimmunoassay confirms hypothyroidism with low triiodothyronine and thyroxine levels.
- Increased TSH level reveals hypothyroidism due to thyroid insufficiency; de-

creased TSH level shows hypothyroidism due to hypothalamic or pituitary insufficiency.
- Elevated levels of serum cholesterol, alkaline phosphatase, and triglycerides are supportive findings.
- Normocytic, normochromic anemia is present.
- In myxedema coma, laboratory tests may also show low serum sodium levels as well as decreased pH and increased partial pressure of carbon dioxide, indicating respiratory acidosis.

Treatment
- Therapy for hypothyroidism consists of gradual thyroid hormone replacement with levothyroxine and, occasionally, liothyronine. The TSH level is the most reliable marker to follow in primary hypothyroidism. It should be kept within the normal range.
- During myxedema coma, effective treatment supports vital functions while restoring euthyroidism. To support blood pressure and pulse rate, treatment includes I.V. administration of levothyroxine and hydrocortisone to correct possible pituitary or adrenal insufficiency. Hypoventilation requires oxygenation and respiratory support.
- Other supportive measures include fluid replacement and antibiotics for infection.

Nursing considerations
- Provide a high-bulk, low-calorie diet, and encourage activity to combat constipation and promote weight loss. Administer cathartics and stool softeners as needed.
- Monitor the patient for symptoms of hyperthyroidism, such as restlessness, sweating, and excessive weight loss after thyroid replacement therapy begins.

- Tell the patient to report signs of aggravated cardiovascular disease, such as chest pain and tachycardia.
- Explain the importance of continuing the course of thyroid medication even if symptoms subside.
- Warn the patient to report infection immediately and to make sure any physician who prescribes drugs for him knows about the underlying hypothyroidism.
- Treatment of myxedema coma requires supportive care:
  - Check frequently for signs of decreasing cardiac output (such as falling urine output).
  - Monitor temperature until stable. Provide extra blankets and clothing and a warm room to compensate for hypothermia. Rapid rewarming may cause vasodilation and vascular collapse.
  - Record intake and output and daily weight. As treatment begins, urine output should increase and body weight should decrease.
  - Turn the edematous bedridden patient every 2 hours, and provide skin care, particularly around bony prominences, at least once per shift.
  - Avoid sedation when possible or reduce the dose because hypothyroidism delays metabolism of many drugs.
  - Maintain a patent I.V. line. Monitor serum electrolyte levels carefully when administering I.V. fluids.
  - Monitor vital signs carefully when administering levothyroxine because rapid correction of hypothyroidism can cause adverse cardiac effects. Report chest pain or tachycardia immediately. Watch for hypertension and heart failure in the elderly patient.
  - Check arterial blood gas values for indications of hypoxia and respiratory acidosis to determine whether the patient needs ventilatory assistance.
  - Because myxedema coma may have been precipitated by an infection, check possible sources of infection, such as blood or urine, and obtain sputum cultures.

Hypothyroidism in children

Deficiency of thyroid hormone secretion during fetal development and early in infancy results in infantile cretinism (congenital hypothyroidism). The characteristic signs and symptoms may not appear until 3 to 6 months after birth.

Untreated hypothyroidism is characterized in infants by respiratory difficulties, persistent jaundice, and hoarse crying and in older children by stunted growth (dwarfism), bone and muscle dystrophy, and mental deficiency.

Cretinism is three times more common in girls than in boys. Early diagnosis and treatment allow the best prognosis; infants treated before age 3 months usually grow and develop normally. Athyroid children who remain untreated beyond age 3 months and children with acquired hypothyroidism who remain untreated beyond age 2 years suffer irreversible mental retardation; their skeletal abnormalities are reversible with treatment.

Causes

- Antithyroid drugs taken during pregnancy
- Chronic autoimmune thyroiditis (children older than age 2)
- Congenital absence or underdevelopment of the thyroid gland
- Inherited enzymatic defect in the synthesis of thyroxine (T_4) caused by an autosomal recessive gene

Signs and symptoms

- Abnormal deep tendon reflexes

- Abnormal facial features: a short forehead, wrinkled eyelids, a dull expression, periorbital edema (puffy, wide-set eyes), and a broad, short, upturned nose
- Anemia
- Below normal body temperature
- Cold and mottled skin
- Constipation
- Delayed eruption of teeth
- Dry, brittle, and dull hair
- Dyspnea on exertion
- Excessive sleeping
- Feeding difficulties
- Hypotonic abdominal muscles and a protruding abdomen
- Jaundice
- Large, protruding tongue that obstructs respiration, making breathing loud and noisy and forcing him to open his mouth to breathe
- Slow pulse rate
- Slow, awkward movements

Diagnostic tests
- A high serum level of thyroid-stimulating hormone (TSH) is associated with low triiodothyronine and T_4 levels. Because early detection and treatment can minimize the effects of hypothyroidism, measurement of infant thyroid hormone levels at birth is mandatory in all 50 states.
- Thyroid scan and ^{131}I uptake tests show decreased uptake levels and confirm the absence of thyroid tissue in athyroid children.
- Increased gonadotropin levels are compatible with sexual precocity in older children and may coexist with hypothyroidism.
- Hip, knee, and thigh X-rays reveal the absence of the femoral or tibial epiphyseal line and delayed skeletal development that's markedly inappropriate for the child's chronological age.
- A low T_4 level associated with a normal TSH level suggests hypothyroidism

secondary to hypothalamic or pituitary disease, a rare condition.

Treatment
- Replacement therapy is initiated using oral levothyroxine, beginning with moderate doses. Dosage gradually increases to levels sufficient for lifelong maintenance. (Rapid increase in dosage may precipitate thyrotoxicity.) Doses are proportionately higher in children than in adults because children metabolize thyroid hormone more quickly.

Nursing considerations
- Prevention, early detection, comprehensive parent teaching, and psychological support are essential. Know the early signs. Be especially wary if parents emphasize how good and how quiet their new baby is.
- Monitor blood pressure and pulse rate; report hypertension and tachycardia immediately. Remember, however, that the normal infant heart rate is about 120 beats/minute. If the infant's tongue is unusually large, position him on his side and observe him frequently to prevent airway obstruction. Check rectal temperature every 2 to 4 hours. Keep the infant warm and his skin moist.
- Explain to the parents that the child will require lifelong treatment with thyroid supplements. Teach them to recognize the signs of overdose, such as rapid pulse rate, irritability, insomnia, fever, sweating, and weight loss. Stress the need to comply with the treatment regimen to prevent further mental impairment.
- Provide support to help the parents deal with a child who may be mentally retarded. Help them adopt a positive but realistic attitude and focus on their child's strengths rather than his weaknesses. Encourage them to provide stimulating activities to help the child reach

his maximum potential. Refer them to appropriate community resources for support.

Hypovolemic shock

In hypovolemic shock, reduced intravascular blood volume causes circulatory dysfunction and inadequate tissue perfusion. Without sufficient blood or fluid replacement, hypovolemic shock syndrome may lead to irreversible cerebral and renal damage, cardiac arrest and, ultimately, death. (See *What happens in hypovolemic shock.*) Hypovolemic shock requires early recognition of signs and symptoms and prompt, aggressive treatment to improve the prognosis.

Causes
- Acute blood loss: about one-fifth of the total volume from GI bleeding, internal hemorrhage (hemothorax and hemoperitoneum), or external hemorrhage (accidental or surgical trauma) or from any condition that reduces circulating intravascular plasma volume or other body fluids such as in severe burns
- Acute pancreatitis
- Ascites and dehydration from excessive perspiration
- Diabetes insipidus
- Diuresis
- Inadequate fluid intake
- Intestinal obstruction
- Peritonitis
- Severe diarrhea or protracted vomiting

Signs and symptoms
- Cold, pale, clammy skin
- Decreased sensorium
- Disseminated intravascular coagulation (DIC)
- Hypotension with narrowing pulse pressure
- Metabolic acidosis
- Rapid, shallow respirations
- Reduced urine output
- Tachycardia

Diagnostic tests
- Diagnosis is confirmed by elevated potassium, sodium, lactate, dehydrogenase, creatinine, and blood urea nitrogen levels.
- Studies also reveal increased urine specific gravity (greater than 1.020) and urine osmolality.
- The patient may have decreased blood pH and partial pressure of arterial oxygen and increased partial pressure of arterial carbon dioxide.
- Gastroscopy, aspiration of gastric contents through a nasogastric tube, and X-rays identify internal bleeding sites.
- Coagulation studies may detect coagulopathy from DIC.

Treatment
- Give supplemental oxygen as needed.
- Identification of bleeding site and control of bleeding is accomplished by direct measures (such as application of pressure and elevation of an extremity) or surgery.
- For severe cases, a pneumatic antishock garment may be helpful.
- Start cardiopulmonary resuscitation (CPR) if the patient develops cardiopulmonary arrest.

Nursing considerations
ACTION STAT!

 Emergency treatment measures must include prompt and adequate blood and fluid replacement to restore intravascular volume and raise blood pressure. Administer normal saline solution or lactated Ringer's solution, as prescribed, and then possibly plasma proteins (albumin) or other plasma expanders until packed red blood cells can be matched. A rapid solution

What happens in hypovolemic shock

In hypovolemic shock, vascular fluid volume loss causes extreme tissue hypoperfusion. Internal fluid losses can result from hemorrhage or third-space fluid shifting. External fluid loss can result from severe bleeding or from severe diarrhea, diuresis, or vomiting.

Inadequate vascular volume leads to decreased venous return and cardiac output. The resulting drop in arterial blood pressure activates the body's compensatory mechanisms in an attempt to increase vascular volume. If compensation is unsuccessful, decompensation and death may occur.

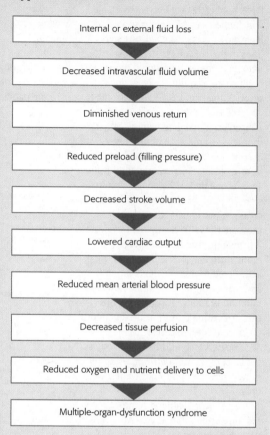

Internal or external fluid loss

Decreased intravascular fluid volume

Diminished venous return

Reduced preload (filling pressure)

Decreased stroke volume

Lowered cardiac output

Reduced mean arterial blood pressure

Decreased tissue perfusion

Reduced oxygen and nutrient delivery to cells

Multiple-organ-dysfunction syndrome

infusion system can provide these crystalloids or colloids at high flow rates.

■ Management of hypovolemic shock necessitates prompt, aggressive supportive measures and careful assessment and monitoring of vital signs. Follow these steps:

– Check for a patent airway and adequate circulation. If blood pressure and heart rate are absent, start CPR.

– Record blood pressure, pulse rate, peripheral pulses, respiratory rate, and other vital signs every 15 minutes, and monitor the electrocardiogram continuously. If blood pressure drops below 80 mm Hg, increase the oxygen flow rate, and notify the practitioner immediately. A progressive drop in blood pressure accompanied by a thready pulse generally signals inadequate cardiac output from reduced intravascular volume. Notify the practitioner, and increase the infusion rate, as prescribed.

– Start I.V. lines with normal saline or lactated Ringer's solution, using a large-bore catheter (14G to 18G), which allows easier administration of later blood transfusions. Don't start I.V. lines in the legs of a patient in shock who has suffered abdominal trauma because infused fluid may escape through the ruptured vessel into the abdomen.

– Insert an indwelling urinary catheter if ordered to measure hourly urine output. If output is less than 30 ml/hour in adults, increase the fluid infusion rate as prescribed, but watch for signs of fluid overload such as an increase in pulmonary artery wedge pressure (PAWP). Notify the physician if urine output doesn't improve. An osmotic diuretic, such as mannitol, may be ordered to increase renal blood flow and urine output. Determine how much fluid to give by checking blood pressure, urine output, central venous pressure (CVP), or PAWP. To increase accuracy, CVP should be measured at the level of the right atrium, using the same reference point on the chest each time.

– Draw an arterial blood sample to measure arterial blood gas (ABG) values. Give oxygen by face mask or airway to ensure adequate oxygenation of tissues. Adjust the oxygen flow rate to a higher or lower level as ABG measurements indicate.

– Draw venous blood for complete blood count and electrolyte, type and crossmatch, and coagulation studies.

– During therapy, assess skin color and temperature and note changes. Cold, clammy skin may be a sign of continuing peripheral vascular constriction, indicating progressive shock. Watch for signs of impending coagulopathy (petechiae, bruising, and bleeding or oozing from the gums or venipuncture sites).

– Explain all procedures and their purpose. Throughout these emergency measures, provide emotional support to the patient and his family.

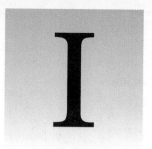

Idiopathic thrombocytopenic purpura

Idiopathic thrombocytopenic purpura (ITP) is a form of thrombocytopenia that results from immunologic platelet destruction. ITP may be acute (postviral thrombocytopenia) or chronic (Werlhof's disease, purpura hemorrhagica, essential thrombocytopenia, autoimmune thrombocytopenia). Acute ITP usually affects children between ages 2 and 6; chronic ITP mainly affects adults younger than age 50, especially females between ages 20 and 40.

The prognosis for acute ITP is excellent; nearly four out of five patients recover without treatment. The prognosis for chronic ITP is good; remissions lasting weeks or even years are common, especially among females.

In acute ITP, which is common in children, the onset is usually sudden and without warning. The onset of chronic ITP is insidious.

Causes

- Autoimmune response
- Drug reactions (chronic ITP)
- Immunization with a live virus vaccine
- Immunologic disorders, such as systemic lupus erythematosus or human immunodeficiency virus infection (chronic ITP)
- Viral infection, such as rubella and chickenpox

Signs and symptoms

- Easy bruising, epistaxis, and bleeding gums (acute ITP)
- Ecchymoses
- Hemorrhage (rare)
- Lesions in vital organs (such as the lungs, kidneys, or brain—may prove fatal)
- Mucosal bleeding from the mouth, nose, and GI tract
- Petechiae

Diagnostic tests

- Platelet count is less than 20,000/mm^3, and bleeding time is prolonged.
- Platelet size and morphologic appearance may be abnormal; anemia may be present if bleeding has occurred.
- As in thrombocytopenia, bone marrow studies show an abundance of megakaryocytes and a shortened circulating platelet survival time (hours or days).
- Occasionally, platelet antibodies may be found in vitro, but ITP is usually inferred from platelet survival data and the absence of an underlying disease.
- Immunoglobulin G level may be increased.

Recognizing impetiginous vesicles

When impetiginous vesicles break, crust forms from the exudate. This infection is especially contagious among young children.

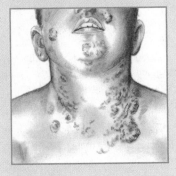

Treatment

- Acute ITP may be allowed to run its course without intervention or may be treated with a glucocorticoid or immune globulin.
- For chronic ITP, a corticosteroid may be the first treatment of choice. Patients who fail to respond within 1 to 4 months or who need high steroid dosage are candidates for splenectomy, which has an 85% success rate.
- Alternative treatments include immunosuppression and high-dose I.V. gamma globulin.

Nursing considerations

- Administer blood, blood components, or vitamin K as prescribed to correct anemia and coagulation defects.
- Provide routine postoperative care if splenectomy is necessary: give pain medication as needed and prescribed, turn the patient every 2 hours, and assist with coughing and deep breathing exercises and incentive spirometry.

- Teach the patient to watch for petechiae, ecchymoses, and other signs of recurrence.
- Monitor him for signs of bone marrow depression, infection, mucositis, GI ulcers, and severe diarrhea or vomiting if the patient is receiving an immunosuppressant.
- Tell the patient to avoid aspirin, ibuprofen, and other nonsteroidal anti-inflammatory drugs.
- Encourage him to contact the Platelet Disorder Support Association.

Impetigo

A contagious, superficial skin infection, impetigo (also known as *impetigo contagiosa*) occurs in nonbullous and bullous forms. This vesiculopustular eruptive disorder spreads most easily among infants, young children, and the elderly. (See *Recognizing impetiginous vesicles*.)

Causes

- Coagulase-positive *Staphylococcus aureus*
- Group A beta-hemolytic streptococci

Predisposing factors

- Anemia
- Malnutrition
- Poor hygiene
- Warm climate

Signs and symptoms
Common nonbullous impetigo

- Burning
- Pruritus
- Regional lymphadenopathy
- Satellite lesions with autoinoculation
- Small red macule developing into a vesicle and becoming pustular with a honey-colored crust within hours

Bullous impetigo
- Thin-walled vesicle with a thin, clear crust upon eruption

Diagnostic tests
- Microscopic visualization of the causative organism in a Gram stain of vesicle fluid usually confirms *S. aureus* infection and justifies antibiotic therapy.
- Culture and sensitivity testing of fluid or denuded skin may indicate the most appropriate antibiotic, but therapy shouldn't be delayed for laboratory results, which can take 3 days.
- The white blood cell count may be elevated if the patient has an infection.

Treatment
- Broad-spectrum, systemic antibiotic (usually a penicillinase-resistant penicillin, cephalosporin, or erythromycin) treatment is typically given for 10 days.
- A topical antibiotic, such as mupirocin (Bactroban) ointment, may be used for minor infections.
- Remove exudate by washing the lesions with soap and water two or three times every day. For stubborn crusts, apply warm soaks or compresses of normal saline or a diluted soap solution.

Nursing considerations
- Urge the patient not to scratch because this spreads impetigo. Advise parents to cut the child's fingernails.
- Give medications as prescribed; remember to check for penicillin allergy. Stress the need to continue prescribed medications as ordered, even after the lesions have healed.
- Teach the patient or his family how to care for impetiginous lesions. To prevent further spread of this highly contagious infection, encourage frequent bathing using an antibacterial soap.
- Tell the patient not to share towels, washcloths, or bed linens with family members. Emphasize the importance of following proper hand-washing technique.
- Assess family members for impetigo. If the patient attends school, notify the school.

▌Inclusion conjunctivitis

Inclusion conjunctivitis, or *chlamydia keratoconjunctivitis,* is an acute ocular inflammation resulting from infection by *Chlamydia trachomatis*—serotypes A through C (trachoma) and D through K (inclusion conjunctivitis). Trachoma is a major cause of worldwide blindness. Although inclusion conjunctivitis occasionally becomes chronic, the prognosis is usually good with treatment. If untreated, it may last 3 to 9 months.

Because contaminated cervical secretions infect the eyes of the neonate during birth, inclusion conjunctivitis is an important cause of ophthalmia neonatorum.

Inclusion conjunctivitis may persist for weeks or months, possibly with superficial corneal involvement.

Causes
- *C. trachomatis*
- Hand-to-eye transfer of the organism from the genitourinary tract (autoinfection; rare)

Signs and symptoms
- Inclusion conjunctivitis: develops 5 to 10 days after contamination
- In children and adults: follicles appearing inside the lower eyelids; preauricular lymphadenopathy and possibly, otitis media and interstitial pneumonia
- In neonates: lower eyelids redden with a thick, purulent discharge and, possibly pseudomembranes (can lead to conjunctival scarring)

Diagnostic tests

- Giemsa-stained conjunctival scraping reveals cytoplasmic inclusion bodies in conjunctival epithelial cells, many polymorphonuclear leukocytes, and a negative culture for bacteria.

Treatment

- Infants are treated with 1% tetracycline eyedrops, erythromycin ophthalmic ointment, or sulfonamide eyedrops 5 to 6 times per day for 2 weeks.
- Adults are given oral tetracycline or erythromycin for 3 weeks.
- Adults with severe disease may also require systemic sulfonamide therapy. Sexual partners should also be examined and treated.
- In neonates, prophylactic tetracycline or erythromycin ointment is applied once, within 1 hour after delivery.

Nursing considerations

- Keep the patient's eyes as clean as possible, using aseptic technique. Clean the eyes from the inner to the outer canthus. Apply warm soaks as needed. Record the amount and color of drainage.
- Remind the patient not to rub his eyes, which can irritate them.
- If the patient's eyes are sensitive to light, keep the room dark or suggest that he wear dark glasses.
- Wash your hands thoroughly before and after giving eye medications to prevent further spread of inclusion conjunctivitis.
- Suggest a pelvic examination for the mother of an infected neonate or for an adult with inclusion conjunctivitis.
- Obtain a history of recent sexual partners so they can be examined for inclusion conjunctivitis.

Influenza

Also called *the grippe* or *the flu,* influenza is an acute, highly contagious infection of the respiratory tract that results from any of three types of *Myxovirus influenzae.* It occurs sporadically or in epidemics (usually during the colder months). Epidemics tend to peak within 2 to 3 weeks after initial cases and last 2 to 3 months.

Although influenza affects all age-groups, its incidence is highest in school children. Its severity is greatest in the very young, the elderly, and those with chronic disease. In these groups, influenza may even lead to death.

One remarkable feature of the influenza virus is its capacity for antigenic variation. Such variation leads to infection by strains of the virus to which little or no immunologic resistance is present in the population at risk. Antigenic variation is characterized as *antigenic drift* (minor changes that occur yearly or every few years) and *antigenic shift* (major changes that lead to pandemics). Influenza viruses are classified into three groups:

- Type A, the most prevalent, strikes every year, with new serotypes causing epidemics every 3 years.
- Type B also strikes annually, but only causes epidemics every 4 to 6 years.
- Type C is endemic and causes only sporadic cases.

The virus invades the epithelium of the respiratory tract, causing inflammation and desquamation.

Causes

- Indirect contact, such as using a contaminated drinking glass
- Inhalation of a respiratory droplet from an infected person

Signs and symptoms
After 24 to 48 hours' incubation

- Cervical adenopathy and croup (in children)
- Chills (sudden onset)
- Headache
- Laryngitis, hoarseness, conjunctivitis, rhinitis, and rhinorrhea (occasionally)
- Malaise (possibly persisting for weeks, especially in elderly patients)
- Myalgia (particularly in the back and limbs)
- Nonproductive cough (possibly persisting past 3 to 5 days)
- Temperature of 101° to 104° F (38.3° to 40° C)
  - higher in children than in adults
  - duration longer than 3 to 5 days indicating complications (myositis, worsening of chronic obstructive pulmonary disease, Reye's syndrome, and primary viral pneumonia or secondary bacterial pneumonia)

Diagnostic tests

- The isolation of M. *influenzae* through the inoculation of chicken embryos (with nasal secretions from infected patients) is essential at the first sign of an epidemic.
- Nose and throat cultures and increased serum antibody titers help confirm the diagnosis.
- Uncomplicated cases show a decreased white blood cell count with an increased lymphocyte count.
- A rapid antigen test for influenza A and B is now available, allowing practitioners and emergency departments to confirm a diagnosis of influenza within 30 minutes.

Treatment

- Treatment focuses on relieving signs and symptoms and includes bed rest, adequate fluid intake, and acetamino-phen (in children) or aspirin to relieve fever and muscle pain.
- Guaifenesin (Mucinex) or another expectorant to relieve nonproductive coughing.
- Saline nasal spray may help relieve nasal congestion.
- Analgesic gargle may lessen sore throat.
- Amantadine (Symmetrel) and rimantadine (Flumadine) (antiviral drugs) have proven effective in reducing the duration of signs and symptoms in influenza A infection.
- Neuramidase inhibitors zanamivir (Relenza) and oseltamivir (Tamiflu) are available for influenza A and B.
- Supportive care (fluid and electrolyte supplements, oxygen, and assisted ventilation) and treatment of bacterial superinfection with appropriate antibiotics are necessary if complicated by pneumonia.

Nursing considerations

- Advise the patient to use mouthwash and to increase his fluid intake.
- Provide warm baths or heating pads to relieve myalgia.
- Give a nonnarcotic analgesic and an antipyretic as prescribed.
- Screen visitors to protect the patient from bacterial infection and the visitors from influenza. Use respiratory precautions.
- Teach the patient proper disposal of tissues and proper hand-washing technique to prevent the virus from spreading.
- Watch for signs and symptoms of developing pneumonia, such as crackles, another temperature rise, and coughing accompanied by purulent or bloody sputum. Help the patient gradually return to his normal activities.
- Teach patients about influenza immunizations. For high-risk patients and

health care personnel, annual inoculations at the start of the flu season (late autumn) are recommended. Remember that such vaccines are made from chicken embryos and must not be given to people who are hypersensitive to eggs, feathers, or chickens. The vaccine administered is based on the previous year's virus and is usually about 75% effective.

DRUG CHALLENGE

 All people receiving the influenza vaccine should be made aware of its adverse effects (discomfort at the vaccination site, fever, malaise and, rarely, Guillain-Barré syndrome). Although the vaccine hasn't been proven harmful to the fetus, it isn't recommended for pregnant women, except those with chronic diseases who are highly susceptible to influenza. For people who are hypersensitive to eggs, amantadine is an effective alternative to the vaccine.

Inguinal hernia

A hernia occurs when all or part of a viscus protrudes from a normal location in the body. Most hernias are protrusions of part of the abdominal viscus through the abdominal wall. Although many kinds of abdominal hernias are possible, inguinal hernias are most common. In these hernias, the large or small intestine, omentum, or bladder protrudes into the inguinal canal. Hernias can be reducible, incarcerated, or strangulated.

An inguinal hernia may be indirect or direct. An indirect inguinal hernia, the more common hernia, results from weakness in the fascial margin of the internal inguinal ring. This type of hernia enters the inguinal canal through the internal inguinal ring and emerges through the external inguinal ring. The hernia extends down the inguinal canal into the scrotum or labia. An indirect inguinal hernia may develop at any age, is three times more common in males, and is especially prevalent in infants younger than age 1.

A direct inguinal hernia results from a weakness in the fascial floor of the inguinal canal. Portions of the bowel or omentum protrude through the floor of the inguinal canal to emerge through the external ring extending above the inguinal ligament. Instead of entering the canal through the internal ring, the hernia passes through the posterior inguinal wall, protrudes directly through the fascia transversalis of the canal (in an area known as *Hesselbach's triangle*), and comes out at the external ring.

Causes
- Improper closing of the peritoneal sac in males
- Increased intra-abdominal pressure (due to heavy lifting, exertion, pregnancy, obesity, excessive coughing, or straining with defecation)
- Weak abdominal muscles (due to congenital malformation, traumatic injury, or aging)

Signs and symptoms
Inguinal hernia
- Lump over the herniated area when the patient stands or strains (disappears when the patient is in a supine position)
- Severe pain with strangulation (possibility for partial or complete bowel obstruction and even intestinal necrosis)
- Sharp, steady pain in the groin (fades when the hernia is reduced)

Partial bowel obstruction
- Anorexia
- Diminished bowel sounds

- Irreducible mass
- Pain and tenderness in the groin
- Vomiting

Complete bowel obstruction

- Absent bowel sounds
- Bloody stools
- High fever
- Shock

Diagnostic tests

- No diagnostic tests are available to confirm inguinal hernia; diagnosis is made by physical examination. (See *Physical examination of the patient with an inguinal hernia.*)
- A suspected bowel obstruction requires X-rays and a white blood cell count (which may be elevated).

Treatment

- Hernia reduction may temporarily relieve pain; however, it shouldn't be attempted if the hernia is incarcerated because reduction could lead to bowel perforation.
- A truss may keep the abdominal contents from protruding into the hernial sac, although it won't cure the hernia. This device is especially beneficial for an elderly or a debilitated patient for whom surgery is potentially hazardous.
- Herniorrhaphy, the treatment of choice, returns the contents of the hernial sac to the abdominal cavity and closes the opening. This procedure is commonly performed laparoscopically under local anesthesia as an outpatient procedure.
- Hernioplasty reinforces the weakened area with steel mesh, fascia, or wire. Complications include urine retention, wound infection, hydrocele formation, and scrotal edema.
- Bowel resection if the hernia is strangulated or necrotic. Rarely, an extensive resection may require temporary

---

Physical examination of the patient with an inguinal hernia

In a patient with a large hernia, physical examination reveals an obvious swelling or lump in the inguinal area. In a patient with a small hernia, the affected area may simply appear full. Palpation of the inguinal area while the patient is performing Valsalva's maneuver confirms the diagnosis.

To detect a hernia in a male patient, the patient is asked to stand with his ipsilateral leg slightly flexed and his weight resting on the other leg. The examiner inserts an index finger into the lower part of the scrotum and invaginates the scrotal skin so the finger advances through the external inguinal ring to the internal ring (1½" to 2" [4 to 5 cm] through the inguinal canal). The patient is then told to cough. If the examiner feels pressure against the fingertip, an indirect hernia exists; if pressure is felt against the side of the finger, a direct hernia exists.

A patient history of sharp or "catching" pain when lifting or straining may help confirm the diagnosis. Many symptomatic inguinal hernias go undiagnosed in women because they're nonpalpable.

---

colostomy. In either case, resection lengthens postoperative recovery and requires an antibiotic, parenteral fluid, and electrolyte replacement.

Nursing considerations

- Apply a truss only after hernia reduction. For best results, apply it in the morning, while the patient is in bed.
- Watch for signs of incarceration and strangulation.

■ Before surgery, monitor the patient's vital signs. Give I.V. fluids and an analgesic for pain as needed if prescribed. Control fever with acetaminophen (Tylenol) or tepid sponge baths as needed.

■ After surgery, evaluate the patient's ability to void. Check the incision at least three times per day for drainage, inflammation, and swelling. Check for normal bowel sounds and fever.

■ Observe the patient carefully for postoperative scrotal swelling. To reduce such swelling, support the scrotum with a rolled towel and apply an ice bag.

■ Encourage fluid intake to maintain hydration and prevent constipation. Teach deep-breathing exercises, and show the patient how to splint the incision before coughing.

■ Warn the patient against lifting or straining. Also, tell him to watch for signs of infection at the incision site and to keep the incision clean and covered until the sutures are removed.

Insect and arachnid bites and stings

Among the most common traumatic complaints are insect and arachnid bites and stings, the more serious of which include those of ticks, brown recluse

(Text continues on page 326.)

Comparing insect and arachnid bites and stings

Insect or arachnid	Signs and symptoms	Treatment	Nursing considerations
Tick ■ Common in woods and fields throughout the United States ■ Attaches to host in any of its life stages (larva, nymph, adult); fastens to host with its teeth, then secretes a cementlike material to reinforce attachment ■ Flat, brown, speckled body about ¼" (6.5 mm) long; eight legs ■ Also transmits Rocky Mountain spotted fever and Lyme disease	■ Itching may be only symptom; or after several days, host may develop tick paralysis (acute flaccid paralysis, starting as paresthesia and pain in legs and resulting in respiratory failure from bulbar paralysis).	■ Removal of tick ■ Local antipruritics for itching papule ■ Mechanical ventilation for respiratory failure	■ To remove a tick, cover it with a tissue or gauze pad soaked in alcohol or mineral, salad, or machine oil. This blocks the tick's breathing pores and causes it to withdraw from the skin. If the tick doesn't disengage after the pad has been in place for 30 minutes, carefully remove it with tweezers, taking care to remove all parts. ■ To reduce the risk of being bitten, teach the patient to keep away from wooded areas, to wear protective clothes, and to carefully examine his body for ticks after being outdoors. ■ Teach patients how to safely remove ticks.

Comparing insect and arachnid bites and stings *(continued)*

Insect or arachnid	Signs and symptoms	Treatment	Nursing considerations
Brown recluse (violin) spider ▪ Common to south-central United States; usually found in dark areas (outdoor privy, barn, woodshed) ▪ Dark brown violin on its back; three pairs of eyes; female more dangerous than male ▪ Most bites between April and October	▪ Venom is coagulotoxic. Reaction begins 2 to 8 hours after bite. ▪ Localized vasoconstriction causes ischemic necrosis at bite site. Small, reddened puncture wound forms a bleb and becomes ischemic. In 3 to 4 days, center becomes dark and hard. Within 2 to 3 weeks, an ulcer forms. ▪ Minimal initial pain increases over time. ▪ Other symptoms include fever, chills, malaise, weakness, nausea, vomiting, edema, seizures, joint pain, petechiae, cyanosis, and phlebitis. ▪ Rarely, thrombocytopenia and hemolytic anemia develop, leading to death within first 24 to 48 hours (usually in a child or a patient with a history of cardiac disease). Prompt and appropriate treatment results in recovery.	▪ No known specific treatment ▪ Combination therapy with corticosteroids, antibiotics, antihistamines, tranquilizers, I.V. fluids, and tetanus prophylaxis ▪ Lesion excision in first 10 to 12 hours to relieve pain (A split-thickness skin graft closes the wound. Without grafting, healing may take 6 to 8 weeks.) ▪ Skin grafting for large chronic ulcer	▪ Clean the lesion with a 1:20 Burow's aluminum acetate solution, and apply antibiotic ointment as ordered. ▪ Take a complete patient history, including allergies and other preexisting medical problems. ▪ Reassure the patient with a disfiguring ulcer that skin grafting can improve his appearance. ▪ To prevent brown recluse bites, tell patients to spray or wear gloves and heavy clothes when working around woodpiles or sheds, to inspect outdoor working clothes for spiders before use, and to discourage children from playing near infested areas.

(continued)

Comparing insect and arachnid bites and stings *(continued)*

Insect or arachnid	Signs and symptoms	Treatment	Nursing considerations
Black widow spider ■ Common throughout the United States, particularly in warmer climates; usually found in dark areas (outdoor privy, barn, woodshed) ■ Female is coal black with red or orange hourglass on ventral side; female larger than male (male doesn't bite) ■ Mortality less than 1% (increased risk among the elderly, infants, and those with allergies)	■ Venom is neurotoxic. Age, size, and sensitivity of patient determine the severity and progression of symptoms. ■ Pinprick sensation, followed by dull, numbing pain (may go unnoticed). ■ Edema and tiny, red bite marks appear. ■ Rigidity of stomach muscles and severe abdominal pain occur (10 to 40 minutes after bite). ■ Muscle spasms in extremities occur. ■ Ascending paralysis develops, causing difficulty swallowing and labored, grunting respirations. ■ Other symptoms include extreme restlessness, vertigo, sweating, chills, pallor, seizures (especially in children), hyperactive reflexes, hypertension, tachycardia, thready pulse, circulatory collapse, nausea, vomiting, headache, ptosis, eyelid edema, urticaria, pruritus, and fever.	■ Neutralization of venom using antivenin I.V., preceded by desensitization when skin or eye tests show sensitivity to horse serum ■ Calcium gluconate I.V. to control muscle spasms ■ Muscle relaxants such as diazepam for severe muscle spasms ■ Frequent vital signs checks during the first 12 hours ■ Epinephrine or antihistamines ■ Oxygen by nasal cannula or mask ■ Tetanus immunization ■ Antibiotics to prevent infection	■ Take a complete patient history, including allergies and other preexisting medical problems. ■ Have epinephrine and emergency resuscitation equipment on hand in case of anaphylactic reaction to antivenin. ■ Keep the patient quiet and warm and immobilize the affected part. ■ Clean the bite site with an antiseptic; apply ice to relieve pain and swelling and to slow circulation. ■ Check vital signs frequently during the first 12 hours after the bite. Report changes to the physician. Symptoms usually subside in 3 to 4 hours. ■ When giving analgesics, monitor respiratory status. ■ To prevent black widow spider bites, tell the patient to spray areas of infestation with creosote at least every 2 months, to wear gloves and heavy clothing when working around woodpiles or sheds, to inspect outdoor working clothes for spiders before putting them on, and to discourage children from playing near infested areas.

Comparing insect and arachnid bites and stings *(continued)*

Insect or arachnid	Signs and symptoms	Treatment	Nursing considerations
Scorpion • Common throughout the United States (30 different species); two deadly species in southwestern states • Curled tail with stinger on end; eight legs; about 3" (7.5 cm) long • Most stings occur during warmer months. • Mortality less than 1% (increased risk among elderly patients and children)	*Local reaction* • Local swelling and tenderness, sharp burning sensation, skin discoloration, paresthesia, and lymphangitis with regional gland swelling occur. *Systemic reaction (neurotoxic)* • Immediate sharp pain; hyperesthesia; drowsiness; itching of nose, throat, and mouth; impaired speech (due to sluggish tongue); and generalized muscle spasms, including jaw muscle spasms, laryngospasms, incontinence, seizures, nausea, vomiting, and drooling occur. • Symptoms last from 24 to 78 hours; the bite site recovers last. • Anaphylaxis is rare. • Death may follow cardiovascular or respiratory failure. • The prognosis is poor if symptoms progress rapidly in first few hours.	• Antivenin (made from cat serum), if available (Contact Antivenin Lab, Arizona State University, Tempe, Arizona.) • Calcium gluconate I.V. for muscle spasm • Phenobarbital I.M. for seizures • Emetine subcutaneously to relieve pain (Opiates such as morphine and codeine are contraindicated because they enhance the venom's effects.)	• Take a complete patient history, including allergies and other pre-existing medical conditions. • Immobilize the patient, and apply a tourniquet proximal to the sting. • Pack the area extending beyond the tourniquet in ice. After 5 minutes, remove the tourniquet. • Monitor vital signs. Watch closely for signs of respiratory distress. (Keep emergency resuscitation equipment available.)

(continued)

Comparing insect and arachnid bites and stings *(continued)*

Insect or arachnid	Signs and symptoms	Treatment	Nursing considerations
Bee, wasp, and yellow jacket ■ Honeybee (rounded abdomen) and bumblebee (over 1" [2.5 cm] long; furry, rounded abdomen): leave stinger in victim after sting ■ Wasp and yellow jacket (slender with elongated abdomen): scrape it off and retain stinger after sting	*Local reaction* ■ Painful wound (protruding stinger from bees), edema, urticaria, and pruritus can occur. *Systemic reaction (neurotoxic)* ■ Symptoms of hypersensitivity usually appear within 20 minutes and may include weakness, chest tightness, dizziness, nausea, vomiting, abdominal cramps, and throat constriction. The shorter the interval between the sting and systemic symptoms, the worse the prognosis. Without prompt treatment, symptoms may progress to cyanosis, coma, and death.	■ Atropine to counteract parasympathetic effects of venom if needed ■ Antihistamines and corticosteroids (in urticaria) ■ Tetanus prophylaxis ■ In anaphylaxis, oxygen by nasal cannula or mask and epinephrine 1:1,000 subcutaneously or I.M. ■ In bronchospasm, albuterol and corticosteroids ■ In hypotension, epinephrine and isoproterenol	■ If the stinger is in place, scrape it off. Don't pull it; this action releases more toxin. ■ Clean the site and apply ice. ■ Watch the patient carefully for signs of anaphylaxis. Keep emergency resuscitation equipment available. ■ Tell a patient who's allergic to bee stings to wear medical identification jewelry or carry a card and to carry an anaphylaxis kit. Teach him how to use the kit, and refer him to an allergist for hyposensitization. ■ To prevent bee stings, tell the patient to avoid wearing bright colors and going barefoot, to avoid flowers and fruit that attract bees, and to use insect repellent.

spiders, black widow spiders, scorpions, bees, wasps, and yellow jackets. (See *Comparing insect and arachnid bites and stings*, pages 322 to 326.)

Causes

The toxic effects of the injected venom or hypersensitivity response to it cause reactions to insect and arachnid bites and stings.

Signs and symptoms

See *Comparing insect and arachnid bites and stings*, pages 322 to 326.

Diagnostic tests

See *Comparing insect and arachnid bites and stings*, pages 322 to 326.

Treatment

See *Comparing insect and arachnid bites and stings*, pages 322 to 326.

Nursing considerations

See *Comparing insect and arachnid bites and stings,* pages 322 to 326.

▌Intestinal obstruction

An intestinal obstruction is a partial or complete blockage of the lumen in the small or large bowel. A small-bowel obstruction is more common (90% of patients) and usually is more serious. A complete obstruction in any part of the bowel, if untreated, can cause death within hours from shock and vascular collapse. Intestinal obstructions are most likely to occur from adhesions caused by previous abdominal surgery, an external hernia, volvulus, Crohn's disease, radiation enteritis, an intestinal wall hematoma (after trauma or anticoagulant therapy), or a neoplasm.

The three forms of intestinal obstruction are:

▪ simple—blockage prevents intestinal contents from passing with no other complications
▪ strangulated—blood supply to part or all of the obstructed section is cut off in addition to blockage of the lumen
▪ closed looped—both ends of a bowel section are occluded, isolating it from the rest of the intestine.

The physiologic effects are similar in all three forms. When intestinal obstruction occurs, fluid, air, and gas collect near the site. Peristalsis increases temporarily as the bowel tries to force its contents through the obstruction, injuring intestinal mucosa and causing distention at and above the site of the obstruction. This distention blocks the flow of venous blood and halts normal absorptive processes. As a result, the bowel begins to secrete water, sodium, and potassium into the fluid pooled in the lumen. This results in further distention and enormous amounts of fluid in the gut.

An obstruction in the upper intestine results in metabolic alkalosis from dehydration and loss of gastric hydrochloric acid; a lower obstruction causes slower dehydration and loss of intestinal alkaline fluids, resulting in metabolic acidosis. Ultimately, an intestinal obstruction may lead to ischemia, necrosis, and death.

Causes
Small-bowel obstruction
▪ Adhesions
▪ Strangulated hernias

Large-bowel obstruction
▪ Carcinomas

Mechanical intestinal obstruction
▪ Compression of the bowel wall due to stenosis, intussusception, volvulus of the sigmoid or cecum, tumors, or atresia.
▪ Foreign body (fruit pits, gallstones, or worms)

Nonmechanical intestinal obstruction
▪ Electrolyte imbalance
▪ Neurogenic abnormality (spinal cord lesions)
▪ Paralytic ileus (see *Paralytic ileus,* page 328)
▪ Thrombosis or embolism of mesenteric vessels
▪ Toxicity (uremia or generalized infection)

Signs and symptoms
Partial small-bowel obstruction
▪ Abdominal distention
▪ Abdominal tenderness with moderate distention

Paralytic ileus

Paralytic (adynamic) ileus is a physiologic form of intestinal obstruction that may develop in the small bowel after abdominal surgery. It causes decreased or absent intestinal motility that usually disappears spontaneously after 2 to 3 days.

Causes

Paralytic ileus can develop as a result of trauma, toxemia, peritonitis, electrolyte deficiency (especially hypokalemia), or the use of certain drugs, such as pain medications, ganglionic blockers, or anticholinergics. It can also result from vascular causes, such as thrombosis and embolism.

Signs and symptoms

Signs and symptoms of paralytic ileus include severe, continuous abdominal discomfort with nausea and vomiting. Abdominal distention is also present. Bowel sounds are diminished or absent. The patient may be severely constipated or may pass flatus and small, liquid stools.

Treatment

Paralytic ileus that lasts longer than 48 hours necessitates intubation for decompression and nasogastric suctioning. Isotonic fluids should be administered to restore intravascular volume and correct electrolyte disorders.

When paralytic ileus results from surgical manipulation of the bowel, treatment may also include administration of a prokinetic drug, such as metoclopramide, erythromycin, or cisapride.

Nursing considerations

If the patient is receiving a cholinergic, alert him that he may experience paradoxical adverse reactions, such as intestinal cramps and diarrhea. Check frequently for returning bowel sounds.

- Borborygmi, and rushes on auscultation (occasionally loud enough to be heard without a stethoscope)
- Colicky pain
- Constipation
- Dehydration
- Hypovolemic shock (late stages)
- Nausea
- Rebound tenderness (if the obstruction has caused strangulation with ischemia)
- Vomiting

Complete small-bowel obstruction
- Constipation
- Mild tenderness
- Passage of small amounts of mucus and blood
- Pronounced abdominal distention
- Vigorous peristaltic rushes and high-pitched tinkles accompanying paroxysms of epigastric or periumbilical pain; peristalsis that propels bowel contents toward the mouth instead of the rectum, possibly occurring every 3 to 5 minutes and lasting about 1 minute each
- Vomiting (earlier and more severe with higher obstruction)

Partial large-bowel obstruction
- Abdominal distention
- Colicky abdominal and hypogastric pain
- Leakage of liquid stools around partial obstruction

Complete large-bowel obstruction
- Constipation (may be the only symptoms for days)
- Colicky abdominal pain

- Continuous hypogastric pain and nausea (typically without vomiting)
- Dramatic abdominal distention (loops of large bowel visible on the abdomen)
- Leakage of liquid stools around the obstruction
- Slower onset of symptoms than in small-bowel obstruction

Diagnostic tests

- Plain abdominal x-rays confirm the diagnosis. Small-bowel obstruction must be distinguished from adynamic ileus. Pancreatitis, acute gastroenteritis, appendicitis, and acute mesenteric ischemia must also be ruled out.
- Abdominal films show the presence and location of intestinal gas or fluid. With small-bowel obstructions, a typical "stepladder" pattern emerges, with alternating fluid and gas levels apparent in 3 to 4 hours.
- With large-bowel obstructions, a barium enema reveals a distended, air-filled colon or a closed loop of sigmoid with extreme distention (sigmoid volvulus).
- Laboratory results that support this diagnosis include:
  – decreased serum sodium, chloride, and potassium levels (due to vomiting)
  – slightly elevated white blood cell count (with necrosis, peritonitis, or strangulation)
  – increased serum amylase level (possibly from irritation of the pancreas by a bowel loop).

Treatment

- Initial therapy involves correcting fluid and electrolyte imbalances, resting the bowel by decompressing it to relieve vomiting and distention, maintaining nothing-by-mouth status, and treating shock and peritonitis.
- A strangulated obstruction usually necessitates blood replacement as well as I.V. fluid administration. Nasogastric

tube suction is necessary to relieve vomiting and abdominal distention.
- Close monitoring of the patient's condition determines the duration of treatment; if the patient fails to improve or if his condition deteriorates, surgery is needed.
- Surgery is performed on all patients with large-bowel obstruction.
- Total parenteral nutrition may be appropriate if the patient suffers a protein deficit from chronic obstruction, postoperative or paralytic ileus, or infection.
- Medication includes an analgesic and a sedative (but not opiates because they inhibit GI motility).
- A broad-spectrum antibiotic is given for peritonitis due to bowel strangulation or infarction, to provide anaerobic and gram-negative coverage.

Nursing considerations

- Monitor the patient's vital signs frequently. A drop in blood pressure may indicate reduced circulating blood volume due to blood loss from a strangulated hernia. Remember, as much as 10 L of fluid can collect in the small bowel, drastically reducing plasma volume. Observe the patient closely for signs of shock (pallor, rapid pulse, and hypotension).
- Assess the patient for signs of metabolic alkalosis (changes in sensorium; slow, shallow respirations; hypertonic muscles; and tetany) or acidosis (shortness of breath on exertion, disorientation and, later, deep and rapid breathing, weakness, and malaise).
- Watch for signs and symptoms of secondary infection, such as fever and chills.
- Monitor urine output carefully to assess renal function and circulating blood volume; the distended intestine may compress the bladder, thus causing urine retention. If you suspect bladder compression, catheterize the patient for residual urine. Also, measure abdominal

girth frequently to detect progressive distention.

■ Provide mouth care. Observe for signs of dehydration (thick, swollen tongue; dry, cracked lips; and dry oral mucous membranes).

■ Record the amount and color of drainage from the decompression tube. Irrigate the tube with normal saline solution to maintain patency. If a weighted tube has been inserted, check periodically to make sure it's advancing. Help the patient turn from side to side (or ambulate) to facilitate passage of the tube.

■ Maintain the patient in semi-Fowler's position as much as possible to promote ventilation and ease respiratory distress from abdominal distention.

■ Auscultate for bowel sounds, and observe him for signs of returning peristalsis (passage of flatus and mucus through the rectum).

■ Explain all diagnostic and therapeutic procedures to the patient, and answer questions he may have. Inform him that these procedures are necessary to relieve the obstruction and reduce pain.

■ Prepare the patient and his family for the possibility of surgery, and provide emotional support and positive reinforcement afterward. Arrange for an enterostomal therapist to visit the patient who has had an ostomy.

▌Intussusception

With intussusception, a portion of the bowel telescopes (invaginates) into an adjacent distal portion. Intussusception may be fatal, especially if treatment is delayed for a strangulated intestine. When a bowel segment (the intussusceptum) invaginates, peristalsis propels it along the bowel, pulling more bowel along with it; the receiving segment is the intussuscipiens. This invagination produces edema, hemorrhage from venous engorgement, incarceration, and obstruction. If treatment is delayed for longer than 24 hours, strangulation of the intestine usually occurs, with gangrene, shock, perforation, and possible death.

Intussusception is most common in infants and is three times more common in males than in females. About 87% of children with intussusception are younger than age 2; about 70% of these children are between 4 and 11 months old.

Causes
■ Unknown
■ Alterations in intestinal motility (children)
■ Benign or malignant tumors (adults)
■ Possible link to viral infections (because of seasonal peaks)

Signs and symptoms
In an infant or a child
■ "Currant jelly" stools containing a mixture of blood and mucus
■ Intermittent, severe, colicky abdominal pain with pallor, diaphoresis and, possibly, grunting respirations
■ Lethargy or somnolence between bouts of colic
■ Tender, distended abdomen, with a palpable, sausage-shaped right upper quadrant mass
■ Vomiting of stomach contents (initially); vomiting of bile-stained or fecal material (later)

In adults
■ Bloody stools
■ Colicky abdominal pain (usually localized in the right lower quadrant, radiating to the back and increasing with eating) and tenderness
■ Diarrhea (occasionally constipation)
■ Strangulation with excruciating pain, abdominal distention, and tachycardia (possibly)

- Vomiting
- Weight loss

Diagnostic tests

- Barium enema confirms colonic intussusception when it shows the characteristic coiled-spring sign; it also delineates the extent of intussusception.
- Upright abdominal X-rays may show a soft-tissue mass and signs of complete or partial obstruction with dilated loops of bowel.
- White blood cell count up to 15,000/mm^3 indicates obstruction; more than 15,000/mm^3, strangulation; more than 20,000/mm^3, bowel infarction.

Treatment

- In children, therapy may include hydrostatic reduction or surgery. Surgery is indicated for children with recurrent intussusception, for those who show signs of shock or peritonitis, and for those in whom symptoms have been present longer than 24 hours.
- In adults, surgery is always the treatment of choice.
- During hydrostatic reduction, the radiologist drips a barium solution into the rectum from a height of not more than 3′ (0.9 m); fluoroscopy traces the barium's progress. If the procedure is successful, contrast flows freely into the ileum and the mass disappears. Inability to show this suggests incomplete reduction and necessitates surgical exploration.
- During surgery, manual reduction is attempted first. After compressing the bowel above the intussusception, the surgeon attempts to milk the intussusception back through the bowel. If manual reduction fails or if the bowel is gangrenous or strangulated, the surgeon performs a resection of the affected bowel segment. An incidental appendectomy is also performed.

Nursing considerations

- Monitor the patient's vital signs before and after surgery. A change in temperature may indicate sepsis; an infant may become hypothermic at the onset of infection. Tachycardia and hypotension may be signs of peritonitis.
- Monitor the patient's fluid intake and output. Watch for signs of dehydration and bleeding. Administer I.V. fluids, blood, or blood products as prescribed.
- Insert a nasogastric (NG) intubation as prescribed to decompress the intestine and minimize vomiting. Monitor NG drainage, and replace lost volume as ordered.
- Monitor the patient who has undergone hydrostatic reduction for passage of stools and barium, a sign that the reduction was successful. Keep in mind that intussusception may recur, usually within the first 36 to 48 hours after the reduction.
- Postoperatively, give broad-spectrum antibiotics as prescribed and provide meticulous wound care. Monitor the incision for inflammation, drainage, and suture separation (dehiscence).
- Encourage the patient to deep-breathe and cough productively, to use incentive spirometry, and to assume the semi-Fowler position when doing so. Teach him to splint the incision when he coughs.
- Offer oral fluids postoperatively when bowel sounds and peristalsis resume; advance the diet as tolerated.
- Monitor the patient for abdominal distention after he resumes a normal diet.
- Offer reassurance and emotional support to the child and his parents. This condition is considered a pediatric emergency, and many parents are unprepared for their child's hospitalization

and possible surgery; they may feel guilty for not seeking medical attention sooner.

- Encourage the parents to participate in their child's care as much as possible to minimize the stress of hospitalization.

Iron deficiency anemia

With iron deficiency anemia, an inadequate supply of iron for optimal formation of red blood cells (RBCs) results in smaller (microcytic) cells with less color on staining. Body stores of iron, including plasma iron, decrease, as does transferrin, which binds with and transports iron. Insufficient body stores of iron lead to a depleted RBC mass and, in turn, a decreased hemoglobin (Hb) level (hypochromia) and decreased oxygen-carrying capacity of the blood. A common disease worldwide, iron deficiency anemia affects 10% to 30% of adults in the United States.

Iron deficiency anemia is most common in premenopausal females, infants (particularly premature and low-birth-weight infants), children, and adolescents (especially females).

Causes

- Blood loss secondary
- Inadequate dietary intake of iron (less than 2 mg/day)
- Intravascular hemolysis
- Iron malabsorption
- Mechanical erythrocyte trauma (caused by a prosthetic heart valve or vena cava filters)
- Pregnancy

Signs and symptoms
Early stage
- No symptoms

Advanced stages
- Decreased Hb level
- Exertional dyspnea
- Fatigue
- Headache
- Inability to concentrate
- Irritability
- Listlessness
- Pallor
- Susceptibility to infection
- Tachycardia

Chronic iron deficiency anemia
- Cracking of the corners of the mouth
- Dysphagia
- Neuralgic pain
- Numbness and tingling of the extremities
- Smooth tongue
- Spoon-shaped and brittle nails

Diagnostic tests
- Characteristic blood study results include:
  - low Hb levels (males, less than 12 g/dl; females, less than 10 g/dl)
  - low hematocrit (males, less than 42%; females, less than 36%)
  - low serum iron levels, with high iron-binding capacity
  - low serum ferritin levels
  - low RBC count, with microcytic and hypochromic cells (in early stages, RBC count may be normal, except in infants and children)
  - decreased mean corpuscular Hb level (in patients with severe anemia).
- Bone marrow studies reveal depleted or absent iron stores (done by staining) and normoblastic hyperplasia.

Treatment
- The first priority is to determine the underlying cause of anemia. Then iron replacement is initiated.

Injecting iron solutions

For deep I.M. injections of iron solutions, use the Z-track technique to avoid subcutaneous irritation and discoloration from leaking medication:

Choose a 19G to 20G 2″ to 3″ needle. After drawing up the solution, change to a fresh needle to avoid tracking the solution through to subcutaneous tissue. Draw 0.5 cc of air into the syringe as an "air-lock."

After cleaning the area and putting on gloves, displace the skin and fat at the injection site (in the upper outer quadrant of the buttocks or the ventrogluteal site only) firmly to one side about ½″ (1 cm).

Insert the needle into the muscle at a 90-degree angle. Aspirate to check for entry into a blood vessel. Inject the solution slowly, followed by the 0.5 cc of air in the syringe. Keep the tissues displaced with your finger, wait 10 seconds, and release the tissues. Pull the needle straight out.

Apply direct pressure to the site, but don't massage it. Caution the patient against vigorous exercise for 15 to 30 minutes.

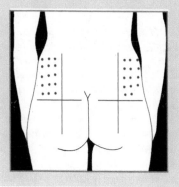

1. Normal position.

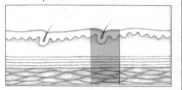

2. Displace tissues.

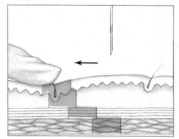

3. Inject and wait 10 seconds.

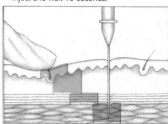

4. Remove needle and release tissues.

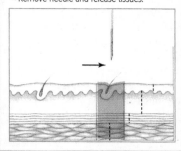

Supportive management in anemia

Nutritional needs

If the patient:
- is fatigued, urge her to eat small, frequent meals throughout the day.
- has oral lesions, suggest that she eat soft, cool, bland foods.
- has dyspepsia, advise her to eliminate spicy foods and to include dairy products in her diet.
- is anorexic and irritable, encourage her family to bring her favorite foods from home (unless her diet is restricted) and to keep her company during meals, if possible.

Activities

- Monitor the patient closely during physical activity. If her pulse accelerates rapidly and she develops hypotension with hyperpnea, diaphoresis, light-headedness, palpitations, shortness of breath, or weakness, stop the activity.
- Tell the patient to pace her activities and allow for frequent rest periods.

Infection precautions

- Instruct the patient to avoid crowds and other sources of infection. Encourage her to practice good hand-washing technique.
- Stress the importance of receiving necessary immunizations and prompt medical treatment for any sign of infection.

Diagnostic tests

- Explain erythropoiesis, the function of blood, and the purpose of diagnostic and therapeutic procedures.

Complications

- Alert the patient to those sources of bleeding that may exacerbate anemia, including urine, stool, gums, and ecchymotic areas.
- If the patient is confined to strict bed rest, teach her and her family how to perform range-of-motion exercises. Stress the importance of frequent turning, coughing, and deep breathing.
- Warn the patient to move about and change positions slowly to minimize dizziness induced by cerebral hypoxia.

- The treatment of choice is an oral preparation of iron or a combination of iron and ascorbic acid (which enhances iron absorption).
- Iron must be given parenterally if the patient is noncompliant to the oral preparation, if she needs more iron than she can take orally, if malabsorption prevents adequate iron absorption, or if a maximum rate of Hb regeneration is desired. (See *Injecting iron solutions*, page 333.)

DRUG CHALLENGE

 Because a total-dose I.V. infusion of supplemental iron is painless and requires fewer injections, it's usually preferred over I.M. administration. Pregnant patients and elderly patients with severe anemia, for example, should receive a total-dose infusion of iron dextran in normal saline solution over 8 hours. To minimize the risk of an allergic reaction to iron, an I.V. test dose of 0.5 ml should be given first.

Nursing considerations

- Review guidelines for managing anemia with the patient and her family. (See *Supportive management in anemia.*)
- Monitor the patient's compliance with the prescribed iron supplement therapy. Advise her not to stop therapy, even if she feels better, because replacement of iron stores takes time.
- Advise the patient that milk and antacids interfere with iron absorption, but that vitamin C can increase it. Instruct her to drink liquid supplemental iron through a straw to avoid staining her teeth.
- Tell the patient to report adverse reactions—such as nausea, vomiting, diarrhea, constipation, fever, and severe stomach pain—which may necessitate a dosage adjustment.
- Monitor the iron infusion rate carefully, if given I.V., and observe for an allergic reaction. If the patient shows signs of such a reaction, stop the infusion and begin supportive treatment immediately. Also, watch for dizziness and headache and for thrombophlebitis around the I.V. site.
- Use the Z-track injection method when administering iron I.M. to prevent skin discoloration, scarring, and irritating iron deposits in the skin.
- Explain the importance of regular checkups because iron deficiency may recur.
- Teach the basics of a nutritionally balanced diet—red meats, green vegetables, eggs, whole wheat, iron-fortified bread, cereals, and milk. (No single food contains enough iron to treat iron deficiency anemia; an average-sized person with anemia would have to eat at least 10 lb [4.5 kg] of steak daily to receive therapeutic amounts of iron.)
- Emphasize the need for high-risk individuals—such as premature neonates, children younger than age 2, and pregnant females—to receive prophylactic oral iron, as ordered by a practitioner. (Children younger than age 2 should also receive supplemental cereals and formulas high in iron.)
- Assess a family's dietary habits for iron intake and note the influence of childhood eating patterns, cultural food preferences, and family income on adequate nutrition.
- Encourage families with deficient iron intake to eat meat, fish, and poultry; whole and enriched grains; and foods high in ascorbic acid.
- Assess the patient's drug history because certain drugs, such as pancreatic enzymes and vitamin E, may interfere with iron metabolism and absorption and because aspirin, steroids, and other drugs may cause GI bleeding.

Irritable bowel syndrome

Also referred to as *spastic colon, spastic colitis, or mucous colitis,* irritable bowel syndrome is marked by chronic abdominal pain, alternating constipation and diarrhea, and abdominal distention. This disorder is extremely common, although 20% of patients never seek medical attention.

Symptoms of irritable bowel syndrome are two to three times more common in females than in males; 80% of patients with a more severe form of the disorder are female. Symptoms first emerge before age 40. The prognosis is good.

Causes

- Anxiety
- Dietary factors: fiber, raw fruits, coffee, alcohol, and cold, highly seasoned, or laxative-acting foods

- Stress

Signs and symptoms
- Abdominal distention and bloating
- Constipation alternating with diarrhea (one of greater incidence than the other)
- Intermittent, crampy lower abdominal pain intensifying 1 to 2 hours after meals (commonly relieved by defecation or passage of flatus)
- Mucus passed through the rectum

Diagnostic tests
- Sigmoidoscopy or colonoscopy shows spastic contractions without evidence of colon cancer or inflammatory bowel disease.
- Barium enema may show colon spasm and tubular appearance of descending colon without evidence of cancer or diverticulosis.
- Stool examination for blood, parasites, and bacteria rules out infection.

Treatment
- Counseling helps the patient understand the relation between stress and her illness.
- Strict dietary restrictions aren't beneficial, but food irritants should be investigated and the patient instructed to avoid them.
- The patient should increase water intake to 8 to 10 glasses of fluid to regulate the consistency of stools and promote balanced hydration.
- Rest and heat applied to the abdomen are helpful.
- Increase bulk in the diet to control diarrhea.
- Drug therapy, if required, may include:
  – antidiarrheals, such as loperamide (Imodium) and diphenoxylate with atropine sulfate (Lomotil) to control diarrhea
  – laxatives to relieve constipation

  – anticholinergic, antispasmodic drugs such as dicyclomine (Bentyl) and propantheline bromide (Pro-Banthine) to reduce intestinal hypermotility and pain
  – antiemetics such as metoclopramide (Reglan) to relieve heartburn, epigastric discomfort, and after-meal fullness.

Nursing considerations
- Because a patient with irritable bowel syndrome isn't hospitalized, focus your care on patient teaching.
- Instruct the patient to avoid irritating foods, and encourage her to develop regular bowel habits.
- Help the patient deal with stress, and warn her against depending on sedatives or antispasmodics.
- Encourage regular checkups because irritable bowel syndrome is associated with a higher-than-normal incidence of diverticulitis and colon cancer.
- For the patient older than age 40, emphasize the need for a yearly flexible sigmoidoscopy and rectal examination.

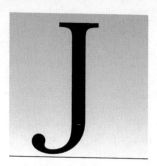

Juvenile rheumatoid arthritis

Affecting children younger than age 16, juvenile rheumatoid arthritis (JRA), also known as *juvenile chronic arthritis*, is an immune-mediated inflammatory disorder of the connective tissues characterized by joint swelling and pain or tenderness. It may also involve such organs as the skin, heart, lungs, liver, spleen, and eyes, producing extra-articular signs and symptoms. The prognosis for JRA is usually good, although disabilities can occur.

JRA has three major types: systemic (Still's disease or acute febrile type), polyarticular, and pauciarticular. Depending on the type, this disease can occur as early as age 6 weeks—although rarely before 6 months—with peaks of onset between ages 1 and 3, and between ages 8 and 12. JRA is considered the major chronic rheumatic disorder of childhood; overall incidence is twice as high in girls, with variation among the types.

With systemic JRA, the child may experience mild, transient arthritis or frank poly-arthritis associated with fever and rash. Joint involvement may not be evident at first, but the child's behavior may clearly suggest joint pain and fatigue.

With polyarticular JRA, the child may be seronegative or seropositive for rheumatoid factor (RF). Seropositive polyarticular JRA, the more severe type, usually occurs late in childhood and can cause destructive arthritis that mimics adult RA.

Pauciarticular JRA, divided into three subtypes, typically involves no more than four joints—usually the knees and other large joints. It accounts for 45% of cases.

Common to all types of JRA is joint stiffness in the morning or after periods of inactivity. Growth disturbances may also occur, resulting in overgrowth or undergrowth adjacent to inflamed joints.

Causes

- Unknown; possible genetic and immune factors

Precipitating factors

- Emotional stress
- Trauma
- Viral or bacterial (particularly streptococcal) infection

Signs and symptoms
Systemic JRA

- Behavior clearly suggestive of joint pain (child may want to constantly sit in a flexed position, may not walk much, or may refuse to walk at all)

- Evanescent rheumatoid rash: small, pale or salmon pink macules, most commonly on the trunk and proximal extremities and occasionally on the face, palms, and soles (with fever); intensifies with massage or application of heat
- Fever (sudden onset, spiking to 103° F [39.4° C] or higher once or twice per day—usually in the late afternoon—rapidly returning to normal or subnormal)
- Hepatosplenomegaly
- Irritability
- Listlessness
- Lymphadenopathy
- Myocarditis
- Nonspecific abdominal pain
- Pericarditis
- Pleuritis

Polyarticular JRA

- Developmental retardation
- Hepatosplenomegaly
- Involves five or more joints and usually develops insidiously
- Listlessness
- Low-grade fever with daily peaks
- Lymphadenopathy
- Subcutaneous nodules on the elbows or heels
- Swollen, stiff, tender joints (most commonly the wrists, elbows, knees, ankles, small joints of the hands and feet and, possibly, the temporomandibular joints and those of the cervical spine, hips, and shoulders)
- Weight loss

Pauciarticular JRA

- *With chronic iridocyclitis:* most commonly affects girls younger than age 6
  - Knees, elbows, ankles, or iris
  - Highest risk for eye complications in young girls who test positive for antinuclear antibodies (ANAs)
  - Typically asymptomatic inflammation of the iris and ciliary body (but possible pain, redness, blurred vision, and photophobia)
- *With sacroiliitis:* usually affects boys (9:1) older than age 8 and human leukocyte antigen (HLA)-B27-positive
  - Lower-extremities; hip, sacroiliac, heel, and foot pain; and Achilles tendinitis
  - Sacroiliac and lumbar arthritis characteristic of ankylosing spondylitis (later)
  - Acute iritis possible but not as common as with the first subtype.
- *With joint involvement but negative for ANAs and HLA-B27 and without iritis:* any age during childhood
  - Asymmetrical involvement of large or small joints
  - Progression to polyarticular disease (possible)

Diagnostic tests

- Laboratory tests are useful for ruling out other inflammatory or even malignant diseases that can mimic JRA and for monitoring disease activity and response to therapy.
- Complete blood count shows decreased hemoglobin levels, neutrophilia, and thrombocytosis.
- Erythrocyte sedimentation rate, complement (C)-reactive protein, haptoglobin, immunoglobulin, and C3 levels may be elevated.
- Test results may be positive for ANAs in patients who have pauciarticular JRA with chronic iridocyclitis.
- RF is present in 15% of patients with JRA, as compared with 85% of patients with RA.
- Positive HLA-B27 test result may forecast later development of ankylosing spondylitis.
- Early X-ray changes include soft-tissue swelling, effusion, and periostitis in affected joints. Later, osteoporosis and accelerated bone growth may appear, fol-

lowed by subchondral erosions, joint space narrowing, bone destruction, and fusion.

Treatment

■ Successful management of JRA usually involves administration of an anti-inflammatory, physical therapy, carefully planned nutrition and exercise, and regular eye examinations. The child and his parents must be involved in therapy.

■ A nonsteroidal anti-inflammatory drug (NSAID)—such as aspirin, ibuprofen, or naproxen (Aleve)—is used to reduce pain and swelling. If this proves ineffective, a disease-modifying antirheumatic drug (DMARD) such as methotrexate (Trexall) is a useful second-line agent. In addition, gold salts, hydroxychloroquine (Plaquenil), auranofin (Ridaura), etanercept (Enbrel), or sulfasalazine (Azulfidine) may be considered. Responses to individual drugs may differ among the various subtypes of JRA.

■ Because of adverse effects, systemic steroids are usually reserved for treatment of systemic complications that are resistant to NSAIDs and DMARDS, such as pericarditis and iritis. However, an intra-articular steroid can be effective in managing pauciarticular and polyarticular JRA.

■ Joint rest (by splinting) used for up to 3 days after joint injections with a corticosteroid may improve anti-inflammatory response.

■ Corticosteroids and mydriatics are commonly used for iridocyclitis. Low-dose cytotoxic drug therapy is currently being investigated.

■ Physical therapy promotes regular exercise to maintain joint mobility and muscle strength, thereby preventing contractures, deformity, and disability. Good posture, gait training, and joint protection are also beneficial.

■ Splints help reduce pain, prevent contractures, and maintain correct joint alignment.

■ Surgery is usually limited to soft-tissue releases to improve joint mobility. Joint replacement is delayed until the child has matured physically and can handle vigorous rehabilitation.

Nursing considerations

■ Encourage the child to be as independent as possible and to develop a positive attitude toward school, social development, and vocational planning.

■ Explain the importance of regular slit-lamp examinations to help ensure early diagnosis and treatment of iridocyclitis.

■ Reinforce the need for exams every 3 months during periods of active disease and every 6 months during remissions if the child has pauciarticular JRA with chronic iridocyclitis.

■ Stress the need for regular eye examinations, even in the absence of joint symptoms. Iridocyclitis may be asymptomatic and, if undiagnosed and untreated, can lead to vision loss.

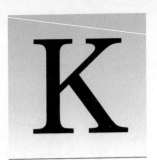

Kaposi's sarcoma

Kaposi's sarcoma, a cancer of the lymphatic cell wall, affects tissues under the skin or mucous membranes that line the mouth, nose, and anus. In recent years, the incidence of Kaposi's sarcoma has risen dramatically along with the incidence of acquired immunodeficiency syndrome (AIDS). It's now the most common AIDS-related cancer.

Kaposi's sarcoma causes structural and functional damage. When associated with AIDS, it progresses aggressively, involving the lymph nodes, the viscera and, possibly, GI structures. The most common extracutaneous sites are the lungs and GI tract (esophagus, oropharynx, and epiglottis).

Causes
- Unknown
- Possibly immunosuppression or hereditary predisposition.

Signs and symptoms
Cutaneous
- Lesions appearing on the skin, buccal mucosa, hard and soft palates, lips, gums, tongue, tonsils, conjunctivae, and sclerae
  - Colors ranging from red-brown to dark purple
  - May appear as large, ulcerative masses (if untreated)
  - May join to form one large plaque (in advanced disease)
  - Varying shapes and sizes

Extracutaneous
- Digestive problems (with metastasis)
- Dyspnea
- Edema
- Pain (if advanced beyond early stages, with breakage of lesion, or impingement on nerves or organs)
- Respiratory distress
- Wheezing

Diagnostic tests
- Tissue biopsy identifies the lesion's type and stage.
- Computed tomography scan can detect and evaluate possible metastasis.

Treatment
- Treatment is indicated only for patients with cosmetically offensive, painful, or obstructive lesions of rapidly progressing disease.
- Radiation therapy alleviates signs and symptoms, including pain from obstructing lesions in the oral cavity or extremities and edema caused by lymphatic blockage. It may also be used for cosmetic improvement.

- Combinations of three or more anti-human immunodeficiency (HIV) drugs may control HIV as well as flatten, shrink, or fade Kaposi's sarcoma lesions.
- A derivative of vitamin A, 9-cis-retinoic acid, can be applied directly to skin lesions.
- Chemotherapy includes combinations of doxorubicin (Rubex), vinblastine, vincristine, and etoposide (Vepesid) to treat internal, widespread Kaposi's sarcoma.
- Biotherapy with interferon alfa-2b may be administered for HIV-related Kaposi's sarcoma. The treatment reduces the number of skin lesions but is ineffective in patients with advanced disease.

Nursing considerations
- Provide emotional support to the patient and his family.
- Allow the patient to participate in self-care decisions whenever possible, and encourage him to participate in self-care measures as much as he can.
- Inspect the patient's skin, looking for new lesions and skin breakdown. If he has painful lesions, help him into a more comfortable position.
- Give pain medication as prescribed. Suggest distractions, explore alternative therapies, and help the patient with relaxation techniques.
- Encourage the patient to share his feelings to help him adjust to changes in his appearance.
- Monitor the patient's weight daily.
- Supply the patient with high-calorie, high-protein meals. If he can't tolerate regular meals, provide him with frequent smaller meals. Consult with the dietitian, and plan meals around the patient's treatment.
- Administer I.V. fluids and parenteral or enteral nutrition as prescribed if the patient is unable to take food by mouth.

Provide an antiemetic and a sedative as prescribed.
- Be alert for adverse reactions to radiation therapy or chemotherapy—such as anorexia, nausea, vomiting, and diarrhea—and take steps to prevent or alleviate them.
- Reinforce the explanation of treatments. Make sure the patient understands which adverse reactions to expect and how to manage them. For example, during radiation therapy, instruct the patient to keep irradiated skin dry to avoid breakdown and subsequent infection.
- Explain about prescribed medications, including possible adverse effects and drug interactions.
- Explain infection-prevention techniques and, if necessary, demonstrate basic hygiene measures to prevent infection. Advise the patient not to share his toothbrush, razor, or other personal items that may be contaminated with blood. These measures are especially important if the patient also has HIV infection.
- Help the patient plan daily periods of alternating activity and rest to help him cope with fatigue. Teach energy-conservation techniques. Encourage him to set priorities, accept the help of others, and delegate nonessential tasks.
- Stress the need for ongoing treatment and care.
- Refer the patient to support groups or hospice care as appropriate.
- Explain the benefits of initiating and executing advance directives and a durable power of attorney.

Keratitis

Keratitis, also known as *inflammation of the cornea,* may be acute or chronic, superficial or deep and usually affects only one eye. Superficial keratitis is fairly common and may develop at any age. The prognosis depends on the cause. Untreated, recurrent keratitis may lead to blindness.

Causes

- Bacterial or fungal infection (less common)
- Congenital syphilis (rarely)
- Corneal trauma
- Exposure (as in Bell's palsy where the eyelids don't close)
- Herpes simplex virus, type 1 (known as *dendritic keratitis* because of a characteristic branched lesion of the cornea resembling the veins of a leaf)
- Wearing contact lenses for prolonged periods (overnight)

Signs and symptoms

- Blurred vision
- Corneal opacities (if left untreated)
- Pain
- Photophobia
- Tearing

Diagnostic tests

- A slit-lamp examination reveals the depth of the keratitis. If it's due to herpes simplex virus, staining the eye with a fluorescein strip produces one or more small branchlike (dendritic) lesions; touching the cornea with cotton reveals reduced corneal sensation.
- Vision testing may show slightly decreased acuity.

Treatment

- With acute keratitis due to herpes simplex virus, treatment consists of vidarabine ophthalmic ointment. A broad-spectrum antibiotic may prevent secondary bacterial infection.
- Chronic dendritic keratitis may respond more quickly to vidarabine. Long-term topical therapy may be nec-

essary. (Corticosteroid therapy is contraindicated in patients with dendritic keratitis or another viral or fungal disease of the cornea.)

- Fungal keratitis requires natamycin (Natacyn).
- Keratitis due to exposure requires application of moisturizing ointment to the exposed cornea and of a plastic bubble eye shield or eye patch.
- Treatment of severe corneal scarring may include keratoplasty (cornea transplantation).

Nursing considerations

- Look for keratitis in the patient predisposed to cold sores. Explain that stress, trauma, fever, colds, and overexposure to the sun may trigger flare-ups.
- Protect the exposed corneas of unconscious patients by cleaning the eyes daily, applying moisturizing ointment, or covering the eyes with an eye shield.

Kidney cancer

Kidney cancer is also known as *nephrocarcinoma, renal cell carcinoma, hypernephroma,* and *Grawitz's tumor.* It usually occurs in older adults, with about 85% of tumors originating in the kidneys and others resulting from metastasis from other primary sites. Renal pelvic tumors and Wilms' tumor occur primarily in children.

Kidney tumors—which are usually large, firm, nodular, encapsulated, unilateral, and solitary—can be separated histologically into clear cell, granular, and spindle cell types. The 5-year survival rate for patients with kidney cancer is about 50%; the 10-year survival rate is lower.

The incidence of this cancer is rising, possibly as a result of exposure to environmental carcinogens as well as increased longevity. Even so, kidney cancer accounts for only about 2% of all adult cancers. It's twice as common in males as in females and usually affects patients older than age 40.

Causes
- Unknown
- Risk factors: heavy cigarette smoking and receiving regular hemodialysis

Signs and symptoms
Coexisting in 10% of patients
- Abdominal or flank pain: constant, possibly dull (acute and colicky with bleeding or blood clots)
- Microscopic or gross hematuria (possibly intermittent)
- Palpable mass (generally smooth, firm and nontender)

Other signs and symptoms
- Bone pain or fracture from a metastatic lesion
- Edema in the legs
- Fever (perhaps from hemorrhage or necrosis)
- Hypercalcemia (rapidly progressing; possibly from ectopic parathyroid hormone production by the tumor)
- Hypertension (from compression of the renal artery with renal parenchymal ischemia)
- Nausea and vomiting
- Urine retention
- Weight loss

Diagnostic tests
- Computed tomography scans, excretory urography, and retrograde pyelography and renal ultrasound identify kidney cancer.
- Cystoscopy rules out associated bladder cancer.
- Nephrotomography or renal angiography distinguishes a kidney cyst from a tumor.

- Results of liver function studies show increased levels of alkaline phosphatase, bilirubin, alanine aminotransferase, and aspartate aminotransferase as well as prolonged prothrombin time. Such results may point to liver metastasis; if metastasis hasn't occurred, however, these abnormalities reverse after the tumor has been resected.
- Routine laboratory findings of hematuria, anemia (unrelated to blood loss), polycythemia, hypercalcemia, and increased erythrocyte sedimentation rate call for more testing to rule out kidney cancer.
- A bone scan rules out skeletal metastasis.

Treatment
- Radical nephrectomy, with or without regional lymph node dissection, offers the only chance of cure.
- Because the disease is radiation-resistant, radiation is used only if the cancer spreads to the perinephric region or the lymph nodes or if the primary tumor or metastatic sites can't be fully excised. In such cases, high doses of radiation are used.
- Chemotherapy has been only erratically effective against kidney cancer.
- Interferon is somewhat effective in advanced disease. Hormone therapy using medroxyprogesterone and testosterone may be tried in advanced cases.
- Biotherapy (lymphokine-activated killer cells with recombinant interleukin-2) shows promise, but causes adverse reactions.

Nursing considerations
- Before surgery, assure the patient that his body will adapt to the loss of a kidney.
- After surgery, encourage coughing and deep breathing and incentive spirometry use.

■ Assist the patient with leg exercises, and turn him every 2 hours.

■ Check dressings often for excessive bleeding. Watch for signs of internal bleeding, such as restlessness, sweating, and increased pulse rate.

■ Place the patient on the operative side to allow the pressure of adjacent organs to fill the dead space at the operative site, improving dependent drainage. If possible, help the patient walk within 24 hours after surgery.

■ Maintain adequate fluid intake, and monitor intake and output. Monitor laboratory results for anemia, polycythemia, or abnormal blood values that may point to bone or liver involvement or that may result from radiation or chemotherapy.

■ Treat adverse reactions to the prescribed drug therapy.

■ Stress the need to comply with the prescribed outpatient treatment regimen.

Kyphosis

Kyphosis, also known as *roundback,* is an anteroposterior curving of the spine that causes a bowing of the back, commonly at the thoracic, but sometimes at the thoracolumbar or sacral, level.

Normally, the spine displays some convexity, but excessive thoracic kyphosis is pathologic. Kyphosis occurs in children and adults. Congenital kyphosis is rare but usually severe, with resultant cosmetic deformity and reduced pulmonary function. Adolescent kyphosis is the most common form of this disorder. Symptomatic adolescent kyphosis is more prevalent in females than in males and usually occurs between ages 12 and 16. Development of adolescent kyphosis is usually insidious, typically occurring after a history of excessive sports activity, and may be asymptomatic except for the obvious curving of the back (sometimes more than 90 degrees).

Causes
Adolescent kyphosis

■ Disk degeneration

■ Growth retardation or a vascular disturbance in the vertebral epiphysis (usually at the thoracic level) during periods of rapid growth or from congenital deficiency in the thickness of the vertebral plates

■ Infection

■ Inflammation

■ Poor posture

■ Stress of weight bearing on the compromised vertebrae

Adult kyphosis

■ Arthritis

■ Compression fracture of the thoracic vertebrae

■ Degeneration of intervertebral disks, atrophy, or osteoporotic collapse of the vertebrae

■ Disk lesions

■ Endocrine disorder, such as hyperparathyroidism or Cushing's disease

■ Metastatic tumor

■ Paget's disease

■ Plasma cell myeloma

■ Polio

■ Poor posture

■ Prolonged steroid therapy

■ Tuberculosis

Signs and symptoms
Adolescent features

■ Fatigue

■ Mild pain at the apex of the curve (about 50% of patients)

■ Prominent vertebral spinous processes at the lower dorsal and upper lumbar levels, with compensatory increased lumbar lordosis and hamstring tightness

- Spastic paraparesis secondary to spinal cord compression or herniated nucleus pulposus (in rare cases)
- Spine curvature present when the patient assumes a recumbent position (if not due to poor posture alone)
- Tenderness or stiffness in the involved area or along the entire spine

Adult features
- Characteristic roundback appearance
- Generalized fatigue
- Local tenderness (usually in patients with senile osteoporosis and a recent compression fracture)
- Pain
- Spine curvature present when the patient assumes a recumbent position (if not due to poor posture alone)
- Weakness of the back

Diagnostic tests
- X-rays may show vertebral wedging, Schmorl's nodes, irregular end plates and, possibly, mild scoliosis of 10 to 20 degrees.
- Vertebral biopsy is used to evaluate other sites of bone disease, primary sites of cancer, and infection.

Treatment
- For kyphosis caused by poor posture alone, treatment may consist of therapeutic exercises, bed rest on a firm mattress (with or without traction), and use of a brace to straighten the kyphotic curve until spinal growth is complete.
- Corrective exercises may include pelvic tilts to decrease lumbar lordosis, hamstring stretches to overcome muscle contractures, and thoracic hyperextensions to flatten the kyphotic curve. These exercises may be performed in or out of the brace.
- Lateral X-rays will be taken every 4 months evaluate correction.

- Gradual weaning from the brace can begin after maximum correction of the kyphotic curve, vertebral wedging has decreased, and the spine has reached full skeletal maturity. Loss of correction indicates that weaning from the brace has been too rapid, and time out of the brace is decreased accordingly.
- Treatment for adolescent and adult kyphosis also includes:
  – measures to correct the underlying cause
  – possible spinal arthrodesis for relief of symptoms
  – surgery, in rare cases, when kyphosis causes neurologic damage, a spinal curve greater than 60 degrees, or intractable and disabling back pain in a patient with full skeletal maturity; preoperative measures may include halofemoral traction
  – corrective surgery with posterior spinal fusion and spinal instrumentation, iliac bone grafting, and plaster immobilization
  – anterior spinal fusion with immobilization in plaster if kyphosis produces a spinal curve greater than 70 degrees.

Nursing considerations
- Provide supportive care for the patient in traction or a brace.
- Provide skillful patient teaching, and sensitive emotional support. (See *Managing kyphosis,* page 346.)
- Explain all preoperative tests thoroughly as well as the need for postoperative traction or casting, if applicable.
- After surgery, check the patient's neurovascular status every 2 to 4 hours for the first 48 hours, and watch for changes.
- Turn the patient often by logrolling him.
- Administer pain medication as prescribed, and monitor its effect.

Managing kyphosis

■ Explain how to perform therapeutic exercises, and emphasize good posture.
■ Tell the patient to use bed rest when pain is severe.
■ Remind the patient to use a firm mattress or bed board for proper support.
■ Explain how to use the brace and encourage compliance with its prescribed use.
■ Teach the patient good skin care to prevent skin breakdown from the brace.
■ Caution the patient that only an orthotist should adjust the brace.
■ Advise the patient to drink plenty of liquids to avoid constipation and to report any illness (especially abdominal pain or vomiting) immediately.
■ Arrange for home visits by a home care nurse.

■ Accurately measure the patient's fluid intake and output, including urine specific gravity.
■ Insert a nasogastric tube and an indwelling urinary catheter as needed.
■ Provide meticulous skin care. Check the skin at the cast edges several times per day; use heel and elbow protectors to prevent skin breakdown.
■ Change dressings as necessary.
■ Assist during the removal of sutures and application of a new cast (usually about 10 days after surgery).
■ Encourage the patient to begin walking again gradually (usually with the use of a tilt-table in the physical therapy department).
■ Provide detailed, written cast care instructions at discharge. Tell the patient to immediately report pain, burning, skin breakdown, loss of feeling, tingling, numbness, or cast odor.

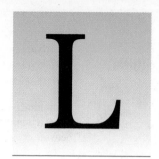

Labyrinthitis

Labyrinthitis, an inflammation of the labyrinth of the inner ear, can incapacitate a patient by producing severe vertigo that lasts for 3 to 5 days; symptoms gradually subside over 3 to 6 weeks. This disorder is rare, although viral labyrinthitis is commonly associated with upper respiratory tract infections.

Causes
- Bacterial or viral infection
- Cholesteatoma
- Chronic otitis media
- Drug toxicity
- Influenza
- Meningitis
- Otitis media
- Trauma

Signs and symptoms
- Giddiness
- Nausea and vomiting
- Purulent drainage (with severe bacterial infection)
- Sensorineural hearing loss
- Severe vertigo:
  - occurs with any movement of the head
  - has gradual onset
  - peaks within 48 hours
  - causes loss of balance and falling in the direction of the affected ear
- Signs of middle ear disease (with cholesteatoma)
- Spontaneous nystagmus, with jerking movements of the eyes toward the unaffected ear

Diagnostic tests
- Culture and sensitivity testing identifies the infecting organism if purulent drainage is present.
- Audiometric testing reveals the extent of sensorineural hearing loss, if any.
- When an infectious cause can't be found, additional testing must be done to rule out a brain lesion or Ménière's disease.
- Computed tomography scanning rules out a brain lesion.

Treatment
- Treatment focuses on relieving symptoms and includes bed rest, with the head immobilized between pillows and oral meclizine (Antivert) to control vertigo.
- Massive doses of an antibiotic are used to combat diffuse purulent labyrinthitis.
- Oral fluids can prevent dehydration from vomiting.
- I.V. fluids may be necessary for severe nausea and vomiting.
- Surgical excision of the cholesteatoma and drainage of the infected areas of the

Managing labyrinthitis

■ Help the patient assess how much his disability will affect his daily life.
■ Work with the patient to identify hazards in the home (such as throw rugs and dark stairways).
■ Discuss the patient's anxieties and concerns about vertigo attacks and decreased hearing.
■ Stress the importance of maintaining or resuming normal diversions or social activities when balance disturbance is absent.
■ Explain the importance of avoiding sudden changes in position.

middle and inner ear may be necessary if conservative treatment fails.
■ Prevention is possible by early and vigorous treatment of predisposing conditions, such as otitis media and a local or systemic infection.

Nursing considerations
■ Keep the side rails up to prevent falls.
■ Give an antiemetic as prescribed for severe vomiting.
■ Record intake and output, and give I.V. fluids as necessary.
■ Tell the patient that recovery may take as long as 6 weeks. During this time, he should limit activities that vertigo may make hazardous.
■ Review steps to manage the condition. (See *Managing labyrinthitis*.)

Laryngeal cancer

The most common form of laryngeal cancer is squamous cell carcinoma (95%); rare forms include adenocarcinoma, sarcoma, and others. Such cancer may be intrinsic or extrinsic.

An *intrinsic* tumor is on the true vocal cord and tends not to spread because underlying connective tissues lack lymph nodes. An *extrinsic* tumor is on some other part of the larynx and tends to spread early. Laryngeal cancer is about nine times more common in males than in females; most patients are between ages 50 and 65.

Laryngeal cancer is classified according to its location:
■ supraglottis (false vocal cords)
■ glottis (true vocal cords)
■ subglottis (downward extension from the vocal cords [rare]).

Causes
■ Unknown

Predisposing factors
■ Alcohol abuse
■ Chronic inhalation of noxious fumes
■ Familial tendency
■ Smoking

Signs and symptoms
Intrinsic laryngeal cancer
■ Hoarseness that persists longer than 3 weeks

Extrinsic laryngeal cancer
■ Lump in the throat
■ Pain or burning in the throat when drinking citrus juice or hot liquid

With metastasis
■ Cough
■ Dysphagia
■ Dyspnea
■ Enlarged cervical lymph nodes
■ Pain radiating to the ear

Diagnostic tests
■ Laryngoscopy is used to visualize the larynx.
■ Xeroradiography, biopsy, laryngeal tomography, computed tomography scan, or laryngography define the borders of the lesion.

- Chest X-ray detects metastasis.

Treatment

- The treatment goal is to eliminate the cancer and preserve speech. If speech preservation is impossible, speech rehabilitation may include esophageal speech or prosthetic devices; surgical techniques to construct a new voice box are still experimental.
- Surgical procedures vary with tumor size and can include cordectomy, partial or total laryngectomy, supraglottic laryngectomy, or total laryngectomy with laryngoplasty.
- Early lesions are treated with laser surgery or radiation.
- Advanced lesions are treated with surgery, radiation, and chemotherapy.
- Chemotherapeutic agents may include methotrexate (Trexall), cisplatin (Platinol), bleomycin (Blenoxane), fluorouracil, and lomustine.

Nursing considerations

- Provide emotional support to the patient and his family.

Before partial or total laryngectomy

- Instruct the patient to maintain good oral hygiene. If appropriate, instruct a male patient to shave off his beard.
- Encourage the patient to express his concerns before surgery. Help him choose a temporary nonspeaking method of communication (such as writing).
- If appropriate, arrange for a laryngectomee to visit him. Explain postoperative procedures (suctioning, nasogastric [NG] tube feeding, and care of laryngectomy tube) and their results (the need to breathe through the neck, altered speech). Also, prepare him for other functional losses: He won't be able to smell, blow his nose, whistle, gargle, sip, or suck on a straw.

After partial laryngectomy

- Administer I.V. fluids and, usually, tube feedings for the first 2 days postoperatively as prescribed; then give the patient oral fluids. Keep the tracheostomy tube (inserted during surgery) in place until edema subsides.
- Keep the patient from using his voice until he has medical permission (usually 2 to 3 days postoperatively). Then caution him to whisper until healing is complete.

After total laryngectomy

- Place him on his side and elevate his head 30 to 45 degrees. When you move him, remember to support his neck.
- Provide laryngectomy tube care until his stoma heals (7 to 10 days). This tube is shorter and thicker than a tracheostomy tube, but requires the same care.
- Watch for crusting and secretions around the stoma, which can cause skin breakdown. To prevent crust formation, provide adequate room humidification. Remove crusting with petroleum jelly, antimicrobial ointment, and moist gauze.
- Teach the patient stoma care.
- Assess the patient for fistula formation (redness, swelling, and secretions on the suture line). A fistula may form between the reconstructed hypopharynx and the skin. This eventually heals spontaneously but may take weeks or months.
- Watch for carotid artery rupture (bleeding), which usually occurs in a patient who has had preoperative radiation, particularly a patient with a fistula that constantly bathes the carotid artery with oral secretions. If carotid rupture occurs, apply pressure to the site, immediately call for help, and take the patient

to the operating room for carotid ligation.

- Watch for tracheostomy stenosis (constant shortness of breath), which occurs weeks to months after laryngectomy; treatment includes fitting the patient with successively larger tracheostomy tubes until he can tolerate a large one.
- Feed the patient through an NG tube if he develops a fistula; otherwise, food will leak through the fistula and delay healing.
- Monitor the patient's vital signs (be especially alert for fever, which indicates infection).
- Record fluid intake and output, and watch for dehydration.
- Provide frequent mouth care.
- Suction gently unless otherwise instructed. Don't attempt deep suctioning, which could penetrate the suture line. Suction through the tube and the patient's nose because he can no longer blow air through his nose; suction his mouth gently.
- Don't stop suction of a drainage catheter until drainage is minimal. After the catheter is removed, check dressings for drainage.
- Administer analgesics as prescribed and as needed.
- Check NG feeding tube placement and elevate the patient's head to prevent aspiration.
- Reassure the patient that speech rehabilitation may help him speak again. Encourage him to contact the International Association of Laryngectomees and other sources of support.

Laryngitis

Laryngitis is a common disorder that involves acute or chronic inflammation of the vocal cords. Acute laryngitis may occur as an isolated infection or as part of a generalized bacterial or viral upper respiratory tract infection. Repeated attacks of acute laryngitis cause inflammatory changes associated with chronic laryngitis.

Causes
Acute laryngitis
- Aspiration of caustic chemicals
- Excessive use of the voice, an occupational hazard in certain vocations (for example, teaching, public speaking, and singing)
- Infection (primarily viral)
- Inhalation of smoke or fumes
- Leisure activities such as cheering at a sports event

Chronic laryngitis
- Alcohol abuse
- Chronic upper respiratory tract disorders (sinusitis, bronchitis, nasal polyps, or an allergy)
- Constant exposure to dust or other irritants
- Mouth breathing
- Smoking

Reflux laryngitis
- Regurgitation of gastric acid into the hypopharynx (see *Managing reflux laryngitis*)

Signs and symptoms
Acute laryngitis
- Dry cough
- Fever
- Hoarseness, ranging from mild to complete loss of voice (typically the first sign)
- Laryngeal edema
- Malaise
- Pain, especially when swallowing or speaking

Chronic laryngitis
- Persistent hoarseness

Managing reflux laryngitis

To prevent gastric reflux, which can lead to laryngitis, instruct the patient on these do's and don'ts.

Do's
■ Elevate the head of the bed (by elevating the mattress). Sleeping on additional pillows won't be sufficient.

■ Take an antacid and a histamine-2 receptor antagonist as prescribed.

Don'ts
■ Don't drink alcohol or coffee or eat foods that cause gastric reflux.
■ Don't eat for 3 to 4 hours before going to bed.

Reflux laryngitis
■ Dysphagia
■ Hoarseness

Diagnostic tests
■ Indirect laryngoscopy shows red, inflamed and, occasionally, hemorrhagic vocal cords, with rounded rather than sharp edges and exudate. Bilateral swelling may be present.
■ In severe cases or if toxicity is a concern, a culture of the exudate is obtained.

Treatment
■ Primary treatment involves resting the voice.
■ For viral infection, symptomatic care includes an analgesic and throat lozenges for pain relief.
■ Bacterial infection requires antibiotic therapy.
■ Severe, acute laryngitis may necessitate hospitalization. When laryngeal edema results in airway obstruction, tracheotomy may be necessary.
■ With chronic laryngitis, effective treatment must eliminate the underlying cause.
■ With reflux laryngitis, postural and dietary changes along with an antacid and a histamine-2 receptor antagonist combine for effective treatment.

Nursing considerations
■ Explain to the patient why he shouldn't talk, and place a sign over the bed to remind others of this restriction. Provide a small chalkboard, slate, or a pad and pencil for communication. Mark the intercom panel so that other facility personnel are aware that the patient can't answer.
■ Minimize the patient's need to talk by trying to anticipate his needs.
■ Suggest that the patient maintain adequate humidification by using a vaporizer or humidifier during winter, by avoiding air conditioning during summer (because it dehumidifies), by using medicated throat lozenges, and by not smoking. Urge him to complete the prescribed antibiotic regimen.
■ Obtain a detailed patient history to help determine the cause of chronic laryngitis. Encourage the patient to modify predisposing habits, such as smoking.

▮ Legionnaires' disease

An acute bronchopneumonia, legionnaires' disease is produced by a fastidious, gram-negative bacillus. This disease may occur epidemically or sporadically, usually in late summer or early fall. Its severity ranges from a mild illness, with or without pneumonitis, to multilobar pneumonia, with a mortality as high as 15%. A milder, self-limiting form (Pontiac fever) subsides within a few days but leaves the patient fatigued for several weeks; this form mimics legionnaires' disease but produces few or no respiratory symptoms, no pneumonia, and no fatalities.

Legionnaires' disease is more common in males than in females and is most likely to affect:
- middle-aged to elderly people
- those who are immunocompromised (particularly those receiving a corticosteroid, for example, after a transplant) or those with lymphoma or other disorders associated with delayed hypersensitivity
- patients with a chronic underlying disease, such as diabetes, chronic renal failure, or chronic obstructive pulmonary disease
- those with alcoholism
- cigarette smokers (three to four times more likely to develop legionnaires' disease than nonsmokers).

Causes
- *Legionella pneumophila,* an aerobic, gram-negative bacillus: probably transmitted by an airborne route (spreads through cooling towers or evaporation condensers in air-conditioning systems but *Legionella* bacilli also flourish in soil and excavation sites)

Signs and symptoms
- After a 2- to 10-day incubation period, nonspecific, prodromal signs and symptoms appear, including:
  - anorexia
  - bradycardia
  - cough (initially nonproductive but possibly leading to production of grayish, nonpurulent and, occasionally, blood-streaked sputum)
  - diarrhea
  - diffuse myalgia
  - disorientation, delirium, mental sluggishness, or mild temporary amnesia
  - dyspnea
  - fine crackles
  - generalized weakness
  - headache
  - malaise
  - nausea and vomiting
  - pleuritic chest pain
  - recurrent chills
  - tachypnea
  - unremitting fever within 12 to 48 hours with a temperature as high as 105° F (40.6° C)
- Complications include:
  - arrhythmias
  - delirium
  - heart failure
  - hypotension
  - pneumonia (may occur with accompanying hypoxia and acute respiratory failure)
  - renal failure
  - seizures
  - shock (usually fatal).

Diagnostic tests
- Chest X-ray shows patchy, localized infiltration, which progresses to multilobar consolidation (usually involving the lower lobes), pleural effusion and, in fulminant disease, opacification of the entire lung.
- Auscultation reveals fine crackles, progressing to coarse crackles as the disease advances.
- Blood studies show leukocytosis, an increased erythrocyte sedimentation rate, an increase in liver enzyme levels (alanine aminotransferase, aspartate aminotransferase, and alkaline phosphatase), hyponatremia, decreased partial pressure of arterial oxygen and, initially, decreased partial pressure of arterial carbon dioxide.

■ Bronchial washings and blood, pleural fluid, and sputum tests rule out other infections.

■ Definitive tests include direct immunofluorescence of respiratory tract secretions and tissue, a culture of *L. pneumophila,* and indirect fluorescent antibody testing of serum comparing acute samples with convalescent samples drawn at least 3 weeks later.

■ A urine specimen for *L. pneumophila* antigen may also be performed.

■ A convalescent serum showing a fourfold or greater rise in antibody titer for *Legionella* confirms this diagnosis.

Treatment

■ Antibiotic therapy (with erythromycin as the drug of choice) begins as soon as legionnaires' disease is suspected and diagnostic material is collected. Rifampin may be used alone or along with erythromycin.

■ Supportive therapy includes administration of an antipyretic, fluid replacement, circulatory support with vasopressor drugs if necessary, and oxygen administration by mask, cannula, or mechanical ventilation.

Nursing considerations

■ Closely monitor the patient's respiratory status. Evaluate chest wall expansion, depth and pattern of respirations, cough, and chest pain.

■ Watch for restlessness, which may indicate that the patient is hypoxemic and requires suctioning, repositioning, or more aggressive oxygen therapy.

■ Continually monitor the patient's vital signs, pulse oximetry or arterial blood gas values, level of consciousness, and dryness and color of his lips and mucous membranes. Watch for signs of shock (decreased blood pressure, thready pulse, diaphoresis, and clammy skin).

■ Keep the patient comfortable. Provide mouth care frequently. If necessary, apply soothing cream to the nostrils.

■ Replace fluid and electrolytes as prescribed. A patient with renal failure may require dialysis.

■ Teach the patient how to cough effectively, and encourage deep-breathing exercises. Stress the need to continue these measures until recovery is complete.

■ Provide mechanical ventilation and other respiratory therapy as needed.

Leukemia, acute

Acute leukemia is a malignant proliferation of white blood cell (WBC) precursors (blasts) in bone marrow or lymph tissue and their accumulation in peripheral blood, bone marrow, and body tissues.

The most common forms are acute lymphoblastic (lymphocytic) leukemia (ALL), characterized by the abnormal growth of lymphocyte precursors (lymphoblasts); acute myeloblastic (myelogenous) leukemia (AML), in which myeloid precursors (myeloblasts) rapidly accumulate; and acute monoblastic (monocytic) leukemia, or Schilling's type, characterized by a marked increase in monocyte precursors (monoblasts). Other variants include acute myelomonocytic leukemia and acute erythroleukemia.

Untreated, acute leukemia is invariably fatal, usually because of complications that result from leukemic cell infiltration of bone marrow or vital organs. With treatment, the prognosis varies.

With ALL, treatment induces remissions in 90% of children (average survival time is 5 years) and in 65% of adults (average survival time is 1 to 2 years). Children ages 2 to 8 have the best survival rate (about 50%) with intensive therapy.

With AML, the average survival time is only 1 year after diagnosis, even with aggressive treatment. With acute monoblastic leukemia, treatment induces remissions lasting 2 to 10 months in 50% of children; adults survive only about 1 year after diagnosis, even with treatment.

Acute leukemia is more common in males than in females, in whites (especially people of Jewish descent), in children between ages 2 and 5 (80% of all leukemias in this age-group are ALL), and in people who live in urban and industrialized areas. Among children, acute leukemia is the most common form of cancer.

Causes
Pathogenesis
■ Accumulation of immature, nonfunctioning WBCs in the tissue where they originate (lymphocytes in lymph tissue, granulocytes in bone marrow)
■ Infiltration of these tissues into the bloodstream and other tissues, leading to organ malfunction due to encroachment or hemorrhage (see *What happens in leukemia*)

Predisposing factors
■ Combination of viruses (viral remnants have been found in leukemic cells)
■ Exposure to radiation and certain chemicals
■ Genetic and immunologic factors

Signs and symptoms
■ Abnormal bleeding
■ Liver or spleen enlargement
■ Lymph node enlargement
■ Malaise
■ Night sweats
■ Pallor
■ Palpitations
■ Sudden onset of high fever
■ Systolic ejection murmur
■ Tachycardia

Diagnostic tests
■ Bone marrow aspirate showing a proliferation of immature WBCs confirms acute leukemia.
■ An aspirate that's dry or free from leukemic cells in a patient with typical signs and symptoms requires a bone marrow biopsy, usually of the posterior superior iliac spine.
■ Blood counts show thrombocytopenia and neutropenia. A differential leukocyte count determines cell type.
■ Lumbar puncture detects meningeal involvement.

Treatment
■ Systemic chemotherapy aims to eradicate leukemic cells and induce remission. Chemotherapy varies according to the type of leukemia:
 – Meningeal leukemia—intrathecal instillation of methotrexate (Trexall) or cytarabine (Depocyt) with cranial radiation is used.
 – ALL—vincristine, prednisone, methotrexate (Trexall), 6-mercaptopurine (Purinethol), and cyclophosphamide (Cytoxan) are used. Intrathecal therapy may be required. Radiation therapy is given for testicular infiltration.
 – AML—a combination of I.V. daunorubicin (Cerubidine) and cytarabine (Depocyt) is used for treatment. If these drugs fail to induce remission, treatment involves some or all of the following: a combination of cyclophosphamide, vincristine, prednisone, or methotrexate; high-dose cytarabine alone or with other drugs; amsacrine; etoposide (Vepesid); and 5-azacytidine (Vidaza) and mitoxantrone (Novantrone).

What happens in leukemia

This illustration shows how white blood cells (agranulocytes and granulocytes) proliferate in the bloodstream in leukemia, overwhelming red blood cells (RBCs) and platelets.

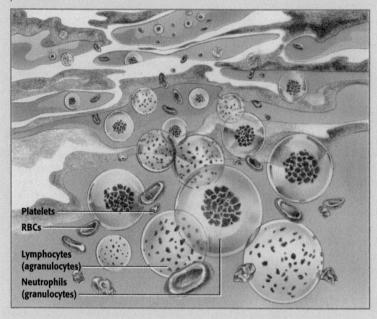

Platelets
RBCs
Lymphocytes (agranulocytes)
Neutrophils (granulocytes)

—Acute monoblastic leukemia—cytarabine and thioguanine with daunorubicin or doxorubicin (Rubex) is used.

- A bone marrow or stem cell transplant may be possible.
- Treatment also may include antibiotic, antifungal, and antiviral drugs and granulocyte injections to control infection.
- Platelet transfusions (to prevent bleeding) and red blood cell transfusions (to prevent anemia) may also be given.

Nursing considerations

- Promote comfort by minimizing the adverse effects of chemotherapy, preserving the veins, managing complications, and providing teaching and psychological support. Because so many of these patients are children, be especially sensitive to their emotional needs and those of their families.

Before treatment

- Explain the course of the disease, treatments, and adverse effects of prescribed drugs.
- Teach the patient and his family how to recognize infection (fever, chills, cough, sore throat) and abnormal bleeding (bruising, petechiae) and how to stop such bleeding (applying pressure and ice to the area).
- Promote good nutrition. Explain that chemotherapy may cause weight loss

and anorexia, so encourage the patient to eat and drink high-calorie, high-protein foods and beverages. However, chemotherapeutic drugs and prednisone may cause weight gain, so dietary counseling and teaching are helpful.

■ Help establish an appropriate rehabilitation for the patient during remission.

For supportive care

■ Watch for signs and symptoms of meningeal leukemia (confusion, lethargy, headache). If these occur, know how to manage care after intrathecal chemotherapy. After such instillation, place the patient in Trendelenburg's position for 30 minutes. Give the patient plenty of fluids, and keep him in a supine position for 4 to 6 hours.

■ Check the lumbar puncture site often for bleeding.

■ If the patient receives cranial radiation, teach him about potential adverse effects, and do what you can to minimize them.

■ Prevent hyperuricemia, which may result from rapid chemotherapy-induced leukemic cell lysis. Give the patient about 2 qt (2 L) of fluids daily, and administer acetazolamide (Diamox), sodium bicarbonate tablets, and allopurinol (Zyloprim). Check urine pH often—it should be above 7.5. Watch for a rash or another hypersensitivity reaction to allopurinol.

■ If the patient receives daunorubicin or doxorubicin, watch for early signs of cardiotoxicity, such as arrhythmias and signs of heart failure.

■ Control infection by placing the patient in a private room and imposing reverse isolation, if necessary. (The benefits of reverse isolation are controversial.) Coordinate patient care so the patient doesn't come in contact with staff who also care for patients with infections or infectious diseases. Avoid using indwelling urinary catheters and giving I.M. injections because they can cause infection. Screen staff and visitors for contagious diseases, and watch for signs of infection.

■ Provide thorough skin care by keeping the patient's skin and perianal area clean, applying mild lotions or creams to keep skin from drying and cracking, and thoroughly cleaning skin before all invasive skin procedures. Use strict aseptic technique and a metal scalp vein needle (metal butterfly needle) when starting I.V. lines. If the patient receives total parenteral nutrition, provide scrupulous subclavian catheter care.

■ Monitor the patient's temperature every 4 hours. A patient with a temperature over 101° F (38.3° C) and a decreased WBC count should receive prompt antibiotic therapy.

■ Watch for bleeding; if it occurs, apply ice compresses and pressure, and elevate the extremity. Avoid giving I.M. injections, aspirin, and aspirin-containing drugs. Also avoid taking rectal temperatures, giving rectal suppositories, and performing digital rectal examinations.

■ Prevent constipation by providing adequate hydration, a high-residue diet, a stool softener, and a mild laxative and by encouraging walking.

■ Control mouth ulceration by checking often for obvious ulcers and gum swelling and by providing frequent mouth care and saline rinses.

■ Tell the patient to use a soft toothbrush and to avoid hot, spicy foods and overuse of commercial mouthwashes. Also, check the rectal area daily for induration, swelling, erythema, skin discoloration, or drainage.

■ Minimize stress by providing a calm, quiet atmosphere that's conducive to rest and relaxation. For children particularly, be flexible with patient care and visiting hours to promote maximum interaction with family and friends and to allow time for schoolwork and play.

▪ For those patients who are refractory to chemotherapy and in the terminal phase of the disease, supportive nursing care aims to provide comfort; management of pain, fever, and bleeding; and patient and family support. Provide the opportunity for religious counseling. Discuss the option of home or hospice care. Support groups, such as the American Cancer Society, may also be helpful.

Leukemia, chronic granulocytic

Chronic granulocytic leukemia (CGL) is also known as *chronic myelogenous (or myelocytic) leukemia*. The disease is characterized by the abnormal overgrowth of granulocytic precursors (myeloblasts, promyelocytes, metamyelocytes, and myelocytes) in bone marrow, peripheral blood, and body tissues.

CGL is most common in young and middle-aged adults and is slightly more common in males than in females; it's rare in children. In the United States, 3,000 to 4,000 cases of CGL develop annually, accounting for about 20% of all leukemias.

The clinical course of CGL proceeds in two distinct phases: the insidious chronic phase, with anemia and bleeding abnormalities, and the acute phase (blastic crisis), in which myeloblasts, the most primitive granulocytic precursors, proliferate rapidly. This disease is invariably fatal. Average survival time is 3 to 4 years after onset of the chronic phase and 3 to 6 months after onset of the acute phase.

Causes
▪ Unknown
▪ Almost 90% of patients have the Philadelphia chromosome (Ph1) (which may be induced by radiation or carcinogenic chemicals)

Signs and symptoms
▪ Anemia (fatigue, weakness, decreased exercise tolerance, pallor, dyspnea, tachycardia, and headache)
▪ Ankle edema
▪ Anorexia
▪ Bleeding and clotting disorders (retinal hemorrhage, ecchymoses, hematuria, melena, bleeding gums, nosebleeds, and easy bruising)
▪ Hepatosplenomegaly, with abdominal discomfort and pain; splenic infarction from leukemic cell infiltration
▪ Low-grade fever
▪ Priapism (rarely)
▪ Prolonged infection
▪ Renal calculi or gouty arthritis
▪ Sternal and rib tenderness from leukemic infiltrations of the periosteum
▪ Vascular insufficiency (rarely)
▪ Weight loss

Diagnostic tests
▪ In patients with typical signs and symptoms, chromosomal analysis of peripheral blood or bone marrow showing the Ph1 and low leukocyte alkaline phosphatase levels confirms CGL.
▪ White blood cell (WBC) abnormalities include leukocytosis (WBC count ranging from 50,000/mm^3 to 250,000/mm^3), occasional leukopenia (WBC count less than 5,000/mm^3), neutropenia (neutrophil count less than 1,500/mm^3) despite a high leukocyte count, and increased circulating myeloblasts.
▪ Hemoglobin level is commonly below 10 g/dl.
▪ Hematocrit is low (less than 30%).

Managing chronic granulocytic leukemia

Because many patients with chronic granulocytic leukemia (CGL) receive outpatient chemotherapy throughout the chronic phase, sound patient teaching is essential.

■ Explain the adverse effects of chemotherapy and the related signs and symptoms.

■ Describe the signs of infection, and advise the patient to promptly contact his practitioner if he experiences any of them.

■ Explain the signs of thrombocytopenia as well as the preventive measures the patient can take (such as avoiding aspirin) to avoid the disorder.

■ Teach the patient what to do if he starts to bleed (such as external pressure).

■ Emphasize the need for adequate rest and a high-calorie, high-protein diet.

■ Platelet count commonly indicates thrombocytosis (more than 1 million/mm³).

■ Serum uric acid level may be more than 8 mg/dl.

■ Bone marrow aspirate or biopsy characteristically shows bone marrow infiltration by significantly increased number of myeloid elements (a biopsy is done only if aspirate is dry); in the acute phase, myeloblasts predominate.

■ Computed tomography scan may identify the organs affected by leukemia.

Treatment

■ Aggressive chemotherapy has so far failed to produce remission in patients with CGL. Consequently, the goal of treatment in the chronic phase is to control leukocytosis and thrombocytosis.

■ The most commonly used oral drugs are busulfan (Myleran) and hydroxyurea (Droxia).

■ Aspirin is commonly given to prevent stroke if the patient's platelet count exceeds 1 million/mm³.

■ Ancillary CGL treatments include:
  – local splenic radiation or splenectomy to increase platelet count and decrease adverse effects related to splenomegaly
  – leukapheresis (selective leukocyte removal) to reduce the WBC count

  – allopurinol to prevent secondary hyperuricemia or colchicine to relieve gout due to elevated serum uric acid levels
  – prompt antibiotic treatment of infections that may result from chemotherapy-induced bone marrow suppression.

■ During the acute phase of CGL, lymphoblastic or myeloblastic leukemia may develop. Treatment is similar to that for acute lymphoblastic leukemia. Remission, if achieved, is commonly short-lived.

■ Bone marrow or stem cell transplantation may help in certain phases of CGL. Despite vigorous treatment, CGL usually progresses after the onset of the acute phase.

Nursing considerations

■ Provide meticulous supportive care, psychological support, and careful patient teaching to help make the most of remissions and minimize complications. (See *Managing chronic granulocytic leukemia*.)

■ Reinforce the explanation of the disease and its treatment to the patient and his family.

During the chronic phase (hospitalization)

- Schedule laboratory tests and physical care with frequent rest periods in between, and assist the patient with walking if necessary.
- Regularly check the patient's skin and mucous membranes for pallor, petechiae, and bruising.
- Suggest a soft-bristled toothbrush, an electric razor, and other safety precautions to minimize bleeding.
- Provide small, frequent meals to minimize the abdominal discomfort of splenomegaly.
- Prevent constipation by administering a stool softener or laxative as prescribed. Ask the dietary department to provide a high-bulk diet, and maintain adequate fluid intake.
- Stress the need for coughing and deep-breathing exercises and incentive spirometry use to prevent atelectasis.

Leukemia, chronic lymphocytic

A generalized, progressive disease that's common in elderly people, chronic lymphocytic leukemia is marked by an uncontrollable spread of abnormal, small lymphocytes in lymphoid tissue, blood, and bone marrow. The prognosis is poor if anemia, thrombocytopenia, neutropenia, bulky lymphadenopathy, or severe lymphocytosis is present.

Nearly all patients with chronic lymphocytic leukemia are males older than age 50. According to the American Cancer Society, chronic lymphocytic leukemia accounts for almost one-third of new leukemia cases annually.

Causes
- Unknown

- Hereditary factors as well as undefined chromosomal abnormalities and certain immunologic defects suspected

Signs and symptoms
Early stages
- Fatigue
- Fever
- Malaise
- Nodal enlargement
- Susceptibility to infection (may be fatal)

Advanced stages
- Anemia, pallor, weakness, dyspnea, tachycardia, palpitations, bleeding, or infection (with bone marrow involvement)
- Bone tenderness
- Edema
- Opportunistic fungal, viral, and bacterial infections (may result in fatal septicemia)
- Pulmonary infiltrates
- Severe fatigue
- Skin infiltrations, manifested by macular to nodular eruptions
- Weight loss

Diagnostic tests
- Routine blood testing shows numerous abnormal lymphocytes in early stages; the white blood cell (WBC) count is mildly but persistently elevated.
- Granulocytopenia is the rule, although the WBC count climbs as the disease progresses.
- Hemoglobin level is below 11 g/dl.
- Hypogammaglobulinemia is present.
- Serum globulin levels are decreased.
- Neutropenia occurs (count is less than 1,500/mm^3).
- Lymphocytosis develops (count is more than 10,000/mm^3).
- Thrombocytopenia is revealed (count is less than 150,000/mm^3).

- Bone marrow aspiration and biopsy show lymphocytic invasion.
- A computed tomography scan identifies affected organs.

Treatment

- Systemic chemotherapy includes an alkylating drug, usually chlorambucil (Leukeran) or cyclophosphamide (Cytoxan), and sometimes a steroid (prednisone) when autoimmune hemolytic anemia or thrombocytopenia occurs.
- When chronic lymphocytic leukemia causes obstruction or organ impairment or enlargement, local radiation treatment can be used to reduce organ size and splenectomy can help relieve the symptoms.
- Allopurinol can be given to prevent hyperuricemia, a relatively uncommon finding.
- Radiation therapy can help relieve symptoms and is generally used to treat enlarged lymph nodes, painful bony lesions, or massive splenomegaly.

Nursing considerations

- Focus patient care on relieving symptoms and preventing infection. Clean the patient's skin daily with mild soap and water. Frequent soaks may be ordered. Monitor the patient for signs and symptoms of infection: temperature over 100° F (37.8° C), chills, redness, or swelling of any body part.
- Watch for signs and symptoms of thrombocytopenia (easy bruising, nosebleeds, bleeding gums, and black, tarry stools) and anemia (pale skin, weakness, fatigue, dizziness, and palpitations).

DRUG CHALLENGE

Advise the patient to avoid aspirin and products containing aspirin. Explain that many medications contain aspirin. Teach him how to recognize aspirin variants on medication labels.

- Explain chemotherapy and its possible adverse effects.
- Tell the patient to avoid coming in contact with obviously ill people, especially children with common contagious childhood diseases.
- Urge the patient to eat high-protein foods and drink high-calorie beverages.
- Stress the importance of follow-up care, frequent blood tests, and taking all medications exactly as prescribed.
- Teach the patient the signs and symptoms of recurrence (swollen lymph nodes in the neck, axillae, and groin; increased abdominal size or discomfort), and tell him to notify his practitioner immediately if he detects any of them.
- Provide emotional support for the patient.
- Explore alternative health measures that may benefit the patient.
- Provide supportive nursing care in terminal stages by managing pain, fever, and bleeding.
- Consult with spiritual care or other support services to help meet patient and family needs.
- Provide appropriate referrals such as home or hospice care if the patient will return home.

▌Liver abscess

A liver abscess occurs when bacteria or protozoa destroy hepatic tissue, producing a cavity, which fills with infectious organisms, liquefied liver cells, and leukocytes. Necrotic tissue then walls off the cavity from the rest of the liver.

Liver abscess carries a mortality of 10% to 20%, despite treatment. Liver abscess affects both sexes and all age-groups, although it's slightly more prevalent in hospitalized children (because of a high rate of immunosuppression) and in females (most commonly those between ages 40 and 60).

Causes

- Biliary tract disease
- Hematogenous spread through the portal bloodstream
- Infection with gram-negative aerobic bacilli, enterococci, streptococci, and anaerobes
- Intra-arterial chemoembolizations or cryosurgery in the liver

Predisposing factors

- Alcoholism
- Diabetes mellitus
- Metastatic cancer to the liver

Signs and symptoms

- Abdominal pain
- Anemia
- Chills
- Diaphoresis
- Dyspnea and pleural pain (if the abscess extends through the diaphragm)
- Fever
- Jaundice (if liver damage)
- Nausea
- Vomiting
- Weight loss

Diagnostic tests

- Ultrasonography and computed tomography (CT) scan with contrast medium can accurately define intrahepatic lesions and allow assessment of intra-abdominal pathology.
- Percutaneous needle aspiration of the abscess can also be performed with diagnostic tests to identify the causative organism.
- Contrast-aided magnetic resonance imaging may also become an accurate method for diagnosing hepatic abscesses.

- Abnormal laboratory values include elevated levels of serum aspartate aminotransferase, alanine aminotransferase, alkaline phosphatase, and bilirubin; an increased white blood cell count; and decreased serum albumin levels.
- With pyogenic abscess, a blood culture can identify the bacterial agent.
- With amebic abscess, a stool culture and serologic and hemagglutination tests can isolate *Entamoeba histolytica.*

Treatment

- Percutaneous drainage either with ultrasound or CT guidance is usually sufficient to evacuate pus.
- Surgery may be performed to drain pus in patients with an unstable condition and continued sepsis (despite attempted nonsurgical treatment) and in patients with a persistent fever (lasting longer than 2 weeks) after percutaneous drainage and appropriate antibiotic therapy.
- Before the causative organism is identified, an antibiotic should be started immediately with aminoglycosides, cephalosporins, clindamycin, or chloramphenicol.
- When the causative organisms are identified, the antibiotic regimen should be modified to match the patient's sensitivities.
- An I.V. antibiotic should be administered for 14 days and then replaced with an oral preparation to complete a 6-week course.

Nursing considerations

- Provide supportive care, monitor vital signs (especially temperature), and maintain fluid and nutritional intake.
- Give an anti-infective and an antibiotic, as prescribed, and watch for possible adverse reactions. Stress the importance of compliance with therapy.

- Explain diagnostic and surgical procedures.
- Watch carefully for complications of abdominal surgery, such as hemorrhage or infection.
- Prepare the patient for I.V. antibiotic administration as an outpatient with home care support.

Liver cancer

A rare form of cancer, liver cancer (primary and metastatic hepatic carcinoma) has a high mortality. It's responsible for roughly 2% of all cancers in the United States and for 10% to 50% in Africa and parts of Asia. Liver cancer is most prevalent in males (particularly in those older than age 60); incidence increases with age. It's rapidly fatal, usually within 6 months, from GI hemorrhage, progressive cachexia, hepatic failure, or metastasis.

Most primary liver tumors (90%) originate in the parenchymatous cells and are hepatomas (hepatocellular carcinoma, primary lower-cell carcinoma). Some primary tumors originate in the intrahepatic bile ducts and are known as *cholangiomas* (cholangiocarcinoma, cholangiocellular carcinoma). Rarer tumors include a mixed-cell type, Kupffer cell sarcoma, and hepatoblastomas (which occur almost exclusively in children and are usually resectable and curable).

The liver is one of the most common sites of metastasis from other primary cancers—particularly those of the colon, rectum, stomach, pancreas, esophagus, lung, or breast—or melanoma. In the United States, metastatic liver cancer is more than 20 times more common than primary cancer and, after cirrhosis, is the leading cause of fatal hepatic disease. At times, liver metastasis may appear as a solitary lesion, the first sign of recurrence after a remission.

Causes
- Unknown
- Congenital in children

Predisposing factors
- Anabolic steroid use
- Chronic infection with hepatitis B or hepatitis C virus
- Cirrhosis
- Environmental exposure to carcinogens, such as the chemical compound aflatoxin (a mold that grows on rice and peanuts), thorium dioxide (a contrast medium formerly used in liver radiography), *Senecio* alkaloids, androgens, or oral estrogens

Signs and symptoms
- Bruit, hum, or rubbing sound if the tumor involves a large part of the liver
- Dependent edema
- Mass in the right upper quadrant
- Occasional evidence of metastasis through the venous system to the lungs, from lymphatics to the regional lymph nodes, or by direct invasion of the portal veins
- Occasional jaundice or ascites
- Severe pain in the epigastrium or the right upper quadrant
- Tender, nodular liver on palpation
- Weight loss, weakness, anorexia, fever

Diagnostic tests
- The confirming test is a needle or open biopsy of the liver. Liver cancer is difficult to diagnose in the presence of cirrhosis, but several tests can help identify it.
- Liver function studies (aspartate aminotransferase, alanine aminotransferase, alkaline phosphatase, lactate dehydrogenase, and bilirubin) show abnormal liver function.

- Alpha-fetoprotein level increases above 500 mcg/ml.
- Chest X-ray may rule out metastasis to the lungs.
- Liver scan may show filling defects.
- Arteriography may define large tumors.
- Electrolyte studies may indicate increased sodium retention (resulting in functional renal failure) and hypoglycemia, leukocytosis, hypercalcemia, or hypocholesterolemia.

Treatment

- A resectable hepatic tumor must be a single tumor in one lobe, without cirrhosis, jaundice, or ascites; few hepatic tumors are resectable. When possible, resection is done by lobectomy or partial hepatectomy.
- Radiation therapy may be used alone or with chemotherapy; both therapies combined produce a better response rate than either therapy used alone.
- Chemotherapeutic drugs include fluorouracil, doxorubicin (Rubex), methotrexate (Trexall), streptozocin (Zanosar), and lomustine I.V. or regular infusion of fluorouracil or floxuridine.
- Liver transplantation is an alternative for some patients.

Nursing considerations

- Provide comprehensive supportive measures and emotional support.
- Monitor the patient's diet throughout because he may need a special diet that restricts sodium, fluids (no alcohol allowed), and protein.
- Weigh the patient daily, and note intake and output accurately. Monitor the patient for signs and symptoms of ascites—peripheral edema, orthopnea, or exertional dyspnea. If ascites are present, measure and record abdominal girth daily.

- Elevate the patient's legs whenever possible to increase venous return and prevent edema.
- Monitor the patient's respiratory function. Note an increase in respiratory rate or shortness of breath. Bilateral pleural effusion (noted on chest X-ray) is common, as is metastasis to the lungs. Watch carefully for signs of hypoxemia from intrapulmonary arteriovenous shunting.
- Institute cooling measures, as tolerated, and administer aspirin suppositories as prescribed if no signs of GI bleeding are apparent. Avoid acetaminophen (Tylenol) because the diseased liver can't metabolize it.
- Provide meticulous skin care. Turn the patient frequently and keep his skin clean to prevent pressure ulcers. Apply lotion to prevent chafing, and give an antipruritic, such as diphenhydramine, for severe itching.
- Monitor the patient for encephalopathy. Many patients develop end-stage signs and symptoms of ammonia intoxication, including confusion, restlessness, irritability, agitation, delirium, asterixis, lethargy and, finally, coma.
- Give lactulose as prescribed if signs of encephalopathy develop.
- Monitor the patient's serum ammonia level and neurologic status. Be prepared to control ammonia accumulation with sorbitol (to induce osmotic diarrhea), neomycin (to reduce bacterial flora in the GI tract), lactulose (to control bacterial elaboration of ammonia), and sodium polystyrene sulfonate (to lower the potassium level).
- Irrigate the transhepatic catheter as prescribed if it's used to relieve obstructive jaundice.
- Monitor the patient's vital signs frequently for an indication of bleeding or infection.

- Give standard postoperative care if surgery is indicated. Watch for intraperitoneal bleeding and sepsis, which may precipitate a coma. Monitor the patient for renal failure by checking urine output, blood urea nitrogen, and creatinine levels hourly.

Lung abscess

A lung abscess is a localized bacterial infection accompanied by pus accumulation and tissue destruction. The abscess may be putrid (due to anaerobic bacteria) or nonputrid (due to anaerobes or aerobes); it commonly has a well-defined border. The availability of effective antibiotics has made lung abscesses much less common than they were in the past.

Complications include rupture into the pleural space, which results in empyema and, rarely, massive hemorrhage. A chronic lung abscess may cause localized bronchiectasis. Failure of an abscess to improve with antibiotic treatment suggests a possible underlying neoplasm or another cause of obstruction.

Causes

- Necrotizing pneumonia
- Poor oral hygiene with dental or gingival (gum) disease
- Septic pulmonary emboli

Signs and symptoms

- Anorexia
- Chills
- Clubbing of fingers
- Cough that may produce bloody, purulent, or foul-smelling sputum
- Diaphoresis
- Dyspnea
- Excessive sweating
- Fever
- Headache
- Malaise
- Pleuritic chest pain
- Weight loss

Diagnostic tests

- Auscultation of the chest may reveal crackles and decreased breath sounds.
- Chest X-ray shows a solid mass or a localized infiltrate with one or more clear spaces, usually containing air-fluid levels.
- Chest computed tomography scan confirms the presence of localized infiltrate or nodular density, occasionally with air-fluid level. Chest imaging may also identify airway masses or foreign bodies that have led to abscess formation.
- Percutaneous aspiration of an abscess or bronchoscopy may be used to obtain cultures to identify the causative organism. Bronchoscopy is only used if abscess resolution is eventful and the patient's condition permits it.
- Blood cultures, Gram stain, and sputum culture are also used to detect the causative organism.
- White blood cell count is commonly elevated.

Treatment

- Antibiotic therapy may last for months until radiographic resolution or definite stability occurs. Symptoms usually disappear in a few weeks.
- Postural drainage may facilitate discharge of necrotic material into upper airways, where expectoration is possible; oxygen therapy may relieve hypoxemia.
- A poor response to therapy requires resection of the lesion or removal of the diseased section of the lung.
- All patients need rigorous follow-up and serial chest X-rays.

Nursing considerations

- Assess the patient's respiratory status frequently.
- Give antibiotics as prescribed.
- Monitor continuous pulse oximetry.
- Provide chest physiotherapy.
- Encourage coughing and deep breathing exercises and incentive spirometry use.
- Encourage the patient to increase his intake of fluids if his condition allows to loosen secretions.
- Provide a quiet, restful atmosphere.
- Provide postoperative care if surgery is needed. Maintain chest tube as prescribed and monitor the closed drainage system for an air leak.

▌Lung cancer

Lung cancer usually develops within the wall or epithelium of the bronchial tree. Its most common types are epidermoid (squamous cell) carcinoma, small cell (oat cell) carcinoma, adenocarcinoma, and large cell (anaplastic) carcinoma.

Although the prognosis is usually poor, it varies with the extent of spread at the time of diagnosis and the growth rate of the specific cell type. Only about 13% of patients with lung cancer survive 5 years after diagnosis. Lung cancer is the most common cause of cancer death in males and is fast becoming the most common cause in females, even though it's largely preventable.

Causes
- Unknown

Predisposing factors
- Exposure to carcinogenic and industrial air pollutants (asbestos, arsenic, chromium, coal dust, iron oxides, nickel, radioactive dust, and uranium)
- Genetics
- Smoking

Signs and symptoms
Early stage
- No symptoms

Late stage
- Anorexia
- Chest pain
- Cough
- Dyspnea
- Fever
- Hemoptysis
- Hoarseness
- Shoulder pain
- Weakness
- Weight loss
- Wheezing

Conditions from tumor-related changes in hormone regulation
- Cushing's and carcinoid syndromes (with small-cell carcinoma)
- Gynecomastia (with large-cell carcinoma)
- Hypercalcemia (with epidermoid tumors)
- Hypertrophic pulmonary osteoarthropathy—bone and joint pain from cartilage erosion due to abnormal production of growth hormone—with large-cell carcinoma or adenocarcinoma

Metastatic signs and symptoms
- Bronchial obstruction: hemoptysis, atelectasis, pneumonitis, and dyspnea
- Cervical thoracic sympathetic nerve involvement: miosis, ptosis, exophthalmos, and reduced sweating
- Chest wall invasion: piercing chest pain, increasing dyspnea, and severe shoulder pain, radiating down the arm
- Esophageal compression: dysphagia

- Local lymphatic spread: cough, hemoptysis, stridor, and pleural effusion
- Pericardial involvement: pericardial effusion, tamponade, and arrhythmias
- Phrenic nerve involvement: dyspnea, shoulder pain, and unilateral paralyzed diaphragm, with paradoxical motion
- Recurrent nerve invasion: hoarseness and vocal cord paralysis
- Vena caval obstruction: venous distention and edema of the face, neck, chest, or back

Diagnostic tests

- Chest X-ray usually shows an advanced lesion, but it can detect a lesion up to 2 years before symptoms appear. It also indicates tumor size and location.
- Sputum cytology analysis, which is 75% reliable, requires a specimen coughed up from the lungs and tracheobronchial tree, not postnasal secretions or saliva.
- Computed tomography (CT) scan of the chest may help to delineate the tumor's size and its relationship to surrounding structures.
- Bronchoscopy can locate the tumor site. Bronchoscopic washings provide material for cytologic and histologic examination. The flexible fiber-optic bronchoscope increases the test's effectiveness.
- A needle biopsy of the lungs uses biplane fluoroscopic visual control or CT guidance to detect peripherally located tumors. This allows a firm diagnosis in 80% of patients.
- Tissue biopsy of accessible metastatic sites includes supraclavicular and mediastinal node and pleural biopsies.
- Thoracentesis allows chemical and cytologic examination of pleural fluid.
- Preoperative mediastinoscopy or mediastinotomy can rule out involvement of

mediastinal lymph nodes (which would preclude curative pulmonary resection).
- Other tests to detect metastasis include a bone scan, positron emission tomography scan, bone marrow biopsy (recommended in small cell carcinoma), and a CT scan of the brain or abdomen.
- After histologic confirmation, staging determines the extent of the disease and helps in planning treatment and predicting the prognosis. (See *Staging lung cancer.*)

Treatment
Surgery

- Unless the tumor is nonresectable or other conditions rule out surgery, excision is the primary treatment for stage I, stage II, or selected stage III squamous cell carcinoma, adenocarcinoma, and large cell carcinoma.
- Excision may include partial removal of a lung (wedge resection, segmental resection, lobectomy, radical lobectomy) or total removal (pneumonectomy, radical pneumonectomy).

Radiation therapy

- Radiation preoperatively may reduce tumor bulk to allow for surgical resection.
- Preradiation chemotherapy helps improve response rates.
- Radiation is ordinarily recommended for stage I and stage II lesions, if surgery is contraindicated, and for stage III lesions when the disease is confined to the involved hemithorax and the ipsilateral supraclavicular lymph nodes.
- It's delayed until 1 month after surgery, to allow the wound to heal, and is then directed to the part of the chest most likely to develop metastasis.
- High-dose radiation therapy or radiation implants may also be used.

Staging lung cancer

Using the tumor, node, metastasis (TNM) classification system, the American Joint Committee on Cancer stages lung cancer as follows:

Primary tumor

TX—primary tumor can't be assessed, or malignant tumor cells detected in sputum or bronchial washings, but undetected by X-ray or bronchoscopy

T0—no evidence of primary tumor

Tis—carcinoma in situ

T1—tumor 3 cm or less in greatest dimension, surrounded by normal lung or visceral pleura; no bronchoscopic evidence of cancer closer to the center of the body than the lobar bronchus

T2—tumor larger than 3 cm; or one that involves the main bronchus and is 2 cm or more from the carina; or one that invades the visceral pleura; or one that's accompanied by atelectasis or obstructive pneumonitis that extends to the hilar region but doesn't involve the entire lung

T3—tumor of any size that extends into neighboring structures, such as the chest wall, diaphragm, or mediastinal pleura; or a tumor in the main bronchus that doesn't involve but is less than 2 cm from the carina; or a tumor that's accompanied by atelectasis or obstructive pneumonitis of the entire lung

T4—tumor of any size that invades the mediastinum, heart, great vessels, trachea, esophagus, vertebral body, or carina; or a tumor with malignant pleural effusion

Regional lymph nodes

NX—regional lymph nodes can't be assessed

N0—no detectable metastasis to lymph nodes

N1—metastasis to the ipsilateral peribronchial or hilar lymph nodes or both

N2—metastasis to the ipsilateral mediastinal or subcarinal lymph nodes or both

N3—metastasis to the contralateral mediastinal or hilar lymph nodes, the ipsilateral or contralateral scalene lymph nodes, or the supraclavicular lymph nodes

Distant metastasis

MX—distant metastasis can't be assessed

M0—no evidence of distant metastasis

M1—distant metastasis

Staging categories

Lung cancer progresses from mild to severe as follows:

Occult carcinoma—TX, N0, M0

Stage 0—Tis, N0, M0

Stage I—T1, N0, M0; T2, N0, M0

Stage II—T1, N1, M0; T2, N1, M0

Stage IIIA—T1, N2, M0; T2, N2, M0; T3, N0, M0; T3, N1, M0; T3, N2, M0

Stage IIIB—any T, N3, M0; T4, any N, M0

Stage IV—any T, any N, M1

Chemotherapy

■ Chemotherapy includes a combinations of drugs, which produce a response rate of about 40%, but have a minimal effect on overall survival.

■ Promising combinations for treating small cell carcinomas include cyclophosphamide with doxorubicin and vincristine; cyclophosphamide with doxorubicin, vincristine, and etoposide; and etoposide with cisplatin, cyclophosphamide, and doxorubicin.

Laser therapy

- In laser therapy, laser energy is directed through a bronchoscope to destroy local tumors.

Immunotherapy

- Immunotherapy is investigational. Nonspecific regimens using bacille Calmette-Guérin (BCG) vaccine or, possibly, *Corynebacterium parvum* offer the most promise.

Nursing considerations
Before surgery

- Supplement and reinforce information about the disease and the surgical procedure.
- Explain expected postoperative procedures, such as the insertion of an indwelling urinary catheter, use of an endotracheal or chest tube (or both), dressing changes, and I.V. therapy.
- Teach the patient how to perform coughing, deep diaphragmatic breathing, and range-of-motion (ROM) exercises.

After thoracic surgery

- Maintain a patent airway, and monitor chest tubes to reestablish normal intrathoracic pressure and prevent postoperative and pulmonary complications.
- Check the patient's vital signs every 15 minutes during the first hour after surgery, every 30 minutes during the next 4 hours, and then every 2 hours. Watch for abnormal respiration and other changes.
- Suction the patient often, and encourage him to begin deep breathing and coughing as soon as possible. Check secretions often. Initially, sputum will be thick and dark with blood, but it should become thinner and grayish yellow within a day.

- Monitor and record closed chest drainage. Keep chest tubes patent and draining effectively.
- Position the patient on the surgical side to promote drainage and lung reexpansion.
- Watch for and report foul-smelling discharge and excessive drainage on the dressing. Usually, the dressing is removed after 24 hours, unless the wound appears infected.
- Monitor the patient's intake and output. Maintain adequate hydration.
- Watch for and treat infection, shock, hemorrhage, atelectasis, dyspnea, mediastinal shift, and pulmonary embolus.
- To help prevent pulmonary embolus, apply antiembolism stockings and encourage ROM exercises.

If the patient is receiving chemotherapy and radiation:
- Explain possible adverse effects of radiation and chemotherapy. Watch for, treat, and (when possible) try to prevent them.
- Ask the dietary department to provide soft, nonirritating foods that are high in protein, and encourage the patient to eat high-calorie between-meal snacks.
- Administer an antiemetic and an antidiarrheal as prescribed and as needed.
- Schedule patient care activities in a way that helps the patient conserve his energy.
- Administer skin care to minimize skin breakdown. If the patient receives radiation therapy in an outpatient setting, warn him to avoid tight clothing, exposure to the sun, and harsh ointments on his chest. Teach him exercises to help prevent shoulder stiffness.

Teach high-risk patients ways to reduce their chances of developing lung cancer:
- Refer smokers who want to quit to local branches of the American Cancer

Society, Smokenders, or other smoking-cessation programs or suggest group therapy, individual counseling, or hypnosis.

- Encourage patients with recurring or chronic respiratory tract infections and those with chronic lung disease who detect a change in the character of a cough to see their practitioner promptly for evaluation.

▌Lupus erythematosus

A chronic inflammatory disorder of the connective tissues, lupus erythematosus appears in two forms: *discoid lupus erythematosus,* which affects only the skin, and *systemic lupus erythematosus* (SLE), which affects multiple organ systems (as well as the skin) and can be fatal. Like rheumatoid arthritis, SLE is characterized by recurring remissions and exacerbations, which are especially common during spring and summer. Onset may be acute or insidious and produce no characteristic clinical pattern.

SLE strikes 8 times more females than males, increasing to 15 times among females of childbearing years. It occurs worldwide, but is most prevalent among Asians and Blacks. The prognosis improves with early detection and treatment, but remains poor for patients who develop cardiovascular, renal, or neurologic complications or severe bacterial infections.

Causes
- Unknown

Predisposing factors
- Abnormal estrogen metabolism
- Drugs such as procainamide, hydralazine, and anticonvulsants
- Exposure to sunlight or ultraviolet light

- Immunization
- Pregnancy
- Streptococcal or viral infection
- Stress

Signs and symptoms
- Aching
- Anorexia
- Chills
- Fatigue
- Fever (low-grade or spiking)
- Malaise
- May involve any organ system (see *Signs and symptoms of systemic lupus erythematosus,* page 370)
- Polyarthralgia
- Rashes
- Weight loss

Joint and skin effects
- Butterfly rash over the nose and cheeks
- Erythematous rash in areas exposed to light
- Painless ulcers of the mucous membranes
- Patchy alopecia
- Raynaud's phenomenon
- Scaly papular rash (mimics psoriasis), especially in sun-exposed areas (see *Discoid lupus erythematosus,* page 371)
- Similar to that in rheumatoid arthritis (usually nonerosive)
- Vasculitis (especially in the digits), possibly leading to infarctive lesions, necrotic leg ulcers, or digital gangrene

Cardiopulmonary effects
- Cardiac: pericardial effusion, pericarditis, myocarditis, endocarditis, and early coronary atherosclerosis
- Pulmonary abnormalities: pleurisy, pleural effusions, pneumonitis, pulmonary hypertension and, rarely, pulmonary hemorrhage

Signs and symptoms of systemic lupus erythematosus

Diagnosing systemic lupus erythematosus (SLE) is difficult because it commonly mimics other diseases, with the signs and symptoms often vague and varying greatly from patient to patient.

For this reason, the American Rheumatism Association has issued a list of criteria for classifying SLE, to be used primarily for consistency in epidemiologic surveys. Usually, four or more of these signs are present at some time during the course of the disease:

- malar or discoid rash
- photosensitivity
- oral or nasopharyngeal ulcerations
- nonerosive arthritis (of two or more peripheral joints)
- pleuritis or pericarditis
- profuse proteinuria (exceeding 0.5 g/day) or excessive cellular casts in the urine
- seizures or psychoses
- hemolytic anemia, leukopenia, lymphopenia, or thrombocytopenia
- anti-double-stranded deoxyribonucleic acid (anti-DNA) or antiSmith antibody test or positive findings of antiphospholipid antibodies (elevated immunoglobulin [Ig] G or IgM anticardiolipin antibodies, positive test for lupus anticoagulant, or false-positive serologic tests for syphilis)
- abnormal antinuclear antibody titer.

Renal effects

- Glomerulonephritis (microscopic hematuria, pyuria, and urine sediment with cellular casts)
- Renal disease (possibly progressing to kidney failure, particularly when untreated)
- Urinary tract infections

Neurologic effects

- Central nervous system (CNS) involvement, possibly with emotional instability, psychosis, and organic brain syndrome
- Headaches, irritability, and depression (common)
- Seizure disorders, peripheral neuropathy, and mental dysfunction

Systemic effects

- Irregular menstrual periods or amenorrhea (during the active phase of SLE)
- Lymph node enlargement (diffuse or local, nontender), abdominal pain, nausea, vomiting, diarrhea, and constipation

Diagnostic tests

- Specific tests for SLE include antinuclear antibody (ANA), anti-DNA, and lupus erythematosus (LE) cell tests, which produce positive findings in most patients with active SLE, but are only marginally useful in diagnosing the disease. The ANA test is sensitive but not specific for SLE, the anti-DNA test is specific for SLE but not sensitive, and the LE test is neither sensitive nor specific for SLE.
- Complete blood cell count with differential may show anemia and a decreased white blood cell (WBC) count.
- Platelet count may be decreased.
- Erythrocyte sedimentation rate may be elevated.
- Serum electrophoresis may show hypergammaglobulinemia.
- Urine studies may show red blood cells and WBCs, urine casts and sedi-

Discoid lupus erythematosus

Discoid lupus erythematosus (DLE) is a form of lupus erythematosus marked by chronic skin eruptions that can lead to scarring and permanent disfigurement if untreated. About 5% of patients with DLE later develop systemic lupus erythematosus (SLE).

Causes

The exact cause of DLE is unknown, but some evidence suggests an autoimmune defect. An estimated 60% of patients with DLE are women in their late 20s or older. This disease is rare in children.

Signs and symptoms

DLE lesions are raised, red, scaling plaques, with follicular plugging and central atrophy. The raised edges and sunken centers give them a coinlike appearance. Although these lesions can appear anywhere on the body, they usually erupt on the face, scalp, ears, neck, and arms or on any part of the body that's exposed to sunlight.

Such lesions can resolve completely or may cause hypopigmentation or hyperpigmentation, atrophy, and scarring. Facial plaques sometimes assume the butterfly pattern characteristic of SLE. Hair tends to become brittle or may fall out in patches; alopecia can be permanent.

Diagnosis

As a rule, the patient history and the appearance of the rash itself are diagnostic. A lupus erythematosus cell test is positive in fewer than 10% of patients. A skin biopsy of lesions reveals immunoglobulins or complement components. SLE must be ruled out.

Treatment

Patients with DLE should avoid prolonged exposure to the sun, fluorescent lighting, or reflected sunlight. They should wear protective clothing, use sunscreen, avoid engaging in outdoor activities during periods of most intense sunlight (between 10 a.m. and 2 p.m.), and report changes in the lesions. Drug treatment consists of topical, intralesional, or systemic medication, as in SLE.

---

ment, and significant protein loss (more than 0.5 g/24 hours).
- Blood studies reveal decreased serum complement (C3 and C4) levels, which indicate active disease.
- Chest X-ray may show pleurisy or lupus pneumonitis.
- Electrocardiography may show a conduction defect with cardiac involvement or pericarditis.
- Kidney biopsy determines the stage of the disease and the extent of renal involvement.
- Some patients show a positive lupus anticoagulant test and a positive anticardiolipin test. Such patients are prone to antiphospholipid syndrome (thrombosis, abortion, and thrombocytopenia).
- Researchers have noted a significant association between the presence of activated protein C resistance and thrombosis in patients with SLE.

Treatment
- Patients with mild disease require little or no medication.
- Nonsteroidal anti-inflammatory drugs, including aspirin, control arthritis symptoms in many patients.

- Skin lesions need topical treatment. Corticosteroid creams, such as hydrocortisone or triamcinolone, are recommended for acute lesions.

 Refractory skin lesions are treated with an intralesional corticosteroid or antimalarial such as hydroxychloroquine. Because hydroxychloroquine can cause retinal damage, such treatment requires ophthalmologic examination every 6 months.

- The treatment of choice, corticosteroids are used for systemic symptoms of SLE, for acute generalized exacerbations, or for serious disease related to vital organ systems, such as pleuritis, pericarditis, lupus nephritis, vasculitis, and CNS involvement.
- Initial doses equivalent to 60 mg or more of prednisone usually bring noticeable improvement within 48 hours.
- As soon as symptoms are under control, steroid dosage is slowly tapered. Rising serum complement levels and decreasing anti-DNA titers indicate that the patient is responding to treatment.
- Diffuse proliferative glomerulonephritis, a major complication of SLE, requires treatment with large doses of steroids and cytotoxic therapy (such as cyclophosphamide).
- Patients with SLE who are on long-term steroid therapy are at particular risk for osteonecrosis of the hips.
- If renal failure occurs, dialysis or a kidney transplant may be necessary.
- Antihypertensives and dietary changes may also be warranted in patients with renal disease.
- In some patients, cytotoxic drugs, such as azathioprine (Imuran), chlorambucil (Leukeran), cyclophosphamide (Neosar), and methotrexate (Trexall), can delay or prevent renal deterioration.

- Joint replacement may be indicated if chronic synovitis and pain are problematic.

Nursing considerations

- Provide supportive care and emotional support.
- Watch for constitutional signs and symptoms, including joint pain or stiffness, weakness, fever, fatigue, and chills. Observe the patient for dyspnea, chest pain, and edema of the extremities.
- Check urine for hematuria, scalp for hair loss, and skin and mucous membranes for petechiae, bleeding, ulceration, pallor, and bruising.
- Provide a balanced diet. Foods high in protein, vitamins, and iron help the patient maintain optimum nutrition and prevent anemia. However, renal involvement may mandate a low-sodium, low-protein diet.
- Urge the patient to get plenty of rest. Schedule diagnostic tests and procedures to allow adequate rest.
- Explain all tests and procedures. Tell the patient that several blood samples are needed initially, then periodically, to monitor her progress.
- Apply heat packs to relieve joint pain and stiffness.
- Encourage regular exercise to maintain full range of motion (ROM) and prevent contractures. Teach ROM exercises as well as body alignment and postural techniques. Arrange for physical therapy and occupational counseling as appropriate.
- Explain the expected benefit of prescribed medications, and watch for adverse reactions, especially when the patient is taking high doses of a corticosteroid.
- Advise the patient receiving cyclophosphamide to drink plenty of fluids.
- Monitor the patient's vital signs, intake and output, weight, and laboratory re-

Managing lupus

Review these educational points with the patient with lupus:

■ Remember to schedule regular check-ups and keep your appointments. Routine blood tests and frequent blood pressure screening can detect a flare-up of lupus in the early stages.

■ Report unexplained signs and symptoms, such as weight loss, fever, extreme fatigue, or persistent fluid retention.

■ Eat a balanced diet and participate in a low-impact exercise program to maintain your energy level and control your weight.

■ Take a calcium supplement and a multivitamin with vitamin D to reduce your risk of osteoporosis if you're taking prednisone. Check with your practitioner for dosage information.

■ Avoid intense sun exposure because it can trigger symptoms. Wear a wide-brimmed hat and long-sleeved clothing outdoors, and stay indoors during the brightest hours of the day. Always apply sunblock and repeat the application for the best protection.

■ Report fever or other sign of infection to your practitioner because antibiotic intervention may be needed.

■ Consult your practitioner before dental or genitourinary procedures because you may need to take an antibiotic first to prevent infection.

■ Check with your practitioner to see if he recommends yearly flu and pneumonia shots for you.

■ Practice effective birth control if you have active lupus (particularly with kidney involvement) or if you're taking a cytotoxic drug. Very active lupus and drug therapy pose significant risks for both mother and child. Some patients with lupus can have successful pregnancies, but planning and discussing with your practitioner is essential.

■ Follow the prescribed drug regimen for the best long-term lupus management.

■ Check with your practitioner or pharmacist regarding special information about your drug regimen (such as taking a drug before, after, or with meals) to derive the most benefit and avoid adverse reactions.

---

ports. Check pulse rates, and watch for orthopnea. Check stools and GI secretions for blood.

■ Observe the patient for hypertension, weight gain, and other signs of renal involvement.

■ Assess the patient for signs of neurologic damage: personality change, paranoid or psychotic behavior, ptosis, or diplopia. Take seizure precautions. If Raynaud's phenomenon is present, warm and protect the patient's hands and feet.

■ Refer the patient to the Lupus Foundation of America and the Arthritis Foundation as necessary.

■ Explain to the patient of childbearing age that available evidence indicates that a woman with SLE can have a safe, successful pregnancy if she has no serious renal or neurologic impairment.

■ Provide patient teaching. (See *Managing lupus.*)

Lyme disease

A multisystemic disorder, Lyme disease is caused by the spirochete *Borrelia burgdorferi,* which is carried by the minute tick *Ixodes dammini* or another tick in the Ixodidae family. Ticks are most active in the spring, summer, and fall.

Lyme disease typically begins with the classic skin lesion called *erythema chronicum migrans*. Weeks or months later, cardiac or neurologic abnormalities sometimes develop, possibly followed by arthritis.

Lyme disease occurs primarily in areas of the United States inhabited by the deer tick, such as:

- in the northeast, from Massachusetts to Maryland
- in the midwest, in Wisconsin and Minnesota
- in the west, in California and Oregon.

Although Lyme disease is endemic to these areas, cases have been reported in all 50 states and 20 other countries, including Germany, Switzerland, France, and Australia.

Causes
- *Borrelia burgdorferi*

Signs and symptoms
Stage 1
- Lesions:
  - Commonly located at the site of a tick bite
  - Hot, itchy
  - May grow to more than 20″ (50 cm) in diameter
  - Red macule or papule

  Also:
- Additional lesions, malar rash, conjunctivitis, or diffuse urticaria (within days of bite)
- Constant malaise and fatigue
- Intermittent headache, fever, chills, achiness, and regional lymphadenopathy
- Meningeal irritation, mild encephalopathy, migrating musculoskeletal pain, and hepatitis (less common)
- Persistent sore throat and dry cough
- Small red blotches (3 to 4 weeks after bite, persisting several more weeks)

Stage 2 (begins weeks to months later)
- Cardiac abnormalities such as a brief, fluctuating atrioventricular heart block
- Facial palsy
- Neurologic abnormalities—fluctuating meningoencephalitis with peripheral and cranial neuropathy (usually resolve after days or months)

Stage 3 (begins weeks or years later)
- Arthritis (may become chronic with severe cartilage and bone erosion)

Diagnostic tests
- Blood tests, including antibody titers to identify *B. burgdorferi*, are the most practical diagnostic tests. The enzyme-linked immunosorbent assay (ELISA) may be ordered because of its greater sensitivity and specificity. ELISAs are confirmed with Western blot analysis. However, serologic test results don't always confirm the diagnosis—especially in the disease's early stages before the body produces antibodies—or seropositivity for *B. burgodorferi*.
- Indirect immunofluorescent antibody tests are marginally sensitive.
- Blood studies show mild anemia and an elevated erythrocyte sedimentation rate, leukocyte count, serum immunoglobulin M level, and aspartate aminotransferase level.

Treatment
- A 28-day course of antibiotic treatment using doxycycline or amoxicillin is generally effective in early disease. Cefuroxime axetil, tetracycline, and ceftriaxone are alternatives.
- Oral penicillin is usually prescribed for children.
- When given in the early stages, these drugs can minimize later complications. When given during the late stages, high-

dose I.V. penicillin or I.V. ceftriaxone may be a successful treatment.

■ Neurologic abnormalities are best treated with I.V. ceftriaxone or I.V. penicillin.

Nursing considerations

■ Take a detailed patient history, asking about travel to endemic areas and exposure to ticks.

■ Check for drug allergies, and carefully administer the prescribed antibiotic.

■ Help with range-of-motion and strengthening exercises if arthritis is present, but avoid overexertion.

■ Assess the patient's neurologic function and level of consciousness frequently. Watch for signs of increased intracranial pressure and cranial nerve involvement, such as ptosis, strabismus, and diplopia.

■ Monitor for cardiac arrhythmias.

Lymphomas, malignant

Also known as *non-Hodgkin's lymphomas* and *lymphosarcomas,* malignant lymphomas are a heterogeneous group of malignant diseases originating in lymph glands and other lymphoid tissue. Nodular lymphomas have a better prognosis than the diffuse form of the disease, but in both, the prognosis is worse than in Hodgkin's disease.

Up to 35,000 new cases appear annually in the United States. Malignant lymphomas are two to three times more common in males than in females and occur in all age-groups.

Although rare in children, these lymphomas occur one to three times more often and cause twice as many deaths as Hodgkin's disease in children under age 15. Incidence rises with age (median age is 50). Malignant lymphomas seem linked to certain races and ethnic

groups, with increased incidence in whites and people of Jewish ancestry.

Causes

■ Unknown

Signs and symptoms

■ Fatigue

■ Fever

■ Malaise

■ Night sweats

■ Nodes on cervical region, with dyspnea and coughing (in children)

■ Swelling of the lymph glands, enlarged tonsils and adenoids, and painless, rubbery nodes in the cervical or supraclavicular areas

■ Weight loss

Diagnostic tests

■ Histologic evaluation of biopsied lymph nodes of tonsils, bone marrow, liver, bowel, or skin or of tissue removed during exploratory laparotomy.

■ A biopsy differentiates malignant lymphoma from Hodgkin's disease.

■ Other tests include chest X-rays; lymphangiography; liver, bone, and spleen scans, computed tomography scan of the abdomen; and excretory urography.

■ Laboratory tests include a complete blood cell count (which may show anemia), uric acid level (elevated or normal), serum calcium level (elevated if bone lesions are present), serum protein level (normal), and liver function studies.

Treatment

■ Radiation therapy is used mainly in the early localized stage of the disease. Total nodal irradiation is usually effective for nodular and diffuse histologies.

■ Chemotherapy is most effective with multiple combinations of antineoplastics; remissions and cures may be induced in this manner.

■ Some cases have required intrathecal chemotherapy.

Nursing considerations

■ Monitor the patient who's receiving radiation or chemotherapy for anorexia, nausea, vomiting, or diarrhea. Plan small, frequent meals scheduled around treatment.

■ Administer I.V. fluids as prescribed if the patient can't tolerate oral intake.

■ Administer an antiemetic and a sedative as prescribed if necessary.

■ Instruct the patient to keep irradiated skin dry.

■ Provide emotional support by informing the patient and his family about the prognosis and diagnosis and by listening to their concerns. If needed, refer the patient and family to the local chapter of the American Cancer Society for information and counseling.

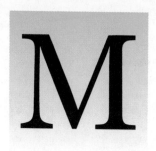

Macular degeneration

Macular degeneration, which is atrophy or degeneration of the macular disk, accounts for about 12% of all cases of blindness in the United States. At least 10% of elderly U.S. residents have irreversible central vision loss from age-related macular degeneration. It affects slightly more women than men.

Two types of age-related macular degeneration occur. The dry, or *atrophic*, form is characterized by atrophic pigment epithelial changes and is usually associated with a slow, progressive distortion of straight lines or edges and central vision loss. The wet, or *exudative*, form causes rapid onset of vision impairment. It's characterized by subretinal neovascularization that causes leakage, hemorrhage, and fibrovascular scar formation, which produce significant loss of central vision.

Causes
- Formation of drusen (clumps of epithelium) or subretinal neovascular membrane in the macular region

Predisposing factors
- Cigarette smoking
- Lack of antioxidants, such as vitamins C and E

Signs and symptoms
- Central vision change such as a blank spot in the center of the page when reading

Diagnostic tests
- Indirect ophthalmoscopy may reveal gross macular changes.
- Amsler grid reveals central visual field distortion.
- I.V. fluorescein angiography may show leaking vessels as fluorescein dye flows into the tissues from the subretinal neovascular net.

Treatment
- Laser photocoagulation reduces the incidence of severe vision loss in patients with subretinal neovascularization.
- Photodynamic therapy with verteporfin, a newer form of laser therapy, is effective in selected patients.

Nursing considerations
- Inform patients who have bilateral central vision loss of the low-vision rehabilitation services that are available to them.
- Explain that special devices, such as low-vision optical aids, are available for patients with good peripheral vision.

Malignant melanoma

Incidence of malignant melanoma, a neoplasm that arises from melanocytes, has increased by 50% in the past 20 years. In particular, an increase in incidence of melanoma in situ suggests that these malignancies are now being detected earlier. The incidence varies in different populations but is about 10 times more common in white than in nonwhite populations. The four types of melanomas are superficial spreading melanoma, nodular malignant melanoma, lentigo maligna melanoma, and acral-lentiginous melanoma.

Melanoma spreads through the lymphatic and vascular systems and metastasizes to the regional lymph nodes, skin, liver, lungs, and central nervous system (CNS). Its course is unpredictable, however, and recurrence and metastasis may occur more than 5 years after resection of the primary lesion. If it spreads to regional lymph nodes, the patient has a 50% chance of survival.

Common sites for melanoma are on the head and neck in men, on the legs in females, and on the backs of people exposed to excessive sunlight. Up to 70% arise from a preexisting nevus. In rare instances, they may appear in the conjunctiva, choroid, pharynx, mouth, vagina, or anus.

Suspect melanoma by using the ABCD Rule of Melanoma:
- *A*symmetry of borders
- *B*leeding or crusting
- *C*olor: blue-black or variegated
- *D*iameter greater than ¼″ (6 mm)

The prognosis varies with tumor thickness. Generally, superficial lesions are curable, whereas deeper lesions tend to metastasize. The Breslow Level Method measures tumor depth from the granular level of the epidermis to the deepest melanoma cell. Melanoma lesions less than 0.76 mm deep have an excellent prognosis, whereas deeper lesions (those 0.76 mm deep or deeper) are at risk for metastasis. The prognosis is better for a tumor on an extremity (which is drained by one lymphatic network) than for one on the head, neck, or trunk (which is drained by several networks).

Causes
- Autoimmune factors
- Excessive exposure to ultraviolet light:
  - Most common in sunny, warm areas
  - Parts of the body exposed to sunlight
  - Blistering sunburn before age 20 (increases risk twofold)
- Genetic factors (increases risk eightfold)
- Hormonal factors (possible increased risk and accelerated growth with pregnancy)
- History of melanoma (10 times the risk of developing second melanoma)
- Skin type:
  - Blond or red hair, fair skin, and blue eyes
  - Prone to sunburn
  - Celtic or Scandinavian descent
  - Rare among blacks (when it does develop, it usually arises in lightly pigmented areas—the palms, plantar surface of the feet, or mucous membranes)

Signs and symptoms
- Superficial spreading melanoma:
  - Develops on sun-exposed areas of the body
  - Horizontal growth may continue for many years
  - Irregular, notched margin
  - Red, white, and blue color over a brown or black background

– Small, elevated tumor nodules that may ulcerate and bleed
– Worsening of prognosis with vertical growth.

- Nodular malignant melanoma:
  – Develops on any area of the body
  – More common in men
  – Most frequently misdiagnosed melanoma (resembles a blood blister or polyp).
- Lentigo maligna melanoma:
  – Develops under the fingernails, on the face, and on the backs of the hands
  – Large (1″ to 2″ [2.5- to 5-cm]), flat freckle of tan, brown, black, whitish, or slate color
  – Scattered black nodules on the surface
  – Slow to develop (usually over many years); ulceration possible
- Acral-lentiginous melanoma:
  – More common in Asian and Black people

Diagnostic tests

- A skin biopsy with histologic examination can distinguish malignant melanoma from a benign nevus, seborrheic keratosis, and pigmented basal cell epithelioma; it can also determine tumor thickness.
- Physical examination, paying particular attention to lymph nodes, can point to metastatic involvement.
- Baseline laboratory studies include a complete blood count with differential, erythrocyte sedimentation rate, platelet count, liver function studies, and urinalysis.
- Depending on the depth of tumor invasion and metastasis, baseline diagnostic studies may also include a chest X-ray and computed tomography (CT) scan of the chest and abdomen.

- Signs of bone metastasis may call for a bone scan; CNS metastasis, a CT scan of the brain.

Treatment

- The extent of surgical resection depends on the size and location of the primary lesion.
- Closure of a wide resection may require a skin graft.
- Surgical treatment may also include regional lymphadenectomy.
- Cutaneous melanoma is nearly 100% curable by excision if diagnosed when malignant cells are confined to the epidermis.
- Deep primary lesions may merit adjuvant chemotherapy and biotherapy or immunotherapy to eliminate or reduce the number of tumor cells.
- Radiation therapy is usually reserved for metastatic disease; gene therapy may also be a treatment option.
- Regardless of the treatment method, melanomas require close, long-term follow-up to detect metastasis and recurrences. About 13% of recurrences develop more than 5 years after the primary surgery.

Nursing considerations

- Provide preoperative teaching, meticulous postoperative care, and emotional support.
- Review the explanation of treatment options. Tell the patient what to expect before and after surgery, what the wound will look like, and what type of dressing he'll have.
- Warn the patient that the donor site for a skin graft may be as painful as the tumor excision site, if not more so. Honestly answer questions he may have about surgery, chemotherapy, and radiation.

- Take steps to prevent infection after surgery. Check dressings often for excessive drainage, foul odor, redness, or swelling.
- Apply an antiembolism stocking if surgery included lymphadenectomy and instruct the patient to keep the extremity elevated.
- Monitor the patient for adverse reactions to chemotherapy during administration and take measures to minimize them.

When preparing for discharge

- Emphasize the need for close follow-up to detect recurrences early. Explain that recurrences and metastasis, if they occur, are commonly delayed, so follow-up must continue for years.
- Tell the patient how to recognize signs of recurrence.
- Provide emotional support. Encourage the patient to verbalize his fears.

With advanced metastatic disease

- Make referrals for home care, social services, and spiritual and financial assistance as needed.
- Stress the detrimental effects of overexposure to solar radiation, especially to fair-skinned, blue-eyed patients. Recommend use of a sunblock or sunscreen.

Mallory-Weiss syndrome

Mild to massive and usually painless bleeding due to a tear in the mucosa or submucosa of the cardia or lower esophagus characterizes Mallory-Weiss syndrome. Such a tear, usually singular and longitudinal, results from prolonged or forceful vomiting. About 60% of these tears involve the cardia; 15%, the termi-

nal esophagus; and 25%, the region across the esophagogastric junction. Mallory-Weiss syndrome is most common in men older than age 40, especially alcoholics.

Causes
- Forceful or prolonged vomiting

Predisposing factors
- Atrophic gastric mucosa
- Childbirth
- Coughing
- Esophagitis
- Gastritis
- Hiatal hernia
- Seizures
- Straining during bowel movements
- Trauma

Signs and symptoms
- Epigastric or back pain, may range from mild to massive but is generally more profuse than in esophageal rupture.
- Massive bleeding—most likely when the tear is on the gastric side, near the cardia—may quickly lead to fatal shock. The blood vessels are only partially severed, preventing retraction and closure of the lumen.
- Vomiting of blood or the passing of large amounts of blood rectally a few hours to several days after normal vomiting.

Diagnostic tests
- Identifying esophageal tears by fiberoptic endoscopy confirms Mallory-Weiss syndrome. These lesions, which usually occur near the gastroesophageal junction, appear as erythematous longitudinal cracks in the mucosa when recently produced and as raised, white streaks surrounded by erythema when older.

■ Angiography (selective celiac arteriography) can determine the bleeding site but not the cause; this is used when endoscopy isn't available.

■ Serum hematocrit helps quantify blood loss.

Treatment

■ Appropriate treatment varies with the severity of bleeding. Usually, GI bleeding stops spontaneously, requiring supportive measures and careful observation but no definitive treatment. However, if bleeding continues, treatment may include:

– angiographic infusion of a vasoconstrictor (vasopressin) into the superior mesenteric artery or direct infusion into a vessel that leads to the bleeding artery

– transcatheter embolization or thrombus formation with an autologous blood clot or other hemostatic material (insertion of artificial material, such as a shredded absorbable gelatin sponge or, less commonly, the patient's own clotted blood through a catheter into the bleeding vessel to aid thrombus formation)

– surgery to suture each laceration (for massive recurrent or uncontrollable bleeding).

Nursing considerations

■ Monitor the patient's respiratory status including pulse oximetry and arterial blood gas measurements

■ Administer oxygen as prescribed.

■ Assess the amount of blood loss, and record related signs, such as hematemesis and melena (including color, amount, consistency, and frequency).

■ Monitor hematologic status (hemoglobin level, hematocrit, red blood cell count). Draw blood for coagulation studies (prothrombin time, partial thromboplastin time, and platelet count) and typing and crossmatching.

■ Try to keep three units of matched packed red blood cells on hand at all times as ordered. Until blood is available, insert a large-bore (14G to 18G) I.V. line, and start a temporary infusion of normal saline solution, as prescribed.

■ Monitor the patient's vital signs, central venous pressure, urine output, and overall clinical status.

■ Give an antiemetic, as prescribed, to prevent postoperative vomiting.

■ Advise the patient to avoid alcohol, aspirin, and other irritating substances.

■ Monitor the patient with portal hypertension for signs of hemorrhage.

▌Ménière's disease

Also known as *endolymphatic hydrops,* Ménière's disease is a labyrinthine dysfunction that produces severe vertigo, sensorineural hearing loss, and tinnitus. It usually affects adults, slightly more males than females, between ages 30 and 60. After multiple attacks over several years, this disorder leads to residual tinnitus and hearing loss.

Causes

■ Autonomic nervous system dysfunction producing a temporary constriction of blood vessels supplying the inner ear

■ Overproduction or decreased absorption of endolymph

■ Premenstrual edema

Signs and symptoms

■ Fullness or blocked feeling in the ear

■ Giddiness

■ Nystagmus

■ Sensorineural hearing loss

■ Severe nausea

■ DO'S & DON'TS

 During a Ménière's disease attack

To ease the effects of a Ménière's disease attack, instruct the patient on these do's and don'ts.

Do's
■ Keep the side rails of the bed up to prevent falls because an attack can begin quite rapidly.
■ Lie on the unaffected ear and look in the direction of the affected ear to decrease signs and symptoms.

Don'ts
■ Don't read or expose yourself to glaring light to reduce dizziness.
■ Don't make sudden position changes or do any tasks that vertigo makes hazardous.
■ Don't get out of bed or walk without assistance.

Managing Ménière's disease

■ Follow a low-sodium diet.
■ Avoid tobacco, alcohol, and caffeine as directed.
■ Practice stress management to help reduce the frequency and severity of vertiginous attacks.
■ Maintain your diversionary and social activities.
■ Try not to let the fear of vertigo stop you from participating in daily activities when vertigo is absent.

■ Severe vertigo
■ Sweating
■ Tinnitus
■ Vomiting

Diagnostic tests
■ Audiometric studies indicate a sensorineural hearing loss and loss of discrimination and recruitment.
■ Electronystagmography, electrocochleography, a computed tomography scan, magnetic resonance imaging, and X-rays of the internal meatus may be needed.

Treatment
Acute management
■ Atropine may stop an attack in 20 to 30 minutes.

■ Epinephrine or diphenhydramine may be necessary in a severe attack.
■ Dimenhydrinate, meclizine, diphenhydramine, or diazepam may be effective in a milder attack.

Long-term management
■ Ongoing therapy includes use of a diuretic or vasodilator and restricted sodium intake (less than 2 g/day). Avoiding high-sugar foods is also helpful.
■ A prophylactic antihistamine or a mild sedative (phenobarbital, diazepam) may also be helpful.
■ If Ménière's disease persists after 2 years of treatment, produces incapacitating vertigo, or resists medical management, surgery may be necessary. Destruction of the affected labyrinth

permanently relieves symptoms but causes irreversible hearing loss.
- Systemic streptomycin is reserved for patients in whom the disease is bilateral and no other treatment can be considered.

Nursing considerations
- Teach the patient what to do and not do during an attack to reduce dizziness and prevent injury. (See *During a Ménière's disease attack.*)

Before surgery
- Record fluid intake and output and characteristics of vomitus if the patient is vomiting. Give an antiemetic, as necessary, and small amounts of fluid frequently.

After surgery
- Record fluid intake and output carefully.
- Tell the patient to expect dizziness and nausea for 1 to 2 days after surgery.
- Give an antibiotic and an antiemetic as prescribed.
- Provide patient teaching information. (See *Managing Ménière's disease.*)

Meningitis

With meningitis, the brain and the spinal cord meninges become inflamed, usually as a result of bacterial infection. Such inflammation may involve all three meningeal membranes—the dura mater, arachnoid, and pia mater.

Meningitis commonly starts out as an inflammation of the pia arachnoid, which may progress to congestion of adjacent tissues and destroy some nerve cells.

The prognosis is good and complications are rare, especially if the disease is recognized early and the infecting organism responds to an antibiotic. However, mortality in patients with untreated meningitis is 70% to 100%. The prognosis is poorer for infants, elderly people, and those who are immunocompromised.

Causes
- Unknown
- Complication of another bacterial infection: bacteremia (especially from pneumonia, empyema, osteomyelitis, and endocarditis), sinusitis, otitis media, tooth abscess, encephalitis, myelitis, or brain abscess (usually caused by *Neisseria meningitidis, Haemophilus influenzae, Streptococcus pneumoniae,* and *Escherichia coli*)
- Complication of existing viral infection

Signs and symptoms
- In infants: possibly asymptomatic but may be fretful, refusing to eat, with copious vomiting leading to dehydration, which prevents a bulging fontanel and thus masks this important sign of increased intracranial pressure (ICP)
- Delirium, deep stupor, and coma
- Increased ICP—headache, vomiting and, rarely, papilledema
- Infection—fever, chills, and malaise
- Irritability
- Meningeal irritation—nuchal rigidity, positive Brudzinski's and Kernig's signs, exaggerated and symmetrical deep tendon reflexes, and opisthotonos (a spasm in which the back and extremities arch backward so that the body rests on the head and heels)
- Photophobia, diplopia, and other vision problems
- Sinus arrhythmias
- Twitching, seizures (in 30% of infants), or coma (with disease progression)

Two telltale signs of meningitis

Brudzinski's sign

To test for *Brudzinski's sign*, place the patient in a dorsal recumbent position, and then put your hands behind his neck and bend it forward. Pain and resistance may indicate meningeal inflammation, neck injury, or arthritis. However, if the patient also flexes the hips and knees in response to this manipulation, chances are he has meningitis.

Kernig's sign

To test for *Kernig's sign*, place the patient in a supine position. Flex his leg at the hip and knee, and then straighten the knee. Pain or resistance points to meningitis.

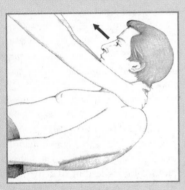

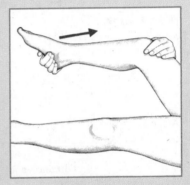

Diagnostic tests

■ A lumbar puncture showing typical findings in cerebrospinal fluid (CSF) and positive Brudzinski's and Kernig's signs usually establish this diagnosis. (See *Two telltale signs of meningitis*.)
■ The lumbar puncture usually indicates elevated CSF pressure from obstructed CSF outflow at the arachnoid villi. The fluid may appear cloudy or milky white, depending on the number of white blood cells present. CSF protein levels tend to be high; glucose levels may be low. (In those with subacute meningitis, CSF findings may vary.)
■ CSF culture and sensitivity tests usually identify the infecting organism, unless it's a virus.

■ Cultures of blood, urine, and nose and throat secretions; a chest X-ray; electrocardiography; and a physical examination, with special attention to skin, ears, and sinuses, can uncover the primary infection site.
■ Blood tests commonly reveal leukocytosis and serum electrolyte abnormalities.
■ Computed tomography scan can rule out cerebral hematoma, hemorrhage, or tumor.

Treatment

■ Vaccination against *H. influenzae* and pneumococcal meningitis begins at age 2 months and has decreased the incidence of these types of meningitis.

■ Usually, an I.V. antibiotic is given for at least 2 weeks and then followed by an oral antibiotic. The antibiotic is specific to the type of meningitis. Examples include ampicillin, cefotaxime, ceftriaxone, and nafcillin.

■ Other drugs include dexamethasone to help stabilize the blood-brain barrier; mannitol to decrease cerebral edema; an anticonvulsant (usually given I.V.) or a sedative to reduce restlessness; and aspirin or acetaminophen to relieve headache and fever.

■ Supportive measures include bed rest, fever reduction, and measures to prevent dehydration. Isolation is necessary if nasal cultures are positive.

■ Treat coexisting conditions, such as endocarditis or pneumonia.

■ To prevent meningitis, a prophylactic antibiotic may be used after ventricular shunting procedures, skull fracture, or penetrating head wounds, but this use is controversial.

Nursing considerations

■ Assess neurologic function often. Observe the patient's level of consciousness, and check for signs of increased ICP (plucking at the bedcovers, vomiting, seizures, a change in motor function and vital signs). Watch for signs of cranial nerve involvement (ptosis, strabismus, diplopia).

■ Watch for deterioration in the patient's condition, which may signal an impending crisis. (See *Ominous signs in meningitis.*)

■ Monitor fluid balance. Maintain adequate fluid intake to avoid dehydration, but avoid fluid overload because of the danger of cerebral edema. Measure central venous pressure and intake and output accurately.

■ Watch for adverse reactions to the I.V. antibiotic and other drugs. To avoid in-

Ominous signs in meningitis

Be especially alert for deterioration in the patient's condition as evidenced by:
■ temperature increase up to 102° F (38.9° C)
■ reduced level of consciousness
■ onset of seizures
■ altered respirations.

filtration and phlebitis, check the I.V. site often, and change the site according to facility policy.

■ Position the patient carefully to prevent joint stiffness and neck pain. Turn him often, according to a planned positioning schedule. Assist with range-of-motion exercises.

■ Maintain adequate nutrition and elimination. It may be necessary to provide small, frequent meals or supplement these meals with nasogastric tube or parenteral feedings.

■ To prevent constipation and minimize the risk of increased ICP resulting from straining during defecation, give the patient a mild laxative or stool softener.

■ Ensure the patient's comfort. Provide mouth care regularly. Maintain a quiet environment. Darkening the room may decrease photophobia.

■ Relieve headache with a nonopioid analgesic, such as aspirin or acetaminophen, as needed. (Opioids interfere with accurate neurologic assessment.)

■ Provide reassurance and support. The patient may be frightened by his illness and frequent lumbar punctures. If he's delirious or confused, attempt to reorient him often.

- Reassure the family that the delirium and behavior changes caused by meningitis usually disappear.
- If a severe neurologic deficit appears permanent, refer the patient to a rehabilitation program as soon as the acute phase of this illness has passed.
- To help prevent meningitis, teach patients with chronic sinusitis or other chronic infections—as well as those exposed to people with meningitis—the importance of quick and proper medical treatment.
- Follow strict aseptic technique when treating patients with head wounds or skull fractures.

Meningococcal infections

Two major meningococcal infections (meningitis and meningococcemia) are usually caused by the gram-negative bacteria *Neisseria meningitidis,* which also causes primary pneumonia, purulent conjunctivitis, endocarditis, sinusitis, and genital infection.

Bacteria are commonly present in upper respiratory flora. Transmission takes place through inhalation of an infected droplet from a carrier (2% to 38% of the population). The bacteria then localize in the nasopharynx.

After an incubation period of 3 to 4 days, the bacteria spread through the bloodstream to the joints, skin, adrenal glands, lungs, and central nervous system. The tissue damage that results (possibly due to the effects of bacterial endotoxins) produces symptoms and, with fulminant meningococcemia and meningococcal bacteremia, progresses to hemorrhage, thrombosis, and necrosis.

Meningococcemia occurs as simple bacteremia, fulminant meningococcemia and, rarely, chronic meningococcemia. It commonly accompanies meningitis. (For more information on meningitis, see "Meningitis," page 383.) Meningococcal infections may occur sporadically or in epidemics; virulent infections may be fatal within a matter of hours.

Meningococcal infections are most common among young children (ages 6 months to 1 year) and military recruits or those enrolled at facilities such as colleges, because of overcrowding.

Causes

- *Streptococcus pneumoniae* and *N. meningitidis*
- Seven serogroups of *N. meningitidis* (A, B, C, D, X, Y, and Z; group A causes most epidemics)

Signs and symptoms

- Arthralgia
- Chills
- Cough
- Headache
- Mild hypotension
- Myalgia (in the back and legs)
- Petechial, nodular, or maculopapular rash
- Seizures
- Sore throat
- Sudden, spiking fever
- Tachycardia
- Tachypnea

Fulminant meningococcemia

- Death from respiratory or heart failure in 6 to 24 hours (if untreated)
- Disseminated intravascular coagulation (DIC)
- Enlargement of skin lesions
- Extreme prostration
- Shock

In neonates and small infants

- Slow, inactive, or irritable; poor appetite and feeding

Chronic meningococcemia

- Enlarged spleen
- Intermittent fever
- Joint pain
- Maculopapular rash

Diagnostic tests

- Isolation of *N. meningitidis* through a positive blood culture, cerebrospinal fluid (CSF) culture, or lesion scraping confirms the diagnosis, except in those with nasopharyngeal infection, because *N. meningitidis* exists as part of the normal nasopharyngeal flora.
- Tests that support the diagnosis include counterimmunoelectrophoresis of the CSF or blood, low white blood cell count and, in patients with skin or adrenal hemorrhages, decreased platelet and clotting levels.
- Diagnostic evaluation must rule out Rocky Mountain spotted fever and vascular purpuras.

Treatment

- As soon as meningococcal infection is suspected, treatment begins with large doses of aqueous penicillin G, ampicillin, or a cephalosporin such as cefoxitin; or, for the patient who is allergic to penicillin, chloramphenicol I.V.
- Therapy may also include mannitol for cerebral edema, heparin I.V. for DIC, dopamine for shock, and digoxin and a diuretic if heart failure develops.
- Supportive measures include fluid and electrolyte maintenance, proper ventilation (patent airway and oxygen if necessary), insertion of an arterial line or a central venous pressure (CVP) line to monitor cardiovascular status, and bed rest.

- Chemoprophylaxis with rifampin or ciprofloxacin is useful for facility workers who come in close contact with the patient; minocycline can also temporarily eradicate the infection in carriers.
- The meningococcal vaccine can be administered to first-year college students living in dormitories as a preventive measure.

Nursing considerations

- Give I.V. antibiotics as prescribed. The dosage of the I.V. antibiotic should be adjusted as necessary to maintain blood and CSF drug levels.
- Enforce bed rest in early stages. Provide a dark, quiet, restful environment.
- Maintain adequate ventilation with oxygen or a ventilator, if necessary. Suction and turn the patient frequently.
- Keep accurate intake and output records to maintain proper fluid and electrolyte levels. Monitor blood pressure, pulse, arterial blood gas levels, and CVP.
- Watch for complications, such as DIC, arthritis, endocarditis, and pneumonia.
- Monitor the patient's complete blood count if he is receiving chloramphenicol.
- Check the patient's drug history for allergies before giving an antibiotic.

To prevent the spread of meningococcal infection

- Vaccines are available to prevent some strains of *N. meningitidis* and many types of *S. pneumoniae*. The vaccine against *Haemophilus influenzae* type B is safe and effective.
- Impose respiratory isolation until the patient has received antibiotic therapy for 24 hours.
- Label all meningococcal specimens. Deliver them to the laboratory quickly

because meningococci are sensitive to changes in humidity and temperature.
- Report all meningococcal infections to public health department officials.

Metabolic acidosis

A physiologic state of excess acid accumulation and deficient base bicarbonate, metabolic acidosis is produced by an underlying pathologic disorder. Symptoms result from the body's attempts to correct the acidotic condition through compensatory mechanisms in the lungs, kidneys, and cells.

Metabolic acidosis is more prevalent among children, who are vulnerable to acid-base imbalance because their metabolic rates are faster and their ratios of water to total body weight are lower. Severe or untreated metabolic acidosis can be fatal.

Causes
- Anaerobic carbohydrate metabolism (pump failure after myocardial infarction, or when pulmonary or hepatic disease, shock, or anemia)
- Diarrhea and intestinal malabsorption
- Excessive burning of fats in the absence of usable carbohydrates (diabetic ketoacidosis, chronic alcoholism, malnutrition, or a low-carbohydrate, high-fat diet)
- Exogenous poisoning, or Addison's disease with an increased excretion of sodium and chloride and the retention of potassium ions (due to a deficiency of glucocorticoids and mineralocorticoids)
- Renal insufficiency and failure (renal acidosis)
- Salicylate intoxication (overuse of aspirin)

Signs and symptoms
- Associated GI distress: anorexia, nausea, vomiting, and diarrhea, possibly leading to dehydration
- Central nervous system depression
- Fruity breath (if underlying diabetes mellitus)
- Headache and lethargy, progressing to drowsiness
- Kussmaul's respirations (as the lungs attempt to compensate by "blowing off" carbon dioxide)
- Stupor
- Coma and death (if untreated)

Diagnostic tests
- Arterial pH below 7.35 confirms metabolic acidosis.
- With severe acidotic states, pH may fall to 7.10 and partial pressure of arterial carbon dioxide may be normal or less than 34 mm Hg as compensatory mechanisms take hold. The bicarbonate level may be less than 22 mEq/L.
- Supportive findings include:
  – urine pH: less than 4.5 in the absence of renal disease
  – serum potassium levels: elevated from chemical buffering
  – glucose level: increased in those with diabetes mellitus
  – serum ketone body level: elevated in those with diabetes mellitus
  – plasma lactic acid level: elevated in those with lactic acidosis
  – anion gap: greater than 14 mEq/L, indicating metabolic acidosis.

  These values result from increased acid production or renal insufficiency. (See *Defining the anion gap.*)

Treatment
- Treatment consists of evaluation and correction of electrolyte imbalances and correction of underlying cause.

- Sodium bicarbonate I.V. must be given for severe cases; oral bicarbonate may be given for chronic metabolic acidosis.

Nursing considerations

- Keep sodium bicarbonate ampules handy for emergency administration. Frequently monitor vital signs, laboratory results, and level of consciousness because changes can occur rapidly.
- If the patient has diabetic acidosis, watch for secondary changes due to hypovolemia, such as decreasing blood pressure.
- Record intake and output accurately to monitor renal function.
- Watch for signs of excessive serum potassium—weakness, flaccid paralysis, and arrhythmias, possibly leading to cardiac arrest. After treatment, check for overcorrection to hypokalemia.
- Prepare for the possibility of seizures by taking seizure precautions.
- Carefully observe patients receiving I.V. therapy or who have intestinal tubes in place, as well as those suffering from shock, hyperthyroidism, hepatic disease, circulatory failure, or dehydration to prevent acidosis.
- Provide teaching for the patient with diabetes.

▮ Metabolic alkalosis

A clinical state marked by decreased amounts of acid or increased amounts of base bicarbonate, metabolic alkalosis causes metabolic, respiratory, and renal responses, producing characteristic symptoms—most notably, hypoventilation. This condition always occurs secondary to an underlying cause. With early diagnosis and prompt treatment, the prognosis is good; however, untreated metabolic alkalosis may lead to coma and death.

Defining the anion gap

The anion gap is the difference between concentrations of serum cations and anions—determined by measuring one cation (sodium) and two anions (chloride and bicarbonate). The normal concentration of sodium is 140 mEq/L; of chloride, 104 mEq/L; and of bicarbonate, 24 mEq/L. Thus, the anion gap between *measured* cations (actually sodium alone) and *measured* anions is about 12 mEq/L (140 minus 128).

Concentrations of potassium, calcium, and magnesium (*unmeasured* cations), or proteins, and phosphate, sulfate, and organic acids (*unmeasured* anions) aren't needed to measure the anion gap. Added together, the concentration of unmeasured cations would be about 11 mEq/L; of unmeasured anions, about 23 mEq/L. Thus, the normal anion gap between unmeasured cations and anions is about 12 mEq/L (23 minus 11)—give or take 2 mEq/L for normal variation.

An anion gap of more than 14 mEq/L indicates *metabolic acidosis*. It may result from the accumulation of excess organic acids or from retention of hydrogen ions, which chemically bond with bicarbonate and decrease bicarbonate levels.

Causes

- Administration of excessive amounts of I.V. fluids with high concentrations of bicarbonate or lactate and respiratory insufficiency—all of which cause chronic hypercapnia from high levels of plasma bicarbonate
- Excessive intake of absorbable alkali (as in milk-alkali syndrome)

- Excessive intake of bicarbonate of soda or other antacids (usually for treatment of gastritis or peptic ulcer)
- Fistulas
- Hyperadrenocorticism—Cushing's disease, primary hyperaldosteronism, and Bartter's syndrome, for example, due to retention of sodium and chloride and urinary loss of potassium and hydrogen
- Loss of acid
- Nasogastric tube drainage or lavage without adequate electrolyte replacement
- Renal mechanisms associated with decreased serum levels of potassium and chloride
- Retention of base
- Steroids and certain diuretics (furosemide, thiazides, and ethacrynic acid)
- Vomiting

Signs and symptoms

- Cardiovascular abnormalities such as atrial tachycardia and respiratory disturbances, such as cyanosis and apnea
- Carpopedal spasm in the hand due to diminished peripheral blood flow during repeated blood pressure checks (a possible sign of impending tetany [Trousseau's sign])
- Confusion
- Diarrhea (which aggravates alkalosis)
- Hypoventilation
- Irritability
- Nausea
- Picking at bedclothes (carphology)
- Seizures and coma (if untreated)
- Twitching
- Vomiting

Diagnostic tests

- A blood pH greater than 7.45 and a bicarbonate level above 29 mEq/L confirm the diagnosis.

- A partial pressure of carbon dioxide greater than 45 mm Hg indicates attempts at respiratory compensation.
- Serum electrolyte levels usually show low potassium, calcium, and chloride levels in patients with metabolic alkalosis.
- Urine pH is usually about 7.
- Urinalysis reveals alkalinity after the renal compensatory mechanism begins to excrete bicarbonate.
- Electrocardiography may show a low T wave merging with a P wave and atrial or sinus tachycardia.

Treatment

- Cautious administration of ammonium chloride I.V. to release hydrogen chloride and restore extracellular fluid and chloride levels.
- Potassium chloride and normal saline solution are usually sufficient to replace losses from gastric drainage, unless the patient has heart failure.
- Replacing potassium chloride and discontinuing diuretics correct metabolic alkalosis resulting from potent diuretic therapy.

Nursing considerations

DRUG CHALLENGE

 When giving ammonium chloride 0.9%, limit the infusion rate to 1 L/4 hours; faster administration may cause hemolysis of red blood cells. Avoid overdosage because it may cause overcorrection to metabolic acidosis. Don't give ammonium chloride to a patient with signs of hepatic or renal disease.

- Dilute potassium when giving I.V. containing potassium salts. Monitor the infusion rate to prevent damage to blood vessels; watch for signs of phlebitis.

- Watch closely for signs of muscle weakness, tetany, or decreased activity.
- Monitor vital signs frequently, and record intake and output to evaluate respiratory, fluid, and electrolyte status. Remember, respiratory rate usually decreases in an effort to compensate for alkalosis. Hypotension and tachycardia may indicate electrolyte imbalance, especially hypokalemia.
- Warn patients against overusing alkaline agents to prevent metabolic alkalosis. Irrigate nasogastric tubes with isotonic saline solution instead of plain water to prevent loss of gastric electrolytes. Monitor I.V. fluid concentrations of bicarbonate or lactate.

Metabolic syndrome

Metabolic syndrome—also called *syndrome X, insulin resistance syndrome, dysmetabolic syndrome,* and *multiple metabolic syndrome*—is a cluster of conditions characterized by abdominal obesity, high blood glucose (type 2 diabetes mellitus), insulin resistance, high blood cholesterol and triglycerides, and high blood pressure. More than 22% of people in the United States meet three or more of these criteria, raising their risk of heart disease and stroke and placing them at high risk for dying of myocardial infarction.

In the normal digestion process, the intestines break down food into its basic components, one of which is glucose. Glucose provides energy for cellular activity, while excess glucose is stored in cells for future use. Insulin, a hormone secreted in the pancreas, guides glucose into storage cells. However, in people with metabolic syndrome, glucose is insulin-resistant and doesn't respond to insulin's attempt to guide it into storage

cells. Excess insulin is then required to overcome this resistance. This excess in quantity and force of insulin causes damage to the lining of the arteries, promotes fat storage deposits, and prevents fat breakdown. This series of events can lead to diabetes, blood clots, and coronary events.

If metabolic syndrome is left untreated, such complications as coronary artery disease, diabetes, hyperlipidemia, and premature death may develop.

Causes
- Genetic predisposition

Predisposing factors
- Abdominal obesity
- High blood pressure
- Insulin resistance and dyslipidemia
- Type 2 diabetes mellitus and a fasting glucose level greater than 110 mg/dl

Signs and symptoms
- Abdominal obesity (evidenced by a waist of more than 40″ [101.6 cm] in males and 35″ [88.9 cm] in females)
- Difficulty losing weight
- Fatigue (especially after eating)
- Hypertension

Diagnostic tests
- Blood studies commonly indicate elevated blood glucose levels, hyperinsulinemia, and elevated serum uric acid.
- Lipid profile studies reveal elevated low-density lipoprotein (LDL) levels, low high-density lipoprotein (HDL) levels, and elevated triglycerides.
- Further diagnostic procedures may be performed to detect hypertension, diabetes, hyperlipidemia, and hyperinsulinemia.

Treatment

- Modest weight reduction through diet and exercise considerably improves glycosylated hemoglobin levels, reduces insulin resistance, improves blood lipid levels, and decreases blood pressure—all elements of metabolic syndrome. In patients with impaired glucose tolerance, losing an average of 7% of body weight can reduce the risk of developing type 2 diabetes by 58%.
- To improve cardiovascular health, a diet rich in vegetables, fruits, whole grains, fish, and low-fat dairy products, combined with regular exercise, is recommended. Moreover, nutrient-dense, low-energy foods should replace low-nutrient, high-calorie foods. Meal replacements and shakes may also reduce risk factors for metabolic syndrome and improve weight loss.
- A regular exercise program of moderate physical activity, in addition to dietary modifications, promotes weight loss, improves insulin sensitivity, and reduces blood glucose levels. According to the Surgeon General's Report on Physical Activity and Health, a person should exercise moderately for a minimum of 30 minutes on most (if not all) days of the week. The selected exercise program should improve cardiovascular conditioning, increase strength through resistance training, and improve flexibility.
- Medications may be used for patients who have a body mass index (BMI) of 27 kg/m^2 or greater as well as other risk factors (such as diabetes, hypertension, and hyperlipidemia) or a BMI of 30 kg/m^2 or greater without other risk factors. Weight loss medications may also be added to lifestyle changes if the patient hasn't achieved significant weight loss after 12 weeks.
- Phentermine (Ionamin) is used for short-term treatment of obesity in conjunction with diet and exercise.
- Orlistat (Xenical) and sibutramine (Meridia) have recently been approved for long-term weight loss.
  – Orlistat decreases the dietary fat absorption by inhibiting pancreatic lipase, which is needed for fat breakdown and absorption. Because of the reduction in absorption of fat-soluble vitamins, the patient may require vitamin supplementation. Obese patients who take orlistat while they're dieting achieve greater weight loss and serum glucose control than those who only diet.
  – Sibutramine promotes weight loss by inhibiting the reuptake of serotonin, norepinephrine, and dopamine and increases the satiety-producing effects of serotonin. It also helps to counteract the drop in metabolic rate that commonly occurs with weight loss.
- Surgical treatment of obesity, such as gastric bypass, produces a greater degree and duration of weight loss than other therapies and improves or resolves most of the factors of metabolic syndrome. Candidates for surgical intervention include patients with a BMI greater than 40 kg/m^2 or those with a BMI greater than 35 kg/m^2 with obesity-related medical conditions. Gastric bypass procedures produce permanent weight loss in the majority of patients.

Nursing considerations

- Monitor the patient's blood pressure and blood glucose, blood cholesterol, and insulin levels.
- Encourage the patient to begin an exercise and weight loss program with a friend or family member. Assist him in exploring options and support his efforts.

- Schedule frequent follow-up appointments with the patient to improve compliance. At that time, review his food diaries and exercise logs. Be positive and promote his active participation and partnership in his treatment plan.

Methicillin-resistant *Staphylococcus aureus*

Methicillin-resistant *Staphylococcus aureus* (MRSA) is a mutation of very common bacterium spread easily by direct person-to-person contact. Previously limited to large teaching hospitals and tertiary care centers, MRSA is now endemic in nursing homes, long-term care facilities, and even community hospitals. Patients most at risk for MRSA include immunosuppressed patients, burn patients, intubated patients, and those with central venous catheters, surgical wounds, or dermatitis.

MRSA enters health care facilities through an infected or colonized patient or a colonized health care worker. Although MRSA has been recovered from environmental surfaces, it's transmitted mainly by health care workers' hands. Many colonized individuals become silent carriers. The most common site of colonization is the anterior nares (40% of adults and most children become transient nasal carriers). Other sites include the groin, axillae, and the gut, although these sites aren't as common. Typically, MRSA colonization is diagnosed by isolating bacteria from nasal secretions.

Others at risk include those with prosthetic devices, heart valves, and postoperative wound infections. Additional risk factors include prolonged hospital stays, extended therapy with multiple or broad-spectrum antibiotics, and proximity to those colonized or infected with MRSA. Patients with acute endocarditis, bacteremia, cervicitis, meningitis, pericarditis, or pneumonia are also at risk.

Causes
- Overuse of antibiotics

Signs and symptoms
- None
- Symptomatic patients exhibit signs and symptoms related to the primary diagnosis.

Diagnostic tests
- MRSA can be cultured from the suspected site with the appropriate culture method. For example, MRSA in a wound infection can be swabbed for culture. Blood, urine, and sputum cultures will reveal sources of MRSA.

Treatment
- Most facilities keep patients in isolation until surveillance cultures are negative.
- Linezolid (Zyvox) (of the oxazolidinedione class of antibiotics) is effective against MRSA.

Nursing considerations
- Wash your hands before and after patient care. Good hand washing is the most effective way to prevent MRSA from spreading.
- Use an antiseptic soap, such as chlorhexidine, because bacteria have been cultured from workers' hands after they've washed with milder soap. One study showed that without proper hand washing, MRSA could survive on health care workers' hands for up to 3 hours.
- Institute contact isolation precautions. A private room should be used, as well as dedicated equipment and disinfection of the environment.

- Change gloves when contaminated or when moving from a "dirty" area of the body to a clean one.
- Instruct family and friends to wear protective clothing when they visit the patient, and show them how to dispose of it.
- Provide teaching and emotional support to the patient and family members.
- Consider grouping infected patients together and having the same nursing staff care for them.
- Don't lay equipment on the patient's bed or bed-side table. Wipe equipment with the appropriate disinfectant before leaving the patient's room.
- Ensure judicious and careful use of antibiotics. Encourage practitioners to limit antibiotic use.
- Instruct the patient to take the antibiotic for the full prescription period, even if he begins to feel better.

Monkeypox

Monkeypox is a rare viral disease identified mostly in the rainforest countries of central and west Africa. The virus was originally discovered in laboratory monkeys in 1958. It was later recovered from an African squirrel, which was thought to be the natural host. It may also infect other rodents, such as rats, mice, and rabbits. The first human cases of monkeypox were reported in remote African locations in 1970. In June 2003, there was an outbreak in the United States involving people who had gotten ill following contact with infected prairie dogs.

The incubation period lasts about 12 days, and the illness lasts 2 to 4 weeks. Although rare, complications may include encephalitis and death.

In Africa, monkeypox is fatal in 10% of those who contract the disease.

Causes
- *Monkeypox virus,* from an infected animal through a bite or direct contact with the animal's blood, body fluids, or lesions

Signs and symptoms
- Backache
- Fever
- General feeling of discomfort and exhaustion
- Headache
- Muscle aches
- Papular rash that begins on the face or other area of the body within 1 to 3 days after onset of the fever (lesions go through several stages before crusting and falling off)
- Swollen lymph nodes

Diagnostic tests
- The virus may be isolated from vesicular fluid to aid in diagnosis and differentiation from other rash-producing viruses.

Treatment
- No specific treatment exists for monkeypox, but the smallpox vaccine appears to reduce the risk of contracting the disease.
- The Centers for Disease Control and Prevention recommends that people who are investigating monkeypox outbreaks and caring for infected individuals or animals should receive smallpox vaccination.
- People exposed to individuals or animals confirmed to have monkeypox should also receive vaccinations (up to 14 days after exposure).
- Vaccinia immune globulin may be considered in some cases, such as in patients who are severely immunocompromised.

- No data are available on the effectiveness of cidofovir (Vistide) in the treatment of human monkeypox cases.

Nursing considerations

- Notify the local health department immediately if you suspect monkeypox.
- Institute a combination of standard, contact, and droplet precautions. Because of the risk of airborne transmission, droplet precautions should be applied whenever possible using a NIOSH-certified N95 (or comparable) filtering disposable respirator that has been fit-tested. Surgical masks may be worn if the respirator isn't available. Isolation should continue until all lesions are crusted over or until the local or state health department advises that isolation is no longer necessary.
- Perform scrupulous hand hygiene after contact with an infected patient or contaminated objects. Teach the patient and his family members proper hand-hygiene practices as well.
- Use eye protection if splash or spray of body fluids is possible.
- Place the patient in a private room. Use a negative pressure room if available.
- Place a mask over the patient's nose and mouth, and cover the exposed skin lesions with a sheet or gown when transporting the patient. If the patient is to remain at home, he should maintain the same precautions.

Mononucleosis

Infectious mononucleosis is an acute infectious disease. It primarily affects young adults and children; in children, however, it's usually so mild that it's commonly overlooked.

Infectious mononucleosis is fairly common in the United States, Canada, and Europe, and both sexes are affected equally. Incidence varies seasonally among college students (most common in early spring and early fall) but not among the general population.

Characteristically, infectious mononucleosis produces fever, sore throat, and cervical lymphadenopathy (the hallmarks of the disease), as well as hepatic dysfunction, increased lymphocytes and monocytes, and development and persistence of heterophil antibodies. The prognosis is excellent, and major complications are uncommon.

Causes

- Epstein-Barr virus (EBV)

Signs and symptoms

After an incubation period of about 4 to 6 weeks in young adults, infectious mononucleosis produces prodromal symptoms:

- Fatigue
- Headache
- Malaise

After 3 to 5 days, patients typically develop these signs and symptoms:

- Cervical lymphadenopathy
- Jaundice
- Maculopapular rash that resembles rubella (in early stage)
- Sore throat
- Splenomegaly, hepatomegaly, stomatitis, exudative tonsillitis, or pharyngitis
- Temperature fluctuations, with an evening peak of 101° to 102° F (38.3° to 38.9° C)

Symptoms usually subside from 6 to 10 days after onset of the disease but may persist for weeks.

Diagnostic tests

- Monospot test is positive for infectious mononucleosis.

- White blood cell (WBC) count increases 10,000 to 20,000/mm^3 during the second and third weeks of illness. Lymphocytes and monocytes account for 50% to 70% of the total WBC count; 10% of the lymphocytes are atypical.
- Heterophil antibodies (agglutinins for sheep red blood cells) in serum drawn during the acute illness and at 3- to 4-week intervals rise to four times normal.
- Indirect immunofluorescence shows antibodies to EBV and cellular antigens. Such testing is usually more definitive than heterophil antibodies.
- Liver function studies are abnormal.

Treatment

- Therapy is supportive: relief of symptoms, bed rest during the acute febrile period, and aspirin or another salicylate for headache and sore throat.
- If severe throat inflammation causes airway obstruction, a steroid can be used to relieve swelling and avoid tracheotomy.
- Splenic rupture, marked by sudden abdominal pain, requires splenectomy.
- About 20% of patients with infectious mononucleosis also have streptococcal pharyngotonsillitis; these patients should receive antibiotic therapy for at least 10 days.

Nursing considerations

- Provide immediate patient teaching because uncomplicated infectious mononucleosis doesn't require hospitalization. Convalescence may take several weeks, usually until the patient's WBC count returns to normal.
- Stress the need for bed rest during the acute illness. If the patient is a student, tell him he may continue less-demanding school assignments and see his friends but should avoid long, difficult projects until after recovery.

- Encourage the patient to drink milk shakes, fruit juices, and broths, and also to eat cool, bland foods to minimize throat discomfort.
- Advise the patient to use saline gargles and aspirin as needed.

█ Multiple myeloma

Multiple myeloma is also known as *malignant plasmacytoma, plasma cell myeloma,* and *myelomatosis.* It's a disseminated neoplasm of marrow plasma cells that infiltrates bone to produce osteolytic lesions throughout the skeleton (flat bones, vertebrae, skull, pelvis, ribs); in late stages, it infiltrates the body organs (liver, spleen, lymph nodes, lungs, adrenal glands, kidneys, skin, GI tract). Multiple myeloma strikes mostly men older than age 40.

The prognosis is usually poor because the disease is commonly diagnosed after it has already infiltrated the vertebrae, pelvis, skull, ribs, clavicles, and sternum. By then, skeletal destruction is widespread and, without treatment, leads to vertebral collapse. Early diagnosis and treatment prolong the lives of many patients by 3 to 5 years. Death usually follows complications, such as infection, renal failure, hematologic disorders, fractures, hypercalcemia, hyperuricemia, or dehydration.

Causes

- Excessive growth and malformation of plasma cells in bone marrow

Signs and symptoms

- Arthritic symptoms: achiness, joint swelling, and tenderness, possibly from vertebral compression
- Back pain
- Fever, malaise, slight evidence of peripheral neuropathy (such as peripheral

paresthesia), pathologic fractures, and easy bruising
▪ Renal complications such as pyelonephritis (caused by tubular damage from large amounts of Bence Jones protein, hypercalcemia, and hyperuricemia) may occur (see *Bence Jones protein*)
▪ Severe, recurrent infection such as pneumonia (with damage to nerves associated with respiratory function)
▪ Symptoms of vertebral compression may become acute, accompanied by anemia, weight loss, thoracic deformities (ballooning), and loss of body height— 5″ (12.7 cm) or more—due to vertebral collapse (with disease progression)

Diagnostic tests
▪ Complete blood count shows moderate or severe anemia. The differential may show 40% to 50% lymphocytes but seldom more than 3% plasma cells. An elevated erythrocyte sedimentation rate results from increased clumping of red blood cells (rouleaux formation) caused by increased concentration of serum immunoprotein.
▪ Urine studies may show Bence Jones protein and hypercalciuria. Absence of Bence Jones protein doesn't rule out multiple myeloma; however, its presence almost invariably confirms the disease.
▪ Bone marrow aspiration detects myelomatous cells (an abnormal number of immature plasma cells).
▪ Serum electrophoresis shows an elevated globulin spike that's electrophoretically and immunologically abnormal.
▪ Urine protein electrophoresis may detect cases that are missed by serum electrophoresis.
▪ X-rays during early stages may show only diffuse osteoporosis. Eventually, they show multiple, sharply circumscribed osteolytic (punched-out) lesions, particularly on the skull, pelvis, and

Bence Jones protein

The hallmark of multiple myeloma, Bence Jones protein (a light chain of gamma globulin), was named for Henry Bence Jones, an English physician who in 1848 noticed that patients with a curious bone disease excreted a unique protein—unique in that it coagulated at 113° to 131° F (45° to 55° C), then redissolved when heated to boiling.

It remained for Otto Kahler, an Austrian, to demonstrate in 1889 that Bence Jones protein was related to myeloma. Bence Jones protein isn't found in the urine of *all* multiple myeloma patients, but it's rarely found in patients without the disease.

spine—the characteristic lesions of multiple myeloma.
▪ Excretory urography can assess renal involvement. To avoid precipitation of Bence Jones protein, iothalamate or diatrizoate is used instead of the usual contrast medium. Also, although oral fluid restriction is usually standard before excretory urography, patients with multiple myeloma receive large quantities of fluid, generally orally but sometimes I.V., before this test is performed.

Treatment
▪ Long-term treatment of multiple myeloma consists mainly of chemotherapy to suppress plasma cell growth and control pain.
▪ Adjuvant local radiation reduces acute lesions, such as collapsed vertebrae, and relieves localized pain.
▪ Other treatment includes melphalan-prednisone combination in high intermittent doses or low continuous daily doses, and an analgesic for pain.

- For spinal cord compression, the patient may require a laminectomy; for renal complications, dialysis. Bone marrow transplantation is sometimes used in younger patients, but the procedure's long-term results are unknown.

- Because the patient may have bone demineralization and may lose large amounts of calcium into blood and urine, he's a prime candidate for renal calculi, nephrocalcinosis and, eventually, renal failure due to hypercalcemia. Hypercalcemia is managed with hydration, a diuretic, a corticosteroid, oral phosphate, and I.V. mithramycin to decrease serum calcium levels.

Nursing considerations

- Monitor the patient's fluid intake and output. (Daily output should be at least 1,500 ml.) Encourage the patient to drink 3,000 to 4,000 ml of fluids daily, as prescribed.

- Encourage the patient to walk. (Immobilization increases bone demineralization and vulnerability to pneumonia.) Give an analgesic, as needed, to lessen pain.

- Never allow the patient to walk unaccompanied; be sure that he uses a walker or other supportive aid to prevent falls. Because the patient is particularly vulnerable to pathologic fractures, he may be fearful. Give reassurance, and allow him to move at his own pace.

- Prevent complications by watching for fever or malaise, which may signal the onset of infection, and for signs of other problems, such as severe anemia and fractures.

- If the patient is bedridden, change his position every 2 hours. Perform passive range-of-motion, and assist with deep-breathing exercises. Promote them as well when he can tolerate active exercise.

- Monitor the patient for adverse effects of chemotherapy or radiation treatments.

- Watch closely for signs of infection if the patient is taking prednisone because this drug commonly masks those signs.

- Get the patient out of bed within 24 hours after laminectomy whenever possible. Check for hemorrhage, motor or sensory deficits, and loss of bowel or bladder function. Position the patient as necessary, maintain alignment, and log-roll when turning.

- Provide emotional support for the patient and his family. Help relieve their anxiety by clearly explaining diagnostic tests (including painful procedures, such as bone marrow aspiration and biopsy), treatments, and the prognosis. If needed, refer them to an appropriate community resource for additional support.

Multiple sclerosis

Multiple sclerosis (MS), an autoimmune disease is characterized by exacerbations and remissions, is a major cause of chronic disability in young adults. MS usually begins between ages 20 and 40 (average age of onset is 27). It's more common in females than in males. Incidence is low in Japan; it's generally higher among urban populations and upper socioeconomic groups. A family history of MS and living in a cold, damp climate increase the risk.

In MS, demyelination of the white matter of the brain and spinal cord and damage to nerve fibers and their targets occurs. Sporadic patches (called *plaques*) of axon demyelination and nerve fiber loss occur throughout the central nervous system, inducing widely disseminated and varied neurologic dysfunction.

Nerve fiber loss may provide an explanation for the invisible neurologic deficits experienced by many patients with MS. The axons decide the presence or absence of function. Loss of myelin doesn't correlate with loss of function.

The prognosis varies. MS may progress rapidly and can disable the patient by early adulthood. It can cause death within months of onset; however, 70% of patients lead active, productive lives with prolonged remissions.

Because early symptoms may be mild, years may elapse between onset of the first signs and the diagnosis.

Forms of MS include:
- Relapsing-remitting—clear relapses (or acute attacks or exacerbations) with full recovery or partial recovery and lasting disability. Between the attacks, there's no worsening of the disease. This type accounts for up to 90% of all MS cases.
- Primary progressive—steady progression or worsening of the disease from the onset with minor recovery or plateaus. This form of MS is uncommon and may involve different brain and spinal cord damage than other forms.
- Secondary progressive—begins as a pattern of clear-cut relapses and recovery but becomes steadily progressive and worsens between acute attacks.
- Progressive relapsing—steadily progressive from the onset but also has clear acute attacks; this form of MS is rare.

Causes
- Unknown

Predisposing factors
- Acute respiratory tract infection
- Emotional stress
- Fatigue
- Overwork
- Pregnancy

Signs and symptoms
- May be transient, or last for hours or weeks; may wax and wane with no predictable pattern, vary from day to day, and be bizarre and difficult for the patient to describe
- Variable with extent and site of myelin destruction, the extent of remyelination, and the adequacy of subsequent restored synaptic transmission
- Vision problems and sensory impairment, such as burning, pins and needles, and electrical sensations (usually initial signs and symptoms)
- Other characteristic changes include:
  – bowel disturbances—involuntary evacuation or constipation
  – dysphagia
  – fatigue—typically the most debilitating symptom
  – muscle dysfunction—weakness, paralysis ranging from monoplegia to quadriplegia, spasticity, hyperreflexia, intention tremor, balance problems, and gait ataxia
  – ocular disturbances—optic neuritis, diplopia, ophthalmoplegia, blurred vision, and nystagmus
  – poorly articulated or scanning speech
  – urinary disturbances—incontinence, frequency, urgency, and frequent infections.

Diagnostic tests
- Magnetic resonance imaging may detect MS lesions.
- EEG is abnormal in one-third of patients.
- Lumbar puncture shows an elevated gamma globulin fraction of immunoglobulin G but normal total cerebrospinal fluid (CSF) protein levels. An elevated CSF gamma globulin level is significant only when serum gamma globulin levels are normal; it reflects hy-

peractivity of the immune system due to chronic demyelination. In addition, the white blood cell count in CSF may be elevated.

■ Electrophoresis can detect oligoclonal bands of immunoglobulin in CSF. Present in most patients, they can be found even when the percentage of gamma globulin in CSF is normal.

Treatment
Acute episodes

■ I.V. methylprednisone followed by oral prednisone is effective in speeding recovery from acute attacks.

■ Antispasmolytics may be used to reduce muscle spasticity.

■ Cholinergics are effective for urinary problems, antidepressants for mood and behavior symptoms, and amantadine for fatigue.

Treating the disease

■ Interferon and glatiramer (a combination of four amino acids) may reduce the frequency and severity of relapses and slow central nervous system damage. These medications, which are available for relapsing-remitting MS, are used to delay disability and decrease injury to the nervous system.

Treating signs and symptoms

■ Spasticity occurs as a result of opposing muscle groups relaxing and contracting at the same time. Baclofen, diazepam, and tizanidine may be prescribed. For severe spasticity, Botox injections, intrathecal injections, nerve blocks, and surgery may be necessary.

■ Stretching and range-of-motion exercises, coupled with correct positioning, are helpful in relaxing muscles and maintaining function.

■ Applying pressure to the contracted area can help with relaxation. Avoid

touching the palm of the hand or sole of the foot. Minimize spasticity by holding the heel of the foot and by folding the hand open from the outer edges.

■ Frequent rest periods, aerobic exercise, and cooling techniques (air conditioning, breezes, water sprays) can minimize fatigue. Amantadine, pemoline, antidepressants, and methylphenidate help to manage fatigue.

■ Treatment of associated bladder problems ranges from simple strategies, such as drinking cranberry juice, to the placement of an indwelling urinary catheter and suprapubic tubes. Intermittent self-catheterization and postvoiding catheterization programs are beneficial.

■ An anticholinergic may be helpful for bladder problems.

■ Increased fiber intake may benefit the patient with associated bowel problems. Bulking agents, such as Metamucil, help to relieve and prevent bowel problems. Daily suppositories and rectal stimulation may be necessary.

■ Sensory symptoms, such as pain, numbness, burning, and tingling, can be managed by a low-dose tricyclic antidepressant, phenytoin, or carbamazepine.

■ Cognitive dysfunction is experienced by 50% of patients with MS. Cognitive problems tend to be minor, with short-term memory loss being the most common symptom. For more severe issues, a neuropsychological consultation may be beneficial.

■ Motor dysfunction, such as problems with balance, strength, and muscle coordination, may be present in MS. Adaptive devices and physical therapy intervention help to maintain mobility.

■ Tremors may be treated with a beta-adrenergic blocker, a sedative, or a diuretic.

■ Dysarthria requires a speech therapy consultation.

- Vertigo may be managed with an anti-histamine, vision therapy, or exercises.
- Vision changes may require vision therapy or adaptive lenses.

Nursing considerations

- Emphasize the need to avoid stress, infections, and fatigue and to maintain independence by developing new ways of performing daily activities.
- Advise the patient to avoid exposure to bacterial and viral infections.
- Stress the importance of eating a nutritious, well-balanced diet that contains sufficient fiber to prevent constipation.
- Encourage adequate fluid intake and regular urination.
- When working with a spastic extremity, never try to force it open. Gently rotate the extremity toward the direction it's being pulled, and then gradually rotate it outward. Repeat, and go a little farther with each attempt.
- Watch for adverse reactions to drug therapy.
- Glatiramer reactions occur immediately after injection. The patient may experience transient flushing, chest pain, palpitations, and dyspnea, which last only a few seconds. Usually no additional treatment is needed.
- Patients receiving interferon require routine laboratory monitoring (complete blood count with differential); blood urea nitrogen, creatinine, and alanine aminotransferase levels; and urinalysis.

DRUG CHALLENGE

 Nonsteroidal anti-inflammatory drugs or acetaminophen given with a bedtime injection of interferon have been helpful in minimizing adverse effects (flulike symptoms, site reactions, suicidal thoughts). Subcutaneous site rotation is necessary. Betaseron injections are given every other day, and the medication must be refrigerated. Glatiramer is given in daily subcutaneous injections.

- Promote emotional stability. Help the patient establish a daily routine to maintain optimal functioning.
- Inform the patient that exacerbations are unpredictable, necessitating physical and emotional adjustments in his lifestyle.
- For more information, refer the patient to the National Multiple Sclerosis Society.

Mumps

Also known as *infectious* or *epidemic parotitis,* mumps is an acute viral disease. It's most prevalent in unvaccinated children between ages 2 and 12, but it can occur in other age-groups. Infants younger than age 1 seldom get this disease because of passive immunity from maternal antibodies. Peak incidence occurs during late winter and early spring. The prognosis for complete recovery is good, although mumps sometimes causes complications.

Epididymo-orchitis and mumps meningitis are complications of mumps. Epididymo-orchitis, which occurs in about 25% of postpubertal males who contract mumps, produces abrupt onset of testicular swelling and tenderness, scrotal erythema, lower abdominal pain, nausea, vomiting, fever, and chills. Swelling and tenderness related to mumps may last for several weeks. Epididymitis may precede or accompany orchitis. In 50% of males with mumps-induced orchitis, the testicles show some atrophy, but sterility is rare.

Mumps meningitis complicates mumps in 10% of patients and affects three to five times more males than fe-

Site of parotid inflammation in mumps

Palpation of the parotid glands can reveal inflammation in mumps, which is commonly accompanied by facial pain.

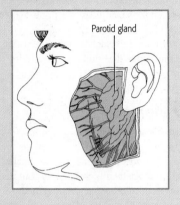

Parotid gland

males. Signs and symptoms include fever, meningeal irritation (nuchal rigidity, headache, and irritability), vomiting, drowsiness, and a lymphocyte count in cerebrospinal fluid ranging from 500 to 2,000/mm³.

Recovery is usually complete. Less-common effects are pancreatitis, deafness, arthritis, myocarditis, encephalitis, pericarditis, oophoritis, and nephritis.

Causes
▪ Paramyxovirus

Signs and symptoms
First 24 hours
▪ Anorexia
▪ Headache
▪ Low-grade fever
▪ Malaise
▪ Myalgia

Later
▪ Earache that's aggravated by chewing
▪ Fever of 101° to 104° F (38.3° to 40° C)
▪ Pain when chewing or when drinking sour or acidic liquids
▪ Parotid gland tenderness and swelling with possible swelling of one or more salivary gland (see *Site of parotid inflammation in mumps*)

Diagnostic tests
▪ Serologic antibody testing can verify the diagnosis when parotid or other salivary gland enlargement is absent.
▪ If comparison between a blood sample obtained during the acute phase of illness and another sample obtained 3 weeks later shows a fourfold rise in antibody titer, the patient most likely had mumps.

Treatment
▪ Analgesics are given for pain; antipyretics, for fever.
▪ Adequate fluid intake prevents dehydration from fever and anorexia.
▪ If the patient can't swallow, I.V. fluid replacement may be necessary.
▪ Avoid giving aspirin to children age 12 and younger with a viral illness because of the risk of Reye's syndrome.

Nursing considerations
▪ Stress the need for bed rest during the febrile period.
▪ Give an analgesic, and apply warm or cool compresses to the neck to relieve pain. Salt-water gargles and a soft-food diet may help relieve symptoms.
▪ Give an antipyretic and tepid sponge baths for fever.
▪ Encourage the patient to drink fluids to prevent dehydration.

■ Advise the patient to avoid spicy, irritating foods and those that require a lot of chewing.

■ Observe the patient closely during the acute phase for signs of central nervous system involvement, such as an altered level of consciousness and nuchal rigidity.

■ Institute respiratory isolation. All personnel who come in contact with the patient should follow standard precautions.

■ Emphasize the importance of routine immunization with live attenuated mumps virus (paramyxovirus) at age 15 months and for susceptible patients (especially males) who are approaching or are past puberty.

■ Remember, immunization within 24 hours of exposure may prevent or attenuate the actual disease. Immunity against mumps lasts at least 12 years.

■ Report all cases of mumps to local public health authorities.

■ Inform the patient that he shouldn't attend school or enter his workplace for 9 days after the onset of mumps.

▋Muscular dystrophy

Muscular dystrophy is actually a group of congenital disorders characterized by progressive symmetrical wasting of skeletal muscles without neural or sensory defects. Paradoxically, these wasted muscles tend to enlarge because of connective tissue and fat deposits, giving an erroneous impression of muscle strength.

Four main types of muscular dystrophy occur: Duchenne's (pseudohypertrophic) muscular dystrophy, which accounts for 50% of all cases; Becker's (benign pseudohypertrophic) muscular dystrophy; facioscapulohumeral (Landouzy-Dejerine) dystrophy; and limb-girdle dystrophy. Emery-Dreifuss muscular dystrophy, myotonic dystrophy, and myotonia congenita are less common.

Duchenne's and Becker's muscular dystrophies affect males almost exclusively. The incidence of Duchenne's muscular dystrophy in males is 13 to 33 per 100,000. Becker's muscular dystrophy occurs in about 1 to 3 males per 100,000. Facioscapulohumeral and limb-girdle dystrophy affect both sexes about equally.

The prognosis varies. Duchenne's muscular dystrophy generally strikes during early childhood and usually results in death within 10 to 15 years. Patients with Becker's muscular dystrophy live into their 40s. Facioscapulohumeral and limb-girdle dystrophies usually don't shorten life expectancy.

Causes
■ Various genetic mechanisms distinguished from one another by the type of inheritance (sex-linked, dominant gene, or recessive gene)

Signs and symptoms
Although the four types of muscular dystrophy cause progressive muscular deterioration, the degree of severity and the age of onset vary.

Duchenne's muscular dystrophy
■ Begins insidiously between ages 3 and 5
■ Leg and pelvic muscles affected initially with spreading to the involuntary muscles
■ Waddling gait, toe-walking, and lordosis
■ Difficulty climbing stairs, frequent falling, inability to run
■ Flaring of scapulae with raised arms

- Enlargement of calf muscles
- Muscle deterioration (rapid progression), followed by contractures
- Confinement to wheelchair by age 9 to 12
- Late in the disease:
  - Cardiomyopathy due to progressive weakening of cardiac muscle
  - Electrocardiogram abnormalities
  - Pulmonary complications
  - Tachycardia
- Death due to sudden heart failure, respiratory failure, or infection

Becker's muscular dystrophy
- Same signs and symptoms as Duchenne's muscular dystrophy; slower progression
- Symptom onset at about age 5 (but patient commonly able to walk well beyond age 15; sometimes past age 40)

Facioscapulohumeral dystrophy
- Onset commonly before age 10
- Slowly progressive and relatively benign
- Muscle weakness of the face, shoulders, and upper arms initially; spreading to all voluntary muscles
- Pendulous lower lip and absence of the nasolabial fold
- Early symptoms: inability to pucker the mouth or whistle, abnormal facial movements, and absence of facial movements when laughing or crying
- Diffuse facial flattening leading to a masklike expression, winging of the scapulae, inability to raise the arms above the head and, in infants, inability to suckle

Limb-girdle dystrophy
- Onset between ages 6 and 10; less commonly, in early adulthood

- Slow course and slight disability (commonly)
- Muscle weakness initially in the upper arm and pelvic muscles
- Winging of the scapulae, lordosis with abdominal protrusion, waddling gait, poor balance, and inability to raise the arms

Emery-Dreifuss dystrophy and myotonic dystrophy
- Variable age of onset
- Hypotonia
- Muscle weakness (variable involvement)

Myotonia congenita
- Infants experience such symptoms as: frequent choking, gagging, or difficulty swallowing
- These same symptoms improve later in life
- Again, these same symptoms occur when a movement is first started. After a few repetitions, the muscle relaxes.

Diagnostic tests
- Electromyography typically demonstrates short, weak bursts of electrical activity in affected muscles.
- Muscle biopsy shows variations in the size of muscle fibers and, in later stages, fat and connective tissue deposits. In Duchenne's muscle dystrophy, a muscle biopsy reveals an absence of dystrophin.
- Immunologic and molecular biological techniques now available in specialized medical centers facilitate accurate prenatal and postnatal diagnosis of Duchenne's and Becker's muscular dystrophies. These techniques also help to identify a person as a carrier. In addition, these newer techniques are replacing muscle biopsy and serum creatine kinase tests as diagnostic procedures.

Treatment

- No treatment stops the progressive muscle impairment of muscular dystrophy.
- Orthopedic appliances as well as exercise, physical therapy, and surgery to correct contractures can help preserve the patient's mobility and independence.
- Treatment for myotonia congenita includes symptomatic relief with mexiletine, phenytoin, procainamide, and quinine.
- Family members who are carriers of muscular dystrophy should receive genetic counseling regarding the risk of transmitting this disease.

Nursing considerations

- Encourage coughing, deep-breathing exercises, and diaphragmatic breathing when respiratory involvement occurs in Duchenne's muscular dystrophy. Teach parents how to recognize early signs of respiratory complications.
- Provide supportive care and emotional support.
- Encourage and assist with active and passive range-of-motion exercises to preserve joint mobility and prevent muscle atrophy.
- Advise the patient to avoid long periods of bed rest and inactivity; if necessary, limit his TV viewing and other sedentary activities.
- Refer the patient for physical therapy. Splints, braces, surgery to correct contractures, trapeze bars, overhead slings, and a wheelchair can help preserve mobility. A footboard or high-topped sneakers and a foot cradle increase comfort and prevent footdrop.
- Encourage adequate fluid intake, increase dietary bulk, and obtain an order for a stool softener because inactivity may cause constipation.

- Help the patient and his family plan a low-calorie, high-protein, high-fiber diet; the patient is prone to obesity because of reduced physical activity.
- Allow the patient plenty of time to perform even simple physical tasks because he's likely to be slow and awkward.
- Encourage communication among family members to help them deal with the emotional strain this disorder produces. Provide emotional support to help the patient cope with continual changes in body image.
- Refer adult patients for sexual counseling, if necessary.
- Refer those who must acquire new job skills for vocational rehabilitation. (Contact the Department of Labor and Industry in your state for more information.)
- Refer patients and their families to the Muscular Dystrophy Association for information on social services and financial assistance.
- Genetic testing can be used to detect the gene that leads to muscular dystrophy in some families. Refer family members for genetic counseling.

▌Myasthenia gravis

Myasthenia gravis produces sporadic but progressive weakness and abnormal fatigability of striated (skeletal) muscles, which are worsened by exercise and repeated movement but improved by anticholinesterase therapy. Usually, this disorder affects muscles innervated by the cranial nerves (face, lips, tongue, neck, and throat), but it can affect any muscle group.

Myasthenia gravis affects 3 in 10,000 people at any age but is more common in young females and older males.

This disease may coexist with immune and thyroid disorders; about 15%

Coping with lifelong myasthenia gravis

To help the patient deal with his condition, remember these patient-teaching tips:

■ Help the patient plan daily activities to coincide with energy peaks.

■ Stress the need for frequent rest periods throughout the day. Emphasize that periodic remissions, exacerbations, and day-to-day fluctuations are common.

■ Teach the patient how to recognize adverse reactions and signs and symptoms of toxic reaction to an anticholinesterase (headaches, weakness, sweating, abdominal cramps, nausea, vomiting, diarrhea, excessive salivation, and bronchospasm) and to a corticosteroid (cushingoid symptoms [swelling of the face, buffalo hump], adrenal insufficiency [fatigue, muscle weakness, dyspnea, anorexia, nausea, and fainting]).

■ Warn the patient to avoid strenuous exercise, stress, infection, and needless exposure to the sun or cold weather, all of which can worsen signs and symptoms.

■ Advise the patient with diplopia that wearing an eye patch or glasses with one frosted lens may help.

■ For more information and an opportunity to meet myasthenic patients who lead full, productive lives, refer the patient to the Myasthenia Gravis Foundation.

persistent myasthenia. The infant appears temporarily weak and may require medications for a few weeks after birth. Usually the baby doesn't develop the disorder, but he must receive follow-up attention.

Myasthenia gravis follows an unpredictable course of periodic exacerbations and remissions. (See *Coping with lifelong myasthenia gravis.*) Onset may be sudden or insidious. There is no known cure. Drug treatment has improved the prognosis and allows patients to lead relatively normal lives, except during exacerbations. When the disease involves the respiratory system, it may be life-threatening.

Causes
■ Failure in transmission of nerve impulses at the neuromuscular junction, possibly due to autoimmune response, ineffective acetylcholine release, or inadequate muscle fiber response to acetylcholine

Signs and symptoms
■ In the early stages: easy fatigability of certain muscles, notably the eye and eyelid muscles and muscles involving swallowing and talking
■ Skeletal muscle weakness and fatigability
■ Muscle weakening throughout the day, especially after exercise
■ Muscle function improvement with short rest periods
■ Full loss of muscle function (occasionally)
■ Muscle weakness intensified during menses and after emotional stress, prolonged exposure to sunlight or cold, or infections
■ Weak eye closure, ptosis, and diplopia
■ Hoarseness or a changing voice

of myasthenic patients have thymomas. Remissions occur in about 25% of patients.

Pregnancy is possible for female patients with myasthenia gravis, although they must be closely supervised. About 20% of infants born to myasthenic mothers have transient, or occasionally

- Difficulty chewing and swallowing; risk for choking
- Eyelid droop leading to impaired vision
- Head bobbing due to weakening of neck muscles
- Decreased tidal volume and vital capacity with weakened respiratory muscles
- Emergency airway and mechanical ventilation with severe respiratory muscle weakness

Diagnostic tests
- Electromyography, with repeated neural stimulation, may help confirm this diagnosis.
- Tensilon test: In myasthenic patients, muscle function improves within 30 to 60 seconds after an I.V. injection of edrophonium or neostigmine, and the improvement lasts up to 30 minutes. Long-standing ocular muscle dysfunction may fail to respond to such testing. This test can differentiate a myasthenic crisis from a cholinergic crisis (caused by acetylcholine overactivity at the neuromuscular junction).
- The acetylcholine receptor antibody titer may be elevated in generalized myasthenia.

Treatment
- Anticholinesterases, such as neostigmine and pyridostigmine, improve communication between nerve and muscle, counteract fatigue and muscle weakness, and allow the return of about 80% of normal muscle function. However, these drugs become less effective as the disease worsens. Decreasing the immune response toward acetylcholine receptors at the neuromuscular junction is the goal of immunosuppressant therapy. Corticosteroids, azathioprine, cyclosporine, and cyclophosphamide are used in a progressive fashion (when the previous drug response is poor, the next one is used).
- To suppress the immune system during acute relapses, gamma globulin may also be used.
- Plasmapheresis is used to treat severe exacerbations or to quickly improve symptoms (for example, preoperatively).
- Patients with thymomas require a thymectomy, which may cause remission in some cases of adult-onset myasthenia.

ACTION STAT!

 Acute exacerbations that cause severe respiratory distress—*myasthenic crises*—necessitate emergency treatment and immediate hospitalization. Tracheotomy, positive-pressure ventilation, and vigorous suctioning to remove secretions usually produce improvement in a few days. Because anticholinesterases aren't effective in patients with myasthenic crisis, this therapy is stopped until respiratory function improves.

Nursing considerations
- Perform a careful baseline assessment to ensure early recognition and treatment of potential crises.
- Provide supportive measures, and thorough patient teaching to help minimize exacerbations and complications.
- Establish an accurate neurologic and respiratory baseline. Thereafter, monitor tidal volume and vital capacity regularly. The patient may need a ventilator and frequent suctioning to remove accumulating secretions.
- Be alert for signs of an impending crisis (increased muscle weakness, respiratory distress, difficulty in talking or chewing).

▪ Space administration of drugs evenly, and give them on time to prevent relapses. Be prepared to give atropine for anticholinesterase overdose or toxicity.

▪ Plan exercise, meals, patient care, and activities to make the most of energy peaks. For example, give medication 20 to 30 minutes before meals to facilitate chewing or swallowing. Allow the patient to participate in self-care.

▪ Give soft, solid foods instead of liquids to lessen the risk of choking when swallowing is difficult.

▪ Try to increase social activity as soon as possible after a severe exacerbation.

DRUG CHALLENGE

 Teach the patient to avoid or closely monitor the effects of certain drugs. Curare-like drugs, local anesthetics, common cold products, tonic water and antiarrhythmics containing quinine, aminoglycoside antibiotics, tetracyclines, morphine sulfate, beta-adrenergic blockers, and calcium channel blockers may worsen muscle weakness by impairing the transmission of impulses across the neuromuscular junction.

▪ Recommend an eye patch if double vision is troublesome.

▪ Advise the patient to avoid stress and excessive heat exposure because they may aggravate symptoms.

Myelitis and acute transverse myelitis

Myelitis, or inflammation of the spinal cord, can result from several diseases. Poliomyelitis affects the cord's gray matter and produces motor dysfunction; leukomyelitis affects only the white matter and produces sensory dysfunction. These types of myelitis can attack any level of the spinal cord, causing partial destruction or scattered lesions.

Acute transverse myelitis, which affects the entire thickness of the spinal cord, produces both motor and sensory dysfunctions. This form of myelitis, which has a rapid onset, is the most devastating, with motor and sensory dysfunctions below the level of spinal cord damage appearing in 1 to 2 days.

The prognosis depends on the severity of cord damage and prevention of complications. If spinal cord necrosis occurs, the prognosis for complete recovery is poor. Even without necrosis, residual neurologic deficits usually persist after recovery. Patients who develop spastic reflexes early in the course of the illness are more likely to recover than those who don't.

Causes

▪ Acute infectious diseases, such as measles or pneumonia

▪ Carbon monoxide, lead, and arsenic: can cause a type of myelitis in which acute inflammation (followed by hemorrhage and possible necrosis) destroys the entire circumference (myelin, axis cylinders, and neurons) of the spinal cord

▪ Chronic adhesive arachnoiditis

▪ Demyelinating diseases, such as acute multiple sclerosis, and inflammatory and necrotizing disorders of the spinal cord, such as hematomyelia.

▪ Parasitic and fungal infections

▪ Poliovirus, herpes zoster, herpesvirus B, or rabies virus

▪ Primary infections of the spinal cord itself, such as syphilis or acute disseminated encephalomyelitis

▪ Smallpox or polio vaccination

▪ Syphilis, abscesses and other suppurative conditions, and tuberculosis

Signs and symptoms

- Flaccid paralysis of the legs (sometimes beginning in just one leg) with loss of sensory and sphincter functions
- Loss of reflexes (early stages) with later reappearance
- Pain in the legs or trunk
- Shock (with severe spinal cord damage)

Diagnostic tests

- Paraplegia of rapid onset usually points to acute transverse myelitis. In such patients, neurologic examination confirms paraplegia or neurologic deficit below the level of the spinal cord lesion and absent or, later, hyperactive reflexes.
- Cerebrospinal fluid usually shows increased lymphocyte or protein levels.
- Neuroimaging studies identify the site and extent of inflammation.
- Diagnostic evaluation must rule out a spinal cord tumor and identify the cause of an underlying infection.

Treatment

- No effective treatment exists for acute transverse myelitis.
- Treatment of underlying infection is appropriate.
- Some patients with postinfectious or multiple sclerosis–induced myelitis have received steroid therapy, but its benefits aren't clear.
- Analgesics are given for pain.

Nursing considerations

- Frequently assess vital signs. Watch carefully for signs of spinal shock (hypotension and excessive sweating).
- Prevent contractures with range-of-motion exercises and proper alignment.
- Watch for signs of urinary tract infections from indwelling urinary catheters.
- Prevent skin infections and pressure ulcers with meticulous skin care. Check pressure points often, and keep skin clean and dry; use a water bed or another pressure-relieving device.
- Provide psychological support to the patient and his family.

Myocarditis

Myocarditis is focal or diffuse inflammation of the cardiac muscle (myocardium). It may be acute or chronic and can occur at any age. Frequently, myocarditis fails to produce specific cardiovascular symptoms or electrocardiogram (ECG) abnormalities, and recovery is usually spontaneous, without residual defects. Occasionally, myocarditis is complicated by heart failure; rarely, it may lead to cardiomyopathy.

Causes

- Autoimmune factors
- Bacterial infections such as diphtheria, tuberculosis, typhoid fever, tetanus, and staphylococcal, pneumococcal, and gonococcal infections
- Chemical poisons such as alcohol
- Helminthic infections such as trichinosis
- Hypersensitive immune reactions
- Medications such as penicillin, ampicillin, hydrochlorothiazide, methyldopa, and sulfonamides
- Parasitic infections such as toxoplasmosis
- Poliomyelitis, influenza, rubeola, rubella
- Radiation therapy
- Rejection syndrome
- Viral infections such as coxsackievirus A and B strains, adenoviruses, and echoviruses

Signs and symptoms

- Fatigue

- Mild, continuous pressure or soreness in the chest (unlike the recurring, stress-related pain of angina pectoris)
- Palpitations
- Right- and left-sided heart failure, with cardiomegaly, jugular vein distention, dyspnea, persistent fever with resting or exertional tachycardia disproportionate to the degree of fever
- Supraventricular and ventricular arrhythmias

With recurrence
- Arrhythmias
- Cardiomyopathy
- Chronic valvulitis (when it results from rheumatic fever)
- Thromboembolism

Diagnostic tests
- A physical examination shows supraventricular and ventricular arrhythmias, third and fourth heart sounds, a faint first heart sound, possibly a murmur of mitral insufficiency (from papillary muscle dysfunction) and, if pericarditis is present, a pericardial friction rub.
- ECG typically shows diffuse ST-segment and T-wave abnormalities (as in pericarditis), conduction defects (prolonged PR interval), and other supraventricular arrhythmias.
- Echocardiography may show a weak heart muscle, valve problems, an enlarged heart, or fluid surrounding the heart.
- Stool and throat cultures may identify the causative bacteria. An endomyocardial biopsy can confirm the diagnosis, but it's rarely performed.
- Laboratory tests can't unequivocally confirm myocarditis, but these findings support this diagnosis:
  - Cardiac enzyme levels (creatine kinase [CK], the CK-MB isoenzyme, aspartate aminotransferase, and lactate dehydrogenase) are elevated.
  - White blood cell count and erythrocyte sedimentation rate are increased.
  - Antibody titers (such as antistreptolysin O titer in rheumatic fever) are elevated.
  - Blood cultures may indicate infection.

Treatment
- Antibiotics are used to treat bacterial infection.
- Modified bed rest decreases the cardiac workload.
- Careful management of complications is necessary.
- Heart failure requires restriction of activity to minimize myocardial oxygen consumption, supplemental oxygen therapy, sodium restriction, a diuretic to decrease fluid retention, and a cardiac glycoside to increase myocardial contractility. However, cardiac glycosides must be administered cautiously because some patients with myocarditis show a paradoxical sensitivity to even small doses.
- Arrhythmias necessitate prompt but cautious administration of antiarrhythmics, which can depress myocardial contractility.
- Thromboembolism requires anticoagulation therapy.
- Treatment with a corticosteroid or other immunosuppressant is controversial and therefore limited to combating life-threatening complications such as intractable heart failure.

Nursing considerations
- Assess cardiovascular status frequently, watching for signs of heart failure, such as dyspnea, hypotension, and tachycardia. Check for changes in cardiac rhythm or conduction.
- Monitor the patient for signs and symptoms of digoxin toxicity (anorexia,

nausea, vomiting, blurred vision, and cardiac arrhythmias) and for complicating factors that may potentiate toxicity, such as electrolyte imbalances or hypoxia.

- Stress the importance of bed rest. Assist with bathing as necessary; provide a bedside commode, which puts less stress on the heart than using a bedpan. Reassure the patient that activity limitations are temporary.
- Instruct the patient on a low-salt diet, if prescribed.
- Recommend that the patient resume normal activities slowly during recovery and avoid competitive sports.

Myringitis

Acute infectious myringitis is characterized by inflammation, hemorrhage, and effusion of fluid into the tissue at the end of the external ear canal and the tympanic membrane. This self-limiting disorder (resolving spontaneously within 3 days to 2 weeks) commonly follows acute otitis media or upper respiratory tract infection and commonly occurs epidemically in children.

Chronic granular myringitis, a rare inflammation of the squamous layer of the tympanic membrane, causes gradual hearing loss. Without specific treatment, this condition can lead to stenosis of the ear canal, as granulation extends from the tympanic membrane to the external ear.

Causes

- Unknown (chronic granular myringitis)
- Bacterial infection
- Viral infection

Signs and symptoms
Acute infectious myringitis

- Bloody discharge with spontaneous rupture of the blebs
- Fever and hearing loss
- Severe ear pain with tenderness over the mastoid process
- Small, reddened, inflamed blebs in the canal, on the tympanic membrane and, with bacterial invasion, in the middle ear

Chronic granular myringitis

- Gradual hearing loss
- Pruritus
- Purulent discharge

Diagnostic tests

- Culture and sensitivity testing of exudate identifies secondary infection.

Treatment
Acute infections myringitis

- Administration of an analgesic, such as aspirin or acetaminophen, and application of heat to the external ear are usually sufficient, but severe pain may necessitate the use of codeine.
- A systemic or topical antibiotic can prevent or treat secondary infection.
- Incision of the blebs and evacuation of serum and blood may relieve pressure and help drain exudate, but these measures don't speed recovery.

Chronic granular myringitis

- Treatment includes systemic antibiotic or local anti-inflammatory antibiotic combination eardrops.
- Surgical excision and cautery are additional treatments.
- If stenosis is present, surgical reconstruction is necessary.

Nursing considerations
- Stress the importance of completing prescribed antibiotic therapy.
- Teach the patient how to instill the topical antibiotic (eardrops). When necessary, explain incision of the blebs.
- Advise early treatment of acute otitis media to help prevent acute infectious myringitis.

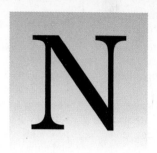

Near drowning

Near drowning refers to surviving—temporarily, at least—the physiologic effects of hypoxemia and acidosis that result from submersion in fluid. Hypoxemia and acidosis are the primary problems in victims of near drowning. Near drowning occurs in three forms:

- Dry: The victim doesn't aspirate fluid but suffers respiratory obstruction or asphyxia (10% to 15% of patients)
- Wet: The victim aspirates fluid and suffers from asphyxia or secondary changes due to fluid aspiration (about 85% of patients)
- Secondary: The victim suffers recurrence of respiratory distress (usually aspiration pneumonia or pulmonary edema) within minutes to 2 days after a near-drowning incident.

Causes

- Blow to the head while in the water
- Boating accident
- Drinking heavily before swimming
- Heart attack while swimming
- Inability to swim
- Panic
- Suicide attempt

Signs and symptoms

- Abdominal distention
- Cough that produces a pink, frothy fluid
- Fever
- Restlessness, irritability, lethargy, confusion, or unconsciousness
- Shallow or gasping respirations, or apnea
- Substernal chest pain
- Tachycardia, bradycardia, or asystole
- Vomiting

Diagnostic tests

- Diagnosis of near drowning relies on patient history rather than diagnostic testing. Characteristic features include auscultation of crackles and rhonchi.
- Arterial blood gas (ABG) analysis reveals hypercarbia, hypoxemia, and metabolic acidosis to confirm the diagnosis.
- Electrocardiography may reveal arrhythmias or myocardial ischemia.
- Chest radiography may show pulmonary edema.

Treatment

ACTION STAT!

 Begin emergency treatment immediately, including cardiopulmonary resuscitation and administration of supplemental oxygen.

- Stabilize the patient's neck until cervical injury has been ruled out.

- Provide intubation and respiratory assistance such as mechanical ventilation with positive end-expiratory pressure, if needed.
- The patient may require nasogastric tube for abdominal decompression. Intubate the patient first if he's unconscious.
- Administer I.V. fluids as indicated.
- Sodium bicarbonate may be given for metabolic acidosis.
- A corticosteroid may be prescribed for the patient with cerebral edema.
- The patient may be given an antibiotic for infection.
- A bronchodilator may be prescribed to ease bronchospasms.

Nursing considerations

- Observe the patient for pulmonary complications and indications of delayed drowning (confusion, substernal pain, adventitious breath sounds).
- Suction the patient as needed.
- Monitor ABG and pulse oximetry values.
- Monitor pulmonary artery catheter readings to assess cardiopulmonary status.
- Monitor vital signs, intake and output, and peripheral pulses. Check for skin perfusion.
- Watch for signs of infection.
- To facilitate breathing, raise the head of the bed slightly, unless contraindicated.

Necrotizing enterocolitis

Neonatal necrotizing enterocolitis (NEC) is a condition characterized by an initial mucosal intestinal injury that may progress to transmural bowel necrosis. Blood shunted from the gut produces mucosal ischemia, leading to swelling of the bowel and breakdown of integrity.

NEC is the leading surgical emergency in neonates in North America and is related to 2% of all infant deaths. Onset usually occurs 1 to 14 days after birth. Infectious complications associated with bowel necrosis include bacterial peritonitis, systemic sepsis, and intra-abdominal abscess formation. Recurrence of NEC and mechanical and functional abnormalities, especially stricture, may develop as late as 3 months postoperatively.

Causes
- Unknown

Risk factors
- Acidosis
- Blood exchange transfusions
- Feeding of concentrated formulas
- Hypothermia
- Infection
- Low birth weight (less than 5 lb [2.3 kg])
- Pharmacologic (cocaine exposure, indomethacin treatment)
- Prematurity (in neonates born at less than 34 weeks' gestation)
- Respiratory failure
- Sepsis
- Significant prenatal stress
- Structural cardiac defects

Signs and symptoms
- Bilious vomitus
- Bloody diarrhea
- Disseminated intravascular coagulation (DIC)
- Distended (especially tense or rigid) abdomen
- Increasing residual gastric contents (which may contain bile)
- Jaundice
- Lethargy
- Metabolic acidosis
- Occult or gross blood in stools

ACTION STAT!

Recognizing the ominous signs of necrotizing enterocolitis

When an infant suffers perinatal hypoxemia, be alert for the following signs and symptoms of gastric distention and perforation:
- Apnea
- Bradycardia
- Cardiovascular shock

- Increasing abdominal tenderness, edema, erythema, or involuntary abdominal rigidity
- Sudden drop in temperature
- Sudden listlessness and ragdoll limpness

- Red or shiny, taut abdomen (may indicate peritonitis)
- Thermal instability

Diagnostic tests

- Abdominal X-rays show nonspecific intestinal dilation and, in later stages of NEC, pneumatosis cystoides intestinalis (gas or air in the intestinal wall). Portal vein gas and fixed or thickened small bowel loops may also be found.
- Platelet count may show thrombocytopenia.
- Clotting studies and hemoglobin levels show DIC.
- Serum sodium levels are decreased.
- Arterial blood gas levels show metabolic acidosis (a result of sepsis).
- Bilirubin levels show infection-induced breakdown of red blood cells.
- Blood and stool cultures identify the infecting organism.
- Guaiac test may show occult blood in stools.

Treatment

- Discontinue oral intake for 7 to 10 days to rest the injured bowel.
- Administer I.V. fluids, including total parenteral nutrition.
- Insert nasogastric (NG) tube for bowel decompression.

- Correct hypoxemia, hypotension, acidosis, and any other reversible medical problems.
- Broad-spectrum antibiotic suppress bacterial flora and prevent bowel perforation.
- Surgery (removal of necrotic and acutely inflamed bowel and formation of temporary colostomy or ileostomy) is indicated in perforation (free intraperitoneal air on X-ray) or symptoms of peritonitis, respiratory insufficiency (caused by severe abdominal distention), progressive and intractable acidosis, or DIC.
- Mechanical ventilation is required after surgery.

Nursing considerations

ACTION STAT!

Be alert for signs of gastric distention and perforation. (See *Recognizing the ominous signs of necrotizing enterocolitis.*)

- Take axillary temperatures to avoid perforating the bowel.
- Prevent cross-contamination by properly disposing of soiled diapers and washing hands after diaper changes.
- Prepare the parents for a potential deterioration in their infant's condition. Explain all treatments, including why feedings are withheld.

Pathophysiology of nephrotic syndrome

```
┌─────────────────────────────┐
│      Hypoalbuminemia        │
└─────────────────────────────┘
              ▼
┌─────────────────────────────┐
│ Reduced intravascular oncotic│
│          pressure           │
└─────────────────────────────┘
              ▼
┌─────────────────────────────┐
│ Loss of fluid into the interstitial│
│            space            │
└─────────────────────────────┘
              ▼
┌─────────────────────────────┐
│    Reduced plasma volume    │
└─────────────────────────────┘
        ▼              ▼
┌──────────────┐ ┌──────────────┐
│  Increased   │ │  Decreased   │
│  aldosterone │ │    renal     │
│  secretion   │ │  function    │
└──────────────┘ └──────────────┘
              ▼
┌─────────────────────────────┐
│  Salt and water retention   │
└─────────────────────────────┘
              ▼
┌─────────────────────────────┐
│  Decreased renal function   │
└─────────────────────────────┘
              ▼
┌─────────────────────────────┐
│           Edema             │
└─────────────────────────────┘
```

- Gently suction secretions, and frequently monitor respirations.
- Replace fluids lost through NG tube and stoma drainage as ordered; monitor drainage losses in output records.
- Weigh the infant daily.
- Obtain a referral for an enterostomal therapy nurse to see an infant with a temporary colostomy or ileostomy to assist in meeting needs.
- Encourage the parents to participate in their infant's physical care.
- Maintain a clean suture line and provide skin care to prevent excoriation

from active enzymes in bowel secretions, which are corrosive.
- Watch for wound disruption, infection, and dehiscence.
- Watch for intestinal malfunction from stricture or short-bowel syndrome.

Nephrotic syndrome

Nephrotic syndrome (or *nephrosis*) is characterized by marked proteinuria, hypoalbuminemia, hyperlipemia, and edema. Major complications are malnutrition, infection, coagulation disorders, thromboembolic vascular occlusion, and accelerated atherosclerosis. Although nephrotic syndrome isn't a disease itself, it results from a specific glomerular defect and indicates renal damage. The prognosis is highly variable, depending on the underlying cause. Some forms may progress to end-stage renal failure. (See *Pathophysiology of nephrotic syndrome*.)

Causes
- Allergic reactions
- Diabetes mellitus and other metabolic diseases
- Heart failure, sickle cell anemia, and other circulatory diseases
- Hereditary nephritis
- Multiple myeloma and other neoplastic diseases
- Nephrotoxins, such as mercury, gold, and nonsteroidal anti-inflammatories
- Preeclampsia toxemia
- Primary (idiopathic) glomerulonephritis (75%)
- Systemic lupus erythematosus, polyarteritis nodosa, and other collagen-vascular disorders
- Tuberculosis, hepatitis B, and other infections

Signs and symptoms
- Anorexia

- Ascites
- Depression
- High blood pressure
- Lethargy
- Mild to severe dependent edema of the ankles or sacrum
- Orthostatic hypotension
- Pallor
- Periorbital edema, especially in children
- Pleural effusion
- Weight gain

Diagnostic tests

- Urinalysis shows consistent proteinuria in excess of 3.5 mg/dl for 24 hours, and an increased number of hyaline, granular, and waxy, fatty casts, and oval fat bodies.
- Laboratory testing reveals increased cholesterol, phospholipid, and triglyceride levels as well as decreased albumin levels.
- Kidney biopsy provides histologic identification of the lesion.

Treatment

- Treatment focuses on correction of the underlying cause, if possible.
- Protein replacement may be instituted with a nutritional diet of 0.6 g protein/kg of body weight and restricted sodium intake.
- A diuretic may be prescribed for edema.
- An antibiotic may be prescribed for infection.
- Some patients respond to an 8-week course of a corticosteroid such as prednisone, followed by maintenance therapy. Others respond better to a combination of prednisone and azathioprine (Imuran) or cyclophosphamide (Cytoxan).
- Chronic nephrotic syndrome unresponsive to conventional therapy may respond to vitamin D replacement.

Nursing considerations

- Treatment for hyperlipidemia is commonly unsuccessful.
- Check urine protein levels frequently. (Urine containing protein appears frothy.)
- Measure blood pressure while the patient is in a supine position and also while he's standing; be alert for a drop in blood pressure that exceeds 20 mm Hg.
- If the patient has had a kidney biopsy, watch for bleeding and shock.
- Monitor intake and output, and check weight at the same time each morning—after the patient voids and before he eats—and while he's wearing the same kind of clothing.
- Ask the dietitian to plan a high-protein, low-sodium diet.
- Provide good skin care because the patient with nephrotic syndrome usually has edema.
- To avoid thrombophlebitis, encourage activity and exercise and provide anti-embolism stockings as needed.
- Offer the patient and his family reassurance and support, especially during the acute phase, when edema is severe and the patient's body image changes.

Neural tube defects

Neural tube defects (NTDs) are serious birth defects that involve the spine or brain; they result from failure of the neural tube to close during the first trimester of pregnancy. The most common forms of NTD are spina bifida (50% of cases), anencephaly (40%), and encephalocele (10%). *Spina bifida occulta* is the most common and least severe spinal cord defect, characterized by incomplete closure of one or more vertebrae without protrusion of the spinal cord or meninges. In more severe forms of spina bifida, incomplete closure of one or more vertebrae causes protrusion of the spinal contents in an external sac or cystic lesion (spina bifida cystica).

Spina bifida cystica has two classifications: myelomeningocele (meningomyelocele) and meningocele. With *myelomeningocele,* the external sac contains meninges, cerebrospinal fluid (CSF), and a portion of the spinal cord or nerve roots distal to the conus medullaris. When the spinal nerve roots end at the sac, motor and sensory functions below the sac are terminated. With *meningocele,* which is less severe than myelomeningocele, the sac contains only meninges and CSF.

With *encephalocele,* a saclike portion of the meninges and brain protrudes through a defective opening in the skull—usually the occipital area but possibly the parietal, nasopharyngeal, or frontal area.

With *anencephaly,* the most severe form of NTD, the closure defect occurs at the cranial end of the neuroaxis and, as a result, part or all of the top of the skull is missing, severely damaging the brain. Portions of the brain stem and spinal cord may also be missing. No diagnostic or therapeutic efforts are helpful; babies with anencephaly are either stillborn or don't survive more than a few hours after birth.

Causes
- Exposure to a teratogen
- Genetic and environmental factors (insufficient folic acid in prenatal diet)
- Part of a multiple malformation syndrome (for example, chromosomal abnormalities such as trisomy 18 or 13 syndrome)

Signs and symptoms
Spina bifida occulta
- Asymptomatic (possibly)
- Depression or dimple, tuft of hair, soft fatty deposits, port wine nevi (or a combination) on the skin over the spinal defect
- Foot weakness or bowel and bladder disturbances

Meningocele
- Asymptomatic (possibly)
- Foot weakness or bowel and bladder disturbances
- Saclike structure over the spine

Myelomeningocele
- Permanent neurologic dysfunction such as flaccid or spastic paralysis; bowel and bladder incontinence (depending on the level of the defect)
- Saclike structure over the spine

Encephalocele
- Mental retardation
- Paralysis and hydrocephalus
- Variable, with the degree of tissue involvement and location of the defect

Anencephaly
- Missing top of skull
- Severe brain damage
- Death

Diagnostic tests
- Alpha-fetoprotein (AFP) screening involves a prenatal blood test performed at 16 to 18 weeks' gestation to measure AFP levels in the blood. AFP indicates the presence of neural tube defects when present in the amniotic fluid.
- If the AFP screen is abnormal, amniocentesis and fetal ultrasound are performed.
- Amniocentesis may detect elevated AFP levels, indicating presence of an open NTD.
- Acetylcholinesterase levels can confirm the diagnosis. (Biochemical testing will usually miss closed NTDs.)
- Fetal karyotype shows chromosomal abnormalities.

- Maternal serum AFP screening in combination with other serum markers (human chorionic gonadotropin [hCG], free beta hCG, or unconjugated estriol) determines fetal risk of neurologic or other disorders.
- Ultrasound may detect neural tube defects or ventral wall defects.
- Spinal X-ray can show bone defects.
- Myelography can differentiate spinal abnormalities, especially spinal cord tumors.
- Skull X-rays, cephalic measurements, and computed tomography (CT) scan demonstrate associated hydrocephalus.
- With encephalocele, X-rays show a basilar bony skull defect. CT scan and ultrasonography further define the defect.

Treatment

- Spina bifida occulta usually requires no treatment.
- Treatment of meningocele consists of surgical closure of the protruding sac and continual assessment of growth and development.
- Treatment of myelomeningocele requires repair of the sac and supportive measures to promote independence and prevent further complications. Surgery doesn't reverse neurologic deficits. Fetal surgery, typically performed at 24 to 30 weeks' gestation, may be used to correct myelomeningocele in utero. The procedure is still considered experimental.
- A shunt may be needed to relieve associated hydrocephalus. If hydrocephalus isn't apparent at the time of initial surgery, the child must be frequently reassessed for its occurrence, because hydrocephalus occurs in about 90% of children with myelomeningocele.
- Treatment of encephalocele includes surgery during infancy to place protruding tissues back in the skull, excise the sac, and correct associated craniofacial abnormalities.

Nursing considerations

- If diagnosed prenatally, refer the parents to a genetic counselor.
- Urge all women of childbearing age to take a vitamin supplement with folic acid until menopause or the end of their childbearing years.
- Coordinate assistance from practitioners, nurses, surgeons, rehabilitation providers, and social workers.

Before surgery

- Prevent local infection by cleaning the defect gently with sterile saline solution or other solutions as ordered.
- Inspect the defect often for signs of infection, and cover it with sterile dressings moistened with sterile saline solution.
- Prevent skin breakdown by placing sheepskin or a foam pad under the infant.
- Give antibiotics as ordered.
- Handle the infant carefully, and don't apply pressure to the defect. Usually, the infant can't wear a diaper or a shirt until after surgical correction because it will irritate the sac, so keep him warm in an infant Isolette. Hold and cuddle the infant; on your lap, position him on his abdomen, and teach the parents to do the same.
- Provide adequate time for parent-child bonding, if possible.
- Measure head circumference daily, and watch for signs of hydrocephalus and meningeal irritation, such as fever or nuchal rigidity. Be sure to mark the spot so you get accurate readings.
- Provide passive range-of-motion exercises and cast care as indicated.
- To prevent hip dislocation, moderately abduct hips with a pad between the knees or with sandbags and ankle rolls.

■ Monitor intake and output. Watch for decreased skin turgor, dryness, or other signs of dehydration. Provide meticulous skin care to genitals and buttocks to prevent infection.

After surgery

■ Watch for hydrocephalus, which can be a complication after surgery. Measure the infant's head circumference as ordered.

■ Monitor vital signs often. Watch for signs of shock, infection, and increased intracranial pressure, such as projectile vomiting. Frequently assess the infant's fontanels. In infants, the most telling sign is bulging fontanels.

■ Change the dressing regularly as ordered, and check and report any signs of drainage, wound rupture, or infection.

■ Place the infant in the prone position to protect and assess the site.

■ Teach the parents to recognize early signs of complications, such as hydrocephalus, pressure ulcers, and urinary tract infections (UTIs).

■ Provide psychological support, and encourage a positive attitude. Help parents work through their feelings of guilt, anger, and helplessness.

■ Encourage parents to begin training their child in a bladder routine by age 3. Emphasize the need for increased fluid intake to prevent UTIs. Teach intermittent catheterization and conduit hygiene as ordered.

■ To prevent constipation and bowel obstruction, stress the need for increased fluid intake, a high-bulk diet, exercise, and a stool softener, as ordered. If possible, teach parents to help empty their child's bowel by telling him to bear down and giving a glycerin suppository as needed.

■ Urge early recognition of developmental lags (a possible result of hydrocephalus). If present, stress the importance of follow-up IQ assessment to help plan realistic educational goals. The child may need to attend a school with special facilities. Also, stress the need for stimulation to ensure maximum mental development. Help parents plan activities appropriate to their child's age and abilities.

■ Refer parents to the Spina Bifida Association of America.

Neuritis, peripheral

Also known as *multiple neuritis,* peripheral neuropathy, and polyneuritis, peripheral neuritis is the degeneration of peripheral nerves. Symptoms depend on the type of nerves affected. Damage to sensory fibers results in changes in usually beginning distally and progressing toward the center of the body. Impaired nervous stimulation due to damage of motor nerve fibers results in weakness, decreased movement, or decreased control of movement. In addition, structural changes occur in muscle, bone, skin, hair, nails, and body organs due to lack of nervous stimulation, disuse of the affected area, immobility, or lack of weight bearing; muscle weakness and wasting also occur. Repeated, unnoticed injury to sensory and motor areas occur due to the inability to feel, causing further injury and can result in infection or structural damage (ulcer formation, poor healing, loss of tissue mass, scarring, and deformity). Peripheral neuritis is associated with a noninflammatory degeneration of the axon and myelin sheaths. Because onset is usually insidious, patients may compensate by overusing unaffected muscles; however, onset is rapid with severe infection. A manifestation of many conditions, peripheral neuritis also can cause damage to the peripheral nerves.

Causes

- Exposure to toxic compounds: sniffing glue or other toxic compounds; nitrous oxide; industrial agents (especially solvents); heavy metals, such as lead, arsenic, and mercury
- Hereditary disorders: Charcot-Marie-Tooth disease, Friedreich's ataxia
- Infectious or inflammatory conditions: acquired immunodeficiency syndrome (AIDS), botulism, Colorado tick fever, diphtheria, Guillain-Barré syndrome, human immunodeficiency virus infection without development of AIDS, leprosy, polyarteritis nodosa, rheumatoid arthritis, sarcoidosis, syphilis, systemic lupus erythematosus, amyloidosis
- Ischemia
- Neuropathy induced by drugs
- Prolonged exposure to cold temperature
- Systemic effects of malignancies: multiple myeloma, lung cancer, lymphoma, leukemia
- Systemic or metabolic disorders: diabetes mellitus, dietary deficiencies, habitual use of alcohol, uremia

Signs and symptoms
Motor and sensory symptoms

- Atrophied muscles (tender or hypersensitive to pressure or palpation)
- Cutaneous manifestations: glossy, red skin and decreased sweating
- Flaccid paralysis
- Footdrop
- Loss of ability to perceive vibratory sensations
- Loss of reflexes; diminished or absent deep tendon reflexes
- Pain of varying intensity
- Paresthesia, hyperesthesia, or anesthesia in the hands and feet
- Wasting

Autonomic symptoms

- Abdominal bloating or swelling
- Anhidrosis (decreased or absence of sweating)
- Blurred or double vision
- Diarrhea or constipation
- Dizziness when standing up
- Early satiety (feeling full after eating a small amount)
- Fainting
- Feeling of incomplete bladder emptying
- Heat intolerance with exertion
- Male impotence
- Nausea and vomiting after meals
- Unintentional weight loss
- Urinary hesitancy
- Urinary incontinence

Diagnostic tests

- The patient history and physical examination delineate the characteristic distribution of motor and sensory deficits.
- Electromyography may show a delayed action potential if this condition impairs motor nerve function.
- Nerve conduction tests and nerve biopsy may reveal abnormalities.

Treatment

- The underlying cause must be identified and corrected.
- Identify and remove the toxic agent if indicated.
- Correct nutritional and vitamin deficiencies with a high-calorie diet rich in vitamins, especially B complex.
- Provide supportive measures to relieve pain.
- Ensure adequate bed rest.
- Provide physical therapy.
- Give analgesics for pain.
- Phenytoin may help some types of neuritic pain, especially that associated with diabetic neuropathy.
- Electrotherapy is advocated for nerve and muscle stimulation.

Nursing considerations

- Perform neurologic assessment and determine level of impairment.
- Relieve pain with correct positioning, administering an analgesic, and monitoring for effect.
- Use safety measures as indicated.
- Instruct the patient to rest, to refrain from using the affected extremity, and to avoid alcohol.
- To prevent pressure ulcers, apply a foot cradle. To prevent contractures, arrange for the patient to obtain splints, boards, braces, or other orthopedic appliances.
- After the pain subsides, passive range-of-motion exercises or massage may be beneficial. Consult with a physical therapist to help determine the most appropriate therapy.
- Use elastic stockings to promote circulation.
- Monitor effects of medications that may be prescribed to relieve autonomic symptoms.
- Monitor urine output. Manually express urine or perform intermittent catheterization if indicated.

Neurogenic arthropathy

Most common in men older than age 40, neurogenic arthropathy (*Charcot's arthropathy*) is a progressively degenerative disease of peripheral and axial joints, resulting from impaired sensory innervation. The loss of sensation in the joints causes progressive deterioration, resulting from unrecognized trauma (especially repeated minor episodes) or primary disease, which leads to laxity of supporting ligaments and eventual disintegration of the affected joints.

Causes

- Alcoholism
- Amyloidosis
- Charcot-Marie-Tooth disease
- Diabetes mellitus (most common)
- Frequent intra-articular injections of a corticosteroid
- Hereditary sensory neuropathy
- Leprosy
- Myelomeningocele (in children)
- Myelopathy of pernicious anemia
- Paraplegia
- Peripheral nerve injury
- Spinal cord trauma
- Syringomyelia (which progresses to neurogenic arthropathy in about 25% of patients)
- Tabes dorsalis (especially among patients ages 40 to 60)

Signs and symptoms

- Joint deformity
- Swelling, warmth, decreased mobility, and instability in a single joint or many joints
- Vertebral neuroarthropathy, progressing to gross spinal deformity (initially, mild, persistent backache)

Diagnostic tests

- X-rays in the early stage show soft-tissue swelling or effusion; in the advanced stage, articular fracture, subluxation, erosion of articular cartilage, periosteal new bone formation, and excessive growth of marginal loose bodies (osteophytosis) or resorption may be seen.
- Vertebral examination shows narrowing of disk spaces, deterioration of vertebrae, and osteophyte formation, leading to ankylosis and deforming kyphoscoliosis.
- Synovial biopsy shows bony fragments and bits of calcified cartilage.
- Neuromuscular tests may reveal motor and sensory deficits and diminished deep tendon reflexes.

Treatment

- Give analgesics or nonsteroidal anti-inflammatory drugs for pain relief.
- Provide immobilization of affected area with crutches, splints, braces, and weight-bearing restrictions.
- In severe disease, surgery may include arthrodesis.
- In those with severe diabetic neuropathy, amputation may be necessary.

Nursing considerations

- Assess the pattern of pain, and monitor the effectiveness of analgesics.
- Check sensory perception, range of motion, alignment, joint swelling, and the status of underlying disease.
- Teach the patient joint protection techniques.
- Advise the patient to avoid physically stressful actions that may cause pathologic fractures, and encourage him to take safety precautions, such as removing throw rugs and clutter that may cause falls.
- Advise the patient to report severe joint pain, swelling, or instability.
- Apply warm compresses to relieve local pain and tenderness.
- Teach the patient the proper technique for using crutches or other orthopedic devices.
- Stress the importance of proper fitting and regular professional readjustment of orthopedic devices and the importance of good skin care.
- Warn that impaired sensation might allow damage from these orthopedic devices without discomfort.
- Emphasize the need to continue regular treatment of the underlying disease.

▌Neurogenic bladder

Also known as *neuromuscular dysfunction of the lower urinary tract, neurologic bladder dysfunction,* and *neuropathic bladder,*

neurogenic bladder refers to all types of bladder dysfunction caused by an interruption of normal bladder innervation. Subsequent complications include urinary incontinence, residual urine retention, urinary tract infection, calculi formation, and renal failure. A neurogenic bladder can be spastic (hypertonic, reflex, or automatic), flaccid (hypotonic, atonic, nonreflex, or autonomous), or uncoordinated (dyssynergic). An upper motor neuron lesion (at or above T12) causes spastic neurogenic bladder, with spontaneous contractions of the detrusor muscles, elevated intravesical voiding pressure, bladder wall hypertrophy with trabeculation, and urinary sphincter spasms. A lower motor neuron lesion (at or below S2) causes flaccid neurogenic bladder, with decreased intravesical pressure, increased bladder capacity and large residual urine retention, and poor detrusor contraction.

Causes

- Acute infectious diseases such as Guillain-Barré syndrome
- Cerebral disorders, such as stroke, brain tumor (meningioma and glioma), Parkinson's disease, multiple sclerosis, and dementia
- Chronic alcoholism
- Collagen diseases such as systemic lupus erythematosus
- Disorders of peripheral innervation, including autonomic neuropathies resulting from endocrine disturbances such as diabetes mellitus (most common)
- Distant effects of cancer such as primary oat cell carcinoma of the lung
- Heavy metal toxicity
- Herpes zoster
- Metabolic disturbances, such as hypothyroidism, porphyria, or uremia (infrequent)
- Sacral agenesis

- Spinal cord disease or trauma, such as spinal stenosis (causing cord compression) or arachnoiditis (causing adhesions between the membranes covering the cord), cervical spondylosis, myelopathies from hereditary or nutritional deficiencies and, rarely, tabes dorsalis
- Vascular diseases such as atherosclerosis

Signs and symptoms
- Changes in initiation or interruption of micturition
- Deterioration or infection in the upper urinary tract
- Hydroureteral nephrosis
- Inability to completely empty the bladder
- Incontinence (variable in degree)
- Vesicoureteral reflux

Spastic neurogenic bladder
- Increased anal sphincter tone
- Involuntary or frequent scanty urination without a feeling of bladder fullness
- Spontaneous spasms of the arms and legs
- Tactile stimulation of the abdomen, thighs, or genitalia precipitating voiding and spontaneous contractions of the arms and legs
- Upper thoracic (cervical) level lesions: hyperactive autonomic reflexes (severe hypertension, bradycardia, headaches) due to bladder distention

Flaccid neurogenic bladder
- Diminished anal sphincter tone
- Greatly distended bladder (evident on percussion or palpation) without feeling of bladder fullness
- Overflow incontinence

Diagnostic tests
- Diagnosis relies on the patient's history, which may reveal an underlying condition or disorder that can cause neurogenic bladder.
- Voiding cystourethrography evaluates bladder neck function, vesicoureteral reflux, and continence.
- Urodynamic studies help evaluate how urine is stored in the bladder, how well the bladder empties, and the rate of movement of urine out of the bladder during voiding. These studies consist of four components:
  - Urine flow study (uroflow) shows diminished or impaired urine flow.
  - Cystometry evaluates bladder nerve supply, detrusor muscle tone, and intravesical pressures during bladder filling and contraction.
  - Urethral pressure profile determines urethral function with respect to the length of the urethra and the outlet pressure resistance.
  - Sphincter electromyelography correlates the neuromuscular function of the external sphincter with bladder muscle function during bladder filling and contraction. This evaluates how well the bladder and urinary sphincter muscles work together.
- Videourodynamic studies are used to correlate visual documentation of bladder function with pressure study results.
- Retrograde urethrography reveals the presence of strictures and diverticula. This test isn't performed on a routine basis.

Treatment
- Techniques of bladder evacuation include Credé's method, Valsalva's maneuver, and intermittent self-catheterization. Credé's method (applying manual pressure over the lower abdomen) and Valsalva's maneuver (performing forced exhalation against a closed glottis) promote complete emptying of the bladder.

Credé's method can result in autonomic dysreflexia in patients with spinal cord injuries. With this medical emergency, blood pressure rises to potentially fatal levels because of stimulation of the sympathetic nervous system.

■ Intermittent self-catheterization allows complete emptying of the bladder.
■ Bethanechol (Duvoid) and phenoxybenzamine (Dibenzyline) facilitate bladder emptying.
■ Propantheline (Pro-banthine), flavoxate (Urispas), dicyclomine (Bentyl), and imipramine (Tofranil) facilitate urine storage.
■ Surgery may be necessary to correct the structural impairment through transurethral resection of the bladder neck, urethral dilatation, external sphincterotomy, or urinary diversion procedures.
■ Implantation of an artificial urinary sphincter may be indicated if permanent incontinence follows surgery for neurogenic bladder.

Nursing considerations

■ Use strict aseptic technique during insertion of an indwelling urinary catheter. Don't interrupt the closed drainage system for any reason.
■ Obtain urine specimens with a needleless device inserted through the aspirating port of the catheter itself (below the junction of the balloon instillation site).
■ Clean the catheter insertion site with soap and water at least twice per day. Don't allow the catheter to become encrusted.

 To prevent backflow of urine into the bladder, keep the drainage bag below the tubing,

and don't raise the bag above the level of the bladder.

■ Clamp the tubing or empty the bag before transferring the patient to a wheelchair or stretcher to prevent accidental urine reflux.
■ If urine output is considerable, empty the bag more frequently than once every 8 hours because bacteria can multiply in standing urine and migrate up the catheter and into the bladder.
■ Watch for signs of infection, including fever and cloudy or foul-smelling urine.
■ Try to keep the patient as mobile as possible.
■ Perform passive range-of-motion exercises, if necessary.
■ If a urinary diversion procedure is to be performed, arrange for consultation with an enterostomal therapist, and coordinate the care.
■ Before discharge, teach the patient and his family evacuation techniques, such as Credé's method and intermittent self-catheterization, as necessary.

■ Norovirus infection

Noroviruses are a group of related viruses that cause acute gastroenteritis, stomach flu, and food poisoning. They're named after the "Norwalk virus," which caused an outbreak of gastroenteritis in a school in Norwalk, Ohio, in 1968. Noroviruses are single-stranded ribonucleic acid, nonenveloped viruses. They have several other names, including norwalklike viruses or caliciviruses (they belong to the virus family *Caliciviridae*) due to their "Star of David" shape with cup-shaped (chalice) indentations. Immunity to norovirus is unclear and may be strain-specific, lasting only a few months. Susceptibility to infection may be genetically determined, with people of O blood group being at greatest risk for severe infection.

An estimated 23 million cases of acute gastroenteritis a year are due to norovirus infection and at least 50% of all food-borne outbreaks can be attributed to the virus.

Noroviruses are very highly contagious and can spread easily from person to person. Outbreaks have occurred in restaurants, day-care centers, and schools. People infected with norovirus are contagious from the moment they begin feeling ill to at least 3 days after recovery; some may be contagious for as long as 2 weeks after recovery.

Symptoms usually start about 24 to 48 hours after the virus is contracted, but they can appear as early as 12 hours after exposure. The average incubation period is 33 to 36 hours.

Causes
- Norovirus

Risk factors
- Contact with feces or vomitus of infected person, or direct contact with an infected person
- Eating food contaminated by food handlers, cold foods (salads, sandwiches, bakery products), or foods such as oysters from a contaminated source
- Sewage contamination of wells and recreational water

Signs and symptoms
- Chills
- Headache
- Low-grade fever
- Malaise
- Muscle aches
- Stomach cramps
- Sudden nausea and vomiting occurring many times per day
- Watery, nonbloody diarrhea

Diagnostic tests
- Reverse transcriptase polymerase chain reaction can be used to test stool and emesis samples, as well as to detect the presence of noroviruses on environmental swabs in special studies.

Treatment
- Treatment is supportive.
- Give oral fluids to prevent dehydration.
- Provide I.V. fluid replacement if necessary.
- Antipyretics are given for fever.
- Analgesics may be prescribed for muscle aches.

Nursing considerations
- Monitor intake and output.
- Encourage intake of fluids in frequent small amounts and increase as tolerated.
- Maintain I.V. patency and monitor hydration status.

ACTION STAT!

 Monitor the patient for signs of dehydration, including decreased skin turgor, slowed capillary refill (more than 2 seconds), tachycardia, decreased blood pressure, and dry mucous membranes. Dehydration is the most common complication of the disease, especially in people who are young or elderly or who have an immunodeficiency.

- Tell the patient that symptoms usually last 24 to 60 hours, after which he can expect to get better and recover.
- Instruct the patient and his family members to frequently wash hands, especially after toilet visits, changing diapers, and before eating or preparing food.
- To avoid future contact with the virus, tell the patient to carefully wash fruits

and vegetables, and steam oysters before eating them.

▪ People infected with norovirus shouldn't prepare food while they have symptoms and for 3 days after they recover from their illness.

▪ Food that may have been contaminated by someone with norovirus infection should be disposed of properly.

▪ Tell the patient and his family to thoroughly clean and disinfect contaminated surfaces immediately after an episode of illness by using a bleach-based household cleaner. Also, clothing that may be contaminated with virus should be removed and washed with soap and hot water.

▪ Flush vomitus and stool down the toilet and make sure that the surrounding area is kept clean.

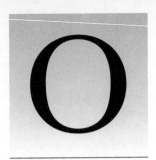

Obesity

Obesity is an excess of body fat with a body mass index (BMI) greater than or equal to 30, which may result from excessive caloric intake and inadequate expenditure of energy. Excessive calorie intake causes nutrients to be converted into fat, which is stored in the body. If the person continues to have excessive caloric intake and decreased energy expenditure, fat continues to accumulate in the body, leading to obesity.

Causes
- Abnormal absorption of nutrients
- Genetic predisposition
- Hypothalamic dysfunction of hunger and satiety centers
- Impaired action of GI and growth hormones and of hormonal regulators such as insulin and hypothyroidism

Signs and symptoms
- BMI of 30 or higher
- Chronic multisystem disorder (in some patients)
- Rashes such as contact dermatoses

Diagnostic tests
- Standard skin thicknesses (subscapular, triceps, biceps and suprailiac) and anthropometric measurements of the waist and hip circumferences are used to determine degree and distribution of obesity.
- Results of a full lipid panel may be normal or elevated.
- Results of a hepatic panel may be normal or abnormal if liver problems exist.
- Thyroid function test results may show primary hypothyroidism.
- A 24-hour urinary free cortisol test may suggest Cushing syndrome or other hypercortisolemic states.
- Fasting glucose and insulin may be elevated.

Treatment
- An increase in activity level facilitates burning of calories.
- Decrease daily calorie intake through a balanced, low-calorie diet that reduces fat and sugar intake.
- Hypnosis, behavior modification techniques, and psychotherapy may be useful for some patients.
- Amphetamines, amphetamine congeners, and sibutramine (Meridia) may be used temporarily to suppress appetite and creating a feeling of well-being.
- Morbid obesity (BMI greater than 40) may be treated with bariatric surgery.

Nursing considerations
- Help the physical therapist develop an exercise plan for the patient that incorporates his preferred activities.

- Monitor calorie counts.
- Consult a nutritional therapist to help the patient formulate a weight-loss diet while meeting dietary requirements.
- Encourage compliance with therapy; discuss advantages of weight loss and discuss complications of obesity (increased incidence of cardiovascular and other systemic problems).
- If a patient undergoes surgery for obesity, micronutrient deficiencies can occur, especially in calcium, vitamin B_{12}, folate, and iron; monitor deficiencies.
- If the patient has surgery, watch for complications, such as uncontrolled diarrhea, potassium or magnesium deficiency, gallstone development, and metabolic encephalopathy.

Osteoarthritis

Osteoarthritis, also known as *hypertrophic osteoarthritis, osteoarthrosis,* and *degenerative joint disease,* is the most common form of arthritis. A chronic disease, it causes deterioration of the joint cartilage and formation of reactive new bone at the margins and subchondral areas of the joints. This degeneration results from a breakdown of chondrocytes, usually in the hips and knees.

Causes
Primary osteoarthritis
- Aging (normal with aging)
- Chemical factors
- Genetic
- Mechanical factors
- Metabolic causes

Secondary osteoarthritis
- Congenital deformity
- Obesity
- Trauma

Signs and symptoms
- Aching during changes in weather (joint pain in rainy weather)
- Altered gait contractures
- Bouchard's nodes on proximal joints (possibly)
- Deep, aching joint pain, particularly after exercise or weight bearing, usually relieved by rest
- "Grating" of the joint during motion
- Heberden's nodes at the distal interphalangeal joints
- Limited movement
- Stiffness in the morning

Diagnostic tests
- X-rays of the affected joint help confirm diagnosis of osteoarthritis but may be normal in the early stages. X-rays may require many views and typically show:
  - narrowing of joint space or margin
  - cystlike bony deposits in joint space and margins
  - sclerosis of the subchondral space
  - joint deformity due to degeneration or articular damage
  - bony growths at weight-bearing areas
  - joint fusion.

Treatment
- Nonsteroidal anti-inflammatory drugs and COX-2 inhibitors are given to help reduce pain caused by inflammation.
- Intra-articular injections of corticosteroids may be given every 4 to 6 months and may delay nodal development in the hands.
- Artificial joint fluid may be injected into the knee for temporary relief of pain for up to 6 months.
- Joint support or stabilization with crutches, braces, cane, walker, cervical collar, or traction may be required.
- Some patients benefit from massage, application of moist heat, and paraffin dips for hands.

- Adequate rest is essential and should be balanced with activity.
- Supervised exercise may decrease muscle spasms and atrophy, and protective techniques prevent undue joint stress.
- Arthroplasty (partial or total), replacement of the deteriorated part of the joint with a prosthetic appliance, may be required.
- Arthrodesis, surgical fusion of bones, is used primarily in the spine (laminectomy).
- Osteoplasty consists of scraping and lavage of deteriorated bone from the joint.
- Osteotomy changes alignment of the bone to relieve stress by excision or cutting of a wedge of bone.

Nursing considerations

- Promote adequate rest, particularly after activity. Plan rest periods during the day, and provide for adequate sleep at night. Teach the patient to "pace" daily activities.
- Assist with physical therapy, and encourage the patient to perform gentle, isometric range-of-motion (ROM) exercises.
- If the patient needs surgery, provide appropriate preoperative and postoperative care.
- Provide emotional support and reassurance to help the patient cope with limited mobility.
- Specific patient care depends on the affected joint:
  – *Hand:* Apply hot soaks and paraffin dips to relieve pain as necessary.
  – *Spine (lumbar and sacral):* Recommend firm mattress (or bed board) to decrease morning pain.
  – *Spine (cervical):* Check cervical collar for constriction; watch for redness with prolonged use.

– *Hip:* Use moist heat pads to relieve pain, and administer an antispasmodic as necessary. Assist with ROM and strengthening exercises, always making sure the patient gets enough rest afterward. Check crutches, cane, braces, and walker for proper fit, and teach the patient how to use them correctly. For example, the patient with unilateral joint involvement should use an orthopedic appliance (such as a cane or walker) on the normal side. Advise the use of cushions when sitting, as well as the use of an elevated toilet seat.
– *Knee:* Twice daily, assist with prescribed ROM exercises, exercises to maintain muscle tone, and progressive resistance exercises to increase muscle strength. Provide elastic supports or braces, if needed.
- Tell the patient to install safety devices at home such as guard rails in the bathroom. The patient's living area may need to be assessed for safety and prevention of injuries.

Osteomyelitis

A pyogenic bone infection, osteomyelitis may be chronic or acute. It commonly results from a combination of local trauma and an acute infection originating elsewhere in the body. Although osteomyelitis may remain localized, it can spread through the bone to the marrow, cortex, and periosteum. Typically, the causative organisms find a culture site in a hematoma from recent trauma or in a weakened area, such as the site of local infection (for example, furunculosis), and spread directly to bone. Acute osteomyelitis is typically a blood-borne disease that usually affects rapidly growing children. Chronic osteomyelitis, although rare, is characterized by multiple draining sinus tracts and metastatic lesions that can persist intermittently for years, flaring up spontaneously after minor trauma. With prompt treatment, the prognosis for acute osteomyelitis is good; for chronic osteomyelitis, which is more prevalent in adults, the prognosis is poor.

Causes
- *Escherichia coli*
- *Pneumococcus*
- *Proteus vulgaris*
- *Pseudomonas aeruginosa*
- *Staphylococcus aureus* (most common)
- *Streptococcus pyogenes*

Signs and symptoms
- Heat
- Malaise
- Nausea
- Restricted movement
- Sudden fever
- Sudden pain in the affected bone
- Swelling
- Tachycardia
- Tenderness

Diagnostic tests
- Bone scan shows infected bone.
- Bone lesion biopsy or culture may reveal the causative organism.
- White blood cell count shows leukocytosis.
- Erythrocyte sedimentation rate and C-reactive protein levels are elevated.
- Blood cultures identify the causative organism.
- Computed tomography scan and magnetic resonance imaging may delineate the extent of infection.
- X-rays may show bone involvement only after the disease has been active for some time—usually 2 to 3 weeks.

Treatment
Acute osteomyelitis
- Large doses of I.V. antibiotics are administered after blood cultures are obtained. A penicillinase-resistant agent, such as nafcillin or oxacillin (Bactocill), is typically given.
- Early surgical drainage relieves pressure buildup and sequestrum formation.
- Immobilization of the affected bone is achieved by plaster cast, traction, or complete bed rest.
- Supportive measures include administration of an analgesic and I.V. fluids.
- An abscess requires incision and drainage, followed by a culture.
- Anti-infective therapy may include:
  – systemic antibiotics
  – intracavitary instillation of an antibiotic through closed-system continuous irrigation with low intermittent suction
  – limited irrigation with a closed drainage system equipped with suction
  – local application of packed, wet, antibiotic-soaked dressings.

Chronic osteomyelitis
- Surgery may be performed to remove dead bone (sequestrectomy) and to promote drainage and decrease pressure (saucerization).
- Resistant chronic osteomyelitis in an arm or leg may necessitate amputation.
- Hyperbaric oxygen increases the activity of naturally occurring leukocytes.
- Free tissue transfers and local muscle flaps fill in dead space and increase blood supply.

Nursing considerations
- Use strict aseptic technique when changing dressings and irrigating wounds.
- If the patient is in skeletal traction for compound fractures, cover the insertion

points of pin tracks with small, dry dressings, and tell him not to touch the skin around the pins and wires.

■ Administer I.V. fluids to maintain adequate hydration as necessary.

■ Provide a diet high in protein and vitamin C.

■ Assess vital signs and wound appearance daily, and monitor daily for new pain, which may indicate secondary infection.

■ Carefully monitor suction equipment. Monitor the amount of solution instilled and suctioned.

■ Support the affected limb in alignment with firm pillows.

■ Provide good skin care. Turn the patient gently every 2 hours, and monitor him for signs of developing pressure ulcers.

■ Provide cast care.

Do's & don'ts

 Check circulation and drainage: If a wet spot appears on the cast, circle it with a marking pen and note the time of appearance (on the cast). Be aware of how much drainage is expected. Check the circled spot at least every 4 hours. Watch for any enlargement.

■ Protect the patient from mishaps, such as jerky movements and falls, which may threaten bone integrity.

Action stat!

 Be alert for sudden pain, crepitus, or deformity. Watch for any sudden malposition of the limb, which may indicate fracture.

■ Before discharge, teach the patient how to protect and clean the wound and, most important, how to recognize signs of recurring infection (increased temperature, redness, localized heat, and swelling).

■ Stress the need for follow-up examinations.

■ Instruct the patient to seek prompt treatment for possible sources of recurrence—blisters, boils, styes, and impetigo.

▌Osteoporosis

In osteoporosis, a metabolic bone disorder, the rate of bone resorption accelerates while the rate of bone formation slows down, causing a loss of bone mass. Bones affected by this disease lose calcium and phosphate salts and thus become porous, brittle, and abnormally vulnerable to fracture. Osteoporosis may be primary or secondary to an underlying disease. Primary osteoporosis is commonly called senile or postmenopausal osteoporosis because it's most common in elderly, postmenopausal women. (See *Osteoporosis in men.*)

Causes
Primary osteoporosis
■ Unknown

Risk factors
■ Declining gonadal adrenal function
■ Faulty protein metabolism due to estrogen deficiency
■ Mild but prolonged negative calcium balance, resulting from an inadequate dietary intake of calcium
■ Sedentary lifestyle

Secondary osteoporosis
■ Alcoholism
■ Bone immobilization or misuse
■ Hyperthyroidism
■ Lactose intolerance
■ Liver disease
■ Malabsorption
■ Malnutrition

- Osteogenesis imperfecta
- Prolonged therapy with steroids or heparin
- Rheumatoid arthritis
- Scurvy
- Sudeck's atrophy (localized to hands and feet, with recurring attacks)

Signs and symptoms
- Colles' fractures after a minor fall
- Hip fracture
- Increasing deformity
- Kyphosis
- Loss of height
- Pain aggravated by movement or jarring
- Pathologic fractures of the neck and femur
- Snapping sound in lower vertebrae when bending over
- Spontaneous wedge fractures
- Sudden pain in the lower back
- Vertebral collapse producing pain that radiates around the trunk

Diagnostic tests
- X-rays show typical degeneration in the lower thoracic and lumbar vertebrae. The vertebral bodies may appear flattened and may look denser than normal.
- Bone mineral density (BMD) testing is performed in dual-energy X-ray absorptiometry (DEXA) to measure the mineralization of bones. Loss of bone mineral becomes evident in later stages.
- Serum calcium, phosphorus, and alkaline phosphatase levels are all within normal limits, but parathyroid hormone level may be elevated.
- Bone biopsy shows bone that's thin and porous but otherwise normal looking.
- A spinal computed tomography (CT) scan shows demineralization. Quantitative CT can evaluate bone density but is

Osteoporosis in men

Osteoporosis in men can be classified in three ways:
- Primary—idiopathic; having no known cause
- Secondary—more common in males than in females; may be due to drug therapy (anticonvulsants, glucocorticoids, long-term heparin or warfarin therapy), lifestyle factors (alcoholism, immobility, smoking), or medical conditions (GI disorders, hypercalciuria, hypogonadism, neoplastic diseases, organ transplantation, rheumatoid arthritis, thyrotoxicosis)
- Senile—occurring after age 70; caused by imbalance in bone breakdown and new bone formation, inadequate calcium and vitamin D intake, and lack of physical activity.

less available and more expensive than DEXA.
- A newer test to help diagnose osteoporosis involves measurement of urinary levels of N-telopeptide.

Treatment
- A physical therapy program emphasizes gentle exercise and activity.
- Sodium fluoride stimulates bone formation.
- Calcium and vitamin D support normal bone metabolism.
- Hormone replacement therapy (HRT) with estrogen and progesterone may retard bone loss and prevent the occurrence of fractures. HRT decreases bone reabsorption and increases bone mass. However, this therapy remains controversial because the potential complications of HRT may outweigh the benefits in some patients.

Testosterone replacement may be used to increase BMD in men with low levels of the hormone, but this treatment is contraindicated in men with prostate cancer. A digital rectal examination and prostate-specific antigen test are performed before therapy and yearly thereafter.

- A back brace supports weakened vertebrae.
- Surgery may be needed to correct pathologic fractures of the femur by open reduction and internal fixation.
- Reduction and plaster cast immobilization for 4 to 10 weeks is the treatment of choice for Colles' fracture.
- Preventive measures include adequate intake of dietary calcium, regular exercise, and avoidance of smoking and excessive alcohol consumption. Medications for maintaining bone health include bisphosphonates (alendronate [Fosamax] and risedronate [Actonel]), calcitonin, estrogens, and raloxifene (Evista). Secondary osteoporosis can be prevented through effective treatment of the underlying disease, as well as by steroid therapy, early mobilization after surgery or trauma, decreased alcohol consumption, careful observation for signs of malabsorption, and prompt treatment of hyperthyroidism.

Nursing considerations

- Focus on the patient's fragility, stressing careful positioning, ambulation, and prescribed exercises.
- Check the patient's skin daily for redness, warmth, and new sites of pain, which may indicate new fractures. Encourage activity; help the patient walk several times daily.
- Perform passive range-of-motion exercises, or encourage the patient to perform active exercises. Make sure she reg-ularly attends scheduled physical therapy sessions.
- Institute safety precautions such as keeping side rails up. Move the patient gently and carefully at all times. Explain to the patient's family and ancillary facility personnel how easily an osteoporotic patient's bones can fracture.
- Provide a balanced diet, high in nutrients that support skeletal metabolism: vitamin D, calcium, and protein. Give an analgesic and provide heat to relieve pain.
- Make sure the patient and her family clearly understand the prescribed drug regimen. Tell them how to recognize significant adverse reactions and to report them immediately. Also tell the patient to report any new pain sites immediately, especially after trauma, no matter how slight.
- Advise the patient to sleep on a firm mattress and to avoid excessive bed rest. Make sure she knows how to wear her back brace.
- Teach the patient good body mechanics—to stoop before lifting anything and to avoid twisting movements and prolonged bending.
- Instruct the female patient taking estrogen in the proper technique for breast self-examination. Tell her to perform this examination at least once per month and to immediately report any lumps. Emphasize the need for regular gynecologic examinations. Tell her to report abnormal bleeding promptly.

▌Otitis externa

Also known as *external otitis* and *swimmer's ear,* otitis externa is an inflammation of the skin of the external ear canal and auricle. It may be acute or chronic, and it's most common in the summer. With treatment, acute otitis externa usually subsides within 7 days (although it may become chronic) and tends to recur.

Causes
- Bacterial infection: *Pseudomonas, Proteus vulgaris,* streptococci, or *Staphylococcus aureus*
- Fungal infection (less common): *Aspergillus niger* or *Candida albicans*

Chronic otitis externa
- Dermatologic conditions, such as seborrhea or psoriasis

Risk factors
- Chronic drainage from a perforated tympanic membrane
- Cleaning the ear canal with a finger or other foreign object
- Exposure to dust, hair care products, or other irritants
- Regular use of earphones, earplugs, or earmuffs (traps moisture in the ear canal, creating a culture medium for infection)
- Swimming in contaminated water (cerumen creates a culture medium for the water-borne organism)

Signs and symptoms
Acute otitis externa
- Fever
- Foul-smelling aural discharge
- Moderate to severe pain exacerbated by manipulating the auricle or tragus, clenching the teeth, opening the mouth, or chewing
- Partial hearing loss
- Regional cellulitis

Chronic otitis externa
- Asteatosis (lack of cerumen; common)
- Aural discharge
- Pruritus
- Scaling and skin thickening with a resultant narrowing of the lumen

Fungal otitis externa
- Asymptomatic
- Black or gray blotting paper–like growth in the ear canal with *A. niger*

Diagnostic tests
- In acute otitis externa, otoscopy reveals a swollen external ear canal (sometimes to the point of complete closure), periauricular lymphadenopathy (tender nodes in front of the tragus, behind the ear, or in the upper neck) and, occasionally, regional cellulitis.
- With chronic otitis externa, physical examination shows thick red epithelium in the ear canal.
- With fungal otitis externa, removal of growth shows thick red epithelium.
- Microscopic examination or culture and sensitivity tests can identify the causative organism and determine antibiotic treatment.
- Audiometric testing may reveal a partial hearing loss.

Treatment
Acute otitis externa
- Clean the ear and remove debris.
- Heat is applied to the periauricular region by using a heat lamp; hot, damp compresses; or a heating pad.
- Aspirin or acetaminophen is given for pain.
- Antibiotic eardrops (with or without hydrocortisone) are administered to treat causative infections.
- If fever persists or regional cellulitis develops, a systemic antibiotic is necessary.

Chronic otitis externa
- Clean the ear and remove debris.
- Antibiotic eardrops are given to treat the causative infection if indicated.
- Application of antibiotic ointment or cream (neomycin, bacitracin, or poly-

myxin, possibly combined with hydrocortisone) may be necessary.

- An ointment that contains phenol, salicylic acid, precipitated sulfur, and petroleum jelly produces exfoliative and antipruritic effects.
- The patient may need to wear specially fitted earplugs while showering, shampooing, or swimming.

Fungal otitis externa

- Carefully clean the affected ear.
- Application of a keratolytic or 2% salicylic acid in cream containing nystatin for treatment of causative organism in candidal infection.
- Instillation of slightly acidic eardrops creates an unfavorable environment in the ear canal for most fungi as well as *Pseudomonas*.

Nursing considerations
Acute otitis externa

- Monitor vital signs, particularly temperature. Watch for and record the type and amount of aural drainage.
- Remove debris, gently clean the ear canal, and then dry gently but thoroughly. (With severe otitis externa, cleaning may be delayed until after initial treatment with antibiotic eardrops.)

<u>DO'S & DON'TS</u>

 To instill eardrops in an adult, pull the pinna upward and backward to straighten the canal. Don't use this same method for children; instead pull the pinna downward and backward. To ensure that the drops reach the epithelium, insert a wisp of cotton moistened with eardrops.

Prevention

- Suggest that the patient use custom-fitted earplugs to keep water out of his ears when showering, shampooing, or swimming.
- Warn the patient against putting any objects in his ears, such as cleaning the ears with cotton swabs or other objects.
- Urge prompt treatment of otitis externa to prevent perforation of the tympanic membrane.
- If the patient is diabetic or immunocompromised, evaluate him for malignant otitis externa (drainage, hearing loss, ear pain, itching, fever). Appropriate treatments include antibiotics and surgical debridement.
- Hearing aid users who are prone to otitis externa should consider having the device vented to improve aeration of the external ear canal.

Otitis media

Inflammation of the middle ear, otitis media may be suppurative or secretory, acute or chronic. Acute otitis media is common in children; its incidence rises during the winter months, paralleling the seasonal rise in nonbacterial respiratory tract infections. With prompt treatment, the prognosis for acute otitis media is excellent; however, prolonged accumulation of fluid within the middle ear cavity causes chronic otitis media, with possible perforation of the tympanic membrane.

Chronic suppurative otitis media may lead to scarring, adhesions, and severe structural or functional ear damage; chronic secretory otitis media, with its persistent inflammation and pressure, may cause conductive hearing loss.

Causes
Suppurative otitis media

- Bacterial infection: beta-hemolytic streptococci, staphylococci, gram-negative bacteria, pneumococci,

Haemophilus influenzae, and *Moraxella catarrhalis*

Risk factors
- Anatomic anomalies
- Genetic factors such as susceptibility to infection
- Normally wider, shorter, more horizontal eustachian tubes and increased lymphoid tissue in children

Chronic suppurative otitis media
- Inadequate treatment of acute otitis episodes
- Resistant strains of bacteria

Secretory otitis media
- Barotrauma
- Eustachian tube dysfunction from viral infection or allergy
- Rapid aircraft descent in a person with an upper respiratory tract infection
- Rapid underwater ascent in scuba diving (barotitis media)

Chronic secretory otitis media
- Edema (allergic rhinitis, chronic sinus infection)
- Inadequate treatment of acute suppurative otitis media
- Mechanical obstruction (adenoidal tissue overgrowth, tumors)

Signs and symptoms
Suppurative otitis media
- Bulging of the tympanic membrane
- Dizziness
- Erythema of tympanic membrane
- Hearing loss (usually mild and conductive)
- Mild to very high fever
- Nausea
- Purulent drainage in the ear canal from tympanic membrane rupture

- Severe, deep, throbbing pain (from pressure behind the tympanic membrane)
- Upper respiratory tract infection (sneezing, coughing)
- Vomiting

Secretory otitis media
- Hearing an echo when speaking
- Popping, crackling, or clicking sounds on swallowing or with jaw movement
- Sensation of fullness in the ear
- Severe conductive hearing loss varies
- Vague feeling of top-heaviness

Chronic otitis media
- Cholesteatoma (a cystlike mass in the middle ear)
- Conductive hearing loss
- Decreased or absent tympanic membrane mobility
- Painless, purulent discharge
- Sudden stoppage of pain with tympanic membrane rupture
- Thickening and scarring of the tympanic membrane

Diagnostic tests
Suppurative otitis media
- Otoscopy reveals obscured or distorted bony landmarks of the tympanic membrane.
- Pneumatoscopy can show decreased tympanic membrane mobility.

Secretory otitis media
- Otoscopic examination reveals tympanic membrane retraction, which causes the bony landmarks to appear more prominent, and clear or amber fluid behind the tympanic membrane.
- If hemorrhage into the middle ear has occurred, the tympanic membrane appears blue-black.

Chronic otitis media
- Otoscopy shows thickening (and sometimes scarring) and decreased mobility of the tympanic membrane.
- Pneumatoscopy shows decreased or absent tympanic membrane movement.
- Mastoid X-rays or computed tomography scans may show spreading infection beyond the middle ear.

Treatment
Suppurative otitis media
- Antibiotics are given for a bacterial infection.
- Nasal spray, nose drops, oral decongestants, or antihistamines may be used to promote drainage of fluid through the eustachian tube.
- Eardrops or analgesics such as ibuprofen (Motrin) or acetaminophen (Tylenol) are given to relieve pain.
- Oral corticosteroids reduce inflammation.
- Severe, painful bulging of the tympanic membrane usually necessitates myringotomy.
- Broad-spectrum antibiotics prevent acute suppurative otitis media in high-risk patients.

DRUG CHALLENGE

 In patients with recurring otitis, antibiotics must be used with discretion to prevent development of resistant strains of bacteria.

Secretory otitis media
- Inflation of the eustachian tube is achieved by performing Valsalva's maneuver several times.
- Nasopharyngeal decongestant therapy is administered for at least 2 weeks—sometimes indefinitely—with periodic evaluation.
- Myringotomy and aspiration of middle ear fluid, followed by insertion of a polyethylene tube into the tympanic membrane, may be used for immediate and prolonged equalization of pressure.
- Treatment should also include correction of the underlying cause, such as elimination of allergens, or adenoidectomy for hypertrophied adenoids.

Chronic otitis media
- Broad-spectrum antibiotics are given for exacerbations of acute otitis media.
- Eustachian tube obstruction, if present, must be cleared.
- Otitis externa must be treated if present.
- Myringoplasty and tympanoplasty are used to reconstruct middle ear structures.
- Mastoidectomy is another treatment used for chronic otitis media.
- Cholesteatoma is excised, if indicated.

Nursing considerations
- Explain all diagnostic tests and procedures to the patient.

DO'S & DON'TS

 After myringotomy, maintain drainage flow. Don't place cotton or plugs deep in the ear canal; sterile cotton may be placed loosely in the external ear to absorb drainage.

- To prevent infection, change the cotton whenever it gets damp, and wash hands before and after giving ear care. Monitor the patient for headache, fever, severe pain, or disorientation.
- After tympanoplasty, reinforce dressings and observe the patient for excessive bleeding from the ear canal. Give an analgesic as needed. Warn the patient against blowing his nose or getting the ear wet when bathing.
- Encourage the patient to complete the prescribed course of antibiotic treat-

ment. Teach correct instillation of ear-drops, if prescribed. Most children will have an effusion present at the completion of a 10- to 14-day course of antibiotic therapy. Effusion may last up to 12 weeks before spontaneous clearance can be expected.

- Suggest that the patient apply heat to his ear, through a warm cloth or a warm-water bottle, to relieve pain.
- Advise the patient to contact his practitioner if symptoms don't improve. Instruct him to watch for and immediately report pain and fever.

Prevention

- Teach the patient to recognize upper respiratory tract infections, and encourage early treatment.
- Instruct parents not to feed their infant in a supine position or put him to bed with a bottle because these actions allow reflux of nasopharyngeal flora.
- To promote eustachian tube patency, instruct the patient to perform Valsalva's maneuver several times daily.
- Identify and treat allergies.

Otosclerosis

The most common cause of conductive deafness, otosclerosis is the slow formation of spongy bone in the otic capsule, particularly at the oval window. Spongy bone in the otic capsule immobilizes the footplate of the normally mobile stapes, disrupting the conduction of vibrations from the tympanic membrane to the cochlea. It occurs in at least 10% of whites, is twice as common in women as in men, and usually occurs between ages 15 and 50. It commonly affects both ears. With surgery, the prognosis is good.

Causes

- Genetic: autosomal dominant trait

- Pregnancy may trigger onset of this condition

Signs and symptoms

- Bilateral deafness
- Paracusis of Willis (hearing conversation better in a noisy environment than in a quiet one)
- Progressive unilateral hearing loss
- Tinnitus

Diagnostic tests

- Rinne test shows bone conduction lasting longer than air conduction (normally, the reverse is true); as otosclerosis progresses, bone conduction also deteriorates.
- Audiometric testing reveals hearing loss ranging from 60 dB, in early stages, to total loss as the disease advances.
- Weber's test detects sound lateralizing to the more affected ear.
- Otoscopic examination reveals a normal tympanic membrane.

Treatment

- Stapedectomy (removal of the stapes) and insertion of a prosthesis restores partial or total hearing.
- Other surgical procedures include fenestration and stapes mobilization; all require normal cochlear function.
- Antibiotics are given postoperatively to prevent infection.
- If surgery isn't possible, hearing aids enable the patient to hear conversation in normal surroundings.

Nursing considerations

- During the first 24 hours after surgery, keep the patient lying flat, with the affected ear facing upward (to maintain the position of the graft).
- Enforce bed rest with bathroom privileges for 48 hours. Because the patient may be dizzy, keep the side rails up and assist him with ambulation.

Otosclerosis: Recovering after surgery

Review the following points with the patient before discharge.

■ Instruct the patient to sneeze and cough with his mouth open for 2 weeks after surgery to avoid dislodging the graft or prosthesis.

■ Inform the patient that he may hear various noises, such as cracking or popping; reassure him that this is normal.

■ Tell the patient that the ear packing or middle ear fluid decreases hearing in the affected ear and that it can seem as if he's talking in a barrel.

■ Reassure the patient that minor ear discomfort is expected, and urge him to take the prescribed pain medication. Stress that excessive ear pain should be reported to the practitioner.

■ Occasionally, a small amount of bleeding from the ear occurs; reassure the patient that this is normal. Excessive ear drainage should be reported to the practitioner.

■ Explain that some patients initially find the improvement in hearing after stapes surgery so great that it causes sensitivity or distress. This usually diminishes as the patient adapts to his improved hearing level.

■ Instruct the patient to avoid loud noises and sudden pressure changes (such as those that occur while diving or flying) until healing is complete (usually 6 months).

■ Advise the patient not to blow his nose for at least 1 week to prevent contaminated air and bacteria from entering the eustachian tube.

■ Stress the importance of protecting the ears against cold; avoiding activities that provoke dizziness, such as straining, bending, or heavy lifting; and, if possible, avoiding contact with anyone who has an upper respiratory tract infection.

■ Teach the patient and his family how to change the external ear dressing (eye pad or gauze pad) and care for the incision.

■ Emphasize the need to complete the prescribed antibiotic regimen and to return for scheduled follow-up care.

■ Assess the patient for pain and vertigo; relieved with repositioning or prescribed medication. (See *Otosclerosis: Recovering after surgery*.)

Ovarian cancer

After cancer of the lung and bronchus, breast, pancreas, and colon, primary ovarian cancer ranks as the fifth leading cause of cancer deaths among American females. In females with previously treated breast cancer, metastatic ovarian cancer is more common than cancer at any other site. The prognosis varies with the histologic type and stage of the disease but is generally poor because ovarian tumors produce few early signs and are usually advanced at diagnosis. Three main types of ovarian cancer exist. Primary epithelial tumors arise in the müllerian epithelium; germ cell tumors, in the ovum itself; and sex cord tumors, in the ovarian stroma (the ovary's supporting framework). Ovarian tumors spread rapidly intraperitoneally by local extension or surface seeding and, occasionally, through the lymphatics and the bloodstream. Generally, extraperitoneal spread is through the diaphragm into the chest cavity, which may cause pleural effusions. Other types of metastasis are rare.

Causes
■ Unknown

Risk factors
- Age older than 55
- Diet high in saturated fats
- Exposure to asbestos, talc, and industrial pollutants
- Family history of ovarian cancer
- Infertility
- Menopausal hormone therapy (estrogen alone) for 10 or more years (suggested by some studies)
- Nulliparity
- Obesity
- Personal history of breast, uterine, colon, or rectal cancer
- Presence of certain genes, including BRCA1 and BRCA2
- Prolonged use of the fertility drug clomiphene citrate (Clomid)

Signs and symptoms
Early signs
- Dyspepsia
- Mild GI disturbances
- Vague abdominal discomfort

Progressive ovarian cancer
- Abdominal distention
- Arrhenoblastomas: virilizing effect
- Constipation
- Granulosa cell tumors: feminizing effect such as bleeding between periods in premenopausal women
- Pain that mimics appendicitis (with tumor rupture, torsion, or infection)
- Pelvic discomfort
- Urinary frequency
- Weight loss

Advanced ovarian cancer
- Ascites
- Pain
- Postmenopausal bleeding
- Symptoms relating to metastatic sites (most commonly pleural effusion)

Diagnostic tests
- Lymph node evaluation and tumor biopsy provides accurate diagnosis and staging.
- Abdominal ultrasonography, computed tomography scan, or magnetic resonance imaging may delineate tumor size.
- Chest X-ray may show distant metastasis and pleural effusion.
- Barium enema (especially in patients with GI symptoms) may reveal obstruction and size of tumor.
- Mammography rules out primary breast cancer.

Treatment
- Occasionally, in a young woman with a unilateral encapsulated tumor who wishes to maintain fertility, a conservative approach may include:
  – resection of the involved ovary
  – biopsies of the omentum and the uninvolved ovary
  – peritoneal washings for cytologic examination of pelvic fluid
  – careful follow-up, including periodic chest X-rays to rule out lung metastasis.
- Aggressive therapy includes:
  – total abdominal hysterectomy and bilateral salpingo-oophorectomy with tumor resection, omentectomy, appendectomy, lymph node biopsies with probable lymphadenectomy, tissue biopsies, and peritoneal washings

DRUG CHALLENGE

 Bilateral salpingo-oophorectomy in a prepubertal girl necessitates hormone replacement therapy, beginning at puberty, to induce the development of secondary sex characteristics.

– I.V. or intraperitoneal chemotherapy, typically with paclitaxel (Taxol) and cisplatin (Platinol)
– radioisotopes as adjuvant therapy (these may cause small-bowel obstructions and stenosis)
– I.V. administration of biological response modifiers, such as interleukin-2, interferon, and monoclonal antibodies.

Nursing considerations
Before surgery
▪ Thoroughly explain all preoperative tests, the expected course of treatment, and surgical and postoperative procedures.
▪ In premenopausal women, explain that bilateral oophorectomy artificially induces early menopause, so they may experience hot flashes, headaches, palpitations, insomnia, depression, and excessive perspiration.

After surgery
▪ Monitor vital signs frequently, maintain I.V. fluids as ordered. Monitor intake and output.
▪ Check the dressing regularly for excessive drainage or bleeding, and watch for signs of infection.
▪ Provide abdominal support, and watch for abdominal distention.
▪ Encourage coughing and deep breathing.
▪ Reposition the patient often, and encourage her to walk shortly after surgery.
▪ Monitor the patient, and treat any adverse reactions of radiation and chemotherapy.

 If the patient is receiving immunotherapy, watch for flulike symptoms that may last 12 to 24 hours after drug administration. Give aspirin or acetaminophen for fever. Keep the patient well covered with blankets, and provide warm liquids to relieve chills. Give an antiemetic as needed.

▪ Enlist the help of a social worker, a chaplain, and other members of the health care team for additional supportive care.

Ovarian cysts
Usually ovarian cysts are nonneoplastic sacs on an ovary that contain fluid or semisolid material. Although these cysts are usually small and produce no symptoms, they require thorough investigation as possible sites of malignant change. Common ovarian cysts include follicular cysts, lutein cysts (granulosa-lutein [corpus luteum] and theca-lutein cysts), and polycystic (or sclerocystic) ovarian disease. Ovarian cysts can develop anytime between puberty and menopause, including during pregnancy. Granulosa-lutein cysts occur infrequently, usually during early pregnancy. The prognosis for nonneoplastic ovarian cysts is excellent.

Causes
▪ Follicular cysts: overdistention of follicles during the menstrual cycle leading to excessive secretion of estrogen during menopause
▪ Granulosa-lutein cysts: excessive accumulation of blood during the hemorrhagic phase of the menstrual cycle
▪ Theca-lutein cysts:
– choriocarcinoma
– hormone therapy (with human chorionic gonadotropin [hCG] or clomiphene citrate)
– hydatidiform mole

Polycystic ovarian disease
▪ Endocrine abnormalities
▪ Stein-Leventhal syndrome

Signs and symptoms

- Torsion or rupture: abdominal tenderness, distention, and rigidity (can mimic appendicitis)

Large or multiple cysts

- Abnormal uterine bleeding secondary to a disturbed ovulatory pattern
- Dyspareunia
- Lower back pain
- Mild pelvic discomfort

Granulosa-lutein cysts

- Delayed menses, followed by prolonged or irregular bleeding (in non-pregnant females)
- Massive intraperitoneal hemorrhage (with rupture)
- Unilateral pelvic discomfort

Polycystic ovarian disease

- Infertility
- Oligomenorrhea
- Secondary amenorrhea

Diagnostic tests

- Visualization of the ovaries through ultrasound, laparoscopy, computed tomography scan, or surgery (commonly for another condition) confirms the presence of ovarian cysts.
- Extremely high hCG titers strongly suggest theca-lutein cysts.

Polycystic ovarian disease

- Urinary 17-ketosteroid levels are slightly elevated in the patient with polycystic ovarian disease.
- Anovulation (shown by basal body temperature graphs and endometrial biopsy) confirms the diagnosis.
- CA-125 is an ovarian cancer marker that can help identify cancerous cysts in women.

Treatment

- Follicular cysts usually don't require treatment because they tend to disappear spontaneously by reabsorption or silent rupture within 60 days. The therapeutic use of hormonal contraception is controversial.
- If granulosa-lutein cysts occur during pregnancy, treatment is symptomatic because they diminish during the third trimester and rarely require surgery.
- Theca-lutein cysts disappear spontaneously after eliminating the hydatidiform mole, destroying the choriocarcinoma, or stopping hCG or clomiphene citrate (Clomid) therapy.
- Treatment of polycystic ovarian disease may include giving clomiphene citrate to induce ovulation, medroxyprogesterone acetate (Provera) for 10 days of every month for the patient who doesn't want to become pregnant, or a low-dose hormonal contraceptive for the patient who needs reliable contraception.
- Surgery (laparoscopy, exploratory laparotomy with possible ovarian cystectomy, oophorectomy) is necessary if an ovarian cyst is found to be persistent or suspicious.

Nursing considerations

- Carefully explain the nature of the particular cyst, the type of discomfort (if any) that the patient is likely to experience, and the amount of time the condition is expected to last.

ACTION STAT!

 Preoperatively, watch for signs of cyst rupture, such as increasing abdominal pain, distention, and rigidity. Monitor vital signs for fever, tachypnea, or hypotension, which may indicate peritonitis or intraperitoneal hemorrhage.

- Postoperatively, encourage frequent movement in bed and early ambulation as ordered. Early ambulation effectively prevents pulmonary embolism.
- Provide emotional support. Offer appropriate reassurance if the patient fears cancer or infertility.
- Before discharge, advise the patient to increase her activities at home gradually—preferably over 4 to 6 weeks.

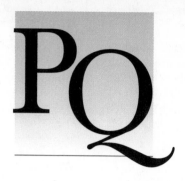

Paget's disease

Also known as *osteitis deformans*, Paget's disease is a slowly progressive metabolic bone disease characterized by an initial phase of excessive bone resorption (osteoclastic phase), followed by a reactive phase of excessive abnormal bone formation (osteoblastic phase). The new bone structure, which is chaotic, fragile, and weak, causes painful deformities of both external contour and internal structure. Paget's disease usually localizes in one or several areas of the skeleton (most commonly the lower torso); however, occasionally, skeletal deformity is widely distributed. It can be fatal, particularly when it's associated with heart failure (widespread disease creates a continuous need for high cardiac output), bone sarcoma, or giant cell tumors. In 5% of the patients, the involved bone will undergo malignant changes.

Causes
- Unknown

Signs and symptoms
- Asymmetrical bowing of the tibia and femur (can reduce height)
- Barrel-shaped chest
- Bony impingement on the cranial nerves may cause blindness and hearing loss with tinnitus and vertigo
- Gout
- Heart failure
- Hypercalcemia
- Hypertension
- Impaired movement
- Kyphosis (spinal curvature due to compression fractures of vertebrae)
- Pagetic sites are warm and tender
- Renal calculi
- Severe and persistent pain that intensifies with weight bearing
- Susceptibility to pathologic fractures after minor trauma (may never completely heal)
- Waddling gait (from softening of pelvic bones)
- With skull involvement, characteristic cranial enlargement over frontal and occipital areas (hat size may increase) and headaches

Diagnostic tests
- X-rays taken before overt symptoms develop show increased bone expansion and density.
- Bone scan (more sensitive than X-rays) clearly shows early pagetic lesions (radioisotope concentrate in areas of active disease).
- Bone biopsy reveals characteristic mosaic pattern.

■ Increased serum alkaline phosphatase (ALP) level is an index of osteoblastic activity and bone formation.

■ Increased 24-hour urine levels for hydroxyproline (amino acid excreted by the kidneys) are an indicator of osteoclastic hyperactivity.

Treatment

■ If the patient is asymptomatic, no treatment is needed.

■ Calcitonin (a hormone, given subcutaneously or I.M.) and etidronate (a bisphosphonate, given orally) reduce serum ALP levels and urinary hydroxyproline secretion and slow bone resorption, which relieves bone lesions.

DRUG CHALLENGE

 Although the patient will need long-term maintenance therapy with calcitonin, the first few weeks of calcitonin produce noticeable improvement; etidronate produces improvement after 1 to 3 months. Other bisphosphonates include alendronate (Fosamax), pamidronate (Aredia), risedronate (Actonel), and tiludronate (Skelid).

■ Plicamycin (Mithracin), a cytotoxic antibiotic, decreases urinary hydroxyproline, serum calcium, and serum ALP levels.

DRUG CHALLENGE

 Plicamycin produces remission of symptoms within 2 weeks and biochemical improvement in 1 to 2 months. However, plicamycin may destroy platelets or compromise renal function, so it's usually given only to patients who have severe disease, require rapid relief, or don't respond to other treatment.

■ Surgery is used to reduce or prevent pathologic fractures, correct secondary deformities, or relieve neurologic impairment. Joint replacement is difficult because bonding material (polymethylmethacrylate) doesn't set properly on pagetic bone.

DRUG CHALLENGE

 To decrease the risk of excessive bleeding due to hypervascular bone, drug therapy with calcitonin and bisphosphonates or plicamycin must precede surgery.

■ Aspirin, indomethacin, or ibuprofen is given to control pain.

Nursing considerations

■ Evaluate the effectiveness of pain control. Assess the patient's pain level daily. Watch for new areas of pain or restricted movements—which may indicate new fracture sites—and sensory or motor disturbances, such as difficulty hearing, seeing, or walking.

■ Monitor serum calcium and ALP levels.

■ If the patient is confined to prolonged bed rest, prevent pressure ulcers by providing good skin care. Reposition the patient frequently, and use a flotation mattress. Provide high-top sneakers to prevent footdrop.

■ Monitor intake and output. Encourage adequate fluid intake to minimize renal calculi formation.

■ Teach the patient how to self-inject calcitonin using proper technique and to rotate injection sites.

■ Warn the patient that he may experience adverse reactions (nausea, vomiting, local inflammatory reaction at injection site, facial flushing, itching of hands, and fever). Reassure him that such reactions are usually mild and infrequent.

■ To help the patient adjust to the changes in lifestyle imposed by this disease, teach him how to pace activities and, if necessary, how to use assistive devices.

■ Encourage the patient to follow a recommended exercise program—avoiding immobilization and excessive activity. Suggest a firm mattress or a bed board to minimize spinal deformities.

■ To prevent falls at home, advise the patient to remove throw rugs and other small obstacles.

■ Emphasize the importance of regular checkups, including those for the eyes and ears.

<u>**D**RUG CHALLENGE</u>

 Tell the patient receiving etidronate to take this medication with fruit juice 2 hours before or after meals (milk or other high-calcium fluids impair absorption), to divide the daily dosage to minimize adverse effects, and to watch for and report stomach cramps, diarrhea, fractures, and increasing or new bone pain.

<u>**D**RUG CHALLENGE</u>

 Tell the patient receiving plicamycin to watch for signs of infection, easy bruising, bleeding, and fever and to report for regular follow-up laboratory testing.

■ Help the patient and his family make use of community support resources, such as a visiting nurse or home health agency. For more information, refer them to the Paget's Disease Foundation.

▌Pancreatic cancer

A deadly GI cancer, pancreatic cancer progresses rapidly. Pancreatic cancer occurs most commonly among blacks, particularly in men ages 35 to 70. Pancreatic tumors are almost always adenocarcinomas and most arise in the head of the pancreas. Tumors of the body and tail of the pancreas and islet cell tumors are rare. (See *Types of pancreatic cancer,* page 448.)

The two main tissue types are cylinder cell and large, fatty, granular cell. The prognosis is poor. Most patients die within 1 year of diagnosis.

Causes
■ Cigarette smoking
■ Hereditary syndromes

Risk factors
■ Chronic alcohol abuse
■ Chronic pancreatitis
■ Diabetes mellitus

Signs and symptoms
■ Abdominal or lower back pain
■ Anorexia
■ Anxiety
■ Bleeding tendencies
■ Depression
■ Diarrhea
■ Emotional disturbances
■ Fever
■ Fluid and electrolyte imbalances
■ Jaundice
■ Premonition of fatal illness
■ Skin lesions (usually on the legs)
■ Steatorrhea
■ Symptoms of diabetes
■ Weight loss

Diagnostic tests
■ Definitive diagnosis requires a laparotomy with a biopsy.

Types of pancreatic cancer

Pathology	Clinical features
Head of pancreas ■ Usually obstructs ampulla of Vater and common bile duct ■ Directly metastasizes to duodenum ■ Adhesions anchor tumor to spine, stomach, and intestines	■ Jaundice (predominant sign)—slowly progressive, unremitting; may cause skin (especially of the face and genitals) to turn olive green or black ■ Pruritus—often severe ■ Weight loss—rapid and severe (as much as 30 lb [13.6 kg]); may lead to emaciation, weakness, and muscle atrophy ■ Slowed digestion, gastric distention, nausea, diarrhea, and steatorrhea with clay-colored stools ■ Liver and gallbladder enlargement from lymph node metastasis to biliary tract and duct wall results in compression and obstruction; gallbladder may be palpable (Courvoisier's sign). ■ Dull, nondescript, continuous abdominal pain radiating to right upper quadrant; relieved by bending forward ■ GI hemorrhage and biliary infection—common
Body and tail of pancreas ■ Large nodular masses become fixed to retropancreatic tissues and spine ■ Direct invasion of spleen, left kidney, suprarenal gland, and diaphragm ■ Involvement of celiac plexus results in thrombosis of splenic vein and spleen infarction	*Body* ■ Pain (predominant symptom)—usually epigastric, develops slowly and radiates to back; relieved by bending forward or sitting up; intensified by lying in a supine position; most intense 3 to 4 hours after eating; when celiac plexus is involved, pain is more intense and lasts longer ■ Venous thrombosis and thrombophlebitis—frequent; may precede other symptoms by months ■ Splenomegaly (from infarction), hepatomegaly (occasionally), and jaundice (rarely) *Tail* Signs and symptoms result from metastasis: ■ Abdominal tumor (most common finding)—produces a palpable abdominal mass; abdominal pain radiates to left hypochondrium and left side of the chest. ■ Anorexia—leads to weight loss, emaciation, and weakness ■ Splenomegaly and upper GI bleeding

■ Ultrasound can identify a mass but not its histology.

■ Computed tomography scan is similar to ultrasound but shows greater detail.

■ Angiography shows vascular supply of tumor.

■ Endoscopic retrograde cholangiopancreatography allows visualization, instillation of contrast medium, and specimen biopsy.

■ Magnetic resonance imaging shows tumor size and location in great detail.

■ Increased serum bilirubin levels support the diagnosis.

■ Serum amylase and serum lipase levels are sometimes elevated.

■ Prothrombin time is prolonged.

- Aspartate aminotransferase and alanine aminotransferase levels are elevated with necrosis of liver cells.
- Alkaline phosphatase level is elevated with biliary obstruction.
- Plasma insulin immunoassay shows measurable serum insulin in the presence of islet cell tumors.
- Hemoglobin level and hematocrit may show mild anemia.
- Fasting blood glucose level may indicate hypoglycemia or hyperglycemia.
- Stool analysis may show occult blood.

Treatment

- Total pancreatectomy may increase survival time.
- Cholecystojejunostomy, choledochoduodenostomy, and choledochojejunostomy may be performed to bypass obstructing common bile duct extensions, decreasing jaundice and pruritus.
- Whipple's operation, or pancreatoduodenectomy, has a high mortality rate but can produce wide lymphatic clearance, except with tumors located near the portal vein, superior mesenteric vein and artery, and celiac axis. This procedure removes the head of the pancreas, the duodenum, gallbladder, end of the common bile duct, and possibly portions of the body and tail of the pancreas and stomach.
- Pancreatic cancer usually responds poorly to chemotherapy, but recent studies using combinations of fluorouracil, streptozocin (Zanosar), ifosfamide, and doxorubicin (Rubex) show a trend toward longer survival time.
- Radiation therapy usually doesn't increase long-term survival, although it may prolong survival time from 6 to 11 months when used as an adjunct to fluorouracil chemotherapy. It can also ease the pain associated with nonresectable tumors.

- Anticholinergics (particularly propantheline [Pro-banthine]) are given to decrease GI tract spasm and motility and reduce pain and secretions.
- Antacids (oral or by nasogastric tube) are used to decrease secretion of pancreatic enzymes and suppress peptic activity, thereby reducing stress-induced damage to gastric mucosa.
- Insulin is given to provide adequate exogenous insulin supply after pancreatic resection.
- Opioids may be given to relieve pain, but only after analgesics fail because morphine, meperidine, and codeine can lead to biliary tract spasm and increase common bile duct pressure.
- Pancreatic enzymes (average dose is 0.5 to 1 mg with meals) are given to assist in the digestion of proteins, carbohydrates, and fats when pancreatic juices are insufficient because of surgery or obstruction.
- If the patient can't tolerate oral feedings, provide total parenteral nutrition and I.V. fat emulsions to correct deficiencies and maintain positive nitrogen balance.
- Blood transfusions combat anemia.
- Vitamin K is used to correct prothrombin deficiency.
- Antibiotics are prescribed to prevent postoperative complications.

Nursing considerations
Before surgery

- Maintain gastric decompression, as necessary.
- Tell the patient about postoperative procedures and adverse effects of radiation and chemotherapy.

After surgery

- Watch for and report complications, such as fistula, pancreatitis, fluid and electrolyte imbalance, infection, hemorrhage, skin breakdown, nutritional deficiency, hepatic failure, renal insufficiency, and diabetes.

- If the patient is receiving chemotherapy, watch for adverse effects.
- Monitor fluid balance, abdominal girth, metabolic state, and weight daily.
- Consult with a nutritional therapist to help meet nutritional needs (high-calorie, low-sodium or fluid-retention diet, as required).
- Provide small, frequent, nutritious meals.
- Give an oral pancreatic enzyme at mealtimes, if needed.
- As necessary, give antacids to prevent stress ulcers.
- To prevent constipation, give laxatives, stool softeners, and cathartics as required; modify diet; and increase fluid intake. To increase GI motility, position the patient properly at mealtime, and help him walk when he can.
- Give pain medication and antipyretics, as ordered, and note the patient's response.
- Watch for signs of hypoglycemia or hyperglycemia; administer glucose or an antidiabetic, as ordered. Monitor blood glucose and urine acetone levels.
- Prevent excoriation in a pruritic patient by clipping his nails and having him wear cotton gloves.
- Watch for signs of upper GI bleeding; test stools and vomitus for occult blood, monitor hemoglobin level and hematocrit.
- To prevent thrombosis, apply antiembolism stockings and assist in range-of-motion exercises.

ACTION STAT!

 If thrombosis occurs, elevate the patient's legs. Prepare to give an anticoagulant or aspirin, as required.

Pancreatitis

Pancreatitis, inflammation of the pancreas, occurs in acute and chronic forms. With pancreatitis, the enzymes that the pancreas normally excretes digest pancreatic tissue (autodigestion). Acute pancreatitis can range from mild self-limiting episodes of abdominal discomfort requiring only simple supportive care (90% of patients) to severe systemic illness associated with significant complications, a lengthy duration, fluid sequestration, metabolic disorder, hypotension, pancreatic hemorrhage or necrosis, sepsis, and death (10% of patients). Complications include heart and kidney failure and adult respiratory distress syndrome. Fulminant pancreatitis causes massive hemorrhage and total destruction of the pancreas, resulting in diabetic acidosis, shock, or coma. (See *Chronic pancreatitis.*)

Causes

- Alcoholism
- Biliary tract disease
- Drugs: glucocorticoids, sulfonamides, chlorothiazide, azathioprine, excessive use of acetaminophen, and hormonal contraceptives
- Duodenal obstruction
- Familial
- Hypercalcemia
- Hyperlipemia
- Hypothermia
- Idiopathic
- Ischemia from vasculitis or vascular disease
- Mumps
- Mycoplasmal pneumonia
- Pancreatic cancer
- Peptic ulcer
- Pregnancy
- Scorpion venom
- Stenosis or obstruction of the sphincter of Oddi

- Surgery
- Trauma
- Viral infections

In children
- Abdominal trauma
- Cystic fibrosis
- Hemolytic uremic syndrome
- Kawasaki disease
- Medication use
- Viral illness (such as mumps and Reye's syndrome)

Signs and symptoms
- Epigastric pain centered close to the umbilicus
- Muscle guarding or tenderness
- Nausea and vomiting
- Periumbilical bruising (Cullen's sign) and bruising of the flanks (Turner's syndrome) with seepage of bloody exudate from the pancreas

In severe attack
- Abdominal rigidity
- Diabetic mellitus or acidosis (if damage occurs to islets of Langerhans)
- Diaphoresis
- Diminished bowel activity (suggesting peritonitis)
- Elevation of the left half of the diaphragm
- Enzyme deficiency
- Extreme malaise and restlessness
- Extreme pain
- Hypoperfusion
- Hypotension
- Hypovolemia
- Mottled skin
- Persistent vomiting
- Right or left pleural effusion
- Sepsis
- Shock
- Tachycardia

Chronic pancreatitis

Usually associated with alcoholism (in more than one-half of all patients), chronic pancreatitis can also follow hyperparathyroidism, hyperlipemia or, infrequently, gallstones, trauma, peptic ulcer, posttraumatic stricture, division of the pancreas, and hereditary or familial pancreatitis. Inflammation and fibrosis cause progressive pancreatic insufficiency and eventually destroy the pancreas.

Symptoms
Chronic pancreatitis is usually associated with constant dull pain with occasional exacerbations, malabsorption, severe weight loss, and hyperglycemia (leading to diabetic symptoms). Relevant diagnostic measures include patient history, abdominal X-rays or computed tomography scans showing pancreatic calcification, elevated erythrocyte sedimentation rate, and examination of stools for steatorrhea.

Treatment
The severe pain of chronic pancreatitis often requires large doses of analgesics or opioids: Addiction is common. Treatment also includes a low-fat diet and oral administration of pancreatic enzymes, such as pancreatin or pancrelipase to control steatorrhea, insulin or oral antidiabetics to curb hyperglycemia and, occasionally, surgical repair of biliary or pancreatic ducts or the sphincter of Oddi to reduce pressure and promote the flow of pancreatic juice. The prognosis is good if the patient can avoid alcohol but poor if he can't.

Diagnostic tests
- Dramatically elevated serum amylase levels—in many patients greater than 500 units/L—confirm pancreatitis; amy-

lase levels return to normal in 48 to 72 hours after the onset of pancreatitis. Persistent elevation of serum amylase levels may indicate pancreatic necrosis, pseudocyst, or abscess.

- Dramatically elevated amylase levels are also found in urine, ascites, or pleural fluid.
- Increased serum lipase levels, which rise more slowly than serum amylase levels, are found.
- Supportive laboratory studies include elevated white blood cell count and serum bilirubin level.
- Blood and urine glucose tests may reveal transient glucosuria and hyperglycemia.
- Abdominal computed tomography scan with contrast is the most sensitive, noninvasive test used to confirm the diagnosis of pancreatitis.
- Abdominal ultrasound and abdominal magnetic resonance imaging may show pancreatic inflammation.
- Abdominal and chest X-rays differentiate pancreatitis from other diseases that cause similar symptoms and detect pleural effusions.
- Endoscopic retrograde cholangiopancreatography shows the anatomy of the pancreas, and is used to differentiate pancreatitis from other disorders such as pancreatic cancer.

Treatment

ACTION STAT!

 Emergency treatment of shock (which is the most common cause of death in early-stage pancreatitis) consists of vigorous I.V. replacement of electrolytes and proteins. Metabolic acidosis that develops secondary to hypovolemia and impaired cellular perfusion requires vigorous fluid volume replacement.

- A nasogastric tube is inserted for abdominal distention.
- An anticholinergic may be administered to reduce vagal stimulation, decrease GI motility, and inhibit pancreatic enzyme secretion.
- Meperidine (Demerol) may be given to relieve abdominal pain. (This drug causes less spasm at the ampulla of Vater than do opiates such as morphine.)
- Diazepam may be given for restlessness and agitation.
- Antibiotics are prescribed to treat bacterial infections.
- Histamine antagonists, such as cimetidine (Tagamet) or ranitidine (Zantac), are given to decrease hydrochloric acid production.
- Hypokalemia, hypocalcemia, hemorrhage, and coagulopathy are treated with appropriate replacement products, such as potassium chloride, I.V. calcium gluconate or chloride, red blood cells, and fresh frozen plasma.
- Hyperglycemia and glycosuria are treated by careful titration of glucose and insulin.
- Treating the underlying condition may prevent recurrent attacks.
- Later, if the patient can't resume oral feedings, total parenteral nutrition may be necessary or nonstimulating enteral feedings.
- Necrotizing pancreatitis requires debridement (usually at 24- to 48-hour intervals) of devitalized tissue and external drainage.

Nursing considerations

- Acute pancreatitis is a life-threatening emergency. Provide supportive care, and continuously monitor the patient.
- Monitor the patient's vital signs and pulmonary artery pressure closely.
- Monitor the patient's fluid intake and output and electrolyte levels.

- Assess the patient for crackles, rhonchi, decreased breath sounds, or respiratory failure.
- Observe the patient for signs of calcium deficiency, such as tetany, carpopedal spasm, cramps, and seizures.

ACTION STAT!

 Serum calcium levels decrease in acute pancreatitis, possibly from fat necrosis, resulting in a binding of calcium with free fatty acids. Muscle twitching, tremors, and irritability are signs of decreased calcium levels.

- Give analgesics, as needed, to relieve the patient's pain and anxiety.

DRUG CHALLENGE

 Observe the patient for adverse reactions to antibiotics: nephrotoxicity with aminoglycosides, pseudomembranous enterocolitis with clindamycin, and blood dyscrasias with chloramphenicol.

- Monitor the patient for complications due to total parenteral nutrition, such as sepsis, hypokalemia, overhydration, and metabolic acidosis.
- Observe the patient for signs of sepsis, such as fever, cardiac irregularities, changes in arterial blood gas measurements, and deep respirations.

Parkinson's disease

Parkinson's disease (also known as *shaking palsy* and *paralysis agitans*) characteristically produces progressive muscle rigidity, akinesia, and involuntary tremor. Deterioration is a progressive process. Death may result from complications, such as aspiration pneumonia or another infection. Parkinson's disease is one of the most common neurologic disorders of the elderly population.

Causes

- Unknown
- Possibly caused by exposure to toxins (such as manganese dust and carbon monoxide, which destroy cells in the substantia nigra).

Signs and symptoms

- Blepharospasm (eyelids are completely closed)
- Bradykinesia or akinesia
- Dementia
- Drooling
- Dysarthria
- Dysphagia
- High-pitched, monotone voice
- Insidious tremor that begins in the fingers (unilateral pill-roll tremor)
- Loss of position sense with postural instability
- Loss of posture control (the patient walks with body bent forward)
- Masklike facial expression
- Muscle rigidity
- Oculogyric crises (eyes are fixed upward, with involuntary tonic movements)
- Tremor decreasing with purposeful movement and sleep
- Tremor increasing during stress or anxiety

Diagnostic tests

- Diagnosis is based on the patient's age and history and on the characteristic clinical picture rather than on specific diagnostic testing.
- Urinalysis may reveal decreased dopamine levels.
- Computed tomography scanning or magnetic resonance imaging may be performed to rule out other disorders such as intracranial tumors. Other causes of tremor must also be ruled out for a conclusive diagnosis.

Treatment

- Levodopa may be given in increasing doses until symptoms are relieved or the patient has an adverse reaction to it.

DRUG CHALLENGE

 Because adverse reactions can be serious, levodopa is commonly given with carbidopa (Sinemet is the combination drug) to halt peripheral dopamine synthesis. When levodopa proves ineffective or too toxic, alternative drug therapy includes anticholinergics such as trihexyphenidyl, antihistamines such as diphenhydramine (Benadryl), and antivirals such as amantadine (Symmetrel).

- Rasagiline (Azilect), a monoamine oxidase–B inhibitor, blocks the breakdown of dopamine and can be used as monotherapy in early Parkinson's disease and as an addition to levodopa in more advanced patients.
- Selegiline (Eldepryl), an enzyme inhibitor, helps conserve dopamine and enhances the therapeutic effect of levodopa.

DRUG CHALLENGE

 Research on the oxidative stress theory has caused a controversy in drug therapy for Parkinson's disease. Although levodopa (with carbidopa) has traditionally been a first-line drug in management of the disease, the drug has also been associated with an acceleration of the disease process. Selegiline followed by levodopa (with carbidopa) may provide increased protection.

DRUG CHALLENGE

 To prevent a dangerous increase in blood pressure when taking rasagiline or selegiline, patients should avoid tyramine-rich foods (and beverages and dietary supplements), such as aged cheeses, air-dried meats, pickled herring, yeast extract, aged red wines, draft beers, sauerkraut, and soy sauce. Symptoms of this reaction include severe headache, blurred vision, difficulty thinking, seizures, chest pain, unexplained nausea or vomiting, or symptoms of a stroke. Patients should seek immediate medical attention if any of these symptoms occur.

- The patient may receive bromocriptine (Parlodel) as an additive to reduce the levodopa dose.
- Catechol-O-methyltransferase inhibitors, such as entacapone (Comtan) and tolcapone (Tasmar) block an enzyme that breaks down peripheral levodopa.
- Stereotactic neurosurgery may be necessary to relieve symptoms.
- Deep brain stimulation may help relieve symptoms.
- Physical therapy maintains normal muscle tone and function.
- Additional therapies include fetal cell transplantation and neurotransplantation.

Nursing considerations

- Carefully monitor drug treatment.
- Encourage independence. The patient with excessive tremor may achieve partial control of his body by sitting on a chair and using its arms to steady himself. Remember that fatigue may cause him to depend more on others.
- Scheduling meals around the time of maximum drug efficiency will help minimize complications and promote good nutrition.
- Help the patient overcome problems related to eating and elimination. For example, if he has difficulty eating, offer

supplementary or small, frequent meals to increase caloric intake.

- Help establish a regular bowel routine by encouraging the patient to drink at least 2,000 ml of liquids daily and to eat high-bulk foods. He may need an elevated toilet seat to assist him from a standing to a sitting position.
- Show the family how to prevent pressure ulcers and contractures with proper positioning.
- Explain that the patient should avoid high-protein meals (this impairs the action of levodopa), and explain household safety measures to prevent accidents.
- Instruct the patient and his family on proper food consistency, correct positioning, and swallowing strategies to decrease dysphagia and avoid aspiration. Also, teach the family how to assess the patient for aspiration.
- Provide emotional support for the patient and his family. Refer to counseling and support groups as appropriate.

Pediculosis

Pediculosis is caused by parasitic forms of lice: *Pediculus humanus* var. *capitis* causes pediculosis capitis (head lice), *Pediculus humanus* var. *corporis* causes pediculosis corporis (body lice), and *Phthirus pubis* causes pediculosis pubis (crab lice). These lice feed on human blood and lay their eggs (nits) in body hairs or clothing fibers. After the nits hatch, the lice must feed within 24 hours or die; they mature in 2 to 3 weeks. When a louse bites, it injects a toxin into the skin that produces mild irritation and a purpuric spot. Repeated bites cause sensitization to the toxin, leading to more serious inflammation. Treatment can effectively eliminate lice.

Causes

- *P. humanus* var. *capitis* (pediculosis of scalp, eyebrows, eyelashes, and beard)
- *P. humanus* var. *corporis* (lives in the seams of clothing and feeds on blood)
- *P. pubis* (typically in pubic hairs, but may extend to the eyebrows, eyelashes, and axillary or body hair)

Risk factors

- Overcrowded conditions
- Poor personal hygiene
- Prolonged wearing of the same clothing (which might occur in cold climates)
- Shared clothing, hats, combs, hairbrushes, bedsheets, or towels harboring lice

Signs and symptoms
Pediculosis capitis

- Excoriation (with severe itching)
- Itching
- Matted, foul-smelling, lusterless hair (in severe cases)
- Occipital and cervical lymphadenopathy
- Oval gray-white nits on hair shafts
- Rash on the trunk (probably due to sensitization)

Pediculosis corporis

- Bacterial infection
- Dry, discolored, thickly encrusted, scaly skin
- Scarring
- Small red papules (usually on the shoulders, trunk, or buttocks)
- Vertical excoriations
- Wheals (probably a sensitivity reaction)

In severe cases

- Fever
- Headache
- Malaise

Pediculosis pubis
- Skin irritation from scratching
- Small gray-blue spots (maculae caeruleae) may appear on the thighs or upper body

Diagnostic tests
- Wood's light examination achieves fluorescence of the adult lice.
- Microscopic examination shows nits visible on the hair shaft.

Treatment
Pediculosis capitis
- Permethrin cream rinse is rubbed into the hair and rinsed after 10 minutes. A single treatment should be sufficient. Alternatives include pyrethrins and lindane shampoo.
- A fine-tooth comb dipped in vinegar removes nits from hair.
- Washing hair with ordinary shampoo removes crusts.

Pediculosis corporis
- Bathing with soap and water removes lice from the body.
- Permethrin cream rinse is rubbed into the hair and skin and rinsed after 10 minutes.
- Lice may be removed from clothes by washing them in hot water, ironing, or dry cleaning.
- Storing clothes for more than 30 days or placing them in dry heat of 140° F (60° C) kills lice.

Pediculosis pubis
- Shampoo the hair with lindane shampoo for 4 minutes, and then repeat in 1 week.
- Clothes and bedsheets must be laundered to prevent reinfestation.

Nursing considerations
- Instruct patients how to use the creams, ointments, powders, and shampoos that can eliminate lice.
- To protect yourself from infestation, avoid prolonged contact with the patient's hair, clothing, and bedsheets.
- Ask the patient with pediculosis pubis for a history of recent sexual contacts so that they can be examined and treated.
- To prevent the spread of pediculosis to other hospitalized persons, examine all high-risk patients on admission, especially elderly patients who depend on others for care, those admitted from nursing homes, or persons living in crowded conditions.

Pelvic inflammatory disease

Pelvic inflammatory disease (PID) is any acute, subacute, recurrent, or chronic infection of the oviducts and ovaries, with adjacent tissue involvement. It includes inflammation of the cervix (cervicitis), uterus (endometritis), fallopian tubes (salpingitis), and ovaries (oophoritis), which can extend to the connective tissue lying between the broad ligaments (parametritis). The most common bacteria found in cervical mucus are staphylococci, streptococci, diphtheroids, chlamydiae, and coliforms, including *Pseudomonas* and *Escherichia coli*. Uterine infection can result from one or several of these organisms or it may follow the multiplication of normally nonpathogenic bacteria in an altered endometrial environment. Early diagnosis and treatment prevents damage to the reproductive system. Untreated PID may cause infertility and may lead to potentially fatal septicemia, pulmonary emboli, and shock.

Causes

- Infection with aerobic or anaerobic organisms (*Neisseria gonorrhoeae*)

Contributing factors

- Abortion
- Chronically infected fallopian tube
- Diverticulitis of the sigmoid colon
- Infection during or after pregnancy
- Insertion of an intrauterine device
- Pelvic abscess
- Pelvic surgery
- Ruptured appendix
- Transfer of contaminated cervical mucus into the endometrial cavity by instrumentation
- Tubal insufflation
- Use of a biopsy curet or an irrigation catheter

Signs and symptoms

- Extreme pain upon movement of the cervix or palpation of the adnexa (see *Forms of pelvic inflammatory disease,* page 458)
- Lower abdominal pain
- Low-grade fever
- Malaise (particularly if gonorrhea is the cause)
- Profuse, purulent vaginal discharge

Diagnostic tests

- Gram stain of secretions from the endocervix or cul-de-sac; culture and sensitivity testing aids selection of the appropriate antibiotic. Urethral and rectal secretions may also be cultured.
- Ultrasonography, magnetic resonance imaging, or computed tomography scanning is used to identify an adnexal or uterine mass.
- Culdocentesis is performed to obtain peritoneal fluid or pus for culture and sensitivity testing.
- C-reactive protein, a blood test to detect inflammation, is highly sensitive for detecting PID and aids diagnosis.

Treatment

- Antibiotic therapy is initiated after culture specimens are obtained and reevaluated when laboratory test results are available (usually after 24 to 48 hours). (Outpatient treatment includes cefoxitin [Mefoxin] plus probenecid given concurrently or a single dose of ceftriaxone [Rocephin]; each regimen given with doxycycline [Vibramycin] for 14 days. Inpatient treatment is doxycycline alone or a combination of clindamycin and gentamicin.)
- Pelvic abscess requires drainage.

ACTION STAT!

 A ruptured abscess is life-threatening. If this complication develops, the patient may need a total abdominal hysterectomy with bilateral salpingo-oophorectomy.

Nursing considerations

- After establishing that the patient doesn't have drug allergies, administer antibiotics and analgesics as necessary.
- Check for fever. If it persists, carefully monitor fluid intake and output, watching the patient for signs of dehydration.
- Watch for abdominal rigidity and distention, possible signs of developing peritonitis.
- Provide frequent perineal care if vaginal drainage occurs.
- To prevent a recurrence, explain the nature and seriousness of PID, and encourage the patient to comply with the treatment regimen.
- Stress the need for the patient's sexual partner to be examined and, if necessary, treated for infection.
- Because PID may cause painful intercourse, advise the patient to consult with her practitioner about sexual activity.

Forms of pelvic inflammatory disease

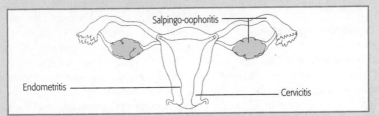

Clinical features

Salpingo-oophoritis
- Acute: sudden onset of lower abdominal and pelvic pain, usually following menses; increased vaginal discharge; fever; malaise; lower abdominal pressure and tenderness; tachycardia; pelvic peritonitis
- Chronic: recurring acute episodes

Cervicitis
- Acute: purulent, foul-smelling vaginal discharge; vulvovaginitis, with itching or burning; red, edematous cervix; pelvic discomfort; sexual dysfunction; metrorrhagia; infertility; spontaneous abortion
- Chronic: cervical dystocia, laceration or eversion of the cervix, ulcerative vesicular lesion (when cervicitis results from herpes simplex virus II)

Endometritis (generally postpartum or postabortion)
- Acute: mucopurulent or purulent vaginal discharge oozing from the cervix; edematous, hyperemic endometrium, possibly leading to ulceration and necrosis (with virulent organisms); lower abdominal pain and tenderness; fever; rebound pain; abdominal muscle spasm; thrombophlebitis of uterine and pelvic vessels (in severe forms)
- Chronic: recurring acute episodes (increasingly common because of widespread use of intrauterine devices)

Diagnostic findings

Salpingo-oophoritis
- Blood studies show leukocytosis or normal white blood cell (WBC) count.
- X-ray may show ileus.
- Pelvic examination reveals extreme tenderness.
- Smear of cervical or periurethral gland exudate shows gram-negative intracellular diplococci.

Cervicitis
- *Chlamydia trachomatis* is the most common organism infecting the cervix, followed by *Neisseria gonorrhoea*.
- Cytologic smears may reveal severe inflammation.
- If cervicitis isn't complicated by salpingitis, WBC count is normal or slightly elevated; erythrocyte sedimentation rate (ESR) is elevated.
- With acute cervicitis, cervical palpation reveals tenderness.
- With chronic cervicitis, causative organisms are usually staphylococci or streptococci.

Endometritis
- With severe infection, palpation may reveal a boggy uterus.
- Uterine and blood samples are positive for the causative organism, usually staphylococcus.
- WBC count and ESR are elevated.

To prevent infection after minor gynecologic procedures, such as dilatation and curettage, tell the patient to immediately report any fever, increased vaginal discharge, or pain. After such procedures, instruct her to avoid douching and intercourse for at least 7 days.

▌Peptic ulcers

Peptic ulcer is a disruption in the gastric or duodenal mucosa when normal defense mechanisms are overwhelmed or impaired by acid or pepsin. Ulcers are circumscribed lesions that extend through the muscularis mucosa. Ulcers are five times more common on the duodenum. Both kinds of ulcers may be asymptomatic or may penetrate the pancreas and cause severe back pain. Other complications of peptic ulcers include perforation, hemorrhage, and pyloric obstruction.

Causes
- Cigarette smoking
- Infection with *Helicobacter pylori*
- Pancreatitis, hepatic disease, Crohn's disease, Zollinger-Ellison syndrome, and preexisting gastritis
- Pathologic hypersecretory states such as Zollinger-Ellison syndrome
- "Type A" personality
- Use of nonsteroidal anti-inflammatory drugs (NSAIDs) and salicylates

Signs and symptoms
Gastric ulcers
- Anorexia
- Nausea
- Pain (constant, but more intense with eating)

Duodenal ulcers
- Peculiar sensation of hot water bubbling in the back of the throat
- Vomiting and other digestive disturbances (rare)
- Weight gain (because the patient eats to relieve discomfort)
- Well-localized midepigastric pain (relieved by food)

Diagnostic tests
- Barium swallow or upper GI and small bowel series help diagnose a peptic ulcer.
- Upper endoscopy or esophagogastroduodenoscopy helps distinguish benign from malignant disease.
- *H. pylori* may be diagnosed with urease breath testing, serologic testing, and by biopsy via upper endoscopy.
- Laboratory analysis may disclose occult blood in stools.
- Hemoglobin level and hematocrit are decreased with GI bleeding.

Treatment
- Medications may include histamine-2 (H_2) receptor antagonists, such as cimetidine (Tagamet) or ranitidine (Zantac), to reduce gastric secretion, or a proton pump inhibitor such as lansoprazole (Prevacid).
- Prostaglandin analogs and antacids are given to protect the mucosa.
- An antisecretory agent, such as misoprostol (Cytotec) is given if the ulceration resulted from NSAID use.
- GI bleeding may be treated by giving H_2-receptor antagonists I.V. as a continuous infusion; an injection of epinephrine or saline (to surround the ulcer) can be administered to stop the bleeding during endoscopy.
- Cautery may be used for hemostasis.
- Vagotomy and pyloroplasty—severing one or more branches of the vagus nerve to reduce hydrochloric acid secretion

and refashioning the pylorus to create a larger lumen and facilitate gastric emptying—may be necessary.

- Distal subtotal gastrectomy (with or without vagotomy) may be necessary and consists of excising the antrum of the stomach, thereby removing the hormonal stimulus of the parietal cells, followed by anastomosis of the remainder of the stomach to the duodenum or the jejunum.

Nursing considerations

- Administer medications as directed.

DRUG CHALLENGE

Observe the patient for adverse reactions to H_2-receptor antagonists and omeprazole (such as dizziness, fatigue, rash, and mild diarrhea). Educate the patient about the potential adverse effects of antibiotic therapy in the treatment of *H. pylori*, which include nausea, vomiting, and diarrhea.

- A patient with a history of cardiac disease or with a sodium-restricted diet should be instructed to take only those antacids that contain low amounts of sodium.
- Advise the patient to avoid taking NSAIDs.
- Warn the patient to avoid stressful situations, excessive intake of coffee, and ingestion of alcoholic beverages during exacerbations of peptic ulcer disease. Counsel the patient to enroll in a smoking cessation program.

After gastric surgery

- Maintain patency of the nasogastric (NG) tube. Don't manipulate the tube. If it isn't functioning, notify the surgeon.
- Monitor intake and output. Record NG tube drainage.
- Assess the patient for bowel sounds.

- Maintain the patient on nothing-by-mouth status until the NG tube is removed or clamped.
- Replace fluids and electrolytes. Assess the patient for signs of dehydration, sodium deficiency, and metabolic alkalosis, which may occur secondary to gastric suction.
- Monitor the patient for possible complications: hemorrhage; shock; iron, folate, or vitamin B_{12} deficiency anemia (from malabsorption or continued blood loss); and dumping syndrome (weakness, nausea, flatulence, diarrhea, distention, and palpitations within 30 minutes after a meal).
- To avoid dumping syndrome, advise the patient to sit upright for up to 2 hours after eating, to drink fluids between meals rather than with meals, to avoid eating large amounts of carbohydrates, and to eat four to six small, high-protein, low-carbohydrate meals throughout the day.

Pericarditis

Pericarditis is an inflammation of the pericardium, the fibroserous sac that envelops, supports, and protects the heart. It occurs in both acute and chronic forms. Acute pericarditis can be fibrinous or effusive, with purulent, serous, or hemorrhagic exudate; chronic constrictive pericarditis is characterized by dense fibrous pericardial thickening. The prognosis depends on the underlying cause but is generally good in acute pericarditis, unless constriction occurs.

Causes

- Aortic aneurysm with pericardial leakage
- Autoimmune disease (acute rheumatic fever, systemic lupus erythematosus, acquired immunodeficiency syndrome)

- Bacterial, fungal, or viral infection (infectious pericarditis)
- Drugs, such as hydralazine, nydrazid, phenytoin, and procainamide
- High-dose radiation to the chest
- Hypersensitivity
- Idiopathic factors (most common in acute pericarditis)
- Myxedema with cholesterol deposits in the pericardium
- Neoplasms (primary or metastases)
- Postcardiac injury (myocardial infarction resulting in Dressler's syndrome; trauma or surgery)
- Rheumatoid arthritis
- Systemic disease
- Uremia

Signs and symptoms
Acute pericarditis
- Diminished or absent apical impulse
- Distant heart sounds
- Dyspnea
- Feeling of fullness in the chest
- Increased cardiac dullness
- Orthopnea
- Pericardial friction rub heard best during forced expiration, with the patient leaning forward or resting on his hands and knees in the bed
- Sharp and sudden pain over the sternum and radiating to the neck, shoulders, back, and arms that increases with deep inspiration and decreases when the patient sits up and leans forward
- Substernal chest pain
- Tachycardia

ACTION STAT!

 If the fluid accumulates rapidly, cardiac tamponade may occur, resulting in pallor, clammy skin, hypotension, paradoxical pulse (a decrease in systolic blood pressure equal to or greater than 10 mm Hg during slow inspiration), jugular vein distention

and, eventually, cardiovascular collapse and death.

Chronic pericarditis
- Ascites
- Fluid retention
- Gradual increase in systemic venous pressure
- Hepatomegaly

Diagnostic tests
- Electrocardiography shows characteristic changes in patients with acute pericarditis (such as elevated ST segments in the limb leads and most precordial leads, diminished QRS complexes, and rhythm changes).
- X-ray, echocardiogram, magnetic resonance imaging, computed tomography, and coronary angiography may show scarring, contracture of the pericardium, or enlargement of the heart.
- In acute pericarditis, an electrocardiogram shows elevation of ST segments in the standard limb leads and most precordial leads lacking the significant changes in QRS-complex morphology.
- In pericardial effusion, echocardiography is diagnostic when it shows an echo-free space between the ventricular wall and the pericardium.
- White blood cell count is normal or elevated, especially in infectious pericarditis.
- Slightly elevated cardiac enzyme levels with associated myocarditis confirm the diagnosis.
- Culture of pericardial fluid obtained by open surgical drainage or cardiocentesis (sometimes identifies a causative organism in bacterial or fungal pericarditis) also confirms the diagnosis.

Treatment
- Bed rest is necessary while fever and pain persist.

- Nonsteroidal anti-inflammatory drugs (NSAIDs), such as aspirin and indomethacin (Indocin), are given to relieve pain and reduce inflammation.
- Corticosteroids are cautiously given to provide rapid, effective relief if symptoms continue after giving NSAIDs.

- Infectious pericarditis requires antibiotics (possibly by direct pericardial injection), surgical drainage, or both.
- Cardiac tamponade may require pericardiocentesis.
- Recurrent pericarditis may necessitate a partial pericardectomy.
- In constrictive pericarditis, a total pericardectomy to permit adequate filling and contraction of the heart may be necessary.
- Treatment of underlying disorders.

Nursing considerations

- Provide complete bed rest.
- Assess pain in relation to respiration and body position to distinguish pericardial pain from myocardial ischemic pain.
- Place the patient in an upright position to relieve dyspnea and chest pain. Provide analgesics and oxygen.
- Reassure the patient with acute pericarditis that his condition is temporary and treatable.

ACTION STAT!

 Monitor the patient for signs of cardiac compression or cardiac tamponade, possible complications of pericardial effusion. Signs include decreased blood pressure, in-

creased central venous pressure, and paradoxical pulse. Because cardiac tamponade requires immediate treatment, keep a pericardiocentesis set handy whenever pericardial effusion is suspected.

- Explain tests and treatments to the patient.
- Provide preoperative and postoperative care as indicated; similar to that with cardiothoracic surgery.

Perirectal abscess and fistula

A perirectal abscess is a localized collection of pus caused by inflammation of the soft tissue outside the anal verge. Such inflammation may produce a fistula in ano—an abnormal opening in the anal skin—that may communicate with the rectum. This disease is three times more common in males than in females. It results from an abrasion or tear in the lining of the anal canal, rectum, or perianal skin, and subsequent infection by *Escherichia coli,* staphylococci, or streptococci.

Causes

- Enema-tip abrasions
- Immunocompromised state
- Infectious dermatitis
- Insertion of foreign objects
- Malignancy
- Preexisting lesions
- Prolapsed thrombotic internal hemorrhoids
- Puncture wounds from ingested eggshells or fishbones
- Radiation
- Ruptured anal hematoma
- Septic lesions in the pelvis (acute appendicitis, acute salpingitis, and diverticulitis)

- Systemic illnesses (ulcerative colitis, Crohn's disease)
- Trauma (for example, from injections for treatment of internal hemorrhoids)

Signs and symptoms
- Chills
- Fever
- Hard, painful lump on one side, preventing comfortable sitting
- Malaise
- Nausea, vomiting
- Painful swelling that's exacerbated by defecation, sitting, coughing
- Pus drainage from abscess
- Tenderness at the site of the abscess
- Throbbing pain

Diagnostic tests
- Culture of drainage identifies infectious organism.

Treatment
- Treatment includes surgical incision and drainage of lesion.
- Fistulas require a fistulotomy—removal of the fistula tract and associated granulation tissue—under general, spinal, or caudal anesthesia.
- If the fistula tract is epithelialized, treatment requires fistulectomy—removal of the fistulous tract—followed by the insertion of drains, which are gradually removed over time.

Nursing considerations
- Provide adequate medication for pain relief.
- Examine the wound frequently to assess proper healing, which should progress from the inside out.
- Inform the patient that complete recovery takes time. Offer encouragement.
- Stress the importance of perianal cleanliness.
- Be alert for the first postoperative bowel movement. The patient may suppress

the urge to defecate because of anticipated pain; the resulting constipation increases pressure at the wound site. Such a patient may benefit from a stool softener.

Peritonitis

Peritonitis is an acute or chronic inflammation of the peritoneum, the membrane that lines the abdominal cavity and covers the visceral organs. Inflammation may extend throughout the peritoneum, or it may be localized as an abscess. Peritonitis commonly decreases intestinal motility and causes intestinal distention with gas. Mortality is 10%, with death usually resulting from bowel obstruction; the mortality was much higher before the introduction of antibiotics.

Causes
- Bacterial invasion in the peritoneum
- Chemical inflammation

Predisposing factors
- Appendicitis
- Diverticulitis
- Gangrenous gallbladder, abdominal neoplasm, or a penetrating wound.
- Peptic ulcer
- Perforated or ruptured gallbladder
- Perforation of the GI tract
- Rupture of a fallopian tube, bladder, gastric ulcer, or release of pancreatic enzymes
- Strangulated obstruction
- Ulcerative colitis
- Volvulus

Signs and symptoms
- Abdominal distention
- Abdominal rigidity
- Altered bowel habits (particularly constipation)
- Anorexia

- Cold skin
- Decreased intestinal motility
- Excessive sweating
- Fever of 103° F (39.4° C) or higher
- Hiccups
- Hypokalemia
- Hypotension
- Nausea, vomiting
- Pain that localizes over the affected area
- Pallor
- Paralytic ileus
- Rebound tenderness
- Shallow breathing
- Shoulder pain
- Signs of dehydration
- Sudden, severe, and diffuse abdominal pain
- Tachycardia
- Weakness

Diagnostic tests

- Abdominal computed tomography scan or X-rays showing edematous and gaseous distention of the small and large bowel support the diagnosis.
- In perforation of a visceral organ, the X-ray shows air in the abdominal cavity.
- Chest X-ray may show elevation of the diaphragm.
- Blood studies reveal leukocytosis (greater than 20,000/µl).
- Paracentesis reveals bacteria, exudate, blood, pus, or urine.
- Laparotomy may be necessary to identify the underlying cause.

Treatment

- Antibiotic therapy is prescribed for specific causative organism.
- To decrease peristalsis and prevent perforation, the patient should receive nothing by mouth; instead, he requires supportive fluids and electrolytes parenterally.
- Analgesics are given to reduce pain.

- Nasogastric (NG) intubation is used to decompress the bowel.
- In perforation, surgery is necessary to eliminate the source of infection by evacuating the spilled contents and repairing any organ perforation.

Nursing considerations

- Monitor vital signs, fluid intake and output, and the amount of NG drainage or vomitus.
- Place the patient in semi-Fowler's position to facilitate comfort.
- Encourage the patient to deep breathe, cough effectively, and use an incentive spirometer.
- Teach the patient how to splint the incision.
- Counteract mouth and nose dryness due to fever and NG intubation with regular cleaning and lubrication.

After surgery

- Give parenteral fluid and electrolytes as ordered. Accurately record fluid intake and output, including drainage from the NG tube and the incision.
- Place the patient in Fowler's position to promote drainage (through drainage tube) by gravity.
- Encourage and assist ambulation as ordered, usually on the first postoperative day.
- Observe for signs of dehiscence and abscess formation.
- Frequently assess for peristaltic activity by listening for bowel sounds and evaluating for passage of flatus, bowel movements, and soft abdomen.
- When peristalsis returns and temperature and pulse rate are normal or when NG output diminishes (less than 200 ml/24 hours), the NG tube is removed.
- Gradually decrease parenteral fluids and increase oral intake.

Pernicious anemia

A megaloblastic anemia, pernicious anemia (also called *Addison's anemia*) is characterized by decreased gastric production of hydrochloric acid and deficiency of intrinsic factor (IF), a substance normally secreted by the parietal cells of the gastric mucosa that's essential for vitamin B_{12} absorption. The resulting vitamin B_{12} deficiency causes serious neurologic, gastric, and intestinal abnormalities. Untreated pernicious anemia may lead to permanent neurologic disability and death.

Causes
- Genetic
- Inherited autoimmune response
- Surgery such as partial gastrectomy

Signs and symptoms
- Jaundiced sclera
- Lips, gums, and tongue appear markedly bloodless
- Numbness and tingling in the extremities
- Pale to bright yellow skin
- Sore tongue
- Susceptibility to infection, especially genitourinary tract
- Weakness

GI signs and symptoms
- Anorexia
- Constipation
- Diarrhea
- Flatulence
- Gingival bleeding
- Nausea, vomiting
- Tongue inflammation
- Weight loss

Central nervous system signs and symptoms
- Altered taste
- Altered vision (diplopia, blurred vision)
- Ataxia
- Delirium
- Depression
- Disturbed position sense
- Headache
- Impaired fine finger movement
- Impotence (in males)
- Irritability
- Lack of coordination
- Light-headedness
- Loss of bowel and bladder control
- Neuritis
- Optic muscle atrophy
- Peripheral numbness and paresthesia
- Poor memory
- Positive Babinski's and Romberg's signs
- Tinnitus
- Weakness in the extremities

Cardiovascular signs and symptoms
- Dyspnea
- Fatigue
- Heart failure
- Light-headedness
- Orthopnea
- Palpitations; premature beats
- Tachycardia
- Weakness
- Wide pulse pressure

Diagnostic tests
- Bone marrow aspiration reveals erythroid hyperplasia (crowded red bone marrow), with increased numbers of megaloblasts but few normally developing red blood cells (RBCs).
- Gastric analysis shows the absence of free hydrochloric acid after histamine or pentagastrin injection.
- Schilling test shows radioactive B_{12} excretion is less than 3% (normal is 7% in first 24 hours via urine). With pernicious anemia, the vitamin remains unabsorbed and is passed in the stool. When

the Schilling test is repeated with IF added, the test shows normal excretion of vitamin B_{12}.
- IF antibodies and antiparietal cell antibodies.
- Blood study results that suggest pernicious anemia include:
  - decreased hemoglobin (Hb) level (4 to 5 g/dl) and decreased RBC count
  - increased mean corpuscular volume (greater than 120/μl) because each larger-than-normal RBC contains increased amounts of Hb; mean corpuscular Hb concentration is also increased
  - low white blood cell and platelet counts and large, malformed platelets
  - serum vitamin B_{12}–assay levels, less than 0.1 mcg/ml
  - elevated serum lactate dehydrogenase levels.

Treatment
- Early I.M. vitamin B_{12} replacement can reverse pernicious anemia and may prevent permanent neurologic damage. An initial high dose of parenteral vitamin B_{12} causes rapid RBC regeneration. Concomitant iron replacement is necessary because rapid cell regeneration increases the patient's iron requirements.

DRUG CHALLENGE

 After the patient's condition improves, the vitamin B_{12} dosage can be decreased to maintenance levels and given monthly. Because such injections must be continued for life, patients should learn how to do the injections themselves.

- Bed rest is necessary until the patient's Hb level rises.
- If the Hb level is dangerously low, blood transfusions may be needed.
- Heart failure is treated with digoxin, diuretic, and a low-sodium diet.

- Antibiotics help combat accompanying infections.

Nursing considerations
- Educate the patient and his family about lifelong vitamin B_{12} replacement therapy.
- If the patient has severe anemia, plan activities, rest periods, and necessary diagnostic tests to conserve energy. Monitor pulse rate often; tachycardia means activities are too strenuous.
- Warn the patient to guard against infections, and tell him to report signs of infection promptly, especially respiratory and urinary tract infections, because the patient's weakened condition may increase susceptibility.
- Provide a well-balanced diet, including foods high in vitamin B_{12} (meat, liver, fish, eggs, and milk). Offer between-meal snacks, and encourage the family to bring favorite foods from home.
- Because a sore mouth and tongue make eating painful, ask the dietitian to avoid giving the patient irritating foods. If these symptoms make talking difficult, supply a pad and pencil or some other aid to facilitate nonverbal communication; explain this problem to the family. Provide diluted mouthwash or, with severe conditions, swab the patient's mouth with tap water or warm saline solution.
- Warn the patient with a sensory deficit not to use a heating pad because it may cause burns.
- If the patient is incontinent, establish a regular bowel and bladder routine. After the patient is discharged, a visiting nurse should follow up on this schedule and make adjustments as needed.
- If neurologic damage causes behavioral problems, assess mental and neurologic status often; if necessary, give a tranquilizer as ordered, and if needed, apply a soft restraint at night.

- Stress to the patient that vitamin B_{12} replacement isn't a permanent cure and that these injections must be continued for life, even after symptoms subside.
- To prevent pernicious anemia, emphasize the importance of vitamin B_{12} supplements for patients who have had extensive gastric resections or those who follow strict vegetarian diets.

Pharyngitis

The most common throat disorder, pharyngitis is an acute or chronic inflammation of the pharynx. It's widespread among adults who live or work in dusty or dry environments, use their voices excessively, habitually use tobacco or alcohol, or suffer from chronic sinusitis, persistent coughs, or allergies. Uncomplicated pharyngitis usually subsides in 3 to 10 days. Some severe forms, such as severe mononucleosis-pharyngitis, may cause airway obstruction.

Causes
Viral
- Adenovirus
- Coronavirus
- Influenza
- Parainfluenza
- Rhinovirus

Bacterial
- Chlamydia
- Group A beta-hemolytic streptococci
- Mycoplasma

Signs and symptoms
- Constant, aggravating urge to swallow
- Coryza
- Exudate confined to the lymphoid areas of the throat
- Generalized redness and inflammation of the posterior wall of pharynx
- Headache
- Large amount of exudate (with bacterial pharyngitis)
- Mild fever
- Muscle and joint pain
- Red, edematous mucous membranes studded with white or yellow follicle
- Rhinorrhea
- Sensation of a lump in the throat
- Slight difficulty in swallowing
- Sore throat

Diagnostic tests
- A throat culture may be performed to identify bacterial organisms that may be the cause of the inflammation.
- Rapid strep tests generally detect group A streptococcal infections, but they miss the fairly common streptococcal groups C and G.
- A white blood cell count (WBC) is used to determine atypical lymphocytes; an elevated total WBC count is present.

Treatment
- Based on the patient's symptoms, treatment for acute viral pharyngitis consists mainly of rest, warm saline gargles, throat lozenges containing a mild anesthetic, and plenty of fluids.
- Analgesics are given as needed for pain.
- If the patient can't swallow fluids, hospitalization may be required for I.V. hydration.
- Antibiotics are prescribed to treat bacterial pharyngitis.
- In chronic pharyngitis, treatment includes eliminating the underlying cause.
- Preventive measures include humidifying the air and avoiding excessive exposure to air conditioning.
- The patient should be urged to stop smoking, if appropriate.

Nursing considerations

- Administer analgesics and warm saline gargles as appropriate.
- Monitor intake and output and watch for signs of dehydration. Assess skin turgor, mucous membranes and, in young children, tearing.
- Encourage the intake of cool fluids to soothe the patient's throat. Also have the patient take normal-size swallows, not sips.
- Provide mouth care to prevent dry lips and oral pyoderma, and maintain a restful environment.
- Elevate the patient's head with three or four pillows.
- Obtain throat cultures, and administer antibiotics as required. If the patient has acute bacterial pharyngitis, emphasize the importance of completing the full course of antibiotic therapy.
- Teach the patient with chronic pharyngitis how to minimize sources of throat irritation in the environment, such as using a bedside humidifier.
- Refer the patient to a self-help group to stop smoking, if appropriate.

∎ Phenylketonuria

Phenylketonuria (PKU) is an inborn error in phenylalanine metabolism that results in the accumulation of high serum levels of the enzyme phenylalanine in the blood. Although blood phenylalanine levels are near normal at birth, they begin to rise within a few days. By the time they reach significant levels (about 30 mg/dl), cerebral damage has begun. Such irreversible damage is probably complete by age 2 or 3. However, early detection and treatment can minimize cerebral damage, and children under strict dietary control can lead normal lives. When left untreated, the disease results in cerebral damage and mental retardation.

Causes

- Autosomal recessive gene

Signs and symptoms

- Abnormal EEG patterns in 80% of cases
- Awkward gait
- Dry, rough skin
- Eczematous skin lesions
- Hyperactive
- Increased muscle tone
- Irritable
- Mental retardation
- Microcephaly
- Musty odor due to skin and urinary excretion of phenylacetic acid
- Normal appearance at birth but beginning to show signs by age 4 months
- Personality disturbances
- Precipitous decrease in IQ in the first year
- Purposeless, repetitive motions
- Seizures (in about one-third of patients; beginning between ages 6 and 12 months)

Diagnostic tests

- An enzyme assay, which is performed on adults, may detect the carrier state.
- Prenatal diagnosis is made with a chorionic villi sample to detect fetal PKU.
- In neonates, PKU screenings (the Guthrie test) are performed on a heel-stick blood sample, a procedure that's mandatory at birth in most states. Because phenylalanine levels may be normal at birth, a neonate should be reevaluated after receiving dietary protein for 24 to 48 hours. Detection of elevated blood levels of phenylalanine confirms the diagnosis.

Treatment

- Restricted dietary intake of the amino acid phenylalanine keeps phenylalanine blood levels between 3 and 9 mg/dl.
- Enzymatic hydrolysate of casein, such as Lofenalac Powder or Pregestimil Powder, is substituted for milk in the diets of affected infants.
- Dietary restrictions should probably continue throughout life. Overzealous dietary restriction can induce phenylalanine deficiency, producing lethargy, anorexia, anemia, rashes, and diarrhea.

Nursing considerations

- Stress the critical importance of adhering to the special diet. The foods to be avoided include breads, cheese, eggs, flour, meat, poultry, fish, nuts, milk, legumes, and aspartame.
- Refer the family to a dietitian trained to assist with this disorder.
- Inform the parents that the child will need frequent tests for urine phenylpyruvic acid and blood phenylalanine levels to evaluate the diet's effectiveness.
- As the child grows older and is supervised less closely, his parents will have less control over what he eats. As a result, deviation from the restricted diet becomes more likely, as does the risk of brain damage. Encourage the parents to allow the child some choices in the kinds of low-protein foods he wants to eat; this will help make him feel trusted and more responsible.
- Teach the parents about normal physical and mental growth and development so that they can recognize any developmental delay that may point to excessive phenylalanine intake.
- Refer parents for genetic counseling as indicated.

■ Pheochromocytoma

A pheochromocytoma is a chromaffin-cell tumor of the adrenal medulla that secretes an excessive amount of the catecholamines epinephrine and norepinephrine, which results in severe hypertension, increased metabolism, and hyperglycemia. Symptomatic episodes may recur as seldom as once every 2 months or as often as 25 times per day. They may occur spontaneously or follow certain precipitating events, such as postural change, exercise, laughing, smoking, induction of anesthesia, urination, change in environmental or body temperature, or the administration of certain medications or intra-arterial radiographic contrast media. This disorder is potentially fatal, but the prognosis is generally good with treatment. Although this tumor is usually benign, it may be malignant in as many as 10% of these patients.

Causes

- Inherited autosomal dominant trait (possibly)

Signs and symptoms

- Abdominal pain
- Absence of signs and symptoms during the latent phase
- Diaphoresis
- Excitation, nervousness
- Feelings of impending doom
- Glycosuria, hyperglycemia
- Headache
- Nausea and vomiting
- Pallor
- Palpitations
- Paradoxical response to antihypertensives
- Paresthesia
- Patient history: acute episodes of hypertension, headache, sweating, and tachycardia, particularly in a patient

with hyperglycemia, glycosuria, and hypermetabolism
- Persistent or paroxysmal hypertension
- Postural hypotension
- Tachycardia
- Tachypnea
- Tremor
- Warmth or flushing

ACTION STAT!

 Pheochromocytoma is commonly diagnosed during pregnancy, when uterine pressure on the tumor induces more frequent attacks; such attacks can prove fatal for both mother and fetus as a result of hypertension and vasoconstriction, which can cause stroke, acute pulmonary edema, cardiac arrhythmias, or hypoxia. For such patients, the risk of spontaneous abortion is high, but most fetal deaths occur during labor or immediately after birth.

Diagnostic tests

- A mass may be seen with iodine-31-metaiodobenzylguanidine scintiscan, abdominal magnetic resonance imaging (MRI), or abdominal computed tomography (CT) scanning.
- An adrenal biopsy detects pheochromocytoma.
- CT scanning or MRI of the adrenal glands is usually successful in identifying the intra-adrenal lesions.
- Increased urinary excretion of total free catecholamines and their metabolites, vanillylmandelic acid (VMA) and metanephrine, as measured by analysis of a 24-hour urine specimen, helps confirm pheochromocytoma.
- Labile blood pressure necessitates urine collection during a hypertensive episode and comparison of this specimen with a baseline specimen. Direct assay of total plasma catecholamines

shows levels 10 to 50 times higher than normal.
- The clonidine suppression test will cause decreased plasma catecholamine levels in normal patients but no change in those with pheochromocytoma.
- Angiography demonstrates an adrenal medullary tumor (but may precipitate a hypertensive crisis).

Treatment

- Surgical removal of the tumor is the treatment of choice.
- To decrease blood pressure, an alpha-adrenergic blocker, such as phentolamine (Regitine) or phenoxybenzamine (Dibenzyline), or metyrosine (Demser), is given from 1 to 2 weeks before surgery.
- Beta-adrenergic blockers (propranolol [Inderal] or atenolol [Tenormin]) may also be used after achieving alpha blockade.
- Postoperatively, to treat hypotension, I.V. fluids, a plasma volume expander, a vasopressor, and a transfusion may be required. Persistent hypertension can also occur in the immediate postoperative period.
- If surgery isn't feasible, alpha- and beta-adrenergic blockers—such as phenoxybenzamine and propranolol, respectively—are beneficial in controlling catecholamine effects and preventing attacks.

ACTION STAT!

 Management of an acute attack or hypertensive crisis requires I.V. phentolamine (push or drip) or nitroprusside (Nitropress) to normalize blood pressure.

Nursing considerations

- To ensure the reliability of urine catecholamine measurements, make sure that the patient avoids foods high in vanillin (such as coffee, nuts, chocolate, and bananas) for 2 days before urine VMA levels are checked.

DRUG CHALLENGE

 Also, be aware that therapy with certain drugs (such as guaifenesin and salicylates) may interfere with the accurate determination of VMA levels. Collect the urine in a special container, with hydrochloric acid, that has been prepared by the laboratory.

- Obtain blood pressure readings often because transient hypertensive attacks are possible. Tell the patient to report headaches, palpitations, diaphoresis, nervousness, or other symptoms of an acute attack.
- If hypertensive crisis develops, monitor the patient's blood pressure and heart rate every 2 to 5 minutes until his blood pressure stabilizes at an acceptable level.
- Check the patient's blood for glucose, and watch for weight loss from hypermetabolism.
- After surgery, the patient's blood pressure may rise or fall sharply. Keep him quiet; provide a private room, if possible, because excitement may trigger a hypertensive episode.
- Postoperative hypertension is common because the stress of surgery and manipulation of the adrenal gland stimulate secretion of catecholamines. Because this excess secretion causes profuse sweating, keep the room cool, and change the patient's clothing and bedding often.

DRUG CHALLENGE

 If the patient receives phentolamine, monitor his blood pressure closely. Also, record adverse reactions to the drug, such as dizziness, hypotension, and tachycardia. The first 24 to 48 hours after surgery are the most critical because blood pressure can drop drastically.

- If the patient is receiving vasopressors I.V., check his blood pressure every 3 to 5 minutes, and regulate the drip to maintain a safe pressure. Arterial pressure lines facilitate constant monitoring.
- Check the patient's dressings and vital signs for indications of hemorrhage (increased pulse rate, decreased blood pressure, cold and clammy skin, pallor, and unresponsiveness).

DRUG CHALLENGE

 Give the patient analgesics for pain as required, but monitor his blood pressure carefully because many analgesics, especially meperidine (Demerol), can cause hypotension. Opioids can also precipitate hypertensive crisis.

- If autosomal dominant transmission of pheochromocytoma is suspected, the patient's family should also be evaluated for this condition.

Pituitary tumors

Constituting 10% of intracranial neoplasms, pituitary tumors typically originate in the anterior pituitary (adenohypophysis). They occur in adults of both sexes, usually between ages 30 and 40. The three tissue types of pituitary tumors are chromophobe adenoma (90%), basophil adenoma, and eosinophil adenoma. The prognosis is fair to good, depending on the extent to which the tumor spreads beyond the sella turcica.

Causes
- Unknown

- Associated with hereditary disorder such as multiple endocrine neoplasia
- Autosomal dominant trait

Chromophobe adenoma may be associated with:
- Growth hormone
- Melanocyte-stimulating hormone
- Production of corticotropin
- Prolactin

Basophil adenoma may be associated with:
- Excessive corticotropin production
- Signs of Cushing's syndrome

Eosinophil adenoma
- Excessive growth hormone

Signs and symptoms
- Amenorrhea
- Blurry vision
- Conjugate deviation of gaze
- Constipation
- Decreased libido and impotence in men
- Dizziness
- Double vision
- Frontal headache
- Head tilting
- Increased fatigability
- Intolerance to cold or heat
- Lethargy
- Lid ptosis
- Limited eye movements
- Nystagmus
- Personality changes or dementia
- Pubic and axillary hair loss
- Rhinorrhea
- Seizures
- Skin changes (waxy appearance, fewer wrinkles)
- Strabismus
- Unilateral blindness
- Weakness

Diagnostic tests
- Magnetic resonance imaging (MRI), cranial computed tomography (CT)

scanning, or skull X-rays with tomography show enlargement of the sella turcica or erosion of its floor if growth hormone secretion predominates.
- X-ray films show enlarged paranasal sinuses and mandible, thickened cranial bones, and separated teeth.
- MRI and CT scan show the location and size of the adenoma.
- Carotid angiography shows displacement of the anterior cerebral and internal carotid arteries if the tumor mass is enlarging; it also rules out intracerebral aneurysm.
- Cerebrospinal fluid (CSF) analysis may show increased protein levels.
- Endocrine function tests may contribute helpful information, but results are often ambiguous and inconclusive.

Treatment
- Surgical options include transfrontal removal of large tumors impinging on the optic apparatus and transsphenoidal resection for smaller tumors confined to the pituitary fossa.
- Radiation is the primary treatment for small, nonsecretory tumors that don't extend beyond the sella turcica and for patients who may be poor postoperative risks; otherwise, it's an adjunct to surgery.
- Postoperative treatment includes hormone replacement with corticosteroids, thyroid and sex hormones; correction of electrolyte imbalance; and, as necessary, insulin therapy.
- Other drug therapy may include bromocriptine (Parlodel), an ergot derivative that shrinks prolactin-secreting and growth hormone-secreting tumors.
- Antiserotonin drugs can reduce increased corticosteroid levels in the patient with Cushing's syndrome.
- Adjuvant radiotherapy is used when only partial removal of the tumor is possible.

- Cryohypophysectomy (freezing the area with a probe inserted by transsphenoidal route) is a promising alternative to surgical dissection of the tumor.

Nursing considerations

- Obtain a comprehensive health history and a physical assessment to establish the onset of neurologic and endocrine dysfunction and provide baseline data for later comparison.
- Make sure that the patient and his family understand that the patient needs lifelong evaluations and, possibly, hormone replacement.
- Reassure the patient that some of the distressing physical and behavioral signs and symptoms caused by pituitary dysfunction (for example, altered sexual drive, impotence, infertility, loss of hair, and emotional lability) will disappear with treatment.
- Maintain a safe, clutter-free environment for the visually impaired or acromegalic patient. Reassure him that he'll probably recover his sight.
- Position patients who have undergone supratentorial or transsphenoidal hypophysectomy with the head of the bed elevated about 30 degrees to promote venous drainage from the head and reduce cerebral edema. (See *Postcraniotomy care.*)
- Place the patient on his side to allow drainage of secretions and prevent aspiration.
- Don't allow a patient who has had transsphenoidal surgery to blow his nose.
- Watch for CSF drainage from the nose. Monitor for signs of infection from the contaminated upper respiratory tract.
- Make sure that the patient understands that he'll lose his sense of smell.
- Regularly compare the patient's postoperative neurologic status with your baseline assessment.

ACTION STAT!

Postcraniotomy care

- Monitor vital signs (especially level of consciousness), and perform a baseline neurologic assessment from which to plan further care and assess progress.
- Maintain the patient's airway; suction as necessary.
- Monitor intake and output carefully.
- Give the patient nothing by mouth for 24 to 48 hours to prevent aspiration and vomiting, which increases intracranial pressure.
- Watch for cerebral edema, bleeding, and cerebrospinal fluid leakage.
- Provide a restful, quiet environment.

- Monitor intake and output to detect fluid imbalances.
- Before discharge, encourage the patient to wear a medical identification bracelet or necklace that identifies his hormone deficiencies and their proper treatment.

Plague

Plague, also known as the *black death,* is an acute infection caused by the gram-negative, nonmotile, nonsporulating bacillus *Yersinia pestis* (formerly called *Pasteurella pestis*). Plague occurs in several forms. Bubonic plague, the most common, causes the characteristic swollen and sometimes suppurative lymph glands (buboes) that give this infection its name. Other forms include septicemic plague, a severe, rapid systemic form; and pneumonic plague, which can be primary or secondary to the other two forms. Without treatment, mortality is about 60% in bubonic plague and approaches 100% in septicemic and pneumonic plagues. With treatment, mortality is about 18%, largely due to the delay between onset and treatment. The patient's age and physical condition are also factors.

Causes
- Bite of a flea from an infected rodent host (rat, squirrel, prairie dog, or hare)
- Handling infected animals or their tissues
- May progress to highly contagious, secondary pneumonic form transmitted by contaminated respiratory droplets
- Inhalation of *Y. pestis* in a laboratory (primary pneumonic form)

Signs and symptoms
Bubonic plague
Milder form
- Malaise
- Pain or tenderness in regional lymph nodes
- Lymph node damage (axillary or inguinal) eventually produces painful, inflamed, and possibly suppurative buboes
- Hemorrhagic areas may become necrotic and appear dark (hence the name "black death")

Rapidly progressing dramatic form
- Abdominal pain
- Chills
- Circulatory collapse
- Constipation followed by diarrhea (frequently bloody)
- Headache
- Insidious onset, possible rapid progression, moribund within hours
- Myalgia
- Nausea, vomiting
- Petechiae
- Prostration
- Rapidly progressing, dramatic form
- Restlessness, disorientation, delirium

- Skin mottling
- Staggering gait
- Sudden high fever of 103° to 106° F (39.4° to 41.1° C)
- Toxemia

Septicemic plague
- Toxicity
- Hyperpyrexia
- Seizures
- Prostration
- Shock
- Disseminated intravascular coagulation (DIC)
- Peritoneal or pleural effusions
- Pericarditis
- Meningitis
- Terminal without prompt treatment

Primary pneumonic plague
- Acute prostration
- Respiratory distress
- Death—typically within 2 to 3 days after onset
- High fever
- Chills
- Severe headache
- Tachycardia
- Tachypnea
- Dyspnea
- Productive cough (first mucoid sputum; later frothy pink or red)

Secondary pneumonic plague
- Cough that produces bloody sputum signal this complication of the pulmonary extension of the bubonic form.

Diagnostic tests
- Characteristic buboes and a history of exposure to rodents strongly suggest bubonic plague. Stained smears and cultures of *Y. pestis* (obtained from a small amount of fluid aspirated from skin lesions) confirm this diagnosis.
- Postmortem examination of a guinea pig inoculated with a sample of blood or

purulent drainage allows isolation of the organism.

■ White blood cell count over 20,000/µl with increased polymorphonuclear leukocytes and hemoagglutination reactions (increased antibody titer) is a laboratory finding with the bubonic plague.

■ Stained smear and blood culture containing Y. *pestis* are diagnostic in septicemic plague.

■ Diagnosis of pneumonic plague requires a chest X-ray to show fulminating pneumonia and stained smear and culture of sputum to identify Y. *pestis*.

■ A rapid diagnostic test for bubonic and pneumonic plague uses monoclonal antibodies to the F antigen of Y. *pestis* and has a sensitivity and specificity of 100%; results are available within 15 minutes and have a shelf life of 21 days at 60° F (15.6° C).

Treatment

■ Streptomycin has proven to be the most effective agent in the treatment of Y. *pestis*. Other effective drugs include gentamicin, doxycycline, and chloramphenicol.

■ Supportive management aims to control fever, shock, and seizures and to maintain fluid balance.

■ Glucocorticoids are used to combat life-threatening toxemia and shock.

■ Diazepam (Valium) can be used to decrease restlessness.

■ Heparin is prescribed to treat DIC.

Nursing considerations

■ Make sure the patient is kept in strict isolation, until at least 48 hours after antimicrobial therapy begins, provided respiratory symptoms don't develop.

■ Use an approved insecticide to rid the patient and his clothing of fleas. Carefully dispose of soiled dressings and linens, feces, and sputum. If the patient has pneumonic plague, wear a gown, mask,

and gloves. Handle all exudates, purulent discharge, and laboratory specimens with rubber gloves. For more information, consult your infection control officer.

DO'S & DON'TS

 Apply hot, moist compresses to buboes. They should never be excised or drained because this could spread the infection.

■ When septicemic plague causes peripheral tissue necrosis, pad the bed's side rails and avoid using restraints or armboards to prevent further injury to necrotic tissue.

■ Obtain a history of patient contacts so that they can be quarantined for 6 days of observation. Administer prophylactic tetracycline as ordered.

■ Report suspected cases of plague to local public health department officials so that they can identify the source of infection.

■ To help prevent plague, discourage contact with wild animals (especially those that are sick or dead), and support programs aimed at reducing insect and rodent populations. Even though the effect of immunization is transient, recommend immunization with the plague vaccine to people who travel to and reside in endemic areas.

▌Pleural effusion and empyema

Pleural effusion is an excess of fluid in the pleural space. Normally, this space contains a small amount of extracellular fluid that lubricates the pleural surfaces. Increased production or inadequate removal of this fluid results in pleural effusion. Empyema is the accumulation of pus and necrotic tissue in the pleural space. Blood (hemothorax) and lymph or chyle (chylothorax) may also collect in this space.

Causes
Transudative pleural effusion
- Disorders resulting in overexpanded intravascular volume
- Heart failure
- Hepatic disease with ascites
- Hypoalbuminemia
- Peritoneal dialysis

Exudative pleural effusion
- Bacterial or fungal pneumonitis or empyema
- Chest trauma
- Collagen disease (lupus erythematosus and rheumatoid arthritis)
- Malignancy
- Myxedema
- Pancreatitis
- Pulmonary embolism (with or without infarction)
- Subphrenic abscess
- Tuberculosis

Empyema
- Carcinoma
- Esophageal rupture
- Idiopathic
- Perforation
- Pneumonitis

Signs and symptoms
- Decreased breath sounds (on auscultation)
- Dullness over the effused area (on percussion; unchanged with respiration)
- Dyspnea
- Fever
- Malaise
- Pleuritic chest pain
- Symptoms related to underlying disorder

Diagnostic tests
- A chest X-ray or thoracic computed tomography scan shows radiopaque fluid in dependent regions.
- Thoracentesis allows analysis of aspirated pleural fluid to show:
  - transudative effusions: usually has a specific gravity less than 1.015 and protein levels less than 3 g/dl
  - exudative effusions: ratio of protein in pleural fluid to serum greater than or equal to 0.5, lactate dehydrogenase (LD) in pleural fluid greater than or equal to 200 IU, and ratio of LD in pleural fluid to LD in serum greater than or equal to 0.6
  - empyema: aspirated fluid contains acute inflammatory white blood cells and microorganisms
  - empyema or rheumatoid arthritis: extremely decreased pleural fluid glucose levels
  - fluid amylase levels higher than serum levels (with pleural effusion due to esophageal rupture or pancreatitis)
  - aspirated fluid may be tested for lupus erythematosus cells, antinuclear antibodies, and neoplastic cells; it may also be analyzed for color and consistency; acid-fast bacillus, fungal, and bacterial cultures; and triglycerides (in chylothorax).
- Cell analysis shows leukocytosis in empyema.
- Negative tuberculin skin test strongly rules against tuberculosis as the cause.
- With exudative pleural effusions in which thoracentesis isn't definitive, pleural biopsy may be done; it's particularly useful for confirming tuberculosis or malignancy.

Treatment
- Thoracentesis is performed to remove fluid or allow careful monitoring of the patient's own reabsorption of the fluid.

- Hemothorax requires drainage to prevent fibrothorax formation.
- Treatment of empyema requires the insertion of one or more chest tubes after thoracentesis to allow the drainage of purulent material and possibly decortication (surgical removal of the thick coating over the lung) or rib resection to allow open drainage and lung expansion.
- Empyema also requires parenteral antibiotics.
- Associated hypoxia requires oxygen administration.

Nursing considerations
- Explain thoracentesis to the patient. Before the procedure, tell the patient to expect a stinging sensation from the local anesthetic and a feeling of pressure when the needle is inserted.
- Instruct the patient to tell you immediately if he feels uncomfortable or has trouble breathing during the procedure.
- Reassure the patient during thoracentesis. Remind him to breathe normally and to avoid sudden movements, such as coughing or sighing. Monitor vital signs, and watch for syncope.

ACTION STAT!

 If fluid is removed too quickly, the patient may develop bradycardia, hypotension, pain, pulmonary edema, or cardiac arrest. Watch for respiratory distress or pneumothorax (sudden onset of dyspnea or cyanosis) after thoracentesis.

- Encourage the patient to do deep-breathing exercises to promote lung expansion. Use an incentive spirometer to promote deep breathing.
- Provide meticulous chest tube care, and use aseptic technique for changing dressings around the tube insertion site in empyema.

- Ensure chest tube patency and record the amount, color, and consistency of any tube drainage.
- Because weeks of such drainage are usually necessary to obliterate the space, make visiting nurse referrals for patients who will be discharged with the tube in place.
- If pleural effusion was a complication of pneumonia or influenza, advise the patient to seek prompt medical attention for chest colds.

Pleurisy

Also known as *pleuritis*, pleurisy is the inflammation of the visceral and parietal pleurae that line the inside of the thoracic cage and envelop the lungs. As the lungs inflate and deflate, the visceral pleura covering the lungs moves against the fixed parietal pleura lining the pleural space, causing pain. This disorder usually begins suddenly.

Causes
- Cancer
- Chest trauma
- Dressler's syndrome
- Pneumonia
- Pulmonary infarction
- Rheumatoid arthritis
- Systemic lupus erythematosus
- Tuberculosis
- Uremia
- Viruses

Signs and symptoms
- Coarse vibration (detectable with palpation)
- Dyspnea
- Pleural friction rub directly over the area of pleural inflammation (detectable with auscultation)
- Sharp, stabbing pain that increases with respiration (may limit movement on the affected side during breathing)

Diagnostic tests

- Diagnosis generally rests on the patient's history and a respiratory assessment.
- A complete blood cell count can help differentiate bacterial from viral infection.
- Chest X-ray and ultrasonography can identify pneumonia and aid in the diagnosis.
- Electrocardiography rules out coronary artery disease as the source of the patient's pain.

Treatment

- Anti-inflammatories are prescribed to reduce inflammation.
- Symptomatic treatment also includes analgesics to reduce pain, and bed rest.
- Severe pain may require an intercostal nerve block of two or three intercostal nerves.
- Pleurisy with pleural effusion calls for thoracentesis as a diagnostic and therapeutic measure.

Nursing considerations

- Stress the importance of bed rest, and plan your care to allow the patient as much uninterrupted rest as possible.
- Administer antitussives and pain medication as necessary, but be careful not to overmedicate the patient.
- Warn a patient who's about to be discharged to avoid the overuse of opioid analgesics because such medications depress coughing and respiration.
- Encourage the patient to cough. To minimize pain, apply firm pressure at the pain site during coughing exercises.

Pneumocystis carinii pneumonia

Associated with human immunodeficiency virus (HIV) infection and other immunocompromising conditions, including organ transplantation, leukemia, and lymphoma, *Pneumocystis carinii* pneumonia (PCP) is an opportunistic infection. Part of the normal flora in most healthy people, *P. carinii* becomes an aggressive pathogen in the immunocompromised patient. Impaired cell-mediated (T-cell) immunity is thought to be more important than impaired humoral (B-cell) immunity in predisposing the patient to PCP; however, the immune defects involved are poorly understood. The organism invades the lungs bilaterally and multiplies extracellularly. As the infestation grows, alveoli fill with organisms and exudate, impairing gas exchange. The alveoli hypertrophy and thicken progressively, eventually leading to extensive consolidation. PCP occurs in up to 90% of patients with HIV infection in the United States at some point during their lifetime and is the leading cause of death in these patients.

Causes

- Infection with *P. carinii*

Signs and symptoms

- Accessory muscle use for breathing
- Anorexia
- Crackles
- Cyanosis
- Decreased breath sounds (in advanced pneumonia)
- Dyspnea
- Generalized fatigue
- Immunocompromising condition (such as HIV infection, leukemia, or lymphoma) or procedure (such as organ transplantation)
- Increasing shortness of breath
- Low-grade, intermittent fever
- Nonproductive cough
- Tachypnea
- Weight loss

Diagnostic tests

- Histologic studies confirm *P. carinii*. In patients with HIV infection, initial examination of a first-morning sputum specimen (induced by inhaling an ultrasonically dispersed saline mist) may be sufficient; however, this technique is usually ineffective in patients without HIV infection.
- Fiber-optic bronchoscopy confirms PCP. Invasive procedures, such as transbronchial biopsy and open-lung biopsy, are less commonly used.
- Chest X-ray may show slowly progressing, fluffy infiltrates and, occasionally, nodular lesions or a spontaneous pneumothorax.
- Gallium scan may show increased uptake over the lungs.
- Arterial blood gas (ABG) studies detect hypoxia and an increased alveolar-arterial gradient.

Treatment

- The drug of choice for all types of PCP is co-trimoxazole (Bactrim) administered orally or I.V.
- Diphenhydramine may be prescribed to reduce adverse effects.
- Pentamidine may be administered I.V. (Pentam) or in aerosol form (Nebupent).

DRUG CHALLENGE

 I.V. pentamidine is associated with a high incidence of severe toxic effects; the inhaled form is usually well tolerated. However, inhaled pentamidine may not effectively reach the lung apices. Adverse reactions associated with inhalation include metallic taste, pharyngitis, cough, bronchospasm, shortness of breath, rhinitis, and laryngitis.

- Supportive measures, such as oxygen therapy, mechanical ventilation, adequate nutrition, and fluid balance are important adjunctive therapies.
- Oral or I.V. morphine sulfate may reduce the respiratory rate and anxiety, enhancing oxygenation.

Nursing considerations

- Implement standard precautions to prevent contagion.
- Frequently assess the patient's respiratory status, and monitor ABG levels every 4 hours.
- Administer oxygen therapy as necessary. Encourage the patient to ambulate and to perform deep-breathing exercises and incentive spirometry to facilitate effective gas exchange.
- Administer antipyretics, as required, to relieve fever.
- Monitor intake and output and daily weight to evaluate fluid balance. Replace fluids as necessary.

DRUG CHALLENGE

 Never give pentamidine I.M. because it can cause pain and sterile abscesses. Give the I.V. form of the drug slowly over 60 minutes to reduce the risk of hypotension.

- Monitor the patient for adverse reactions to antimicrobial drugs.
- Coordinate the efforts of each member of the health care team to allow adequate rest periods between procedures; teach the patient energy conservation techniques.
- Provide nutritional supplements as needed. Encourage the patient to eat a high-calorie, protein-rich diet. Offer small, frequent meals if the patient can't tolerate large amounts of food.
- Reduce anxiety by providing a relaxing environment, eliminating excessive environmental stimuli, and allowing ample time for meals.

- Give emotional support, and help the patient identify and use meaningful support systems.
- Instruct the patient about the medication regimen, especially about possible adverse effects.
- If the patient will require oxygen therapy at home, explain that an oxygen concentrator may be most effective.

Pneumonia

An acute infection of the lung parenchyma, pneumonia often impairs gas exchange. Bronchopneumonia involves distal airways and alveoli; lobular pneumonia, part of a lobe; and lobar pneumonia, an entire lobe. Complications include hypoxemia, respiratory failure, pleural effusion, empyema, lung abscess, and bacteremia, with the spread of infection to other parts of the body resulting in meningitis, endocarditis, and pericarditis. The prognosis is generally good for people with normal lungs and adequate host defenses before the onset of pneumonia. However, pneumonia is the seventh-leading cause of death in the United States, and in 2003, severe acute respiratory syndrome, a new, deadly type of pneumonia, emerged. (See *SARS*.)

Causes
Primary pneumonia
- Bacterial
- Fungal
- Inhalation or aspiration of a pathogen
- Mycobacterial
- Mycoplasmal
- Protozoal
- Rickettsial
- Viral

Secondary pneumonia
- Hematogenous spread of bacteria from a distant focus (see *Types of pneumonia,* pages 482 to 485)
- Initial lung damage from a noxious chemical
- Superinfection

Predisposing factors
- Abdominal and thoracic surgery
- Alcoholism
- Aspiration
- Atelectasis
- Cancer (particularly lung cancer)
- Chronic illness and debilitation
- Chronic respiratory disease (chronic obstructive pulmonary disease [COPD], asthma, bronchiectasis, cystic fibrosis)
- Common colds or other viral respiratory tract infections
- Exposure to noxious gases
- Immunosuppressant therapy
- Influenza
- Malnutrition
- Sickle cell disease
- Smoking
- Tracheostomy

Contributing factors for aspiration pneumonia
- Debilitation
- Decreased level of consciousness
- Impaired gag reflex
- Nasogastric (NG) tube feedings
- Old age
- Poor oral hygiene

Signs and symptoms
- Coughing
- Diffuse, fine crackles
- Fever
- Localized or extensive consolidation
- Pleural effusion
- Pleuritic chest pain
- Shaking chills
- Sputum production

Diagnostic tests

- Chest X-ray shows infiltrates.
- Sputum smear reveals acute inflammatory cells.
- Positive blood cultures in patients with pulmonary infiltrates strongly suggest pneumonia produced by the organisms isolated from the blood cultures.
- Pleural effusions, if present, should be tapped and the fluid analyzed for evidence of infection in the pleural space.
- Transtracheal aspirate of tracheobronchial secretions or bronchoscopy with brushings or washings may be done to obtain material for smear and culture.

Treatment

- Antimicrobial therapy varies with the causative agent.
- Humidified oxygen therapy is administered for hypoxia.
- Mechanical ventilation may be necessary for the patient with respiratory failure.
- High-calorie diet, adequate fluid intake, and bed rest are additional supportive measures.
- An analgesic may be prescribed to relieve pleuritic chest pain.
- Patients with severe pneumonia on mechanical ventilation may require positive end-expiratory pressure to facilitate adequate oxygenation.

Nursing considerations

- Maintain a patent airway and adequate oxygenation. Measure arterial blood gas levels, especially in hypoxic patients. Administer supplemental oxygen as ordered; patients with underlying chronic lung disease should be given oxygen cautiously.
- Teach the patient how to cough and perform deep-breathing exercises to clear secretions, and encourage him to do so often.

SARS

The Centers for Disease Control and Prevention and the World Health Organization are investigating a new disease called severe acute respiratory syndrome (SARS). First reported in China, Vietnam, and Hong Kong in 2003, it has since spread to other countries, including the United States and Canada.

SARS commonly begins with a fever greater than 100.4° (38°C), headache, general discomfort and body aches and, in some patients, mild respiratory symptoms. After 2 to 7 days, SARS patients may develop a dry cough and difficulty breathing. The disease, which is highly contagious, is spread by droplets and through contact with contaminated objects. It's also possible that SARS can be spread more broadly through the air or by other ways that aren't currently known. A new type of coronavirus is the suspected cause.

Treatment for SARS is mostly palliative. Antivirals, such as oseltamivir and ribavirin, and steroids in combination with antivirals have been used in patients with SARS; however, efficacy of these treatments remains unknown.

- For severe pneumonia that requires endotracheal (ET) intubation or tracheostomy with or without mechanical ventilation, provide thorough respiratory care and suction often, using sterile technique, to remove secretions.
- Obtain sputum specimens by suction if the patient can't produce specimens independently. Collect specimens in a sterile container and deliver them promptly to the microbiology laboratory.

(Text continues on page 484.)

Types of pneumonia

Type	Signs and symptoms
Viral	
Influenza (prognosis poor even with treatment; 50% mortality)	▪ Cough (initially nonproductive; later, purulent sputum), marked cyanosis, dyspnea, high fever, chills, substernal pain and discomfort, moist crackles, frontal headache, and myalgia ▪ Death from cardiopulmonary collapse
Adenovirus (insidious onset; generally affects young adults)	▪ Sore throat, fever, cough, chills, malaise, small amounts of mucoid sputum, retrosternal chest pain, anorexia, rhinitis, adenopathy, scattered crackles, and rhonchi
Respiratory syncytial virus (most prevalent in infants and children)	▪ Listlessness, irritability, tachypnea with retraction of intercostal muscles, slight sputum production, fine moist crackles, fever, severe malaise and, possibly, cough or croup
Measles (rubeola)	▪ Fever, dyspnea, cough, small amounts of sputum, coryza, skin rash, and cervical adenopathy
Chickenpox (varicella) (uncommon in children but present in 30% of adults with varicella)	▪ Cough, dyspnea, cyanosis, tachypnea, pleuritic chest pain, hemoptysis, and rhonchi 1 to 6 days after onset of rash
Cytomegalovirus	▪ Difficult to distinguish from other nonbacterial pneumonias ▪ Fever, cough, shaking chills, dyspnea, cyanosis, weakness, and diffuse crackles ▪ In neonates, devastating multisystemic infection; in normal adults, resembles mononucleosis; in immunocompromised hosts, varies from clinically inapparent to devastating
Bacterial	
Streptococcus (*Streptococcus pneumoniae*)	▪ Sudden onset of a single, shaking chill, and sustained temperature of 102° to 104° F (38.9° to 40° C), commonly preceded by upper respiratory tract infection

Diagnostic tests	Treatment
▪ Chest X-ray: diffuse bilateral bronchopneumonia radiating from hilus ▪ White blood cell (WBC) count: normal to slightly elevated ▪ Sputum smears: no specific organisms	▪ Supportive: for respiratory failure, endotracheal intubation and ventilator assistance; for fever, hypothermia blanket or antipyretics; for influenza A, amantadine or rimantadine
▪ Chest X-ray: patchy distribution of pneumonia, more severe than indicated by physical examination ▪ WBC count: normal to slightly elevated	▪ Treat symptoms only ▪ Good prognosis; usually clears with no residual effects
▪ Chest X-ray: patchy bilateral consolidation ▪ WBC count: normal to slightly elevated	▪ Supportive: humidified air, oxygen, antimicrobials commonly given until viral etiology confirmed, aerosolized ribavirin ▪ Complete recovery in 1 to 3 weeks
▪ Chest X-ray: reticular infiltrates, sometimes with hilar lymph node enlargement ▪ Lung tissue specimen: characteristic giant cells	▪ Supportive: bed rest, adequate hydration, antimicrobials, assisted ventilation, if necessary
▪ Chest X-ray: shows more extensive pneumonia than indicated by physical examination, and bilateral, patchy, diffuse, nodular infiltrates ▪ Sputum analysis: predominant mononuclear cells and characteristic intranuclear inclusion bodies with skin rash confirm diagnosis	▪ Supportive: adequate hydration, oxygen therapy in critically ill patients ▪ Therapy with I.V. acyclovir
▪ Chest X-ray: in early stages, variable patchy infiltrates; later, bilateral, nodular, and more predominant in lower lobes ▪ Percutaneous aspiration of lung tissue, transbronchial biopsy or open-lung biopsy: microscopic examination shows intranuclear and cytoplasmic inclusions; virus can be cultured from lung tissue	▪ Supportive: adequate hydration and nutrition, oxygen therapy, bed rest ▪ Generally, benign and self-limiting in mononucleosis-like form ▪ In immunosuppressed patients, disease is more severe and may be fatal, ganciclovir or foscarnet treatment warranted
▪ Chest X-ray: areas of consolidation, often lobar ▪ WBC count: elevated ▪ Sputum culture: may show gram-positive *S. pneumoniae*	▪ Antimicrobial therapy: penicillin G or erythromycin for 7 to 10 days (Such therapy begins after obtaining culture specimen but without waiting for results.)

(continued)

Types of pneumonia *(continued)*

Type	Signs and symptoms
Bacterial *(continued)*	
Klebsiella	■ Fever and recurrent chills; cough producing rusty, bloody, viscous sputum (currant jelly); cyanosis of lips and nail beds due to hypoxemia; and shallow, grunting respirations ■ Likely in patients with chronic alcoholism, pulmonary disease, and diabetes
Staphylococcus	■ Temperature of 102° to 104° F (38.9° to 40° C), recurrent shaking chills, bloody sputum, dyspnea, tachypnea, and hypoxemia ■ Commonly occurs in patients with viral illness, such as influenza or measles, and in patients with cystic fibrosis
Aspiration	
Results from vomiting and aspiration of gastric or oropharyngeal contents into trachea and lungs	■ Noncardiogenic pulmonary edema may follow damage to respiratory epithelium from contact with stomach acid ■ Crackles, dyspnea, cyanosis, hypotension, and tachycardia ■ May be subacute pneumonia with cavity formation; lung abscess possible with presence of foreign body

■ Administer pain medication as needed; record the patient's response to medications.

■ Maintain adequate nutrition to offset high caloric utilization secondary to infection. Ask the dietary department to provide a high-calorie, high-protein diet consisting of soft, easy-to-eat foods. Supplement oral feedings with NG tube feedings or parenteral nutrition as ordered.

■ Monitor fluid intake and output.

■ Provide a quiet, calm environment for the patient, with frequent rest periods.

■ To control the spread of infection, dispose of secretions properly. Tell the patient to sneeze and cough into a disposable tissue; tape a waxed bag to the side of the bed for used tissues.

■ Encourage annual influenza vaccination and Pneumovax for high-risk patients, such as those with COPD, chronic heart disease, or sickle cell disease.

Do's & don'ts

 To prevent aspiration during NG tube feedings, elevate the patient's head, check the tube's position, and administer the formula slowly. Don't give large volumes at one time; this could cause vomiting. If the patient has an ET tube, inflate the tube cuff. Keep the patient's head elevated for at least 30 minutes after the feeding. Check for residual formula at 4- to 6-hour intervals.

Diagnosis	Treatment
• Chest X-ray: typically, but not always, consolidation in the upper lobe that causes bulging of fissures • WBC count: elevated • Sputum culture and Gram stain: may show gram-negative cocci (Klebsiella)	• Antimicrobial therapy: an aminoglycoside and, in serious infections, a cephalosporin
• Chest X-ray: multiple abscesses and infiltrates; high incidence of empyema • WBC count: elevated • Sputum culture and Gram stain: may show gram-positive staphylococci	• Antimicrobial therapy: nafcillin or oxacillin for 14 days if staphylococci are penicillinase producing • Chest tube drainage of empyema
• Chest X-ray: locates areas of infiltrates, which suggest diagnosis	• Antimicrobial therapy: penicillin G or clindamycin • Supportive: oxygen therapy, suctioning, coughing, deep-breathing, adequate hydration, and I.V. corticosteroids

Pneumothorax

With pneumothorax, air or gas accumulates between the parietal and visceral pleurae. The amount of air or gas trapped in the intrapleural space determines the degree of lung collapse. Pneumothorax can also be classified as open or closed. With open pneumothorax (usually the result of trauma), air flows between the pleural space and the outside of the body. With closed pneumothorax, air reaches the pleural space directly from the lung. With a tension pneumothorax, the air in the pleural space is under higher pressure than air in adjacent lung and vascular structures. Without prompt treatment, a tension or a large pneumothorax results in fatal pulmonary and circulatory impairment.

Causes
Spontaneous pneumothorax
- Emphysematous bulla that ruptures
- Interstitial lung disease (eosinophilic granuloma or lymphangiomyomatosis).
- Ruptured congenital blebs
- Tubercular, pneumocystic, or malignant lesions that erode into the pleural space

Traumatic pneumothorax
- Closed pleural biopsy
- Insertion of a central venous line
- Penetrating chest injury (a gunshot or knife wound)
- Thoracentesis

- Thoracic surgery
- Transbronchial biopsy

Signs and symptoms
- Asymmetrical chest wall movement
- Crackling beneath the skin (subcutaneous emphysema)
- Cyanosis
- Decreased or absent breath sounds over the collapsed lung
- Decreased vocal fremitus
- Hyperresonance on the affected side
- Hypotension and tachycardia with tension pneumothorax
- Mediastinal shift and jugular vein distention in tension pneumothorax
- Overexpansion and rigidity of the affected chest side
- Pallor
- Shortness of breath
- Sudden, sharp, pleuritic pain (exacerbated by movement of the chest, breathing, and coughing)
- Weak and rapid pulse

Diagnostic tests
- Chest X-ray films showing air in the pleural space and, possibly, mediastinal shift confirms this diagnosis.
- If the pneumothorax is significant, arterial blood gas analysis reveals pH less than 7.35, partial pressure of arterial oxygen less than 80 mm Hg, and partial pressure of arterial carbon dioxide more than 45 mm Hg.
- Pulse oximetry results may show early decline. Levels of arterial oxygen saturation may decrease initially but typically return to normal within 24 hours.

Treatment
- If lung collapse is less than 30%, treatment consists of bed rest, oxygen administration and, possibly, needle aspiration of air with a large-bore needle attached to a syringe.

- If more than 30% of the lung is collapsed, treatment consists of insertion of a thoracostomy tube in the second or third intercostal space in the midclavicular line, connected to an underwater seal or low-pressure suction.
- Recurring spontaneous pneumothorax may be treated by instilling a sclerosing agent through a thoracostomy tube or during thoracostomy.
- Thoracotomy and pleurectomy may be performed to prevent recurrence by causing the lung to adhere to the parietal pleura.
- Traumatic and tension pneumothoraces require chest tube drainage.
- Traumatic pneumothorax may also require surgical repair.

Nursing considerations
- Watch for pallor, gasping respirations, and sudden chest pain. Carefully monitor vital signs at least every hour for indications of shock, increasing respiratory distress, or mediastinal shift. Listen for breath sounds over both lungs. Falling blood pressure and rising pulse and respiratory rates may indicate tension pneumothorax, which could be fatal without prompt treatment.
- After the chest tube is in place, encourage the patient to cough and breathe deeply (at least once an hour) to facilitate lung expansion. Administer analgesics and instruct the patient in splinting to facilitate breathing.
- In a patient with chest tube drainage, watch for continuing air leakage (bubbling), indicating that the lung defect has failed to close; this may require surgery.
- Watch for increasing subcutaneous emphysema by checking around the neck or at the tube insertion site for crackling beneath the skin.
- If the patient is on a ventilator, watch for difficulty in breathing in time with

the ventilator as well as pressure changes on ventilator gauges.

- Change dressings around the chest tube insertion site as necessary. Be careful not to reposition or dislodge the tube.

- Monitor vital signs frequently after thoracotomy. Also, for the first 24 hours, assess respiratory status by checking breath sounds hourly.
- Observe the chest tube site for leakage, and note the amount and color of drainage.
- Walk the patient as appropriate (usually on the first postoperative day) to facilitate deep inspiration and lung expansion.
- Reassure the patient, and explain what pneumothorax is, what causes it, and which tests and procedures are used to help the diagnosis.
- Make the patient as comfortable as possible. (The patient with pneumothorax is usually most comfortable sitting upright.)

█ Polycystic kidney disease

An inherited disorder, polycystic kidney disease is characterized by multiple, bilateral, grapelike clusters of fluid-filled cysts that grossly enlarge the kidneys, compressing and eventually replacing functioning renal tissue. This disease appears in two distinct forms. The infantile form causes stillbirth or early neonatal death; a few infants survive for 2 years and then develop fatal renal, heart, or respiratory failure. The adult form begins insidiously but usually becomes obvious between ages 30 and 50; renal deterioration is more gradual but progresses relentlessly to fatal uremia. The prognosis in adults varies; after uremic symptoms develop, polycystic kidney disease is usually fatal within 4 years, unless the patient receives treatment with dialysis, a kidney transplant, or both.

Causes
- Infantile: inherited autosomal recessive trait
- Adult type: autosomal dominant trait

Signs and symptoms
Infantile polycystic kidney disease
- Floppy, low-set ears
- Heart failure
- Hepatic fibrosis (portal hypertension, bleeding varices)
- Pointed nose
- Pronounced epicanthal folds
- Renal failure
- Respiratory distress
- Small chin
- Uremia

Adult polycystic kidney disease
- Colicky abdominal pain
- Hypertension
- Life-threatening retroperitoneal bleeding (with ruptured cyst)
- Lumbar pain
- Polyuria
- Proteinuria
- Recurrent hematuria
- Renal failure
- Swollen or tender abdomen worsened by exertion and relieved by lying down
- Uremia
- Urinary tract infection
- Widening girth

Diagnostic tests

- In advanced stages, grossly enlarged and palpable kidneys make the diagnosis obvious.
- Excretory urography or retrograde ureteropyelography reveals enlarged kidneys, with elongation of the renal pelvis, flattening of the calyces, and indentations caused by cysts. Excretory urography of the neonate shows poor excretion of contrast medium.
- Ultrasonography, tomography, and radioisotope scans show kidney enlargement and cysts. Computed tomography scan and magnetic resonance imaging show multiple areas of cystic damage.
- Urinalysis and creatinine clearance tests (nonspecific tests that evaluate renal function) indicate abnormalities.
- Diagnosis must rule out renal tumors.

Treatment

- Treatment includes urine cultures and creatinine clearance tests every 6 months; when a urine culture detects infection, prompt and vigorous antibiotic treatment is needed.
- Progressive renal failure requires treatment similar to that for other types of renal disease, including dialysis or, rarely, a kidney transplant.
- Cystic abscess or retroperitoneal bleeding may require surgical drainage.
- Intractable pain (a rare symptom) may also require surgery.
- Anemia is treated with iron and other supplements, erythropoietin, or blood transfusions
- Because the disease affects both kidneys, nephrectomy usually isn't recommended because it increases the risk of infection in the remaining kidney.

Nursing considerations

- Refer the young adult patient or the parents of an infant with polycystic kidney disease for genetic counseling. Such parents will probably have many questions about the risk to other offspring.
- Provide supportive care to minimize associated symptoms. Carefully assess the patient's lifestyle and his physical and mental status, and determine how rapidly the disease is progressing. Use this information to individualize the patient's care plan.
- Provide care for the patient requiring dialysis and transplantation as indicated; provide appropriate care and patient teaching as the disease progresses.
- Explain all diagnostic procedures. Before beginning excretory urography or other procedures that use an iodine-based contrast medium, determine whether the patient has ever had an allergic reaction to iodine or shellfish. Even if the patient doesn't have a history of allergy, watch for an allergic reaction after performing the procedures.
- Administer antibiotics for urinary tract infection. Stress to the patient the need to take the medication exactly as prescribed, even if symptoms are minimal or absent.

Polycythemia, secondary

Also known as *reactive polycythemia,* secondary polycythemia is a disorder characterized by excessive production of circulating red blood cells (RBCs) due to hypoxia, tumor, or disease. Incidence rises among persons living at high altitudes.

Causes

- Increased production of erythropoietin due to:
  - central nervous system disease (encephalitis, parkinsonism)
  - central or peripheral alveolar hypoventilation (barbiturate intoxication, pickwickian syndrome)

– chronic obstructive pulmonary disease
– endocrine disorders (Cushing's syndrome, Bartter's syndrome, pheochromocytomas)
– heart failure
– hemoglobin (Hb) abnormalities (carboxyhemoglobinemia as seen in heavy smokers)
– low oxygen content at high altitudes.
– neoplasms (renal tumors, uterine myomas, and cerebellar hemangiomas)
– pathologic response to renal disease (such as renal vascular impairment, renal cysts, or hydronephrosis)
– recessive genetic trait (rare)
– transposition of the great vessels

Signs and symptoms

- Clubbing of the fingers (if underlying disease is cardiovascular)
- Emphysema
- Hypertension
- Hypoxemia
- Ruddy cyanotic skin

Diagnostic tests

- Bone marrow biopsies reveal hyperplasia confined to the erythroid series.
  Laboratory findings for secondary polycythemia include:
- increased RBC mass (increased hematocrit, Hb level, mean corpuscular volume, and mean corpuscular Hb level)
- elevated urinary erythropoietin level
- increased blood histamine level
- decreased or normal arterial oxygen saturation.

Treatment

- Treatment focuses on correction of the underlying disease or environmental condition.
- If altitude is a contributing factor, relocation may be advisable.
- If secondary polycythemia has produced hazardous hyperviscosity of the blood or if the patient doesn't respond to treatment of the primary disease, reduction of blood volume by phlebotomy or pheresis may be effective.
- Emergency phlebotomy is indicated for prevention of impending vascular occlusion or before emergency surgery. In the latter case, it's usually advisable to remove excess RBCs and reinfuse the patient's plasma.
- Elective surgery should be avoided until polycythemia is controlled.

Nursing considerations

- Keep the patient as active as possible to decrease the risk of thrombosis due to increased blood viscosity.
- Provide a reduced calorie and sodium diet to counteract the tendency for hypertension.
- Before and after phlebotomy, check blood pressure with the patient lying down. After the procedure, give about 24 oz (710 ml) of water or juice. To prevent syncope, have him sit up for about 5 minutes before walking.
- Emphasize the importance of regular blood studies (every 2 to 3 months), even after the disease is controlled.
- Teach the patient and his family about the underlying disorder. Help them understand its relationship to polycythemia and the measures needed to control both.
- Teach the patient to recognize symptoms of recurring polycythemia, and emphasize the importance of reporting them promptly.

Polycythemia, spurious

Spurious polycythemia has many other names, including *relative polycythemia*, *stress erythrocytosis*, *stress polycythemia*, *benign polycythemia*, *Gaisböck's disease*, and *pseudopolycythemia*. Spurious polycythemia is characterized by increased hematocrit and normal or decreased red blood cell (RBC) total mass; it results from decreasing plasma volume and subsequent hemoconcentration. This disease usually affects middle-aged people and is more common in males than in females.

Causes
- Adrenocortical insufficiency
- Aggressive diuretic therapy
- Burns
- Decreased fluid intake
- Diabetic acidosis
- Elevated serum cholesterol and uric acid levels
- Familial tendency
- Hemoconcentration from nervous stress
- Hypertension
- Increased hematocrit due to high RBC mass and low plasma volume
- Persistent vomiting or diarrhea
- Renal disease
- Thromboembolitic disease

Signs and symptoms
- Cardiac or pulmonary disease
- Claudication
- Diaphoresis
- Dizziness
- Dyspnea
- Fatigue
- Headaches
- Ruddy appearance
- Short neck
- Slight hypertension
- Tendency to hypoventilate when recumbent

Diagnostic tests
- Hemoglobin level, hematocrit, and RBC count are elevated; RBC mass, arterial oxygen saturation, and bone marrow are normal.
- Plasma volume may be decreased or normal.
- Hypercholesterolemia, hyperlipidemia, or hyperuricemia may be present.
- Spurious polycythemia is distinguishable from polycythemia vera by its characteristic normal or decreased RBC mass, elevated hematocrit, and absence of leukocytosis.

Treatment
- Rehydration with appropriate fluids and electrolytes is the primary therapy for spurious polycythemia secondary to dehydration. Therapy must also include appropriate measures to prevent continuing fluid loss.
- Prevent life-threatening thromboembolism.
- To prevent thromboemboli in predisposed patients, regular exercise and a low-cholesterol diet is recommended. Antilipemics may also be necessary.
- Reduced calorie intake may be required for the obese patient.

Nursing considerations
- Carefully monitor intake and output during rehydration to maintain fluid and electrolyte balance.
- Whenever appropriate, suggest counseling about the patient's work habits and lack of relaxation. If the patient is a smoker, make sure that he understands how important it is to stop smoking. Refer him to a smoking cessation program if necessary.
- Emphasize the need for follow-up examinations every 3 to 4 months after leaving the hospital.
- Thoroughly explain spurious polycythemia, all diagnostic measures, and therapy.

Polycythemia vera

Polycythemia vera (also known as *primary polycythemia, erythremia, polycythemia rubra vera, splenomegalic polycythemia,* or *Vaquez-Osler disease*) is a chronic myeloproliferative disorder characterized by increased red blood cell (RBC) mass, leukocytosis, thrombocytosis, and increased hemoglobin concentration, with normal or increased plasma volume. Increased RBC mass results in hyperviscosity and inhibits blood flow to microcirculation. Subsequently, increased viscosity, diminished velocity, and thrombocytosis promote intravascular thrombosis. The prognosis depends on age at diagnosis (usually occurs between ages 40 and 60), the treatment used, and complications. Hemorrhage is a complication of polycythemia vera. Mortality is high if polycythemia is untreated or is associated with leukemia or myeloid metaplasia.

Causes

- Stem cell defect
- Uncontrolled and rapid cellular reproduction and maturation causing proliferation or hyperplasia of all bone marrow cells (panmyelosis)

Signs and symptoms

- Clubbing of the digits
- Dizziness
- Feeling of fullness in the head
- Headache
- Ruddy cyanosis of the nose
- Variable symptoms according to body system affected (see *Clinical features of polycythemia vera,* page 492)

Diagnostic tests

- Laboratory studies confirm polycythemia vera by showing increased RBC mass and normal arterial oxygen saturation in association with splenomegaly or two of the following: thrombocytosis, leukocytosis, elevated alkaline phosphatase level, or elevated serum vitamin B_{12} level or unbound vitamin B_{12}–binding capacity.
- Another common finding is increased uric acid production, leading to hyperuricemia and hyperuricuria.
- Other laboratory results include an increased blood histamine level, a decreased serum iron concentration, and a decreased or absent urinary erythropoietin.
- Bone marrow biopsy reveals panmyelosis.

Treatment

- Phlebotomy can reduce RBC mass promptly; frequency and the amount of blood removed each time depend on the patient's condition. Typically, 350 to 500 ml of blood can be removed every other day until the hematocrit is reduced to the low-normal range.
- After repeated phlebotomies, the patient develops iron deficiency, which stabilizes RBC production and reduces the need for phlebotomy. Pheresis permits the return of plasma to the patient, diluting the blood and reducing hypovolemic symptoms.
- For severe symptoms, myelosuppressive therapy may be used.
- To compensate for increased uric acid production, give additional fluids, administer cyproheptadine and allopurinol, and alkalinize the urine to prevent uric acid calculi.

Nursing considerations

- Check blood pressure, pulse rate, and respirations before and during phlebotomy. During phlebotomy, make sure the patient is lying down comfortably to prevent vertigo and syncope. Stay alert for tachycardia, clamminess, or com-

Clinical features of polycythemia vera

Signs and symptoms	Causes
Eye, ear, nose, and throat	
▪ Vision disturbances (blurring, diplopia, scotoma, engorged veins of fundus and retina) and congestion of conjunctiva, retina, retinal veins, and oral mucous membrane	▪ Hypervolemia and hyperviscosity
▪ Epistaxis or gingival bleeding	▪ Engorgement of capillary beds
Central nervous system	
▪ Headache or fullness in the head, lethargy, weakness, fatigue, syncope, tinnitus, paresthesia of digits, and impaired mentation	▪ Hypervolemia and hyperviscosity
Cardiovascular	
▪ Hypertension	▪ Hypervolemia and hyperviscosity
▪ Intermittent claudication, thrombosis and emboli, angina, and thrombophlebitis	▪ Hypervolemia, thrombocytosis, and vascular disease
▪ Hemorrhage	▪ Engorgement of capillary beds
Skin	
▪ Pruritus (especially after hot bath)	▪ Basophilia (secondary histamine release)
▪ Urticaria	▪ Altered histamine metabolism
▪ Ruddy cyanosis	▪ Hypervolemia and hyperviscosity due to congested vessels, increased oxyhemoglobin levels, and reduced hemoglobin levels
▪ Night sweats	▪ Hypermetabolism
▪ Ecchymosis	▪ Hemorrhage
GI and hepatic	
▪ Epigastric distress	▪ Hypervolemia and hyperviscosity
▪ Early satiety and fullness	▪ Hepatosplenomegaly
▪ Peptic ulcer pain	▪ Gastric thrombosis and hemorrhage
▪ Hepatosplenomegaly	▪ Congestion, extramedullary hemopoiesis, and myeloid metaplasia
▪ Weight loss	▪ Hypermetabolism
Respiratory	
▪ Dyspnea	▪ Hypervolemia and hyperviscosity
Musculoskeletal	
▪ Arthralgia	▪ Increased urate production secondary to nucleoprotein turnover

plaints of vertigo. If these effects occur, the procedure should be stopped.

- Immediately after phlebotomy, check blood pressure and pulse rate. Have the patient sit up for about 5 minutes before allowing him to walk; this prevents vasovagal attack or orthostatic hypotension. Also, administer 24 oz (710 ml) of juice or water.
- Tell the patient to watch for and report signs or symptoms of iron deficiency (pallor, weight loss, weakness, or glossitis).
- Keep the patient active and ambulatory to prevent thrombosis. If bed rest is necessary, prescribe a daily program of both active and passive range-of-motion exercises.
- Watch for complications: hypervolemia, thrombocytosis, and signs and symptoms of an impending stroke (decreased sensation, numbness, transitory paralysis, fleeting blindness, headache, and epistaxis).
- Regularly examine the patient for bleeding. Tell him which bleeding sites are most common (such as the nose, gingivae, and skin) so that he can check for bleeding. Advise him to promptly report any abnormal bleeding.
- If symptomatic splenomegaly is present, suggest or provide small, frequent meals, followed by a rest period, to prevent nausea and vomiting.
- Instruct the patient to immediately report acute abdominal pain; it may signal splenic infarction, renal calculi, or abdominal organ thrombosis.

During myelosuppressive treatment:
- Monitor complete blood count and platelet count before and during therapy. Warn an outpatient who develops leukopenia that his resistance to infection is low; advise him to avoid crowds and watch for the symptoms of infection.

- If leukopenia develops in a hospitalized patient who needs reverse isolation, follow hospital guidelines. If thrombocytopenia develops, tell the patient to watch for signs of bleeding (blood in urine, nosebleeds, and black stools).

DRUG CHALLENGE

 Tell the patient about the adverse effects of alkylating agents (nausea, vomiting, and risk of infection).

 Porphyrias

Porphyrias are metabolic disorders that affect the biosynthesis of heme (a component of hemoglobin) and cause excessive production and excretion of porphyrins or their precursors. Porphyrins, which are present in all protoplasm, figure prominently in energy storage and use. Classification of porphyrias depends on the site of excessive porphyrin production; they may be erythropoietic (erythroid cells in bone marrow), hepatic (in the liver), or erythrohepatic (in bone marrow and liver). (See *Types of porphyrias,* pages 494 and 495.) An acute episode of intermittent hepatic porphyria may cause fatal respiratory paralysis. In the other forms of porphyrias, the prognosis is good with proper treatment.

Causes
- Acute porphyria with menstruation in premenopausal females
- Günther's disease: inherited autosomal recessive trait
- Inherited autosomal dominant traits
- Toxic-acquired porphyria: ingestion of or exposure to lead

Signs and symptoms
- Acute abdominal pain

Types of porphyrias

Types	Signs and symptoms	Treatment
Erythropoietic porphyria		
Günther's disease ■ Usual onset before age 5	■ Red urine (earliest, most characteristic sign); severe cutaneous photosensitivity leading to vesicular or bullous eruptions on exposed areas and, eventually, scarring and ulceration ■ Hypertrichosis ■ Brown- or red-stained teeth ■ Splenomegaly, hemolytic anemia	■ Beta-carotene to prevent photosensitivity reactions ■ Anti-inflammatory ointments ■ Prednisone to reverse anemia ■ Packed red blood cells to inhibit erythropoiesis and excreted porphyrins ■ Hemin for recurrent attacks ■ Splenectomy for hemolytic anemia ■ Topical dihydroxyacetone and sunscreen filter ■ Oral cholestyramine and charcoal to reduce intestinal reabsorption of porphyrins
Erythrohepatic porphyria		
Protoporphyria ■ Usually affects children ■ Most common in males	■ Photosensitive dermatitis ■ Hemolytic anemia ■ Chronic hepatic disease	■ Avoidance of causative factors ■ Beta-carotene to reduce photosensitivity
Toxic-acquired porphyria ■ Usually affects children ■ Significant mortality	■ Acute colicky pain ■ Anorexia, nausea, vomiting ■ Neuromuscular weakness ■ Behavioral changes ■ Seizures, coma	■ Chlorpromazine I.V. to relieve pain and GI symptoms ■ Avoidance of lead exposure
Hepatic porphyria		
Acute intermittent porphyria ■ Most common form ■ Most common in females ages 15 to 40	■ Colicky abdominal pain with fever, general malaise, and hypertension ■ Peripheral neuritis, behavioral changes, possibly leading to frank psychosis ■ Respiratory paralysis can occur	■ Chlorpromazine I.V. to relieve abdominal pain and control psychic abnormalities; meperidine for severe pain ■ Avoidance of barbiturates, alcohol, and fasting ■ Hemin for recurrent attacks ■ High-carbohydrate diet ■ I.V. glucose

Types of porphyrias *(continued)*

Types	Signs and symptoms	Treatment
Hepatic porphyria *(continued)*		
Variegate porphyria ■ Usual onset between ages 30 and 50 ■ Occurs almost exclusively among South African whites ■ Affects males and females equally	■ Skin lesions, extremely fragile skin in exposed areas ■ Hypertrichosis of face and temples ■ Hyperpigmentation ■ Abdominal pain during acute attack ■ Neuropsychiatric manifestations	■ High-carbohydrate diet ■ Avoidance of sunlight, or the wearing of protective clothing when avoidance isn't possible ■ Hemin for recurrent attacks
Porphyria cutanea tarda ■ Most common in men between ages 40 and 60 ■ Highest incidence in South Africans	■ Facial pigmentation ■ Red-brown urine ■ Photosensitive dermatitis ■ Hypertrichosis	■ Avoidance of precipitating factors, such as alcohol, estrogen, sunlight exposure, and iron ■ Phlebotomy at 2-week intervals to lower serum iron level
Hereditary coproporphyria ■ Rare ■ Affects males and females equally	■ Asymptomatic or mild neurologic, abdominal, or psychiatric symptoms	■ Avoidance of barbiturates ■ Hemin for recurrent attacks ■ High-carbohydrate diet

■ Altered pigmentation of lesions
■ Autonomic effects
■ Chronic brain syndrome
■ Constipation
■ Edema
■ Erythema
■ Fatty infiltration of the liver
■ Fever
■ Fluid and electrolyte imbalance
■ Focal hepatocellular necrosis.
■ Hepatic siderosis

■ Hirsutism on the upper cheeks and periorbital areas
■ Itching and burning of skin lesions
■ Labile hypertension
■ Leukocytosis
■ Milia (white papules on the dorsal aspects of the hands)
■ Neuropathy
■ Peripheral neuropathy
■ Photosensitivity
■ Severe colicky lower abdominal pain
■ Tachycardia

Diagnostic tests

▪ Diagnosis requires screening tests for porphyrins or their precursors (such as aminolevulinic acid [ALA] and porphobilinogen [PBG]) in urine, stool, or blood.

▪ The protoporphyrin test measures porphyrins in the blood.

▪ Enzyme assays also help measure porphyrins.

▪ A urinary lead level of 0.2 mg/L confirms toxic-acquired porphyria.

▪ Increased serum iron levels confirm porphyria cutanea tarda.

▪ Leukocytosis, syndrome of inappropriate antidiuretic hormone, and elevated bilirubin and alkaline phosphatase levels are diagnostic for acute intermittent porphyria.

Treatment

▪ Treatment includes avoiding overexposure to the sun.

▪ Beta-carotene may be prescribed to reduce photosensitivity.

▪ Hemin (an enzyme-inhibitor derived from processed red blood cells) is given to control recurrent attacks of acute intermittent porphyria, Günther's disease, variegate porphyria, and hereditary coproporphyria

▪ A high-carbohydrate diet decreases urinary excretion of ALA and PBG.

▪ Restricted fluid intake inhibits the release of antidiuretic hormone.

Nursing considerations

▪ Warn the patient to avoid excessive sun exposure, use a sunscreen when outdoors, and take a beta-carotene supplement to reduce photosensitivity.

▪ Encourage the patient to adhere to a high-carbohydrate diet.

▪ Tell the patient to avoid all alcohol and drugs that may precipitate an attack.

▪ Tell the patient to avoid skin trauma.

▎Potassium imbalance

Potassium, a cation that's the dominant cellular electrolyte, facilitates contraction of both skeletal and smooth muscles—including myocardial contraction—and figures prominently in nerve impulse conduction, acid-base balance, enzyme action, and cell-membrane function. Because the normal serum potassium level has such a narrow range (3.5 to 5 mEq/L), a slight deviation in either direction can produce profound clinical consequences. Paradoxically, both hypokalemia (potassium deficiency) and hyperkalemia (potassium excess) can lead to muscle weakness and flaccid paralysis because both create an ionic imbalance in neuromuscular tissue excitability. Both conditions also diminish excitability and conduction rate of the heart muscle, which may lead to cardiac arrest.

Causes
Hypokalemia

▪ Acid-base imbalances

▪ Certain drugs, especially potassium-wasting diuretics, steroids, and certain sodium-containing antibiotics (carbenicillin)

▪ Chronic renal disease

▪ Cushing's syndrome

▪ Excessive GI or urinary losses (vomiting, gastric suction, diarrhea, dehydration, anorexia, or prolonged laxative use)

▪ Excessive ingestion of licorice

▪ Hyperglycemia

▪ Primary hyperaldosteronism

▪ Prolonged potassium-free I.V. therapy

▪ Severe serum magnesium deficiency

▪ Trauma (injury, burns, or surgery)

Hyperkalemia

▪ Adrenal gland insufficiency

▪ Burns

Clinical features of potassium imbalance

Dysfunction	Hypokalemia	Hyperkalemia
Acid-base balance	▪ Metabolic alkalosis	▪ Metabolic acidosis
Cardiovascular	▪ Dizziness, hypotension, arrhythmias, electrocardiogram (ECG) changes (flattened T waves, elevated U waves, depressed ST segment), cardiac arrest (with serum potassium levels < 2.5 mEq/L)	▪ Tachycardia and later bradycardia, ECG changes (tented and elevated T waves, widened QRS complex, prolonged PR interval, flattened or absent P waves, depressed ST segment), cardiac arrest (with levels > 7 mEq/L)
Central nervous system	▪ Malaise, irritability, confusion, mental depression, speech changes, decreased reflexes, respiratory paralysis	▪ Hyperreflexia progressing to weakness, numbness, tingling, and flaccid paralysis
Gastrointestinal	▪ Nausea and vomiting, anorexia, diarrhea, abdominal distention, paralytic ileus, or decreased peristalsis	▪ Nausea, diarrhea, abdominal cramps
Genitourinary	▪ Polyuria	▪ Oliguria, anuria
Musculoskeletal	▪ Muscle weakness and fatigue, leg cramps	▪ Muscle weakness, flaccid paralysis

▪ Crushing injuries
▪ Decreased urine output
▪ Dehydration
▪ Diabetic acidosis
▪ Excessive amounts of potassium infused I.V. or administered orally
▪ Failing renal function
▪ Potassium-sparing diuretics
▪ Renal dysfunction or failure

Signs and symptoms

See *Clinical features of potassium imbalance.*

Diagnostic tests

▪ In hypokalemia, serum potassium levels are less than 3.5 mEq/L.

▪ In hyperkalemia, serum potassium levels are greater than 5 mEq/L.

Additional tests may be necessary to determine the underlying cause of the imbalance.

Treatment
Hypokalemia

▪ Treatment focuses on replacement therapy with potassium chloride (I.V. or oral supplement).
▪ When diuresis is necessary, spironolactone, a potassium-sparing diuretic, may be administered concurrently with a potassium-wasting diuretic to minimize potassium loss.

- Hypokalemia can be prevented by giving a maintenance dose of potassium I.V. to patients who may not take anything by mouth and to others predisposed to potassium loss.
- Determine the patient's chloride level. As appropriate, give a potassium chloride supplement if the level is low and potassium gluconate if it's normal.

Hyperkalemia

- Treatment consists of withholding potassium and administering a cation exchange resin orally or by enema.
- In an emergency, rapid infusion of 10% calcium gluconate decreases myocardial irritability and temporarily prevents cardiac arrest but doesn't correct serum potassium excess; it's also contraindicated in patients receiving a cardiac glycoside.
- As an emergency measure, sodium bicarbonate I.V. increases pH and causes potassium to shift back into the cells.
- Insulin and 10% to 50% glucose I.V. also move potassium back into the cells.
- Infusions should be followed by dextrose 5% in water because an infusion of 10% to 15% glucose will stimulate the secretion of endogenous insulin.
- Sodium polystyrene sulfonate (Kayexalate) with 70% sorbitol produces an exchange of sodium ions for potassium ions in the intestine.
- Hemodialysis or peritoneal dialysis can also facilitate the removal of excess potassium.

Nursing considerations
For hypokalemia

- Check serum potassium and other electrolyte levels in patients who are likely to develop a potassium imbalance and in those requiring potassium replacement; they risk overcorrection to hyperkalemia.
- Carefully assess intake and output.

- Administer slow-release potassium or dilute oral potassium supplements in 4 oz (118.3 ml) or more of water or other fluid to reduce gastric and small-bowel irritation.

DRUG CHALLENGE

 Give I.V. potassium only after it's diluted in solution; potassium is irritating to vascular, subcutaneous, and fatty tissues and may cause phlebitis or tissue necrosis if it infiltrates.

- Carefully monitor patients receiving a cardiac glycoside because hypokalemia will enhance its action and may produce signs and symptoms of digoxin toxicity (anorexia, nausea, vomiting, blurred vision, and arrhythmias).
- Infuse potassium slowly (no more than 20 mEq/L/hour) to prevent hyperkalemia. Never administer it by I.V. push or bolus; it may cause cardiac arrest.
- Monitor cardiac rhythm, and be alert for irregularities.
- To prevent hypokalemia, instruct patients (especially those predisposed to hypokalemia due to long-term diuretic therapy) to include in their diet foods rich in potassium—oranges, bananas, tomatoes, dark-green leafy vegetables, milk, dried fruits, apricots, and peanuts.

For hyperkalemia

- Frequently monitor serum potassium and other electrolyte levels, and carefully record intake and output.
- Administer sodium polystyrene sulfonate orally or rectally (by retention enema).

DRUG CHALLENGE

 Watch for signs and symptoms of hypokalemia with prolonged use and of hypoglycemia (muscle weakness, syncope, hunger, and diaphoresis) with repeated insulin and glucose treatment.

■ Watch for signs of hyperkalemia in predisposed patients, especially those with decreased urine output or those receiving oral or I.V. potassium supplements.

 Before giving a blood transfusion, check to see how long ago the blood was donated; older blood cell hemolysis releases potassium. Infuse only fresh blood for patients with average to high serum potassium levels.

■ Watch for cardiac arrhythmias.

▎Pressure ulcers

Pressure ulcers, commonly called *pressure sores, decubitus ulcers,* or *bedsores,* are localized areas of cellular necrosis that occur most commonly in the skin and subcutaneous tissue over bony prominences. (See *Pressure points: Common sites of pressure ulcers,* page 500.) The intensity and duration of such pressure govern the severity of the ulcer; pressure exerted over an area for a moderate period (1 to 2 hours) produces tissue ischemia and increased capillary pressure, leading to edema and multiple small-vessel thromboses. An inflammatory reaction gives way to ulceration and necrosis of ischemic cells. In turn, necrotic tissue predisposes the patient to bacterial invasion and subsequent infection. These ulcers may be superficial, caused by local skin irritation with subsequent surface maceration, or deep, originating in underlying tissue. Deep lesions commonly go undetected until they penetrate the skin; however, by then, they have usually caused subcutaneous damage.

Causes
■ Unrelieved pressure over bony prominences

Predisposing factors
■ Altered mobility
■ Edema
■ Fever
■ Inadequate nutrition
■ Incontinence
■ Obesity
■ Pathologic conditions

Signs and symptoms
■ Black eschar around and over the lesion
■ Foul-smelling, purulent discharge
■ Necrosis
■ Shiny, erythematous changes over the compressed area
■ Small blisters or erosions
■ Ulceration

Diagnostic tests
■ Diagnosis is based on physical examination revealing the presence of pressure ulcers rather than diagnostic testing. Pressure ulcers are described according to stages:
  – Stage I: skin is red but not broken
  – Stage II: damage extends through the epidermis and dermis
  – Stage III: damage extends to the subcutaneous tissue
  – Stage IV: involvement reaches muscle and, possibly, bone.
  Testing may include:
■ Wound culture and sensitivity of the exudate identify infecting organism.
■ If severe hypoproteinemia is suspected, total serum protein values and serum albumin studies may be appropriate.

Pressure points: Common sites of pressure ulcers

Pressure ulcers may develop in any of these pressure points. To prevent sores, frequently reposition the patient, and carefully check for any skin changes.

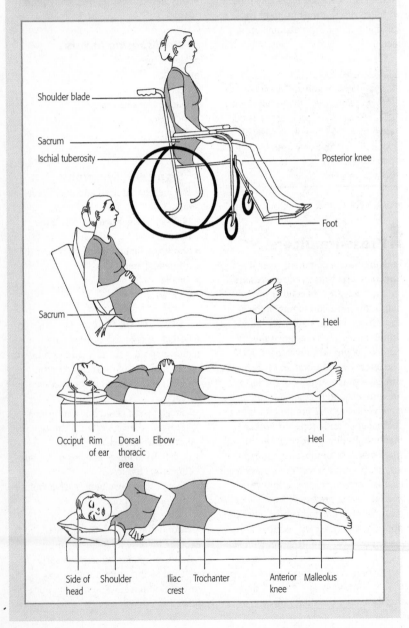

Special aids for preventing and treating pressure ulcers

The following devices and topical agents can help prevent and treat pressure ulcers.

Pressure relief aids

■ *Gel flotation pads* disperse pressure over a greater skin surface area; convenient and adaptable for home and wheelchair use.

■ *Alternating pressure mattress* contains tubelike sections, running lengthwise, that deflate and reinflate, changing areas of pressure. Use mattress with a single untucked sheet because layers of linen decrease its effectiveness.

■ *Spanco mattress* has polyester fibers with silicon tubes to decrease pressure without limiting the patient's position. It has no weight limitation.

■ *Sheepskin* is soft, dry, absorbent, and easy to clean. It should be in direct contact with the patient's skin. It's available in sizes to fit elbows and heels and is adaptable to home use.

■ *Clinitron bed* supports the patient at a subcapillary pressure point and provides warm, relaxing, therapeutic airflow. The bed is filled with beads that move when the air flows. It eliminates friction and maceration.

■ *Low air-loss beds,* such as Flexicare and Accucare, slow the drying of any saline soaks, and elderly patients often experience less disorientation than with high air-loss beds. The head of the bed can be elevated so the chance of aspiration is reduced, especially in patients who require tube feeding. Patients can get out of bed more easily and can be moved more easily on low air-loss surfaces.

Topical agents

■ Gentle soap
■ Dakin's solution
■ Zinc oxide cream
■ Absorbable gelatin sponge
■ Granulated sugar (mechanical irritant to enhance granulation)
■ Dextranomer (inert, absorbing beads)
■ Karaya gum patches
■ Topical antibiotics (only when infection is confirmed by culture and sensitivity tests)
■ Silver sulfadiazine cream (antimicrobial agent) for necrotic areas
■ Water vapor–permeable dressings
■ Duoderm, Tegaderm dressings

Skin-damaging agents to avoid

■ Harsh alkali soaps
■ Alcohol-based products (can cause vasoconstriction)
■ Tincture of benzoin (may cause painful erosions)
■ Hexachlorophene (may irritate the central nervous system)
■ Petroleum gauze

Treatment

■ Prevent pressure ulcer formation with movement and exercise to improve circulation, and adequate nutrition to maintain skin health.
■ Treatment focuses on relieving pressure on the affected area, keeping the area clean and dry, and promoting healing. (See *Special aids for preventing and treating pressure ulcers.*)

Nursing considerations

■ Assess the skin of bedridden patients every 4 hours for possible changes in color, turgor, temperature, and sensation. Examine an existing ulcer for any change in size or degree of damage.

When using pressure relief aids or topical agents, explain their function to the patient.

- Prevent pressure ulcers by repositioning the bedridden patient at least every 2 hours. To minimize the effects of a shearing force, use a footboard and don't raise the head of the bed more than 60 degrees. Also use a draw or pull sheet to turn the patient or to pull him up. Keep the patient's knees slightly flexed for short periods. Perform passive range-of-motion (ROM) exercises, or encourage the patient to do active ROM exercises if possible.

- To prevent pressure ulcers in immobilized patients, use pressure relief aids on their beds.

- Provide meticulous skin care. Keep the skin clean and dry without the use of harsh soaps. Gently massaging the skin around the affected area—not on it—promotes healing. Rub moisturizing lotions into the skin thoroughly to prevent maceration of the skin surface. Change bed linens frequently for patients who are diaphoretic or incontinent. Use a fecal incontinence bag for incontinent patients.

- Clean ulcers with noncytotoxic solutions that don't kill or damage the cells. (Solutions such as sodium hypochlorite, acetic acid, povidone-iodine, and hydrogen peroxide are cytotoxic and shouldn't be used.) Dressings, if needed, should be porous and lightly taped to healthy skin.

- Debridement may be ordered by applying open wet dressings and allowing them to dry on the ulcer. Assist with surgical debridement as indicated.

- Encourage a high-protein diet—supplemented with vitamins, minerals, and fluids—sufficient to maintain body weight and promote healing. Consult with a dietitian regarding a diet that promotes granulation of new tissue. Encourage the debilitated patient to eat frequent, small meals that include protein and calorie-rich supplements. Assist weakened patients with their meals.

Proctitis

Proctitis is an acute or chronic inflammation of the rectal mucosa. The prognosis is good unless massive bleeding occurs.

Causes
- Allergies (especially to milk)
- Bacterial infections
- Chronic constipation
- Emotional upset
- Endocrine dysfunction
- Food poisoning
- Habitual laxative use
- Radiation (especially for cancer of the cervix, uterus, or prostate)
- Rectal injury
- Rectal medications
- Vasomotor disturbance

Predisposing factors
- Autoimmune disorders
- High-risk sexual practices
- Homosexuality

Signs and symptoms
- Constipation
- Cramps in the left abdominal quadrant
- Feeling of rectal fullness
- Intense urge to defecate
- Small amounts of stool that may contain blood and mucus
- Tenesmus

Diagnostic tests
- Sigmoidoscopy shows edematous, bright-red or pink rectal mucosa that's thick, shiny, friable and, possibly, ulcerated.

- In chronic proctitis, sigmoidoscopy shows thickened mucosa, loss of vascular pattern, and stricture of the rectal lumen.
- Supportive tests include biopsy to rule out cancer and a bacteriologic examination to detect the cause.

Treatment

- Treatment focuses on eliminating the underlying cause (fecal impaction, laxatives, or other medications).
- Corticosteroids (in enema or suppository form) may reduce inflammation, as may sulfasalazine (Azulfidine), mesalamine (Asacol), or similar agents.
- Tranquilizers may be appropriate for the patient with emotional stress.

Nursing considerations

- Tell the patient to watch for and report bleeding and other persistent symptoms.
- Fully explain proctitis and its treatment to help the patient understand the disorder and prevent its recurrence.
- As appropriate, offer emotional support and reassurance during rectal examinations and treatment.

Prostate cancer

Prostate cancer is the second most common neoplasm found in males older than age 50. Adenocarcinoma is its most common form; sarcoma occurs only rarely. Most prostatic cancer originate in the posterior prostate gland; the rest, near the urethra. Malignant prostatic tumors seldom result from the benign hyperplastic enlargement that commonly develops around the prostatic urethra in elderly males. Prostatic cancer seldom produces symptoms until it's advanced.

Causes

- Unknown

Signs and symptoms

- Difficulty initiating a urinary stream
- Dribbling
- Hematuria (rarely)
- Unexplained cystitis
- Urine retention

Diagnostic tests

- A digital rectal examination that reveals a small, hard nodule may help diagnose prostatic cancer.
- Biopsy confirms the diagnosis.
- Prostate-specific antigen (PSA) will be elevated.
- Transrectal prostatic ultrasonography may be used for patients with abnormal digital rectal examination and PSA test findings.
- Serum acid phosphatase levels will be elevated in two-thirds of males with metastatic prostatic cancer.
- Magnetic resonance imaging, computed tomography scan, and excretory urography can help define the tumor's extent.
- Elevated alkaline phosphatase levels and a positive bone scan indicate bone metastasis.

Treatment

- Orchiectomy reduces androgen production
- Radical prostatectomy is usually effective for localized lesions without metastasis.
- Radiation therapy is used to cure some locally invasive lesions and to relieve pain from metastatic bone involvement. It may also be used prophylactically for patients with tumors in regional lymph nodes.
- If hormone therapy, surgery, and radiation therapy aren't feasible or successful, chemotherapy (using combinations of cyclophosphamide, doxorubicin, fluo-

rouracil, cisplatin, etoposide, and vinde-sine) may be tried.

Nursing considerations
Before prostatectomy

■ Explain the expected after effects of surgery (such as impotence and inconti-nence) and radiation.
■ Teach the patient to perform perineal (Kegel) exercises 1 to 10 times per hour. Have him squeeze his buttocks together, hold this position for a few seconds, and then relax.

After prostatectomy or suprapubic prostatectomy

■ Regularly check the dressing, incision, and drainage systems for excessive bleeding; monitor the patient for signs of bleeding (pallor, falling blood pres-sure, and rising pulse rate) and infec-tion.
■ Make sure the patient receives plenty of fluids.
■ Give antispasmodics, as necessary, to control postoperative bladder spasms. Also give analgesics as needed.
■ Urinary incontinence is common after surgery; keep the patient's skin clean, dry, and free from drainage and urine.
■ Encourage perineal exercises within 24 to 48 hours after surgery.
■ Provide catheter care—especially if a three-way catheter with a continuous ir-rigation system is in place. Check the tubing for kinks and blockages, espe-cially if the patient reports pain. Warn him not to pull on the catheter.

After transurethral prostatic resection

■ Watch for signs of urethral stricture (dysuria, decreased force and caliber of urinary stream, and straining to urinate) and for abdominal distention (from ure-thral stricture or catheter blockage). Irri-gate the catheter as needed.

After perineal prostatectomy
DO'S & DON'TS

 Avoid taking a rectal tempera-ture or inserting any kind of rec-tal tube. Provide pads to absorb urine leakage, a rubber ring for the pa-tient to sit on, and sitz baths for pain and inflammation.

After perineal or retropubic prostatectomy

■ Explain that urine leakage after catheter removal is normal and will sub-side.

After radiation therapy

■ Watch for common adverse reactions: proctitis, diarrhea, bladder spasms, and urinary frequency. Internal radiation usually results in cystitis within the first 2 to 3 weeks.
■ Urge the patient to drink at least 2 qt (2 L) of fluid daily.
■ Provide analgesics and antispasmodics as ordered.

▌Prostatitis

An inflammation of the prostate gland, prostatitis may be acute or chronic. Acute prostatitis most commonly results from gram-negative bacteria and is easy to recognize and treat. However, chronic prostatitis, the most common cause of recurrent urinary tract infection in males, is less easy to recognize. Organ-isms probably spread to the prostate by the bloodstream or from ascending ure-thral infection, invasion of rectal bacte-ria via lymphatics, reflux of infected bladder urine into prostate ducts.

Causes
- Enterobacter
- *Escherichia coli* (80% of bacterial infections)
- Klebsiella
- Proteus
- Pseudomonas
- Serratia
- Staphylococcus
- Streptococcus

Contributing factors
- Infrequent or excessive sexual intercourse
- Procedures such as cystoscopy or catheterization

Signs and symptoms
- Arthralgia
- Chills
- Cloudy urine
- Dysuria
- Fever
- Lower back pain
- Myalgia
- Nocturia
- Perineal fullness and discomfort
- Tender, indurated, swollen, firm, and warm prostate
- Urinary obstruction
- Urination is frequent and urgent

Chronic bacterial prostatitis
- Asymptomatic (occasionally)
- Hemospermia
- Painful ejaculation
- Persistent urethral discharge
- Same urinary symptoms as the acute form
- Sexual dysfunction

Diagnostic tests
- Urine culture can usually help identify the causative infectious organism.
- Rectal examination findings may suggest prostatitis.
- Urine cultures obtained by triple-void urine specimens are compared: one specimen is collected when the patient starts voiding; another specimen collected midstream; another specimen collected after the patient stops voiding and the physician massages the prostate to express prostate secretions. A significant increase in colony count in the prostatic specimens confirms prostatitis.

Treatment
- Systemic antibiotic therapy (aminoglycosides, in combination with penicillins or cephalosporins may be most effective for severe cases) is initiated to remove causative organism.
- If prostatitis is due to a sexually transmitted disease, ceftriaxone and doxycycline or floxacin are used.
- Supportive therapy includes bed rest, adequate hydration, and administration of analgesics, antipyretics, sitz baths, and stool softeners as necessary.
- In symptomatic chronic prostatitis, regular massage of the prostate is most effective.
- Regular ejaculation may help promote drainage of prostatic secretions.
- Anticholinergics and analgesics may help relieve nonbacterial prostatitis symptoms.
- Alpha-adrenergic blockers and muscle relaxants may relieve prostatodynia.
- Antispasmolytics may be administered for bladder spasms.
- If drug therapy is unsuccessful, treatment may include transurethral resection of the prostate, which requires removal of all infected tissue. However, this procedure usually isn't performed on young adults because it may cause retrograde ejaculation and sterility. Total prostatectomy is curative but may cause impotence and incontinence.

Nursing considerations

- Ensure bed rest and adequate hydration. Provide stool softeners to prevent pain with straining, and administer sitz baths as required.
- Emphasize the need for strict adherence to the prescribed drug regimen. Instruct the patient to drink at least eight 8-oz glasses of water per day.

D RUG CHALLENGE

 Have the patient report adverse drug reactions, such as rash, nausea, vomiting, fever, chills, and GI irritation.

- Teach the patient to avoid food and beverages that could increase prostate secretions, such as alcohol and caffeinated beverages and foods.

▌Protein-calorie malnutrition

One of the most prevalent and serious depletion disorders, protein-calorie malnutrition occurs as marasmus (protein-calorie deficiency), characterized by growth failure and wasting; and as kwashiorkor (protein deficiency), characterized by tissue edema and damage. Both forms vary from mild to severe and may be fatal, depending on accompanying stress (particularly sepsis or injury) and duration of deprivation. Protein-calorie malnutrition increases the risk of death from pneumonia, chickenpox, or measles.

Causes

- Chronic diarrhea
- Chronic metabolic disease
- Defective utilization of nutrients (malabsorption syndrome, short-bowel syndrome, and Crohn's disease)
- Inability to take anything by mouth for an extended period

- Increased protein-calorie requirements (severe burns and injuries, systemic infections, and cancer)
- Insufficient intake of dietary amino acid

Signs and symptoms
Chronic protein-calorie malnutrition

- Anorexia
- Children: small for chronological age
- Dry, "baggy" skin
- Emaciation with no adipose tissue
- Irritability
- Low temperature
- Nausea and vomiting
- Slowed pulse rate and respirations
- Sparse, dull brown or reddish yellow hair
- Weakness

Chronic kwashiorkor

- Diminishing of adipose tissue
- Dry, peeling skin
- Edema masking severe muscle wasting
- Hepatomegaly
- Positive growth in height

Secondary protein-calorie malnutrition

- Loss of immunocompetence
- Similar to chronic protein calorie malnutrition

Diagnostic tests

- Diagnosis is based on clinical features, dietary history, and anthropometry.
- Height and weight less than 80% of standard for the patient's age and sex, and below-normal arm circumference and triceps skinfold confirm the diagnosis.
- Serum albumin level less than 2.8 g/dl (normal: 3.3 to 4.3 g/dl) supports the diagnosis.
- Urinary creatinine (24-hour) level shows lean body mass status by relating

creatinine excretion to height and ideal body weight, to yield creatinine-height index.

- Skin tests with standard antigens indicate degree of immunocompromise by determining reactivity expressed as a percentage of normal reaction.
- The finding of moderate anemia helps support the diagnosis.

Treatment

- Restore fluid and electrolyte balance parenterally.
- Enteral nutrition after anorexia has subsided; the preferred treatment is oral feeding of high-quality protein foods, especially milk, and protein-calorie supplements.
- A patient who's unwilling or unable to eat may require supplementary feedings through a nasogastric tube or total parenteral nutrition (TPN) through a central venous catheter. Cautious realimentation is essential to prevent complications from overloading the compromised metabolic system.
- Accompanying infection must also be treated, preferably with antibiotics that don't inhibit protein synthesis.

Nursing considerations

- Encourage the patient with protein-calorie malnutrition to consume as much nutritious food and fluid as possible. Help the patient eat if necessary. Cooperate closely with the dietitian to monitor intake and provide acceptable meals and snacks.
- If TPN is necessary, observe strict aseptic technique when handling catheters, tubes, and solutions and during dressing changes.
- Watch for protein-calorie malnutrition in patients who have been hospitalized for a prolonged period, have had no oral intake for several days, or have cachectic disease.

- To help eradicate protein-calorie malnutrition in developing countries, encourage prolonged breast-feeding, educate mothers about their children's needs, and provide supplementary foods as needed.
- If the older patient is anorectic, consider asking family members and other visitors to bring in special foods from home that may improve the patient's appetite. In addition, encouraging the family to collaborate on feeding a dependent patient can help promote his recovery, enhance his feelings of well-being, and stimulate him to eat more.

Pseudomembranous enterocolitis

An acute inflammation and necrosis of the small and large intestines, pseudomembranous enterocolitis usually affects the mucosa but may extend into submucosa and, rarely, other layers. Necrosed mucosa is replaced by a pseudomembrane filled with staphylococci, leukocytes, mucus, fibrin, and inflammatory cells. Marked by severe diarrhea, serious complications include such conditions as electrolyte imbalance, hypotension, and shock. It's generally fatal in 1 to 7 days from severe dehydration and from toxicity, peritonitis, or colonic perforation.

Causes

- Change in the flora of the colon and an overgrowth of a toxin-producing strain of *Clostridium difficile*

Contributing factors

- Immunocompromised status (cystic fibrosis, neurologic disease, liver and renal disease, diabetes mellitus, malnutrition, and hematologic disorders)
- Postoperatively in debilitated patients with abdominal surgery

- Treatment with broad-spectrum antibiotics (ampicillin, clindamycin, and cephalosporins)

Signs and symptoms
- Abdominal pain and cramping
- Abdominal tenderness
- Colitis
- Copious watery diarrhea (can be up to 30 stools per day)
- Leukocytosis
- Low-grade fever

Diagnostic tests
- Rectal biopsy through sigmoidoscopy confirms pseudomembranous enterocolitis.
- Stool cultures can identify *C. difficile*.

Treatment
- A patient who's receiving broad-spectrum antibiotic therapy requires immediate discontinuation of the antibiotics.
- If possible, medications that slow peristalsis should be avoided.
- Effective treatment usually includes orally administered metronidazole; oral vancomycin is usually given for severe or resistant cases.
- Treatment also includes maintenance of fluid and electrolyte balance.
- Treat hypotension and shock with pressors, such as dopamine and levarterenol.

Nursing considerations
- Monitor vital signs, skin color, and level of consciousness. Be alert for signs of shock.
- Record fluid intake and output, including fluid lost in stools. Watch for dehydration (poor skin turgor, sunken eyes, and decreased urine output).
- Check serum electrolyte levels daily, and watch for signs and symptoms of

hypokalemia, especially malaise and a weak, rapid, irregular pulse.

Pseudomonas infections

Pseudomonas is a small gram-negative bacillus that produces nosocomial infections, superinfections of various parts of the body, and a rare disease called melioidosis. In elderly patients, *Pseudomonas* infection usually enters through the genitourinary tract; in infants, through the umbilical cord, skin, and GI tract. This bacillus is also associated with bacteremia, endocarditis, and osteomyelitis in drug addicts. Treatment of local *Pseudomonas* infection is usually successful and complications are rare. However, in patients with poor immunologic resistance—premature infants, elderly patients, or those with debilitating disease, burns, or wounds—septicemic *Pseudomonas* infections are serious and sometimes fatal.

Causes
- *P. aeruginosa* (most common)
- *P. acidovorans, P. alcaligenes, P. cepacia, P. fluorescens, P. maltophilia, P. putida, P. putrefaciens, P. stutzeri,* and *P. testosteroni*

Contributing factors
- These organisms are frequently found in liquids that are allowed to stand for a

long time (hospital soaps, saline solution, water in flower vases), incubators, humidifiers, and respiratory therapy equipment

Signs and symptoms
- Drainage with distinct, sickly sweet odor
- Greenish-blue pus crusted on wound

Other signs and symptoms dependent on infection site
- Bacteremia
- Bronchitis, pneumonia, or bronchiectasis
- Corneal ulcers
- Endocarditis
- Infant epidemic diarrhea and other diarrheal illnesses
- Mastoiditis
- Meningitis
- Otitis externa, otitis media
- Skin infections (such as burns and pressure ulcers)
- Urinary tract infection (UTI)

Diagnostic tests
Diagnosis requires isolation of the *Pseudomonas* organism in blood, cerebrospinal fluid, urine, exudate, or sputum culture.

Treatment
- Antibiotic treatment includes aminoglycosides, such as gentamicin or amikacin (Amikin), combined with a *Pseudomonas*-sensitive penicillin, such as piperacillin or ticarcillin.

DRUG CHALLENGE

 An alternative combination is amikacin and a similar penicillin. Such combination therapy is necessary because *Pseudomonas* quickly becomes resistant to carbenicillin alone.

- In UTIs, carbenicillin indanyl sodium can be used alone if the organism is susceptible and the infection doesn't have systemic effects.
- Local *Pseudomonas* infections or septicemia secondary to wound infection require 1% acetic acid irrigations, topical application of colistimethate sodium and polymyxin B, and debridement or drainage of the infected wound.

Nursing considerations
- Observe and record the character of wound exudate and sputum.
- Before administering antibiotics, ask the patient about a history of allergies, especially to penicillin.

DRUG CHALLENGE

 If combinations of carbenicillin or ticarcillin and an aminoglycoside are ordered, schedule the doses 1 hour apart (carbenicillin and ticarcillin may decrease the antibiotic effect of the aminoglycoside). Don't give both antibiotics through the same administration set.

- Monitor the patient's renal function (urine output, blood urea nitrogen, specific gravity, urinalysis, and creatinine) during treatment with aminoglycosides.
- Protect immunocompromised patients from exposure to this infection. Attention to hand washing and aseptic techniques prevent further spread.
- To prevent *Pseudomonas* infection, maintain proper endotracheal and tracheostomy suctioning technique: Use strict sterile technique when caring for I.V. lines, catheters, and other tubes; properly dispose of suction bottle contents; and label and date solution bottles and change them frequently, according to your facility's policy.

Psoriasis

Psoriasis is a chronic, recurrent disease, marked by epidermal proliferation. Its lesions, which appear as erythematous papules and plaques covered with silver scales, vary widely in severity and distribution. It's characterized by recurring partial remissions and exacerbations. Flare-ups are commonly related to specific systemic and environmental factors but may be unpredictable; they can usually be controlled with therapy.

Causes
- Environmental factors (trauma, infections).
- Genetic
- Immune disorder (possibly)

Predisposing factors
- Climate (cold weather)
- Emotional stress
- Endocrine changes
- Pregnancy

Signs and symptoms
- Accumulation of thick, crumbly debris under the nail causing it to separate from the nail-bed (onycholysis)
- Arthritic symptoms, usually in one or more joints of the fingers or toes, in the larger joints, or sometimes in the sacroiliac joints (may progress to spondylitis)
- Erythematous, well-defined plaques (silver scales that flake off easily or appear thickened) on the scalp, chest, elbows, knees, back, and buttocks
- Fine bleeding points with removal of scales (Auspitz sign)
- Itching
- Pain
- Small guttate lesions, typically thin and erythematous with few scales; alone or with plaques
- Small indentations or pits and yellow or brown discoloration of fingernails
- Widespread involvement (exfoliative or erythrodermic psoriasis)

Localized pustular psoriasis
- Pustules on the palms and soles remaining sterile until opened

Generalized pustular (von Zumbusch) psoriasis
- Commonly occurs with fever, leukocytosis, and malaise
- Groups of pustules coalescing to form lakes of pus on red skin

Diagnostic tests
- Diagnosis depends on patient history, appearance of the lesions and, if needed, the results of skin biopsy.
- In severe cases, the serum uric acid level is typically elevated due to accelerated nucleic acid degradation; however, indications of gout are absent.
- Human leukocyte antigens may be present in early-onset familial psoriasis.

Treatment
- Palliative treatment includes exposure to ultraviolet (UV) light (UVB or natural sunlight) to the point of minimal erythema. A thin layer of petroleum jelly may be applied before UVB exposure (the most common treatment for generalized psoriasis). Exposure time can increase gradually.
- Tar preparations or crude coal tar itself may be applied to affected areas about 15 minutes before exposure or may be left on overnight and wiped off the next morning.
- Topical corticosteroids are the treatment of choice for mild to moderate psoriasis of the trunk, arms, and legs. Treatment commonly combines a topical corticosteroid with an emollient, coal tar preparation, and UV light therapy. Topi-

cal vitamin D has been shown to be as effective as topical steroids.

- Small, stubborn plaques may require intralesional steroid injections.

DRUG CHALLENGE

 Anthralin ointment or paste mixture may be used for well-defined plaques but must not be applied to unaffected areas because it causes injury and stains normal skin. Apply petroleum jelly around the affected skin before applying anthralin.

- Calcipotriene ointment, a vitamin D_3 analogue applied topically, works best when alternated with a topical steroid, as noted above with anthralin.
- Low-dose antihistamines, oatmeal bath, emollients, and open wet dressings may help relieve pruritus.
- Aspirin and local heat help alleviate the pain of psoriatic arthritis; severe cases may require nonsteroidal anti-inflammatory drugs.
- Therapy for psoriasis of the scalp consists of a tar shampoo followed by application of a steroid lotion.
- No effective topical treatment exists for psoriasis of the nails.

Nursing considerations

- Make sure that the patient understands his prescribed therapy; provide written instructions to avoid confusion.
- Teach the correct application of prescribed ointments, creams, and lotions. A steroid cream, for example, should be applied in a thin film and rubbed gently into the skin until the cream disappears.
- Warn the patient never to put an occlusive dressing over anthralin. Suggest the use of mineral oil, then soap and water, to remove anthralin.
- Caution the patient to avoid scrubbing his skin vigorously, to prevent Koebner's phenomenon. If a medication has been

applied to the scales to soften them, suggest that the patient use a soft brush to remove them.

DRUG CHALLENGE

 Watch for adverse reactions, especially allergic reactions to anthralin, atrophy and acne from steroids, and burning, itching, nausea, and squamous cell epitheliomas.

- Caution the patient receiving therapy to stay out of the sun on the day of treatment, and to protect his eyes with sunglasses that screen UVA for 24 hours after treatment. Tell him to wear goggles during exposure to this light.
- Be aware that psoriasis can cause psychological problems. Assure the patient that psoriasis isn't contagious, that remissions can occur, and that exacerbations are controllable with treatment. However, make sure that he understands that there is no cure for psoriasis.
- Because stressful situations tend to exacerbate psoriasis, the patient may benefit from stress management techniques and support groups.
- Refer all patients to the National Psoriasis Foundation, which provides information and directs patients to local chapters.

Psoriatic arthritis

Psoriatic arthritis is a rheumatoid-like joint disease associated with psoriasis of the skin and nails. Although the arthritis component of this syndrome may be clinically indistinguishable from rheumatoid arthritis, the rheumatoid nodules are absent, and serologic tests for rheumatoid factor are negative. Some patients develop a more asymmetrical oligoarthritis affecting large or small joints. Psoriatic arthritis is usually mild, with intermittent flare-ups; however, in rare cases it may progress to crippling arthritis mutilans.

Causes
- Hereditary (human leukocyte antigen-B27-positive status in 20% to 50% of patients)
- Streptococcal infection
- Trauma

Signs and symptoms
- Arthritis involving one or several joints asymmetrically or symmetrically
- Eye involvement
- Fever
- General malaise
- Joint and skin lesions (possibly simultaneous)
- Nail changes (pitting, transverse ridges, onycholysis, keratosis, yellowing, destruction)
- Psoriatic lesions preceding the arthritic component
- Sausagelike appearance of the distal interphalangeal joints of the hands (characteristic)
- Spinal involvement

Diagnostic tests
- Inflammatory arthritis in a patient with psoriatic skin lesions suggests psoriatic arthritis.
- X-rays confirm joint involvement and show marginal erosion at interphalangeal joints with areas of thin, "fluffy" new bone formation; "whittling" of the distal end of the terminal phalanges; "pencil-in-cup" deformity of the distal interphalangeal joints; absence of osteoporosis; sacroiliitis; atypical spondylitis with syndesmophyte formation, resulting in hyperostosis and paravertebral ossification, which may lead to vertebral fusion.
- Blood studies indicate negative rheumatoid factor and elevated erythrocyte sedimentation rate and uric acid levels.

Treatment
- For mild psoriatic arthritis, treatment includes immobilization through joint rest or splints, isometric exercises, paraffin baths, and heat therapy.
- Aspirin and other non-steroidal anti-inflammatory drugs may be prescribed for pain.
- A low-dose systemic corticosteroid or topical steroids may help control skin lesions.
- More severe arthritis requires treatment with disease-modifying antirheumatic drugs.

Nursing considerations
- Explain the disease and its treatment to the patient and his family.
- Reassure the patient that psoriatic plaques aren't contagious. Avoid showing revulsion at the sight of psoriatic patches—doing so will only reinforce the patient's fear of rejection.
- Encourage exercise, particularly swimming, to maintain strength and range of motion.
- Teach the patient how to apply skin care products and medications correctly; explain possible adverse reactions.
- Stress the importance of adequate rest and protection of affected joints.
- Encourage regular, moderate exposure to the sun.
- Refer the patient to the Arthritis Foundation for self-help and support groups.

▌Pulmonary edema

With pulmonary edema, fluid accumulates in the extravascular spaces of the lung. With cardiogenic pulmonary edema, fluid accumulation results from elevations in pulmonary venous and capillary hydrostatic pressures. A common complication of cardiac disorders, pulmonary edema can occur as a chronic condition or develop quickly and rapidly become fatal. The compromised left ventricle requires increased filling pressures to maintain adequate output; these pressures are transmitted to the left atrium, pulmonary veins, and pulmonary capillary bed. This increased pulmonary capillary hydrostatic force promotes transmission of intravascular fluids into the pulmonary interstitium, decreasing lung compliance and interfering with gas exchange.

Causes

- Left-sided heart failure possibly due to:
  - Arteriosclerosis
  - Cardiomyopathic heart disease
  - Hypertension
  - Valvular heart disease

Predisposing factors

- Decreased serum colloid osmotic pressure (nephrosis, burns, hepatic disease, nutritional deficiency)
- Impaired lung lymphatic drainage (Hodgkin's disease, obliterative lymphangitis)
- Infusion of excessive volumes of I.V. fluids
- Left atrial myxoma
- Mitral stenosis
- Pulmonary veno-occlusive disease

Signs and symptoms
Early signs and symptoms

- Coughing
- Dependent crackles
- Diastolic (S_3) gallop
- Exertional dyspnea
- Jugular vein distention
- Orthopnea
- Paroxysmal nocturnal dyspnea
- Tachycardia
- Tachypnea

Later signs and symptoms

- Arrhythmias
- Cold, clammy, diaphoretic, and cyanotic skin
- Confusion
- Decreased cardiac output
- Depressed level of consciousness
- Diffuse crackles
- Frothy, bloody sputum
- Hypotension
- Increased tachycardia
- Labored and rapid respiration
- Thready pulse

Diagnostic tests

- Arterial blood gas (ABG) analysis shows hypoxia; partial pressure of arterial carbon dioxide varies. Profound respiratory alkalosis and acidosis may occur. Metabolic acidosis occurs when cardiac output is low.
- Chest X-ray films show diffuse haziness of the lung fields and, often, cardiomegaly and pleural effusions.
- Pulmonary artery catheterization identify left-sided heart failure by showing an elevated pulmonary artery wedge pressure.
- An echocardiogram may reveal weak heart muscle, leaking or narrow heart valves, or fluid surrounding the heart.

Treatment

- Administration of high concentrations of oxygen (by a cannula, face mask and, if the patient fails to maintain an acceptable partial pressure of arterial oxygen, assisted ventilation).
- Diuretics (furosemide, bumetanide) to promote diuresis, and mobilize extravascular fluid.
- Cardiac glycoside or a vasopressor increases cardiac contractility.
- Antiarrhythmics may also be given, particularly in arrhythmias related to decreased cardiac output.

■ Arterial vasodilators (nitroprusside) decrease peripheral vascular resistance, preload, and afterload.
■ Morphine reduces anxiety and dyspnea and dilates the systemic venous bed, promoting blood flow from the pulmonary circulation to the periphery.

Nursing considerations

■ Carefully monitor the vulnerable patient for early signs of pulmonary edema, especially tachypnea, tachycardia, and abnormal breath sounds. Check for peripheral edema, which may also indicate that fluid is accumulating in pulmonary tissue.
■ Administer oxygen as ordered and monitor for effect.
■ Monitor vital signs every 15 to 30 minutes while administering nitroprusside in dextrose 5% in water by I.V. drip.

DRUG CHALLENGE

 Protect nitroprusside from light by wrapping the bottle or bag with aluminum foil. Nitroprusside increases blood cyanide levels and may result in toxicity. Monitor levels and watch for adverse effects, including ineffective oxygenation levels despite adequate cardiac output.

■ Watch for arrhythmias in patients receiving a cardiac glycoside and for marked respiratory depression in those receiving morphine.
■ Assess the patient's condition frequently, and record his response to treatment.
■ Monitor ABG levels, oral and I.V. fluid intake, urine output and, in the patient with a pulmonary artery catheter, pulmonary end-diastolic and wedge pressures. Check the cardiac monitor often.

Pulmonary embolism and infarction

Pulmonary embolism is an obstruction of the pulmonary arterial bed by a dislodged thrombus or foreign substance. Types of emboli include air emboli, amniotic fluid emboli, fat emboli, talc emboli (from drugs intended for oral administration that are injected I.V. by addicts), and tumor cell emboli. More than half of such thrombi arise in the deep veins of the legs and are usually multiple. Although pulmonary infarction (tissue death) may be so mild as to be asymptomatic, massive embolism (more than 50% obstruction of pulmonary arterial circulation) and infarction can be rapidly fatal.

Causes

■ Dislodged thrombi (from trauma, sudden muscular action, or a change in peripheral blood flow)

Predisposing factors

■ Advanced age
■ Burns
■ Chronic pulmonary disease
■ Heart failure or atrial fibrillation
■ Hormonal contraceptives
■ Long-term immobility
■ Lower-extremity fractures or surgery
■ Malignancy
■ Obesity
■ Pregnancy
■ Recent surgery
■ Thrombophlebitis, polycythemia vera, thrombocytosis, autoimmune hemolytic anemia, and sickle cell disease
■ Varicose veins and vascular injury

Signs and symptoms

■ Angina or pleuritic chest pain
■ Circulatory collapse (weak, rapid pulse; hypotension)
■ Crackles at the site of embolism

- Cyanosis
- Dyspnea
- Hypoxia (restlessness)
- Jugular vein distention
- Leg edema
- Low-grade fever
- Massive hemoptysis
- Pleural effusion
- Pleural friction rub
- Productive cough (sputum may be blood-tinged)
- Right-sided ventricular S_3 gallop and increased intensity of the pulmonic component of S_2
- Splinting of the chest
- Syncope
- Tachycardia

Diagnostic tests

- Chest X-ray helps to rule out other pulmonary diseases; it also shows areas of atelectasis, an elevated diaphragm, pleural effusion, a prominent pulmonary artery and, occasionally, the characteristic wedge-shaped infiltrate suggestive of pulmonary infarction.
- Spiral computed tomography scan may identify a thrombus in the pulmonary vasculature.
- Lung scan shows perfusion defects in areas beyond occluded vessels; it doesn't rule out microemboli.
- Pulmonary angiography reveals emboli.
- In extensive embolism, the electrocardiogram may show right-axis deviation; right bundle-branch block; tall, peaked P waves; ST-segment depression and T-wave inversions (indicating right heart strain); and supraventricular tachyarrhythmias.
- Arterial blood gas (ABG) analysis showing decreased partial pressures of arterial oxygen and carbon dioxide are characteristic but don't always occur.

Treatment

- Treatment includes initiation of oxygen therapy, as needed.
- Anticoagulation with heparin inhibits new thrombus formation; this treatment is monitored by daily coagulation studies (partial thromboplastin time [PTT]). Low-molecular-weight heparin has been used successfully for intramuscular injections.
- Long-term therapy with oral anticoagulants, such as warfarin (Coumadin), is used to prevent recurrence.
- Patients with massive pulmonary embolism and shock may need fibrinolytic therapy with urokinase, streptokinase, or a tissue plasminogen activator to enhance fibrinolysis of the pulmonary emboli and remaining thrombi.
- Emboli that cause hypotension may require the use of vasopressors.
- Treatment of septic emboli requires antibiotics, not anticoagulants, and evaluation for the infection's source, particularly endocarditis.
- Surgery (which shouldn't be done without angiographic evidence of pulmonary embolism) consists of vena caval ligation, plication, or insertion of a device (umbrella filter) to filter blood returning to the heart and lungs.
- To prevent postoperative venous thromboembolism, a combination of heparin and dihydroergotamine may be given.

Nursing considerations

- Administer oxygen as ordered; monitor ABG levels and pulse oximetry for trends.
- Be prepared to provide endotracheal intubation with assisted ventilation if breathing is severely compromised.
- Administer heparin, as needed, through I.V. push or continuous drip. Monitor coagulation studies daily. Effec-

tive heparin therapy raises PTT to 1.5 to 2.5 times normal.

■ After the patient's condition is stable, encourage him to move about frequently, and assist with isometric and range-of-motion exercises.

■ Check pedal pulses, temperature, and color of the feet to detect venostasis. Never vigorously massage the patient's legs.

■ Use incentive spirometry to assist in deep breathing.

■ Warn the patient not to cross his legs because it promotes thrombus formation.

DRUG CHALLENGE

 Watch closely for nosebleed, petechiae, and other signs of abnormal bleeding; check stools for occult blood. Tell the patient to prevent bleeding by shaving with an electric razor and by brushing his teeth with a soft toothbrush. Advise patients taking anticoagulants to watch for signs of bleeding (bloody stools, blood in urine, large ecchymoses), to take the prescribed medication exactly as ordered, and to avoid taking any additional medication (even for headaches or colds) or changing doses of medication without consulting their practitioners.

■ Stress the importance of follow-up laboratory tests (prothrombin time) to monitor anticoagulant therapy.

■ To prevent pulmonary emboli in patients predisposed to this condition, encourage early ambulation. With close medical supervision, low-dose heparin may be useful prophylactically.

■ Pulmonary hypertension

Pulmonary hypertension occurs when pulmonary artery pressure (PAP) rises above normal and isn't attributable to the effects of aging or altitude. In both the rare primary form and the more common secondary form, a resting systolic PAP greater than 30 mm Hg and a mean PAP greater than 18 mm HG indicates pulmonary hypertension. Primary, or idiopathic, pulmonary hypertension is rare; secondary pulmonary hypertension results from existing cardiac or pulmonary disease. Primary pulmonary hypertension begins as hypertrophy of the small pulmonary arteries. The medial and intimal muscle layers of these vessels thicken, decreasing distensibility and increasing resistance. This disorder then progresses to vascular sclerosis and obliteration of small vessels. Secondary pulmonary hypertension results from diseases producing alveolar destruction and increased pulmonary vascular resistance. The prognosis depends on the severity of the underlying disorder.

Causes
Primary pulmonary hypertension
■ Altered immune mechanisms

Secondary pulmonary hypertension
■ Hypoxemia from an underlying disease process, including:
 – alveolar hypoventilation (chronic obstructive pulmonary disease , sarcoidosis, diffuse interstitial pneumonia, pulmonary metastasis, scleroderma)
 – atrial or ventricular septal defect
 – kyphoscoliosis
 – mitral stenosis
 – obesity
 – obstructive sleep apnea
 – patent ductus arteriosus
 – rheumatic valvular disease
 – vascular obstruction (pulmonary embolism, vasculitis, left atrial myxoma,

idiopathic veno-occlusive disease, fibrosing mediastinitis, mediastinal neoplasm).

Signs and symptoms

- Fatigability
- Increasing dyspnea on exertion
- Signs of right-sided heart failure (peripheral edema, ascites, jugular vein distention, and hepatomegaly)
- Syncope
- Variable with underlying disorder
- Weakness

Diagnostic tests

- Arterial blood gas (ABG) analysis reveals hypoxemia (decreased partial pressure of oxygen).
- In right ventricular hypertrophy, electrocardiography shows right-axis deviation and tall or peaked P waves in inferior leads.
- Cardiac catheterization shows increased PAP—pulmonary systolic pressure above 30 mm Hg; pulmonary artery wedge pressure (PAWP) is increased if the underlying cause is left-sided myxoma, mitral stenosis, or left-side failure.
- Pulmonary angiography detects filling defects in pulmonary vasculature, such as those that develop in patients with pulmonary emboli.
- In underlying obstructive disease, pulmonary function tests may show decreased flow rates and increased residual volume; in underlying restrictive disease, total lung capacity may decrease.

Treatment

- Oxygen therapy is initiated to decrease hypoxemia and resulting pulmonary vascular resistance.
- For patients with right-sided heart failure, treatment also includes fluid restriction, cardiac glycosides to increase cardiac output, and diuretics.

- Treatment also includes correction of the underlying cause. If that isn't possible and the disease progresses, the patient may need a heart-lung transplant.
- Epoprostenol (PGI2) may be given as a continuous home infusion in patients with primary pulmonary hypertension.

Nursing considerations

- Administer oxygen therapy as required, and observe the response. Be alert for signs of increasing dyspnea so that treatment can be adjusted accordingly.
- Monitor ABG levels for acidosis and hypoxemia. Watch for changes in level of consciousness.
- When caring for a patient with right-sided heart failure, especially one receiving diuretics, record weight daily, carefully measure intake and output, and explain all medications and diet restrictions.
- Check for increasing jugular vein distention, which may indicate fluid overload.
- Monitor vital signs, especially blood pressure and heart rate. Watch for hypotension and tachycardia. If the patient has a pulmonary artery catheter, check PAP and PAWP as required and watch for any changes.
- Advise against overexertion and suggest frequent rest periods between activities.
- Refer the patient to the social services department if special equipment (such as oxygen equipment) is needed for home use.
- Make sure that the patient understands the prescribed diet and medications.

▌Pyelonephritis, acute

One of the most common renal diseases, acute pyelonephritis (also known as *acute infective tubulointerstitial nephritis*)

Chronic pyelonephritis

Chronic pyelonephritis is a persistent kidney inflammation that can scar the kidneys and may lead to chronic renal failure. Its cause may be bacterial, metastatic, or urogenous. This disease is most common in patients who are predisposed to recurrent acute pyelonephritis, such as those with urinary obstruction or vesicoureteral reflux.

Clinical features

Patients with chronic pyelonephritis may have a childhood history of unexplained fevers or bedwetting. Signs and symptoms may include flank pain, anemia, low urine specific gravity, proteinuria, leukocytes in urine and, especially in late stages, hypertension. Uremia rarely develops from chronic pyelonephritis unless structural abnormalities exist in the excretory system. Bacteriuria may be intermittent. When no bacteria are found in the urine, diagnosis depends on excretory urography (renal pelvis may appear small and flattened) and renal biopsy.

Treatment

Effective treatment of chronic pyelonephritis requires control of hypertension, elimination of the existing obstruction (when possible), and long-term antimicrobial therapy.

is a sudden inflammation caused by bacteria that primarily affects the interstitial area and the renal pelvis or, less often, the renal tubules. Typically, the infection spreads from the bladder to the ureters, then to the kidneys, as in vesicoureteral reflux. Vesicoureteral reflux may result from congenital weakness at the junction of the ureter and the bladder. Pyelonephritis occurs more commonly in females, probably because of a shorter

urethra and the proximity of the urinary meatus to the vagina and rectum (both of which allow bacteria to reach the bladder more easily) and a lack of the antibacterial prostatic secretions produced in the male. With treatment and continued follow-up, the prognosis is good and extensive permanent damage is rare. (See *Chronic pyelonephritis.*)

Causes

- Contamination from instrumentation (catheterization, cystoscopy, or urologic surgery)
- *Escherichia coli, Proteus, Pseudomonas, Staphylococcus aureus,* and *Streptococcus faecalis*
- Hematogenic infection (septicemia or endocarditis)
- Inability to empty the bladder (neurogenic bladder)
- Lymphatic infection.
- Urinary obstruction (tumors, strictures, or benign prostatic hyperplasia)
- Urinary stasis

Predisposing factors

- Age
- Bacterial growth in the urine due to glycosuria
- Neurogenic bladder
- Other renal diseases
- Pregnancy
- Sexually active female

Signs and symptoms

- Anorexia
- Burning during urination
- Cloudy urine with ammonia or fishy odor
- Dysuria
- Flank pain
- General fatigue
- Hematuria (usually microscopic but may be gross)
- Nocturia
- Shaking chills

Preventing acute pyelonephritis

Review these teaching points with your patient to help prevent acute pyelonephritis.
■ Instruct female patients to prevent bacterial contamination by wiping the perineum from front to back after defecation.

■ Advise routine checkups for patients with a history of urinary tract infections.
■ Teach patients to recognize signs and symptoms of infection, such as cloudy urine, burning on urination, urgency, and frequency, especially when accompanied by a low-grade fever.

■ Temperature of 102° F (38.9° C) or higher
■ Urinary frequency and urgency

Diagnostic tests
■ Diagnosis requires urinalysis and culture. Typical findings include:
– pyuria (pus in urine)—urine sediment reveals the presence of leukocytes singly, in clumps, and in casts; and, possibly, a few red blood cells
– significant bacteriuria—more than 100,000 organisms/µl of urine revealed in urine culture
– low specific gravity and osmolality, resulting from a temporarily decreased ability to concentrate urine
– slightly alkaline urine pH
– proteinuria, glycosuria, and ketonuria (less common).
■ X-ray films of the kidneys, ureters, and bladder may reveal calculi, tumors, or cysts in the kidneys and urinary tract.
■ Excretory urography may show asymmetrical kidneys.

Treatment
■ Treatment consists of administration of I.V. antibiotics; chronic pyelonephritis may require long-term antibiotic therapy. Commonly used antibiotics include sulfa drugs, amoxicillin, cephalosporins, levofloxacin, and ciprofloxacin.
■ Urinary analgesics such as phenazopyridine are also appropriate.

■ Follow-up treatment includes reculturing urine after drug therapy stops.
■ In obstruction or vesicoureteral reflux treatment may necessitate surgery to relieve the obstruction or correct the anomaly.
■ Patients at high risk for recurring urinary tract and kidney infections—such as those with prolonged use of an indwelling urinary catheter or maintenance antibiotic therapy—require long-term follow-up.

Nursing considerations
■ Administer antipyretics for fever.
■ Make sure the patient receives plenty of fluids so that he achieves urine output of more than 2,000 ml/day. This helps to empty the bladder of contaminated urine. Don't encourage the intake of more than 3 qt (3 L) of fluids because this may decrease the effectiveness of the antibiotics.
■ Teach proper technique for collecting a clean-catch urine specimen. Be sure to refrigerate or culture a urine specimen within 30 minutes of collection to prevent overgrowth of bacteria.
■ Stress the need to complete prescribed antibiotic therapy, even after symptoms subside. Encourage long-term follow-up care for high-risk patients.
■ Provide patient teaching on disease prevention. (See *Preventing acute pyelonephritis*.)

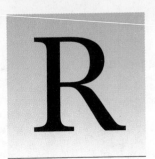

Rabies

Usually transmitted by an animal bite, rabies (hydrophobia) is an acute central nervous system (CNS) infection caused by a ribonucleic acid virus.

The incubation period ranges from 10 days to 7 years, with an average of 3 to 7 weeks. In the United States, dog vaccinations have reduced rabies transmission to humans. Wild animals—such as raccoons, skunks, foxes, and bats—account for 70% of rabies cases.

If symptoms occur, rabies is almost always fatal. Treatment soon after a bite, however, may prevent fatal CNS invasion. After an animal bite, the virus begins to replicate in the striated muscle cells at the bite site. It next spreads up the nerve to the CNS and replicates in the brain. Finally, it moves through the nerves into other tissues, including the salivary glands. Occasionally, airborne droplets and infected tissue transplants can transmit the virus.

Causes
- Bite from an infected animal

Signs and symptoms
Local and prodromal (after 1 to 3 months' incubation)
- Local or radiating pain or burning
- Sensation of cold, pruritus, and tingling at the bite site
- Slight fever (100° to 102° F [37.8° to 38.9° C])
- Malaise
- Headache
- Anorexia
- Nausea
- Sore throat
- Persistent loose cough
- Nervousness, anxiety, and irritability
- Hyperesthesia
- Photophobia
- Sensitivity to loud noises
- Pupillary dilation
- Tachycardia
- Shallow respirations
- Excessive salivation
- Lacrimation
- Perspiration

From 2 to 10 days after onset of prodromal symptoms
- Agitation and marked restlessness
- Anxiety and apprehension
- Cranial nerve dysfunction that causes ocular palsies, strabismus, asymmetrical pupillary dilation or constriction, absent corneal reflexes, weakened facial muscles, and hoarseness
- Tachycardia or bradycardia
- Cyclic respirations
- Urine retention
- Temperature of about 103° F (39.4° C)

- Hydrophobia (literally, "fear of water"), during which forceful, painful pharyngeal muscle spasms expel liquids from the mouth and cause dehydration and, possibly, apnea, cyanosis, and death
- Difficulty swallowing, causing frothy saliva to drool from the patient's mouth
- Eventually, even the sight, mention, or thought of water causing uncontrollable pharyngeal muscle spasms and excessive salivation
- Between episodes of excitation and hydrophobia, the patient commonly cooperative and lucid

Terminal phase (about 3 days after excitation and hydrophobia subside)
- Gradual, generalized, flaccid paralysis
- Peripheral vascular collapse
- Coma and death

Diagnostic tests
- Virus is isolated from the patient's saliva or throat, and blood tests show fluorescent rabies antibody (FRA).
- The white blood cell count is elevated, with increased polymorphonuclear and large mononuclear cells.
- Urinary glucose, acetone, and protein levels are elevated.
- Confinement of the suspected animal for 10 days of observation by a veterinarian also helps support this diagnosis.
- The animal's brain tissue can be tested for FRA and Negri bodies (oval or round masses that conclusively confirm rabies).

Treatment
- All bite wounds and scratches are thoroughly washed with soap and water. (See *First aid for animal bites*.)
- Check the patient's immunization status, and administer tetanus-diphtheria prophylaxis if needed.

ACTION STAT!

First aid for animal bites

Take these actions if a patient is bitten by an animal:
- Immediately wash the site of the bite vigorously with soap and water for at least 10 minutes to remove the animal's saliva.
- Flush the wound with a viricidal agent, followed by a clear-water rinse.
- Apply a sterile dressing when you're sure the wound is clean.
- Don't immediately stop the bleeding (unless it's massive) because blood flow helps to clean the wound.
- Ask the patient about the bite episode. Find out whether he provoked the animal (if so, chances are it isn't rabid) and whether he can identify it or its owner (the animal may need to be confined for observation).
- Consult local health authorities for treatment information.

- Antibiotics are given, as prescribed, to control bacterial infection.
- If the wound requires suturing, special treatment and suturing techniques must be used to allow proper wound drainage.

Nursing considerations
- Rotate injection sites on the upper arm or thigh when injecting the rabies vaccine. Watch for and treat symptoms of redness, itching, pain, and tenderness at the injection site.
- Cooperate with public health authorities to determine the vaccination status of the animal. If the animal is proven rabid, help identify others at risk.
- Provide aggressive supportive care (even after the onset of coma) to make

probable death less agonizing if rabies develops.
- Monitor the patient's cardiac and pulmonary function continuously.
- Start contact and droplet precautions to prevent the spread of infection. Wear a gown, gloves, eye protection, and a mask when handling saliva and articles contaminated with saliva. Take precautions to avoid being bitten by the patient during the excitation phase.
- Keep the room dark and quiet.
- Provide emotional support to the patient and his family to help them cope with the patient's symptoms and probable death.
- Stress the need for vaccination of household pets that may be exposed to rabid wild animals to help prevent this dreaded disease. Tell pet owners that if a wild animal bites a pet, they should seek veterinary assistance immediately. Warn people to avoid touching wild animals, especially if they appear ill or overly docile (a possible sign of rabies).
- Recommend prophylactic rabies vaccination to high-risk people, such as farm workers, forest rangers, spelunkers (cave explorers), and veterinarians.

Raynaud's disease

One of several primary arteriospastic disorders, Raynaud's disease is characterized by episodic vasospasm in the small peripheral arteries and arterioles, precipitated by exposure to cold or stress. This condition occurs bilaterally and usually affects the hands or, less commonly, the feet.

Raynaud's disease is most prevalent in women, particularly between late adolescence and age 40. A benign condition, it requires no specific treatment and has no serious after-effects.

Raynaud's *phenomenon*, however, a condition usually associated with several connective tissue disorders—such as scleroderma, systemic lupus erythematosus, and polymyositis—has a progressive course, leading to ischemia, gangrene, and amputation. Differentiating the two disorders is difficult because some patients who experience mild symptoms of Raynaud's disease for several years may later develop overt connective tissue disease—most commonly, scleroderma.

Causes
- Unknown

Signs and symptoms
- Cutaneous gangrene (uncommon)
- Numbness and tingling
- Skin on the fingers blanches, then becomes cyanotic before changing to red and before changing from cold to normal temperature after exposure to cold or stress
- Trophic changes, such as sclerodactyly, ulcerations, or chronic paronychia (in long-standing disease)

Diagnostic tests
- Cold stimulation test produces symptoms.
- Other tests should rule out secondary disease processes, such as chronic arterial occlusive disease or connective tissue disease.

Treatment
- Initially, treatment consists of avoidance of cold, mechanical, or chemical injury, smoking cessation, and reassurance that symptoms are benign.
- Calcium channel blockers may be prescribed to reduce arterial spasm.
- Vasodilators relax the walls of the blood vessels (for unusually severe symptoms).
- Drug therapy may include phenoxybenzamine (Dibenzyline) or reserpine.

- Sympathectomy may be helpful when conservative treatment fails to prevent ischemic ulcers (occurs in less than 25% of patients).
- Practicing a stress reduction technique, such as medication, biofeedback, or yoga, may be helpful.

Nursing considerations

- Warn the patient against becoming exposed to the cold. Tell the patient to wear mittens or gloves in cold weather or when handling cold items or defrosting the freezer.
- Advise the patient to avoid stressful situations and to stop smoking.
- Instruct the patient to inspect the skin frequently and to seek immediate care for signs of skin breakdown or infection.
- Teach the patient about calcium channel blockers or vasodilators, their use, and their adverse effects.

<small>**DRUG CHALLENGE**</small>

 Some drugs can aggravate Raynaud's disease by increasing blood vessel spasm. Examples include beta-adrenergic blockers, hormonal contraceptives, and over-the-counter medications, such as cough and cold preparations and diet drugs that contain phenylpropanolamine or pseudoephedrine.

- Provide psychological support and reassurance to allay the patient's fear of amputation and disfigurement.

■ Renal calculi

Although renal calculi (or kidney stones) may form anywhere in the urinary tract, they usually develop in the renal pelvis or the calyces of the kidneys. Such formation follows precipitation of substances normally dissolved in urine (calcium oxalate, calcium phosphate, magnesium ammonium phosphate or, occasionally, urate or cystine).

Renal calculi vary in size and may be solitary or multiple. They may remain in the renal pelvis or enter the ureter and may damage renal parenchyma; large calculi cause pressure necrosis. In certain locations, calculi cause obstruction, with resultant hydronephrosis, and tend to recur.

About 1 in 1,000 Americans require hospitalization for renal calculi. They're more common in males than in females and are rare in blacks and children.

Causes

- Unknown
- Genetic factors

Predisposing factors

- Dehydration and resultant decreased urine production (causes calculus-forming substances to become concentrated)
- Infection in tissue (provides a site for calculus development)
- Metabolic factors such as hyperparathyroidism, renal tubular acidosis, elevated uric acid levels (usually with gout), defective oxalate metabolism, genetic defect in cystine metabolism, and excessive intake of vitamin D or dietary calcium
- pH changes (provide a favorable medium for calculus formation, especially for magnesium ammonium phosphate or calcium phosphate calculi)
- Urinary stasis (as in immobility from spinal cord injury; may produce an obstruction that could form calculi)

Signs and symptoms

- Abdominal distention
- Anuria (rarely)
- Fever and chills
- Flank, back, or abdominal pain depending on the location of the calculi

- Hematuria
- Nausea and vomiting
- Pyuria

Diagnostic tests
- Kidney-ureter-bladder radiography reveals most renal calculi.
- Excretory urography, retrograde pyelography, abdominal computed tomography scan, or abdominal or kidney magnetic resonance imaging reveals tumors or obstructions of the ureter. These tests help confirm the diagnosis and determine the size and location of calculi.
- Calculus analysis shows mineral content.
- Kidney ultrasonography, an easily performed noninvasive, nontoxic test, helps detect obstructive changes such as unilateral or bilateral hydronephrosis.
- Urine culture of midstream specimen may indicate urinary tract infection.
- A 24-hour urine collection is evaluated for calcium oxalate, phosphorus, and uric acid excretion levels; three separate collections, along with blood samples, are needed for accurate testing.
- Serial blood calcium and phosphorus levels help detect hyperparathyroidism and show an increased calcium level in proportion to the normal level of serum protein.
- Blood protein level measures the level of free calcium unbound to protein.
- Blood chloride and bicarbonate levels may show renal tubular acidosis.
- Increased blood uric acid levels may indicate gout as the cause.
- Other tests must rule out appendicitis, cholecystitis, peptic ulcer, and pancreatitis as potential sources of pain.

Treatment
- Treatment usually involves encouraging the natural passage of renal calculi through vigorous hydration because 90% of them are smaller than 5 mm in diameter.
- Antimicrobial therapy (varying with the cultured organism) is used to treat infection.
- Analgesics, such as meperidine (Demerol) or morphine, may be prescribed for pain.
- A diuretic may be given, as ordered, to prevent urinary stasis and further calculus formation. (Thiazides decrease calcium excretion into urine.)
- Prevention of calculus formation includes a low-calcium diet, often combined with oxalate-binding cholestyramine, for absorptive hypercalciuria; parathyroidectomy for hyperparathyroidism; and allopurinol (Zyloprim) and urinary alkalinization for uric acid calculi.
- Surgical removal may be required if calculi are too large for natural passage.
- Percutaneous ultrasonic lithotripsy and extracorporeal shock-wave lithotripsy shatter the calculus into fragments for removal by suction or natural passage.
- Preventive measures include hydration, early mobilization of patients, repositioning, and exercise for immobilized patients or those with inadequate mobility.

Nursing considerations
- Maintain a 24- to 48-hour record of urine pH with nitrazine pH paper, strain all urine through gauze or a tea strainer, and save all solid material recovered for analysis to aid diagnosis.
- Encourage the patient to walk, if possible, to facilitate spontaneous passage. To help prevent future stones, promote sufficient intake of fluids to maintain a urine output of 3 to 4 L/day (urine should be very diluted and colorless). Use caution in the patient with a history of cardiac disease because he may not be

able to tolerate these large volumes of fluid.

▪ Offer fruit juices, particularly cranberry juice, to help acidify urine. If the patient can't drink the required amount of fluid, supplemental I.V. fluids may be given. Record intake and output and daily weight to assess fluid status and renal function.

▪ Stress the importance of proper diet and compliance with drug therapy. For example, if the patient's stone was caused by a hyperuricemic condition, advise him or whoever prepares his meals which foods are high in purine. (See *Preventing recurrence of renal calculi.*)

▪ Provide reassurance if surgery is necessary. The patient is apt to be fearful, especially if surgery involves removing a kidney, so emphasize that the body can adapt well to having one kidney. If he's to have an abdominal or flank incision, teach deep-breathing and coughing exercises.

▪ Provide indwelling urinary catheter or nephrostomy tube care after surgery. Expect bloody drainage from the catheter.

▪ Check dressings regularly for bloody drainage, and know how much drainage to expect. Watch closely for signs of suspected hemorrhage (such as excessive drainage and rising pulse rate). Use sterile technique when changing dressings.

▪ Watch for signs and symptoms of infection (such as rising fever and chills), and administer an antibiotic as prescribed.

▪ Encourage frequent position changes and ambulation as soon as possible to prevent pneumonia. Have the patient hold a small pillow over the operative site to splint the incision and thereby facilitate deep-breathing and coughing exercises and incentive spirometer use.

Preventing recurrence of renal calculi

Before discharge, your patient needs to learn how to prevent a recurrence of renal calculi. Teach him to:
▪ closely follow the prescribed dietary and medication regimens
▪ increase fluid intake
▪ check his urine pH, if appropriate, and keep a daily record
▪ immediately report symptoms of acute obstruction (pain and the inability to void).

▌Renal failure, acute

Obstruction, reduced circulation, and renal parenchymatous disease can all cause sudden interruption of kidney function. Acute renal failure is usually reversible with medical treatment; otherwise, it may progress to end-stage renal disease, uremic syndrome, and death. About 5% of all hospitalized patients develop acute renal failure.

Acute renal failure can be classified as prerenal, intrarenal (intrinsic or parenchymatous), or postrenal.

Causes

▪ Prerenal failure from diminished blood flow to the kidneys, which may result from:
– autoimmune disorders such as scleroderma
– blood loss
– cardiovascular disorders, such as heart failure, arrhythmias, and tamponade
– disorders of the blood, such as idiopathic thrombocytopenic purpura, transfusion reactions, and other hemolytic disorders
– disorders resulting from childbirth-like bleeding (associated with placen-

tal abruption or placenta previa) that can damage the kidneys
- embolism
- hypovolemia
- malignant hypertension
- pooling of fluid in ascites or burns
- sepsis
- shock
■ Intrarenal renal failure from damage to the kidneys, which may result from:
- acute poststreptococcal glomerulonephritis
- acute pyelonephritis
- acute tubular necrosis
- bilateral renal vein thrombosis
- ischemia
- nephrotoxins
- renal myeloma
- sickle cell disease
- systemic lupus erythematosus
- vasculitis
■ Postrenal failure from a bilateral obstruction of urine outflow, which may result from:
- benign prostatic hyperplasia
- clots
- papillae from papillary necrosis
- renal calculi
- strictures
- tumors
- urethral edema from catheterization

Signs and symptoms
■ Early signs: oliguria, azotemia and, rarely, anuria
■ Fever and chills, indicating infection, a common complication
■ Later signs: electrolyte imbalances, metabolic acidosis, and other severe effects as the patient becomes increasingly uremic and renal dysfunction disrupts other body systems:
- Cardiovascular—early in the disease, hypotension; later, hypertension, arrhythmias, fluid overload, heart failure, systemic edema, anemia, altered clotting mechanisms

- Central nervous system (CNS)—headache, drowsiness, irritability, confusion, peripheral neuropathy, seizures, coma
- Cutaneous—dryness, pruritus, pallor, purpura; rarely, uremic frost
- GI—anorexia, nausea, vomiting, diarrhea or constipation, stomatitis, bleeding, hematemesis, dry mucous membranes, uremic breath
- Respiratory—Kussmaul's respirations, pulmonary edema

Diagnostic tests
■ Blood test results indicating intrinsic acute renal failure include elevated urea nitrogen, creatinine, and potassium levels; low bicarbonate and hemoglobin (Hb) levels; and low pH and hematocrit (HCT).
■ Urine specimens show casts, cellular debris, decreased specific gravity and, in glomerular diseases, proteinuria and urine osmolality close to serum osmolality. The urine sodium level is less than 20 mEq/L if oliguria results from decreased perfusion and more than 40 mEq/L if it results from an intrinsic problem.
■ Other studies include renal ultrasonography, kidney-ureter-bladder radiography, excretory urography, renal scan, retrograde pyelography, computed tomography, and nephrotomography.

Treatment
■ Identify and treat reversible causes, such as nephrotoxic drug therapy, obstructive uropathy, and volume depletion.
■ Supportive measures include a diet high in calories and low in protein, sodium, and potassium, with supplemental vitamins and restricted fluids.
■ Meticulous electrolyte monitoring is essential to detect hyperkalemia. As ordered, give I.V. hypertonic glucose and

insulin—and oral or rectal potassium exchange resin—to remove potassium from the body if hyperkalemia occurs.

■ Hemodialysis or peritoneal dialysis may be necessary if measures fail to control hyperkalemia and uremic symptoms.

■ Continuous renal replacement therapy may be used for patients who can't tolerate hemodialysis or who are hemodynamically unstable.

Nursing considerations

■ Measure and record intake and output, including all body fluids, such as wound drainage, nasogastric output, and diarrhea. Weigh the patient daily.

■ Assess HCT and Hb level, and replace blood components as needed. *Don't* use whole blood if the patient is prone to heart failure and can't tolerate extra fluid volume.

■ Monitor the patient's vital signs. Watch closely for signs and symptoms of pericarditis (such as pleuritic chest pain, tachycardia, and pericardial friction rub), inadequate renal perfusion (such as hypotension), and acidosis.

■ Monitor electrolyte levels to detect hyperkalemia. Strictly monitor potassium levels. Signs and symptoms of hyperkalemia include malaise, anorexia, paresthesia, muscle weakness, and electrocardiogram changes (such as tall, peaked T waves; widening QRS complex; and disappearing P waves). Don't give any drug that contains potassium.

■ Assess the patient frequently, especially during emergency treatment to lower his potassium level. If the patient receives hypertonic glucose and insulin infusions, monitor his potassium level. If you give sodium polystyrene sulfonate (Kayexalate) rectally, make sure the patient doesn't retain it and become constipated, which could lead to bowel perforation.

■ Maintain nutritional status. Provide a high-calorie, low-protein, low-sodium, low-potassium diet, with vitamin supplements. Give the patient with anorexia small, frequent meals.

■ Prevent complications of immobility by encouraging frequent coughing and deep breathing and by performing passive range-of-motion exercises. Help the patient walk as soon as possible. Add lubricating lotion to the patient's bathwater to combat skin dryness.

■ Provide frequent mouth care to prevent dry mucous membranes. If stomatitis occurs, the patient may need an antibiotic solution. Have the patient swish the solution around in his mouth before swallowing.

■ Use appropriate safety measures, such as side rails and restraints; the patient with CNS involvement may be dizzy or confused.

■ Provide emotional support to the patient and his family. Reassure them by clearly explaining all procedures.

■ During peritoneal dialysis, position the patient carefully. Elevate the head of the bed to reduce pressure on the diaphragm and aid respiration. Stay alert for bleeding and signs of infection, such as cloudy drainage and elevated temperature. Measure intake and output, including the dialysate solution, and record any discrepancies in the amount of the dialysate returned.

■ Reduce the amount of dialysate if pain occurs. If the patient has diabetes, periodically monitor his blood glucose level, and administer insulin as needed. Watch for complications, such as peritonitis, atelectasis, hypokalemia, pneumonia, and shock.

■ Check the blood access site (an arteriovenous fistula or a subclavian or femoral catheter) every 2 hours for patency and signs of clotting if the patient requires hemodialysis. Don't use the arm with the shunt or fistula for taking blood pressure or drawing blood. Weigh the patient before beginning dialysis.

■ During dialysis, monitor the patient's vital signs, clotting times, blood flow, the function of the vascular access site, and arterial and venous pressures. Watch for complications, such as septicemia, embolism, hepatitis, and rapid fluid and electrolyte loss.

■ Monitor the patient's vital signs and the vascular access site, weigh the patient, and watch for signs of fluid and electrolyte imbalances after dialysis.

Renal failure, chronic

Although chronic renal failure is usually the result of a gradually progressive loss of renal function, it occasionally results from a rapidly progressive disease of sudden onset. Few symptoms develop until after more than 75% of glomerular filtration is lost, then the remaining normal parenchyma deteriorates progressively, and symptoms worsen as renal function decreases.

Chronic renal failure may progress through the following stages:

■ reduced renal reserve (glomerular filtration rate [GFR] 45% to 50% of normal)

■ renal insufficiency (GFR of 20% to 35% of normal)

■ renal failure (GFR of 20% to 25% of normal)

■ end-stage renal disease (GFR less than 20% of normal).

If chronic renal failure continues unchecked, uremic toxins accumulate and produce potentially fatal physiologic changes in all major organ systems. If the patient can tolerate it, maintenance dialysis or kidney transplantation can sustain life.

Causes

■ Acute renal failure that fails to respond to treatment

■ Chronic glomerular disease such as glomerulonephritis

■ Chronic infection, such as chronic pyelonephritis or tuberculosis

■ Collagen disease such as systemic lupus erythematosus

■ Congenital anomaly such as polycystic kidneys

■ Endocrine disease such as diabetic neuropathy

■ Nephrotoxic drug therapy such as long-term aminoglycoside therapy

■ Obstructive process such as calculi

■ Vascular disease, such as renal nephrosclerosis or hypertension

Signs and symptoms
Cardiovascular

■ Cardiomyopathy

■ Heart failure

■ Hypertension and arrhythmias, including life-threatening ventricular tachycardia or fibrillation

■ Pericardial effusion (and possibly cardiac tamponade)

■ Peripheral edema

■ Uremic pericarditis

Cutaneous

■ Dry, brittle hair that may change color and fall out easily

■ Ecchymoses

■ Pallid, yellowish bronze, dry, and scaly skin

■ Petechiae

■ Purpura

■ Severe itching

■ Thin, brittle fingernails with characteristic lines

■ Uremic frost (most common in critically ill or terminal patients)

Endocrine changes

- Amenorrhea and cessation of menses in women
- Impaired carbohydrate metabolism (causing increased blood glucose levels similar to those found with diabetes mellitus)
- Impotence and decreased sperm production in men
- Increased aldosterone secretion (related to increased renin production)
- Infertility and decreased libido in both sexes
- Stunted growth in children (even with elevated growth hormone levels)

GI

- Anorexia, nausea, and vomiting
- Inflammation and ulceration of GI mucosa causing stomatitis, gum ulceration and bleeding and, possibly, parotitis, esophagitis, gastritis, duodenal ulcers, lesions on the small and large bowel, uremic colitis, pancreatitis, and proctitis
- Metallic taste in the mouth
- Uremic fetor (ammonia smell to breath)

Hematopoietic changes

- Anemia
- Blood loss from dialysis and GI bleeding
- Decreased red blood cell (RBC) survival time
- Increased bleeding and clotting disorders, demonstrated by purpura, hemorrhage from body orifices, easy bruising, ecchymoses, and petechiae.
- Mild thrombocytopenia
- Platelet defects

Neurologic

- Apathy
- Coma
- Confusion
- Drowsiness

- EEG changes indicating metabolic encephalopathy
- Irritability
- Muscle cramping and twitching
- Restless leg syndrome, one of the first symptoms of peripheral neuropathy; eventually, progressing to paresthesia and motor nerve dysfunction (usually bilateral footdrop) unless dialysis is initiated
- Seizures
- Shortened memory and attention span

Renal and urologic

- Decreased urine output; urine very dilute and containing casts and crystals
- Fluid overload and metabolic acidosis
- Initially, hypotension, dry mouth, loss of skin turgor, listlessness, fatigue, and nausea; later, somnolence and confusion
- Muscle irritability and then muscle weakness as the potassium level rises
- Sodium retention and overload

Respiratory

- Dyspnea from heart failure
- Kussmaul's respirations as a result of acidosis
- Pleural friction rub and effusions
- Pleuritic pain
- Pulmonary edema
- Reduced pulmonary macrophage activity with increased susceptibility to infection
- Uremic pleuritis and uremic lung (or uremic pneumonitis)

Skeletal changes

- Arterial calcification, which may produce coronary artery disease
- Calcium-phosphorus imbalance and consequent parathyroid hormone imbalances, causing muscle and bone pain, skeletal demineralization, pathologic fractures, and calcifications in the brain, eyes, gums, joints, myocardium, and blood vessels

■ Renal osteodystrophy (renal rickets) in children

Diagnostic tests

■ Blood studies show elevated blood urea nitrogen, creatinine, sodium, and potassium levels; decreased arterial pH and bicarbonate levels; and low hemoglobin (Hb) level and hematocrit (HCT).

■ Creatinine clearance tests show a gradual deterioration of renal function.

■ Kidney biopsy allows histologic identification of underlying pathology.

■ Renal or abdominal X-ray, abdominal computed tomography scan, magnetic resonance imaging, or ultrasonography shows reduced kidney size.

■ Urine specific gravity becomes fixed at 1.010; urinalysis may show proteinuria, glycosuria, erythrocytes, leukocytes, and casts, depending on the cause.

■ X-ray studies include kidney-ureter-bladder radiography, excretory urography, nephrotomography, renal scan, and renal arteriography.

Treatment

■ A low-protein diet reduces the level of protein metabolism end products, which the kidneys can't excrete. (A patient receiving continuous peritoneal dialysis should receive a high-protein diet.)

■ A high-calorie diet prevents ketoacidosis and the negative nitrogen balance that results in catabolism and tissue atrophy. The diet should also restrict sodium and potassium.

■ Maintaining fluid balance requires careful monitoring of the patient's vital signs, weight changes, and urine volume.

■ Loop diuretics, such as furosemide (Lasix) (if some renal function remains), and fluid restriction can reduce fluid retention.

■ A cardiac glycoside, such as digoxin (Lanoxin), may be used to mobilize edema fluids.

■ An angiotensin-converting enzyme inhibitor may be given to decrease blood pressure and associated edema.

■ An antiemetic taken before meals may relieve nausea and vomiting; famotidine (Pepcid), omeprazole (Prilosec), or ranitidine (Zantac) may decrease gastric irritation.

■ Methylcellulose (Citrucel) or docusate (Colace) can help prevent constipation.

■ Anemia necessitates iron and folate supplements; severe anemia requires infusion of fresh frozen packed cells or washed packed cells. However, transfusions relieve anemia only temporarily.

■ Synthetic erythropoietin (epoetin alfa) may be given to stimulate the division and differentiation of cells within the bone marrow to produce RBCs. Androgen therapy (testosterone or nandrolone [Bolandione]) may increase RBC production.

■ Antipruritics, such as trimeprazine or diphenhydramine (Benadryl), relieve itching; aluminum hydroxide gel lowers serum phosphate level.

■ The patient may benefit from supplementary vitamins (particularly B vitamins and vitamin D) and essential amino acids.

■ Carefully monitor serum potassium levels to detect hyperkalemia.

ACTION STAT!

 Emergency treatment for severe hyperkalemia includes dialysis therapy and administration of 50% hypertonic glucose I.V., regular insulin, calcium gluconate I.V., and cation exchange resins such as sodium polystyrene sulfonate (Kayexalate).

ACTION STAT!
Cardiac tamponade resulting from pericardial effusion may require emergency pericardial tap or surgery.

■ Hemodialysis or peritoneal dialysis (particularly continuous ambulatory peritoneal dialysis and continuous cyclic peritoneal dialysis) can help control most manifestations of end-stage renal disease. (See *Continuous ambulatory peritoneal dialysis,* page 532.)

■ Kidney transplantation may be helpful for some patients with end-stage renal disease.

Nursing considerations

■ Provide good skin care. Bathe the patient daily, using superfatted soaps, oatmeal baths, and skin lotion to ease pruritus. Give good perineal care, using mild soap and water. Turn the patient often, and use an airflow mattress to prevent skin breakdown.

■ Provide good oral hygiene. Brush the patient's teeth often with a soft brush or sponge-tipped applicator.

■ Offer small, palatable meals that are also nutritious; try to provide favorite foods within dietary restrictions. Encourage intake of high-calorie foods. Instruct the outpatient to avoid high-sodium, high-protein, and high-potassium foods.

■ Encourage adherence to fluid and protein restrictions. To prevent constipation, stress the need for exercise and sufficient dietary fiber.

■ Watch for hyperkalemia, indicated by cramping of the legs and abdomen and diarrhea. As potassium levels rise, watch for muscle irritability and a weak pulse rate. Monitor electrocardiogram results for indications of hyperkalemia—tall, peaked T waves; widening QRS complex; prolonged PR interval; and disappearance of P waves.

■ Carefully assess the patient's hydration status. Check for jugular vein distention, and auscultate the lungs for crackles. Measure daily intake and output carefully, including all drainage, vomitus, diarrhea, and blood loss. Record daily weight, presence or absence of thirst, axillary sweat, dryness of tongue, hypertension, and peripheral edema.

■ Monitor the patient for bone and joint complications. Prevent pathologic fractures by turning him carefully and ensuring his safety. If the patient is bedridden, provide passive range-of-motion exercises.

■ Encourage deep breathing and coughing to prevent pulmonary congestion. Listen often for crackles, rhonchi, and decreased breath sounds. Stay alert for signs and symptoms of pulmonary edema, such as dyspnea, restlessness, and crackles. Administer a diuretic and other medications as prescribed.

■ Carefully observe and document seizure activity. Infuse sodium bicarbonate for acidosis and a sedative or an anticonvulsant for seizures. Pad the side rails, and keep an oral airway and suction setup at the bedside. Assess the patient's neurologic status periodically, and check for Chvostek's and Trousseau's signs, indicators of low serum calcium levels.

■ Observe the patient for signs of bleeding. Watch for prolonged bleeding at puncture sites and at the vascular access site used for hemodialysis. Monitor Hb level and HCT, and check stools, urine, and vomitus for blood.

■ Watch for signs of pericarditis, such as a pericardial friction rub and chest pain. Also, watch for the disappearance of friction rub, with a drop of 15 to 20 mm Hg in blood pressure during inspiration

Continuous ambulatory peritoneal dialysis

For patients with renal failure, continuous ambulatory peritoneal dialysis (CAPD) is a useful alternative to hemodialysis in a special treatment center. It's a simple, easily taught procedure that allows the patient greater independence.

Using the peritoneum as a dialysis membrane, CAPD allows almost uninterrupted exchange of dialysis solution. Each day, four to six exchanges of fresh dialysis solution are infused. A Tenckhoff catheter is surgically implanted in the abdomen, just below the umbilicus. A bag of dialysis solution is aseptically attached to the tube, and the fluid is allowed to flow into the peritoneal cavity (as shown at top left). This takes about 10 minutes.

The dialyzing fluid remains in the peritoneal cavity for 4 to 6 hours (8 to 10 hours for overnight exchanges). During this time, the bag may be rolled up and placed under a shirt or blouse (as shown at bottom left), and the patient can go about normal activities while dialysis takes place.

The fluid is then drained out of the peritoneal cavity through gravity flow by unrolling the bag and suspending it below the pelvis (as shown at right). Drainage takes about 20 minutes.

After the fluid drains, the patient aseptically connects a new bag of dialyzing solution and fills the peritoneal cavity again. He repeats this procedure four to six times per day.

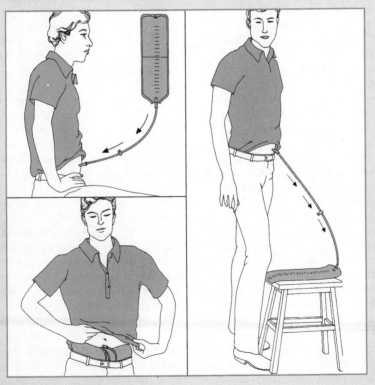

Caring for the patient requiring hemodialysis

Do's

■ Check the vascular access site every 2 hours for patency and the extremity for adequate blood supply and intact nervous function (temperature, pulse rate, capillary refill time, and sensation).

■ If a fistula is present, palpate for a thrill and listen for a bruit. Use a gentle touch to avoid occluding the fistula. Note signs of clotting.

■ Check the patient's hepatitis antigen status. If it's positive, he's a carrier of hepatitis B, and stool, needle, blood, and excretion precautions should be instituted.

■ Monitor hemoglobin level and hematocrit. Assess the patient's tolerance of his levels; he may be more sensitive to lower levels than others. Instruct the anemic patient to conserve energy and to rest frequently.

■ After dialysis, check for disequilibrium syndrome, a result of sudden correction of blood chemistry abnormalities. Signs and symptoms range from a headache to seizures. Also, check for excessive bleeding from the dialysis site. Apply a pressure dressing or absorbable gelatin sponge as indicated. Monitor blood pressure carefully after dialysis.

■ A patient undergoing dialysis is under a great deal of stress, as is his family. Refer them to appropriate counseling agencies for assistance in coping with chronic renal failure.

Don'ts

■ Don't use the arm with the vascular access site to take blood pressure readings, draw blood, or give injections; these procedures may rupture the fistula or cause scarring that occludes blood flow.

■ Withhold the 6 a.m. (or morning) dose of antihypertensive on the morning of dialysis, and instruct the outpatient to do the same.

■ Don't occlude the fistula when palpating for a thrill.

(paradoxical pulse)—an early sign of pericardial tamponade.

■ Schedule medications carefully. Give iron before meals, aluminum hydroxide gels after meals, and an antiemetic, as necessary, 30 minutes before meals. Also give an antihypertensive as prescribed.

■ Apply an emollient to soothe the perianal area before rectal instillation of sodium polystyrene sulfonate if prescribed. Make sure that the sodium polystyrene sulfonate enema is expelled; otherwise, it will cause constipation and won't lower the potassium level.

■ Prepare the patient by fully explaining the procedure if the patient requires dialysis. Make sure that he understands how to protect and care for the arteriovenous shunt, fistula, or other vascular access. (See *Caring for the patient requiring hemodialysis*.)

 # Renal infarction

Renal blood vessel occlusion results in renal infarction—the formation of a coagulated, necrotic area in one or both kidneys. The location and size of the infarction depend on the site of vascular occlusion. Most commonly, infarction affects the renal cortex, but it can extend into the medulla. (See *Sites of renal infarction*, page 534.) Residual renal function after infarction depends on the extent of the damage from the infarction.

Sites of renal infarction

Infarction may occur in the renal cortex or medulla or within the renal blood vessels.

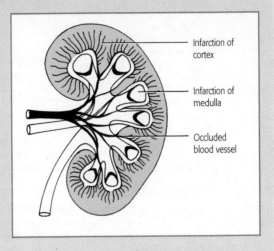

Infarction of cortex

Infarction of medulla

Occluded blood vessel

Causes
- Atherosclerosis
- Renal artery embolism
- Thrombus from flank trauma, sickle cell anemia, scleroderma, or arterionephrosclerosis

Signs and symptoms
- Possibly asymptomatic
- Anorexia, nausea, and vomiting
- Costovertebral tenderness
- Fever
- Renovascular hypertension
- Severe upper abdominal pain or gnawing flank pain and tenderness
- Small nonpalpable kidney (when caused by arterial occlusion)

Diagnostic tests
- Urinalysis reveals proteinuria and microscopic hematuria.
- Urine enzyme levels, especially lactate dehydrogenase (LD) and alkaline phosphatase, are typically elevated as a result of tissue destruction.
- Blood studies may reveal elevated serum enzyme levels, especially aspartate aminotransferase, alkaline phosphatase, and LD. Blood studies may also reveal leukocytosis and an increased erythrocyte sedimentation rate.
- Excretory urography shows absent or reduced excretion of contrast dye, indicating vascular occlusion or urethral obstruction.
- Isotopic renal scan, a noninvasive technique, demonstrates absent or reduced blood flow to the kidneys.
- Renal arteriography provides absolute proof of an existing infarction but is used as a last resort because it's a high-risk procedure.
- Computed tomography pinpoints areas of occlusion and the extent of infarction.

Treatment
- Infection in the infarcted area or significant hypertension may require surgical repair of the occlusion or nephrectomy.

- Surgery to establish collateral circulation to the area can relieve renovascular hypertension.
- Persistent hypertension may respond to antihypertensive therapy and a low-sodium diet.
- Additional treatments include administration of intra-arterial streptokinase (Streptase), blood clot lysis, catheter embolectomy, and heparin therapy.

Nursing considerations
- Assess the degree of renal function, and offer supportive care to maintain homeostasis.
- Monitor the patient's intake and output, vital signs (particularly blood pressure), electrolyte levels, and daily weight.
- Watch for signs of fluid overload, such as dyspnea, tachycardia, jugular vein distention, crackles on auscultation, and electrolyte imbalances.
- Carefully explain all diagnostic procedures.
- Provide reassurance and emotional support for the patient and his family.
- Encourage the patient to return for a follow-up examination, which usually includes excretory urography or a renal scan to assess regained renal function.

Renal tubular acidosis

A syndrome of persistent dehydration, hyperchloremia, hypokalemia, metabolic acidosis, and nephrocalcinosis, renal tubular acidosis (RTA) results from the kidneys' inability to conserve bicarbonate. This disorder occurs as distal (type I or classic) RTA or proximal (type II) RTA. The prognosis is usually good but depends on the severity of renal damage that precedes treatment.

Distal RTA results from an inability of the distal tubule to secrete hydrogen ions against established gradients across the tubular membrane. This leads to decreased excretion of titratable acids and ammonium, increased loss of potassium and bicarbonate in urine, and systemic acidosis. Prolonged acidosis causes mobilization of calcium from bone and eventually hypercalciuria, predisposing the patient to the formation of renal calculi.

Distal RTA may be classified as primary or secondary:
- Primary distal RTA may occur sporadically or through a hereditary defect and is most prevalent in females, older children, adolescents, and young adults.
- Secondary distal RTA has been linked to many renal and systemic conditions, such as starvation, malnutrition, hepatic cirrhosis, and several genetically transmitted disorders.

Proximal RTA results from defective bicarbonate reabsorption in the proximal tubule. This causes bicarbonate to flood the distal tubule, which normally secretes hydrogen ions, and leads to impaired formation of titratable acids and ammonium for excretion. Ultimately, metabolic acidosis results.

Proximal RTA occurs in two forms:
- With primary proximal RTA, the reabsorptive defect is idiopathic and is the only disorder present.
- With secondary proximal RTA, the reabsorptive defect may be one of several defects and results from proximal tubular cell damage from a disease such as Fanconi's syndrome.

Causes
- Defect in the kidneys' normal tubular acidification of urine

Signs and symptoms
In infants
- Anorexia
- Apathy

- Constipation
- Dehydration
- Growth retardation
- Nephrocalcinosis
- Occasional fever
- Polyuria
- Rickets
- Tissue wasting
- Vomiting
- Weakness

In children and adults
- Growth problems (in children)
- Rickets
- Urinary tract infection

Diagnostic tests
- Impaired urine acidification with systemic metabolic acidosis confirms distal RTA.
- Bicarbonate wasting due to impaired reabsorption confirms proximal RTA.
- Other relevant laboratory test results show:
  - decreased bicarbonate, pH, potassium, and phosphorus levels
  - increased chloride and alkaline phosphatase levels
  - alkaline pH, with low titratable acids and ammonium content in urine; and increased urinary bicarbonate and potassium levels, with low specific gravity.
- X-rays may show nephrocalcinosis (in later stages).

Treatment
- Supportive treatment of patients with RTA requires replacement of the substances being abnormally excreted, especially bicarbonate. It may include sodium bicarbonate tablets or Shohl's solution to control acidosis, and oral potassium to treat dangerously low potassium levels. Vitamin D and calcium supplements aren't usually given because the tendency toward nephrocalci-

nosis persists even after bicarbonate therapy.
- An antibiotic is prescribed if pyelonephritis occurs.
- Treatment of renal calculi secondary to nephrocalcinosis varies and may include supportive therapy until the calculi pass or until surgery for severe obstruction is performed.

Nursing considerations
- Urge compliance with the prescribed drug regimen. Inform the patient and his family that the prognosis for RTA and bone lesion healing is directly related to the adequacy of treatment.
- Monitor laboratory values, especially potassium levels, for signs of hypokalemia.
- Test urine for pH and strain it for calculi.
- If rickets develops, explain the disorder and its treatment to the patient and his family.
- Teach the patient how to recognize signs and symptoms of calculi (hematuria and low abdominal or flank pain). Advise him to report such signs and symptoms immediately.
- Instruct the patient with low potassium levels to eat foods with a high potassium content, such as bananas, oranges and orange juice, and baked potatoes.
- Encourage family members to seek genetic counseling or screening for RTA.

Renal vein thrombosis

Clotting in the renal vein results in renal congestion, engorgement and, possibly, infarction. Renal vein thrombosis may affect both kidneys and may be acute or chronic.

Chronic thrombosis usually impairs renal function, causing nephrotic syndrome. Abrupt onset of thrombosis that causes extensive damage may precipitate rapidly fatal renal infarction.

If thrombosis affects both kidneys, the prognosis is poor. However, less severe thrombosis that affects only one kidney or gradual progression that allows development of collateral circulation may preserve partial renal function.

Causes
- Back or abdominal trauma
- Complication of amyloidosis, systemic lupus erythematosus, diabetic nephropathy, or membranoproliferative glomerulonephritis
- Heart failure
- Periarteritis
- Severe dehydration from diarrhea (in infants)
- Stricture (scar formation)
- Thrombophlebitis of the inferior vena cava
- Tumor that obstructs the renal vein (usually hypernephroma)

Signs and symptoms
Acute
- Enlarged and easily palpable kidneys
- Fever
- Hematuria
- Hypertension (rare)
- Leukocytosis
- Oliguria and other uremic signs (with bilateral obstruction)
- Pallor
- Peripheral edema
- Proteinuria
- Severe lumbar pain and tenderness in the epigastric region and costovertebral angle

Chronic
- Hyperlipidemia
- Hypoalbuminemia
- Nephrotic syndrome symptoms
- Peripheral edema (possible)
- Proteinuria

In infants
- Enlarged kidneys, oliguria, and renal insufficiency that may progress to acute or chronic renal failure

Diagnostic tests
- Abdominal X-ray, computed tomography scanning, magnetic resonance imaging, or ultrasonography shows occlusion of the renal vein.
- Excretory urography provides reliable diagnostic evidence.
  - With acute renal vein thrombosis, the kidneys appear enlarged and excretory function diminishes. The contrast medium seems to "smudge" necrotic renal tissue.
  - With chronic thrombosis, ureteral indentations resulting from collateral venous channels may be present.
- Renal arteriography and kidney biopsy may confirm the diagnosis.
- Urinalysis reveals gross or microscopic hematuria, proteinuria (more than 2 g/ day in chronic disease), casts, and oliguria.
- Blood studies show leukocytosis, hypoalbuminemia, and hyperlipidemia.
- Venography confirms the presence of the occluding thrombosis.

Treatment
- Anticoagulant therapy with heparin or warfarin (Coumadin) may be given to prevent formation of new clots.
- Thrombolytic therapy, using streptokinase (Streptase) or alteplase (Activase), is also effective.
- Conservative treatment may be ordered; the patient may be placed on bed rest or limited activity for a brief period, allowing the thrombosis to resolve over time.
- Surgery must be performed within 24 hours of thrombosis, but even then it has only limited success because thrombi commonly extend into the small

veins. Extensive intrarenal bleeding and severe hypertension in an atrophic kidney may necessitate nephrectomy.

- Patients who survive abrupt thrombosis with extensive renal damage develop nephrotic syndrome and require treatment of renal failure, such as dialysis and possible transplantation.
- Some infants with renal vein thrombosis recover completely after rehydration and heparin therapy or surgery; others suffer irreversible kidney damage.

Nursing considerations

- Assess the patient's renal function regularly. Monitor his vital signs, intake and output, daily weight, and electrolyte levels.
- Administer a diuretic for edema, as ordered, and enforce dietary restrictions, such as limited sodium and potassium intake.
- Monitor the patient closely for signs and symptoms of pulmonary emboli, such as chest pain and dyspnea.

DRUG CHALLENGE

If heparin is given by constant I.V. infusion, frequently monitor partial thromboplastin time to determine the patient's response to it. Dilute the drug; administer it by infusion pump so the patient receives the least amount necessary.

- During anticoagulant therapy, watch for signs of bleeding, such as tachycardia, hypotension, hematuria, bleeding from the nose or gums, ecchymoses, petechiae, and black, tarry stools.
- Instruct the patient on maintenance warfarin therapy to use an electric razor and a soft toothbrush and to avoid situations that place him at risk for trauma. Suggest that he wear a medical identification bracelet, and tell him to avoid aspirin, which aggravates bleeding tenden-

cies. Stress the need for close medical follow-up.

▌Respiratory acidosis

An acid-base disturbance characterized by reduced alveolar ventilation and manifested by hypercapnia (partial pressure of arterial carbon dioxide [$PaCO_2$] greater than 45 mm Hg), respiratory acidosis can be acute (from a sudden failure in ventilation) or chronic (as in long-term pulmonary disease). The prognosis depends on the severity of the underlying disturbance and on the patient's general condition.

Hypoventilation compromises excretion of carbon dioxide produced through metabolism. The retained carbon dioxide then combines with water to form excess carbonic acid, decreasing the blood pH. As a result, the concentration of hydrogen ions in body fluids, which directly reflects acidity, increases.

Causes

- Airway obstruction
- Asthma
- Chronic bronchitis
- Chronic obstructive pulmonary disease (COPD)
- Extensive pneumonia
- Large pneumothorax
- Parenchymal lung disease
- Pulmonary edema
- Severe respiratory distress syndrome

Predisposing factors

- Central nervous system (CNS) trauma: medullary injury (may impair ventilatory drive)
- Chronic metabolic alkalosis (causes reduced alveolar ventilation in attempt to normalize pH)
- Drugs: opioids, anesthetics, hypnotics, and sedatives (decrease the sensitivity of the respiratory center)

- Neuromuscular disease (such as myasthenia gravis, Guillain-Barré syndrome, and poliomyelitis): respiratory muscles unable to respond properly to respiratory drive, reducing alveolar ventilation

Signs and symptoms
Cardiovascular abnormalities
- Atrial and ventricular arrhythmias
- Hypertension
- Hypotension with vasodilation (bounding pulses and warm periphery) (in severe acidosis)
- Tachycardia

CNS disturbances
- Apprehension
- Coma
- Confusion
- Dyspnea and tachypnea, with papilledema and depressed reflexes
- Headaches
- Hypoxemia
- Restlessness
- Somnolence, with a fine or flapping tremor (asterixis)

Diagnostic tests
- Arterial blood gas (ABG) analysis confirms respiratory acidosis. $PaCO_2$ exceeds the normal level of 45 mm Hg, pH is below the normal range of 7.35 to 7.45, and bicarbonate level is normal in the acute stage but elevated in the chronic stage.
- Chest X-ray, computed tomography scan, or pulmonary function test may help diagnose lung disease.

Treatment
- The underlying condition causing the alveolar hypoventilation must be corrected.
- Significantly reduced alveolar ventilation may require mechanical ventilation until the underlying condition can be treated.

- In a patient with COPD, treatment includes a bronchodilator, oxygen, a corticosteroid and, commonly, an antibiotic. An elevated $PaCO_2$ level may persist despite optimal treatment.
- Drug therapy is necessary for patients with conditions such as myasthenia gravis.
- Foreign bodies must be removed from the airway.
- Antibiotics are prescribed for pneumonia.
- Dialysis is needed to treat drug toxicity.
- Metabolic alkalosis must be corrected.

Nursing considerations
- Closely monitor the patient's blood pH. If it drops below 7.15, profound CNS and cardiovascular deterioration may result, requiring administration of I.V. sodium bicarbonate.

DRUG CHALLENGE

 Administration of sodium bicarbonate should be reserved for only the most critical cases because it can cause a paradoxical worsening of CNS effects.

- Stay alert for critical changes in the patient's respiratory, CNS, and cardiovascular functions. Also, watch closely for ABG value variations, and monitor electrolyte status. Maintain adequate hydration.
- Maintain a patent airway and provide adequate humidification if acidosis requires mechanical ventilation. Perform tracheal suctioning regularly and vigorous chest physiotherapy if needed. Continuously monitor ventilator settings and the patient's respiratory status.
- Closely monitor the patient with COPD and chronic carbon dioxide retention for signs of respiratory acidosis. Also, administer oxygen at low flow

rates, and closely monitor the patient if he's receiving an opioid or a sedative.
- Instruct the patient who has received a general anesthetic to turn, use the incentive spirometer, and cough, and perform deep-breathing exercises frequently to prevent the onset of respiratory acidosis.

Respiratory alkalosis

Caused by alveolar hyperventilation, respiratory alkalosis is a condition marked by a decrease in partial pressure of arterial carbon dioxide ($PaCO_2$) to below 35 mm Hg. Uncomplicated respiratory alkalosis leads to a decrease in hydrogen ion concentration, which causes elevated blood pH. Hypocapnia occurs when the elimination of carbon dioxide by the lungs exceeds the production of carbon dioxide at the cellular level.

Causes
Nonpulmonary
- Anxiety
- Aspirin toxicity
- Central nervous system (CNS) disease (inflammation or tumor)
- Fever
- Hepatic failure
- Metabolic acidosis
- Pregnancy
- Sepsis

Pulmonary
- Acute asthma
- Interstitial lung disease
- Pneumonia
- Pulmonary vascular disease

Signs and symptoms
- Agitation
- Cardiac arrhythmias that fail to respond to conventional treatment (severe respiratory alkalosis)
- Carpopedal spasms
- Circumoral and peripheral paresthesia
- Deep, rapid breathing, possibly exceeding 40 breaths/minute
- Light-headedness or dizziness
- Muscle weakness
- Seizures (severe respiratory alkalosis)
- Twitching (possibly progressing to tetany)

Diagnostic tests
- Arterial blood gas (ABG) analysis confirms respiratory alkalosis and rules out respiratory compensation for metabolic acidosis. Findings include:
  - bicarbonate level that's normal in the acute stage but below normal in the chronic stage
  - $PaCO_2$ below 35 mm Hg
  - pH that's elevated in proportion to the fall in $PaCO_2$ in the acute stage but that drops toward normal in the chronic stage.

Treatment
- Treat the underlying condition. (For example, remove ingested toxins or treat fever, sepsis, or CNS disease.)
- The patient may be instructed to breathe into a paper bag, which helps relieve acute anxiety and increases carbon dioxide levels in severe respiratory alkalosis.
- Monitor ABG values, and adjust dead space or minute ventilation volume to prevent hyperventilation in patients receiving mechanical ventilation.

Nursing considerations
- Watch for and report changes in neurologic, neuromuscular, or cardiovascular function.
- Help the patient breathe into a paper bag if necessary.
- Monitor ABG and serum electrolyte levels closely, watching for variations.
- Monitor for arrhythmias if respiratory alkalosis is severe.

Respiratory distress syndrome

Also called *hyaline membrane disease* and *infant respiratory distress syndrome,* respiratory distress syndrome (RDS) is the most common cause of neonatal mortality and a major component of neonatal morbidity.

The severity and prognosis for RDS are directly related to the gestational age of the neonate. An inverse relationship exists between gestational age and RDS; the lower the gestational age the greater potential for RDS. It commonly affects premature infants born before the 37th gestational week (and about 60% of those born before the 28th week). It's more common in neonates of diabetic mothers and in neonates born with acidosis such as those delivered under stressful conditions—for example, by cesarean birth or suddenly after antepartum hemorrhage.

Although alveolar development has begun by 25 to 27 weeks' gestation, the alveoli are insufficient for effective respiration. Also, the intercostal muscles are weak, and the alveoli and capillary blood supply are immature. In RDS, the premature neonate develops widespread alveolar collapse because of lack of surfactant, a lipoprotein present in alveoli and respiratory bronchioles. Surfactant normally lowers surface tension and aids in maintaining alveolar patency, preventing collapse, particularly at end expiration.

Aggressive management using mechanical ventilation improves the prognosis.

Causes

- Surfactant deficiency

Signs and symptoms

- Audible expiratory grunting
- Frothy sputum
- Hypotension
- Intercostal, subcostal, or sternal retractions
- Low body temperature
- Nasal flaring
- Oliguria
- Pallor
- Peripheral edema
- Rapid, shallow respirations within minutes or hours of birth

In severe disease

- Apnea
- Bradycardia
- Cyanosis

Diagnostic tests

- Chest X-ray may be normal for the first 6 to 12 hours (in 50% of neonates with RDS) but later shows a fine reticulonodular pattern and dark streaks, indicating air-filled, dilated bronchioles.
- Arterial blood gas (ABG) analysis shows decreased partial pressure of arterial oxygen (PaO_2); normal, decreased, or increased partial pressure of arterial carbon dioxide; and decreased pH (from respiratory or metabolic acidosis or both).
- When a cesarean birth is necessary before 36 weeks' gestation, amniocentesis allows determination of the lecithin-sphingomyelin ratio, which helps to assess prenatal lung development and the risk of RDS.

Treatment

- Natural lung surfactant, such as beractant (Survanta), is given by an endotracheal (ET) tube as soon as possible after birth.
- Vigorous respiratory support includes warm, humidified, oxygen-enriched gases administered by oxygen hood or, if such treatment fails, by mechanical ventilation.

- Severe cases require mechanical ventilation with positive end-expiratory pressure (PEEP) or continuous positive airway pressure (CPAP), administered by a tightly fitting face mask or, when necessary, ET intubation.
- A radiant infant warmer or Isolette is used for thermoregulation.
- I.V. fluids and sodium bicarbonate are prescribed to control acidosis and maintain fluid and electrolyte balance.
- Tube feedings or total parenteral nutrition may be needed if the neonate is too weak to eat.

Nursing considerations

- Closely monitor ABG levels as well as fluid intake and output. If the neonate has an umbilical catheter (arterial or venous), check for arterial hypotension or abnormal central venous pressure.
- Watch for such complications as infection, thrombosis, or decreased circulation to the legs.
- If the neonate is attached to a transcutaneous PaO_2 monitor (an accurate method for determining PaO_2), change the site of the lead placement every 2 to 4 hours to avoid burning the skin.
- Weigh the neonate once or twice daily. To evaluate his progress, assess skin color, rate and depth of respirations, severity of retractions, nostril flaring, frequency of expiratory grunting, frothing at the lips, and restlessness.
- Regularly assess the effectiveness of oxygen or ventilator therapy. Evaluate every change in the fraction of inspired oxygen and PEEP or CPAP by monitoring oxygen saturation or ABG levels. Be sure to adjust PEEP or CPAP as indicated, based on findings.
- When the neonate is receiving mechanical ventilation, watch carefully for signs of barotrauma (increase in respiratory distress or subcutaneous emphysema) and accidental disconnection from

the ventilator. Frequently check ventilator settings.
- Stay alert for signs of complications of PEEP or CPAP therapy, such as decreased cardiac output, pneumothorax, and pneumomediastinum. Mechanical ventilation increases the risk of infection in premature neonates, so preventive measures are essential.
- As needed, arrange for follow-up care with a neonatal ophthalmologist to check for retinal damage.
- Teach the parents about their neonate's condition and, if possible, let them participate in his care (using sterile technique) to encourage normal parent-infant bonding. Advise parents that full recovery may take up to 12 months. When the prognosis is poor, prepare the parents for the neonate's impending death, and offer emotional support.
- Help reduce mortality in RDS by detecting respiratory distress early. Recognize intercostal retractions and grunting, especially in a premature neonate, as signs of respiratory distress syndrome, and make sure that the neonate receives immediate treatment.

Respiratory syncytial virus infection

A subgroup of the myxoviruses resembling paramyxovirus causes respiratory syncytial virus (RSV) infection. RSV is the leading cause of lower respiratory tract infections in infants and young children; it's the major cause of pneumonia, tracheobronchitis, and bronchiolitis in this age-group and a suspected cause of many fatal respiratory diseases of infancy.

Rates of illness are highest in infants age 1 to 6 months; incidence peaks between ages 2 and 3 months. RSV also causes repeated infections throughout life, usually associated with moderate to severe coldlike symptoms, and may predispose a child to asthma. Severe lower respiratory tract disease can occur, especially among elderly people and those with compromised cardiac, pulmonary, or immune systems. This virus creates annual epidemics during winter and spring.

Infants and children with a history of neonatal respiratory distress syndrome are at especially high risk for developing RSV as are those who are exposed to tobacco smoke, attend day-care centers, live in crowded conditions, or have school-age siblings. Antibody titers seem to indicate that few children younger than age 4 escape contracting some form of RSV, even if it's mild. In fact, RSV is the only viral disease that has its maximum impact during the first few months of life.

RSV has also been identified in patients with various central nervous system disorders, such as meningitis and myelitis.

Causes
- Virus transmitted from person to person by respiratory secretions

Signs and symptoms
- Bronchiolitis or bronchopneumonia
- Coughing
- Dyspnea
- Inflamed mucous membranes in the nose and throat
- Malaise
- Otitis media (common complication in infants)
- Pharyngitis
- Severe, life-threatening lower respiratory tract infections (rarely)
- Wheezing

Diagnostic tests
- Cultures of nasal and pharyngeal secretions may show RSV; however, the

virus is very labile, so cultures aren't always reliable.
- Serum antibody titers may be elevated, but before age 4 months, maternal antibodies may affect test results.
- Serology results (from indirect immunofluorescence and the enzyme-linked immunosorbent assay) are positive for RSV.
- Chest X-rays help detect pneumonia or bronchiolitis.

Treatment
- Mild cases may resolve without treatment.
- Severe infections require hospitalization to provide supplemental oxygen, humidified air, and hydration by I.V. fluids.
- Respiratory support using mechanical ventilation may be needed.
- Ribavirin (Virazole) aerosol may be used in those who have severe RSV or are immunocompromised; however, many studies show no association with improvement in clinical outcome from the use of this agent.
- Palivizumab (Synagis), a monoclonal antibody preparation, can be given prophylactically to infants and children at high risk for RSV infection. RSV I.V. immune globulin may also be given during RSV season, although palivizumab is typically preferred because of its easy I.M. administration route.

Nursing considerations
- Monitor the patient's respiratory status. Observe the rate and pattern; watch for nasal flaring or retraction, cyanosis, pallor, and dyspnea; and auscultate for wheezing, rhonchi, or other signs of respiratory distress. Monitor arterial blood gas values.
- Maintain a patent airway, and be especially watchful when the patient has periods of acute dyspnea. Perform per-

cussion and provide drainage and suction when necessary. Provide a high-humidity atmosphere. Semi-Fowler's position may help prevent aspiration of secretions.

■ Monitor intake and output carefully. Observe the patient for signs of dehydration such as decreased skin turgor. Encourage the patient to drink plenty of high-calorie fluids, and administer I.V. fluids as needed.

■ Promote bed rest, allowing for as much uninterrupted rest as possible.

■ Hold and cuddle infants; talk to and play with toddlers. Offer diversionary activities suitable to the child's condition and age. Foster parental visits and cuddling. Restrain a child only as necessary.

■ Impose droplet isolation precautions. Patients hospitalized with RSV should ideally be placed in rooms with negative-pressure ventilation. Maintain strict hand washing, and instruct family members to do so as well.

▋Retinal detachment

When the sensory retina splits from the retinal pigment epithelium, retinal detachment occurs, creating a subretinal space. This space then fills with fluid, called subretinal fluid. Retinal detachment usually involves only one eye but may involve the other eye later. The condition is twice as common in males as in females.

Surgical reattachment is usually successful, but the prognosis for good vision depends on the area of the retina that's been affected.

Causes
In adults
■ Degenerative changes
■ Retinal tear or hole

■ Seepage of fluid into the subretinal space

In children
■ Heredity
■ Retinopathy of prematurity
■ Trauma
■ Tumors (retinoblastomas)

Signs and symptoms
Initially
■ Floating spots
■ Recurrent flashes of light

Later
■ Gradual, painless vision loss (may be described as a veil, curtain, or cobweb that eliminates a portion of the visual field)

Diagnostic tests
■ Ophthalmoscopy after full pupil dilation shows the usually transparent retina as gray and opaque; with severe detachment, it reveals folds in the retina and a ballooning out of the area.
■ Indirect ophthalmoscopy is used to detect retinal tears.
■ Ocular ultrasonography is performed if the patient has an opaque lens.

Treatment
■ Restriction of eye movements and complete bed rest is advised to prevent further detachment. The patient's head is positioned to allow gravity to pull the detached retina into closer contact with the choroid.
■ A hole in the peripheral retina can be treated with cryotherapy; a hole in the posterior portion, with laser therapy.
■ Surgical interventions are scleral buckling to reattach the retina and, possibly, replacement of the vitreous with oil, air, gas, or silicone.

Nursing considerations

- Provide emotional support; the patient may be distraught because of his decreased vision.
- Wash the patient's face with baby shampoo to prepare for surgery. Administer an antibiotic and cycloplegic-mydriatic eyedrops.
- After surgery, instruct the patient to lie in the position that facilitates the gas or oil to tamponade the retina. This may be a prone position. Discourage straining during defecation, bending down, and coughing hard, sneezing, or vomiting, which can raise intraocular pressure. Administer an antiemetic, as prescribed, if necessary. Discourage activities that increase the risk of bumping the eye.
- Gently clean the eye with cycloplegic eyedrops and steroid-antibiotic eyedrops after removing the protective patch.
- Use cold compresses to decrease swelling (postoperative edema) and pain.
- Administer an analgesic, such as acetaminophen (Tylenol), as needed, noting persistent pain.
- Teach the patient how to properly instill eyedrops, and emphasize the need for compliance and follow-up care.
- Encourage the patient to wear dark glasses to compensate for sensitivity to light.

▌Reye's syndrome

An acute childhood illness, Reye's syndrome causes fatty infiltration of the liver with concurrent hyperammonemia, encephalopathy, and increased intracranial pressure (ICP). With Reye's syndrome, damaged hepatic mitochondria disrupt the urea cycle, which normally changes ammonia to urea for its excretion from the body. This results in hyperammonemia, hypoglycemia, and an increase in serum short-chain fatty

acids, leading to encephalopathy. Simultaneously, fatty infiltration is found in renal tubular cells, neuronal tissue, and muscle tissue, including the heart.

Reye's syndrome affects children from infancy to adolescence and occurs equally in boys and girls. It affects Whites older than age 1 more often than it does Blacks. The prognosis depends on the severity of central nervous system depression. Previously, mortality was as high as 90%. Today, ICP monitoring and, consequently, early treatment of increased ICP—along with other treatment measures—have cut mortality to about 5%. Death is usually a result of cerebral edema or respiratory arrest. Most comatose patients who survive may have some residual brain damage.

Causes

- Aspirin use
- Follows within 1 to 3 days of an acute viral infection, such as an upper respiratory tract infection or infection from *Haemophilus influenzae* type B or varicella (chickenpox).

Signs and symptoms

- Develops in five stages; the severity of the child's signs and symptoms varying with the degree of encephalopathy and cerebral edema
- Brief recovery period after the initial viral infection
- A few days later: intractable vomiting, lethargy, rapidly changing mental status that may progress to coma, hyperactive reflexes, and rising blood pressure, respiratory rate, and pulse rate
- As the coma deepens: seizures, followed by decreased tendon reflexes and, commonly, respiratory failure
- Increased ICP from cerebral edema, which may result from acidosis, increased cerebral metabolic rate, or impaired autoregulatory mechanism

- Atypical presentation possible in infants

Diagnostic tests

- Liver function studies show aspartate aminotransferase and alanine aminotransferase levels elevated to twice normal; the bilirubin level is usually normal.
- Liver biopsy reveals fatty droplets uniformly distributed throughout cells.
- Cerebrospinal fluid (CSF) analysis reveals a white blood cell count of less than 10 mm^3; with coma, CSF pressure increases.
- Coagulation studies result in prolonged prothrombin time and partial thromboplastin time.
- Blood values show elevated serum ammonia levels; normal or, in 15% of cases, low serum glucose levels; and increased serum fatty acid and lactate levels.
- Testing the serum salicylate level rules out aspirin overdose.

Treatment

- The stage of the syndrome dictates the type of treatment necessary. (See *Stages of treatment for Reye's syndrome.*)

Nursing considerations

DRUG CHALLENGE

 Advise parents against the use of aspirin or aspirin-containing over-the-counter medications in children under age 18. Use of analgesics and antipyretics may include acetaminophen (Tylenol) or ibuprofen (Motrin) rather than aspirin. Because of the associated risk of Reye's syndrome, parents should be taught to never give aspirin to children unless it's specifically prescribed.

Stages of treatment for Reye's syndrome

Signs and symptoms

Stage I
Vomiting, lethargy, hepatic dysfunction

Stage II
Hyperventilation, delirium, hepatic dysfunction, hyperactive reflexes

Stage III
Coma, hyperventilation, decorticate rigidity, hepatic dysfunction

Stage IV
Deepening coma; decerebrate rigidity; large, fixed pupils; minimal hepatic dysfunction

Stage V
Seizures, loss of deep tendon reflexes, flaccidity, respiratory arrest, ammonia level > 300 mg/dl

Baseline treatment	**Baseline intervention**
■ To decrease intracranial pressure (ICP) and brain edema, give I.V. fluids at two-thirds of the maintenance dose. Also give an osmotic diuretic or furosemide (Lasix). ■ To treat hypoprothrombinemia, give vitamin K; if vitamin K proves unsuccessful, give fresh frozen plasma. ■ Monitor serum ammonia and blood glucose levels and plasma osmolality every 4 to 8 hours to check progress.	■ Monitor the patient's vital signs, and check his level of consciousness for increasing lethargy. Take his vital signs more often as his condition deteriorates. ■ Monitor fluid intake and output to prevent fluid overload. Maintain urine output at 1 ml/kg/hour, plasma osmolality at 290 mOsm, and blood glucose at 150 mg/dl. (*Goal:* Keep glucose levels high, osmolality normal to high, and ammonia levels low.) Also, restrict protein.
■ Continue baseline treatment.	■ Maintain seizure precautions. ■ Watch closely for signs of coma that require invasive or supportive therapy such as intubation. ■ Keep the head of the bed raised 30 degrees.
■ Continue baseline and seizure treatment. ■ Monitor ICP. ■ Provide endotracheal intubation and mechanical ventilation to control partial pressure of carbon dioxide ($Paco_2$). A paralyzing agent, such as I.V. pancuronium, may help maintain ventilation. ■ Give I.V. mannitol (Osmitrol).	■ Monitor ICP (should be < 20 mm Hg before suctioning), or give a barbiturate I.V. as needed; hyperventilate the patient as necessary. ■ When ventilating the patient, maintain $Paco_2$ between 25 and 30 mm Hg and partial pressure of arterial oxygen between 80 and 100 mm Hg. ■ Closely monitor cardiovascular status with a pulmonary artery catheter or central venous pressure line. ■ Perform good skin and mouth care, and perform range-of-motion exercises.
■ Continue baseline and supportive care. ■ If all previous measures fail, some pediatric centers use barbiturate coma, decompressive craniotomy, hypothermia, or an exchange transfusion.	■ Check the patient for loss of reflexes and signs of flaccidity. ■ Give the family members the extra support they need, considering their child's poor prognosis.
■ Continue baseline and supportive care.	■ Help the family to face the patient's impending death.

- Monitor the patient's vital signs and neurologic status frequently, and report changes immediately.
- Assess the patient's respiratory status, and maintain a patent airway.
- Institute seizure precautions.
- Monitor intake and output closely.
- Refer parents to the National Reye's Syndrome Foundation for more information.

Rhabdomyolysis

Rhabdomyolysis results from the toxicity of destroyed muscle cells, causing kidney damage or failure. In the United States, rhabdomyolysis affects 8% to 15% of patients with acute renal failure; about 5% of cases result in death.

Rhabdomyolysis follows direct injury to the muscle fibers, specifically the sarcolemma, which then release myoglobin into the bloodstream. The myoglobin alters filtration in the kidneys, resulting in damage and failure.

Causes

- Blunt trauma
- Exposure to extreme cold
- Extensive burn injury
- Heatstroke
- Heavy exercise in children
- Metabolic or genetic factors
- Near electrocution or near drowning
- Prolonged immobilization
- Shaken-baby syndrome
- Snakebite
- Toxins
- Viral, bacterial, or fungal infection (such as legionnaires' disease or, especially, *Haemophilus influenzae* type A or B infection)

Predisposing factors

- Alcohol abuse
- Recent soft-tissue compression

Signs and symptoms

- Dark urine
- Fatigue
- Fever
- Joint pain
- Malaise
- Myalgia or muscle pain (especially in the thighs, calves, or lower back)
- Nausea
- Seizures
- Tenderness
- Vomiting
- Weakness
- Weight gain

Diagnostic tests

- Creatine kinase levels 100 times normal or higher suggest rhabdomyolysis.
- Urine test results are positive for hemoglobin or myoglobin.
- Serum potassium may be elevated (potassium is released from cells into the bloodstream when cell breakdown occurs).

Treatment

- Early, aggressive hydration may prevent complications from rhabdomyolysis by rapidly eliminating myoglobin from the kidneys. I.V. hydration and diuretics promote diuresis. Diuretics, such as mannitol or furosemide (Lasix), may aid in flushing the pigment out of the kidneys.
- Bicarbonate may be given to prevent myoglobin from breaking down into toxic compounds in the kidney.
- Dialysis and, in severe cases, kidney transplantation may be necessary.

Nursing considerations

- Monitor intake and output, vital signs, electrolyte levels, daily weight, and laboratory results.
- Watch for signs of renal failure (such as decreasing urine output and increasing urine specific gravity), fluid overload

(such as dyspnea and tachycardia), pulmonary edema, and electrolyte imbalances (such as serum potassium).

▪ Provide reassurance and emotional support for the patient and family.

▪ Ensure adequate hydration, monitor the patient for adverse reactions to any of his prescribed drugs, and monitor blood transfusion carefully to help prevent rhabdomyolysis.

▪ Provide care accordingly if the patient develops acute renal failure. (See "Renal failure, acute," pages 525 to 528.)

Rheumatic fever and rheumatic heart disease

Commonly recurrent, acute rheumatic fever is a systemic inflammatory disease of childhood that follows a group A beta-hemolytic streptococcal infection. Rheumatic heart disease refers to rheumatic fever's cardiac involvement; it may affect the endocardium, myocardium, or pericardium in the early acute phase and may cause chronic valvular disease later. Valvular disease may eventually result in chronic valvular stenosis and insufficiency, including mitral stenosis and insufficiency and aortic insufficiency. In children, mitral insufficiency remains the major after-effect of rheumatic heart disease.

Long-term antibiotic therapy can minimize recurrence of rheumatic fever, reducing the risk of permanent cardiac damage and eventual valvular deformity.

Although rheumatic fever tends to run in families, this may merely reflect contributing environmental factors. In lower socioeconomic groups, incidence is highest in children between ages 5 and 15, probably resulting from malnutrition and crowded living conditions. The disease usually strikes during cool, damp weather in winter and early spring. In the United States, it's most common in the northern states.

Causes

▪ Hypersensitivity to group A beta-hemolytic streptococcal infection

Signs and symptoms

▪ Carditis
– Pericarditis: pericardial friction rub, occasionally pain and effusion
– Myocarditis: characteristic lesions called Aschoff bodies (in the acute stages); cellular swelling and fragmentation of interstitial collagen, leading to formation of a progressively fibrotic nodule and interstitial scars
– Endocarditis: valve leaflet swelling; erosion along the lines of leaflet closure; and blood, platelet, and fibrin deposits, which form beadlike vegetations (usually affects the mitral valve in females and the aortic valve in males)
– Severe rheumatic carditis: heart failure with dyspnea, right upper quadrant pain, tachycardia, tachypnea, significant mitral and aortic murmurs, hacking nonproductive cough

▪ Firm, movable, nontender, subcutaneous nodules ⅛" to ¾" (0.5 to 2 cm) in diameter, usually near tendons or bony prominences of joints

▪ Migratory joint pain or polyarthritis

▪ Skin lesions such as erythema marginatum (rarely)

▪ Swelling, redness, and signs of effusion in the knees, ankles, elbows, or hips

▪ Temperature of at least 100.4° F (38° C)

▪ Transient mild to severe chorea up to 6 months after the original streptococcal infection, which always resolves without residual neurologic damage
– Mild chorea: hyperirritability, deterioration in handwriting, inability to concentrate

– Severe chorea: purposeless, non-repetitive, involuntary muscle spasms; poor muscle coordination; weakness

Typical murmurs

- Diastolic murmur of aortic insufficiency (less common than other two types)
- Midsystolic murmur caused by stiffening and swelling of the mitral leaflet
- Systolic murmur of mitral insufficiency (high-pitched, blowing, holosystolic, loudest at apex, possibly radiating to the anterior axillary line)

Diagnostic tests

- White blood cell count and erythrocyte sedimentation rate may be elevated (during the acute phase); blood studies show slight anemia from suppressed erythropoiesis during inflammation.
- C-reactive protein test result is positive (especially during the acute phase).
- Cardiac enzyme levels may be increased in those with severe carditis.
- Antistreptolysin O titer is elevated in 95% of patients within 2 months of onset. (Rising anti-DNase B test results can also detect recurrent streptococcal infection.)
- Electrocardiography changes aren't diagnostic, but the PR interval is prolonged in 20% of patients.
- Chest X-rays show normal heart size, except with myocarditis, heart failure, or pericardial effusion.
- Echocardiography helps evaluate valvular damage, chamber size, ventricular function, and the presence of a pericardial effusion.
- Cardiac catheterization evaluates valvular damage and left ventricular function in those with severe cardiac dysfunction.

Treatment

In acute phase

- Low doses of antibiotics, such as penicillin or erythromycin (E-Mycin) are given.
- Salicylates, such as aspirin, can help relieve fever and minimize joint swelling and pain; if carditis is present or the salicylate fails to relieve pain and inflammation, corticosteroids may be used.
- Supportive treatment requires strict bed rest for about 5 weeks during the acute phase with active carditis, followed by a progressive increase in physical activity, depending on clinical and laboratory findings and the patient's response to treatment.

Preventive treatment

- The patient should be maintained on low-dose antibiotic therapy indefinitely, but especially during the first 5 to 10 years after the initial episode of rheumatic fever, to prevent recurrence.
- Patients older than age 18 who contract rheumatic fever without carditis may need only 5 years of prophylactic antibiotics; antibiotics may continue indefinitely in patients with frequent potential exposure to group A streptococcus.
- Additional antibiotic prophylaxis is required before invasive procedures, including dental and surgical procedures.

Surgery and other measures

- Heart failure necessitates continued bed rest and diuretic therapy.
- Severe mitral or aortic valvular dysfunction causing persistent heart failure requires corrective valvular surgery, including commissurotomy (separation of the adherent, thickened leaflets of the mitral valve), valvuloplasty (inflation of a balloon within a valve), or valve replacement (with a prosthetic valve).

Corrective valvular surgery is rarely necessary before late adolescence.

Nursing considerations

- Teach the patient and his family about this disease and its treatment.
- Before giving penicillin, ask the parents if the child has ever had a hypersensitivity reaction to it. Even if the patient has never had a reaction to penicillin, warn that such a reaction is possible.
- Tell the parents that if the child develops a rash, fever, chills, or other signs or symptoms of allergy at any time during penicillin therapy, they should stop the drug and immediately contact the practitioner.
- Instruct the parents to watch for and report early signs of heart failure, such as dyspnea and a hacking, nonproductive cough.
- Stress the need for bed rest during the acute phase, and suggest appropriate, physically undemanding diversions.
- After the acute phase, encourage family and friends to spend as much time as possible with the child to minimize boredom. Advise the parents to secure a tutor to help the child keep up with schoolwork during his long convalescence.
- Tell the parents that failure to seek treatment for streptococcal infection is common because the illness may seem no worse than a cold.
- If the child has severe carditis, help parents prepare for permanent changes in the child's lifestyle.
- Warn the parents to watch for and immediately report signs and symptoms of recurrent streptococcal infection—sudden sore throat, diffuse throat redness and oropharyngeal exudate, swollen and tender cervical lymph nodes, pain on swallowing, a temperature of 101° to 104° F (38.3° to 40° C), headache, and

nausea. Urge them to keep the child away from people with respiratory tract infections.
- Explain the importance of good dental hygiene in preventing gingival infection.
- Make sure that the child and his family understand the need to comply with prolonged antibiotic therapy and follow-up care and the need for additional antibiotics during dental surgery.
- Arrange for a visiting nurse to oversee home care if necessary.

Rheumatoid arthritis

A chronic, systemic inflammatory disease, rheumatoid arthritis (RA) primarily attacks peripheral joints and surrounding muscles, tendons, ligaments, and blood vessels. Partial remissions and unpredictable exacerbations mark the course of this potentially crippling disease.

RA occurs worldwide, striking nearly three times more women than men. It can occur at any age, but peak incidence is ages 35 to 50.

This disease usually requires lifelong treatment and, sometimes, surgery. In most patients, it follows an intermittent course and allows normal activity, although 10% suffer total disability from severe articular deformity, associated extra-articular symptoms, or both. The prognosis worsens with the development of nodules, vasculitis, and high titers of rheumatoid factor (RF).

If unarrested, the inflammatory process within the joints occurs in four stages:
- First stage: Synovitis develops from congestion and edema of the synovial membrane and joint capsule. Infiltration by lymphocytes, macrophages, and neutrophils perpetuates the local inflammatory response. These cells as well as fibroblast-like synovial cells produce en-

zymes that help to degrade bone and cartilage.

- Second stage: Pannus (thickened layers of granulation tissue) is formed, covering and invading cartilage and eventually destroying the joint capsule and bone.
- Third stage: Fibrous ankylosis (fibrous invasion of the pannus and scar formation that occludes the joint space) occurs. Bone atrophy and malalignment cause visible deformities and disrupt the articulation of opposing bones, causing muscle atrophy and imbalance and, possibly, partial dislocations or subluxations.
- Fourth stage: Fibrous tissue calcifies, resulting in bony ankylosis and immobility.

Causes
- Unknown
- Possible influence of infection (bacterial or viral) and hormonal factors

Signs and symptoms
Early stage
- Anorexia
- Fatigue
- Malaise
- Persistent low-grade fever
- Vague articular symptoms
- Weight loss

Late stage
- Cardiopulmonary lesions
- Carpal tunnel syndrome
- Destruction of the odontoid process (part of the second cervical vertebra)
- Diminished joint function
- Infection
- Joints that are tender and painful, at first only when the patient moves them but eventually even at rest
- Joints that feel hot to the touch
- Lymphadenopathy
- Myositis

- Osteoporosis
- Pericarditis
- Peripheral neuritis, producing numbness or tingling in the feet or weakness and loss of sensation in the fingers
- Pleuritis
- Pulmonary nodules or fibrosis
- Rheumatoid nodules—subcutaneous, round or oval, nontender
- Scleritis and episcleritis
- Spindle-shaped fingers resulting from marked edema and congestion in the joints
- Stiff, weak, or painful muscles, especially after inactivity and on rising in the morning
- Temporomandibular joint disease, which impairs chewing and causes earaches
- Vasculitis, possibly leading to skin lesions, leg ulcers, and multiple systemic complications

Diagnostic tests
- X-rays in early stages show bone demineralization and soft-tissue swelling; later, loss of cartilage and narrowing of joint spaces; and finally, cartilage and bone destruction and erosion, subluxations, and deformities.
- RF is positive in 75% to 80% of patients, as indicated by a titer of 1:160 or higher.
- Synovial fluid analysis shows increased volume and turbidity but decreased viscosity and elevated white blood cell counts (commonly greater than 10,000/mm^3).
- Serum protein electrophoresis may show elevated serum globulin levels.
- Erythrocyte sedimentation rate and C-reactive protein level are elevated in 85% to 90% of patients (may be useful to monitor response to therapy because elevation typically parallels disease activity).

■ Complete blood count usually shows moderate anemia, slight leukocytosis, and thrombocytosis.

Treatment

■ Salicylates, particularly aspirin, are the mainstay of RA therapy, because they decrease inflammation and relieve joint pain.

■ Nonsteroidal anti-inflammatory drugs (such as indomethacin [Indocin], fenoprofen [Nalfon], and ibuprofen [Motrin]), antimalarials (hydroxychloroquine [Plaquenil]), sulfasalazine (Azulfidine), gold salts, and corticosteroids (prednisone) may also be used. (See *Drug therapy for arthritis,* pages 554 and 555.)

■ Immunosuppressants—such as methotrexate (Trexall), cyclophosphamide (Cytoxan), and azathioprine (Imuran)—are also therapeutic; they're used more commonly early in the disease process.

■ COX-2 inhibitor, such as celecoxib (Celebrex), significantly reduce the risk of GI bleeding.

■ Cyclophosphamide (Cytoxan), which suppresses the immune system and is associated with toxic adverse effects, may be used in patients who have been unsuccessful with other therapies.

■ Other drugs for RA therapy include:
– Etanercept (Enbrel), an injectable agent, and infliximab (Remicade), given I.V. every 2 months, inhibit the inflammatory protein tumor necrosis factor.
– Leflunomide (Arava) blocks the growth of new cells.
– Anakinra (Kinerel), an injectable agent, blocks another inflammatory protein, interleukin-1.

■ Supportive measures include 8 to 10 hours of sleep every night, frequent rest periods between daily activities, and splinting to rest inflamed joints.

■ A physical therapy program, including range-of-motion exercises and carefully individualized therapeutic exercises, forestalls loss of joint function.

■ Application of heat relaxes muscles and relieves pain. Moist heat usually works best for patients with chronic disease. Ice packs are effective during acute episodes.

■ Early intervention, under the guidance of an occupational therapist, with splinting and joint protection devices can effectively delay the progression of joint deformities.

■ Advanced disease may require synovectomy, joint reconstruction, or total joint arthroplasty. (See *When arthritis requires surgery,* page 556.)

■ Metatarsal head and distal ulnar resectional arthroplasty, insertion of a Silastic prosthesis between metacarpophalangeal and proximal interphalangeal joints, and arthrodesis (joint fusion) are useful surgical procedures. Arthrodesis sacrifices joint mobility for stability and relief of pain.

■ Synovectomy (removal of destructive, proliferating synovium, usually in the wrists, knees, and fingers) may halt or delay the course of the disease.

■ Osteotomy (the cutting of bone or excision of a wedge of bone) can realign joint surfaces and redistribute stresses.

■ Tendons may rupture spontaneously, requiring surgical repair. Tendon transfers may prevent deformities or relieve contractures.

■ Apheresis may slow down RA or stop it from worsening.

Nursing considerations

■ Provide appropriate teaching and postoperative care if the patient requires knee or hip arthroplasty.

■ Carefully assess all joints. Look for deformities, contractures, immobility, and

(*Text continues on page 556.*)

Drug therapy for arthritis

Drug and adverse effects	Clinical considerations
Aspirin ■ Prolonged bleeding time; GI disturbances, including nausea, dyspepsia, anorexia nervosa, ulcers, and hemorrhage; hypersensitivity reactions ranging from urticaria to anaphylaxis; and salicylism (mild toxicity: tinnitus, dizziness; moderate toxicity: restlessness, hyperpnea, delirium, marked lethargy; severe toxicity: coma, seizures, severe hyperpnea)	■ Don't use in patients with GI ulcers, bleeding, or hypersensitivity or in neonates. ■ Give with food, milk, antacid, or a large glass of water to minimize adverse GI reactions. ■ Monitor the salicylate level. Remember that toxicity can develop rapidly in febrile, dehydrated children. ■ Teach the patient to reduce dose, one tablet at a time, if tinnitus occurs. ■ Teach the patient to watch for signs of bleeding, such as bruising, melena, and petechiae.
Cyclosporine ■ Nephrotoxicity (rise in blood urea nitrogen [BUN] and creatinine levels), hypertension, bone marrow suppression, nausea, vomiting, paresthesia, and bone pain	■ Avoid use in patients with preexisting hypertension or renal disease. ■ Monitor blood pressure closely. ■ Monitor BUN and creatinine levels. ■ Be aware that levels of cyclosporine may be increased by other medications that are metabolized by the liver.
Fenoprofen, ibuprofen, naproxen, piroxicam, sulindac, and tolmetin ■ Prolonged bleeding time; central nervous system abnormalities (headache, drowsiness, restlessness, dizziness, tremor); GI disturbances, including hemorrhage and peptic ulcer; and increased BUN and liver enzyme levels	■ Don't use in patients with renal disease, in asthmatics with nasal polyps, or in children. ■ Use cautiously if the patient has a GI disorder or cardiac disease or if he's allergic to other nonsteroidal anti-inflammatory drugs. ■ Give with milk or meals to minimize adverse GI reactions. ■ Tell the patient that the drug's effect may be delayed for 2 to 3 weeks. ■ Monitor kidney, liver, and auditory functions in long-term therapy. Stop drugs if abnormalities develop. ■ Use cautiously in elderly patients; they may experience severe GI bleeding without warning.
Gold (oral and parenteral) ■ Dermatitis, pruritus, rash, stomatitis, nephrotoxicity, and blood dyscrasias; with oral form, GI distress and diarrhea	■ Watch for adverse reactions. Observe the patient for nitritoid reaction, indicated by flushing, fainting, and sweating. ■ Check urine for blood and albumin before each dose. If positive, drug may need to be withheld. Stress the need for regular follow-up, including blood and urine testing.

Drug therapy for arthritis (continued)

Drug and adverse effects	Clinical considerations
Gold (oral and parenteral) (continued)	■ To avoid local nerve irritation, mix drug well and give by deep I.M. injection in the buttock. ■ Advise the patient not to expect improvement for 3 to 6 months. ■ Instruct the patient to report rash, bruising, bleeding, hematuria, or oral ulcers.
Hydroxychloroquine ■ Blood dyscrasias, GI irritation, corneal opacities, and keratopathy or retinopathy	■ The drug is contraindicated in patients with retinal or visual field changes. ■ Use cautiously in patients with hepatic disease, alcoholism, glucose-6-phosphate dehydrogenase deficiency, or psoriasis. ■ Perform complete blood count (CBC) and liver function tests before therapy and during maintenance therapy. The patient should also have a regular ophthalmologic examination. ■ Tell the patient to take the drug with food or milk. ■ Warn the patient that dizziness may occur.
Methotrexate ■ Tubular necrosis, bone marrow depression, leukopenia, thrombocytopenia, pulmonary interstitial infiltrates, stomatitis, hyperuricemia, rash, pruritus, dermatitis, alopecia, diarrhea, dizziness, cirrhosis, and hepatic fibrosis	■ Don't give if the patient is breast-feeding, pregnant, or an alcoholic. ■ Monitor uric acid (UA) levels, CBC, and liver function test results. ■ Monitor intake and output. ■ Warn the patient to promptly report unusual bleeding (especially GI) or bruising. ■ Warn the patient to avoid alcohol. ■ Advise the patient to follow the prescribed regimen.
Prednisone ■ Hyperglycemia, hypertension, fluid retention and weight gain, acne, cataracts, dyspepsia, muscle weakness, osteoporosis, mental status changes, insomnia, psychosis, and Cushing's syndrome	■ Give as an initial high dose to suppress inflammation, followed by slow tapering to the lowest possible dose. ■ Advise the patient not to stop the drug suddenly because this can lead to adrenal insufficiency. ■ Monitor glucose level and blood pressure.
Sulfasalazine ■ Nausea, vomiting, abdominal pains, rash, bone marrow suppression, headache, and hypersensitivity reaction	■ Give in divided doses. ■ Don't give if the patient has a known sulfa allergy. ■ Monitor CBC, UA, and liver enzyme levels. ■ Caution the patient not to take sulfasalazine at the same time as an antacid, which interferes with absorption.

When arthritis requires surgery

Arthritis severe enough to necessitate total knee or total hip arthroplasty calls for comprehensive preoperative teaching and postoperative care.

Before surgery

■ Explain preoperative and surgical procedures. Show the patient the prosthesis to be used, if available.

■ Teach the patient postoperative exercises (such as isometrics), and supervise his practice. Also teach deep-breathing and coughing exercises that will be necessary after surgery.

■ Explain that total hip or knee arthroplasty requires frequent range-of-motion exercises of the leg after surgery; total knee arthroplasty requires frequent leg-lift exercises.

■ Show the patient how to use a trapeze to move himself about in bed after surgery, and make sure that he has a fracture bedpan handy.

■ Tell the patient what kind of dressings to expect after surgery. After total knee arthroplasty, the patient's knee may be placed in a constant passive motion device to increase postoperative mobility and prevent emboli. After total hip arthroplasty, he'll have an abduction pillow between the legs to help keep the hip prosthesis in place.

After surgery

■ Closely monitor and record the patient's vital signs. Watch for complications, such as steroid crisis and shock if the patient is receiving a steroid. Monitor distal leg pulses often, marking them with a waterproof marker to make them easier to find.

■ As soon as the patient awakens, make sure he can perform active dorsiflexion. Supervise isometric exercises every 2 hours. After total hip arthroplasty, check traction for pressure areas and keep the head of the bed raised 30 to 45 degrees.

■ Change or reinforce dressings as needed, using sterile technique. Check wounds for hematoma, excessive drainage, color changes, or foul odor—all possible signs of hemorrhage or infection. (Wounds on rheumatoid arthritis patients may heal slowly.) Avoid contaminating dressings while helping the patient use the urinal or bedpan.

■ Administer blood replacement products, an antibiotic, and pain medication as needed. Monitor serum electrolyte and hemoglobin levels and hematocrit.

■ Have the patient turn, cough, and deep-breathe every 2 hours, and then percuss his chest.

■ After total knee arthroplasty, keep the patient's leg extended and slightly elevated.

■ After total hip arthroplasty, keep the patient's hip in abduction to prevent dislocation. Watch for an inability to rotate the hip or bear weight on it, increased pain, or a leg that appears shorter—all may indicate dislocation.

■ As soon as he's allowed, help the patient get out of bed and sit in a chair, keeping his weight on the unaffected side. When he's ready to walk, consult with the physical therapist for walking instruction and aids.

inability to perform everyday activities.

■ Monitor the patient's vital signs, and note weight changes, sensory disturbances, and level of pain. Administer an analgesic, and watch for adverse reactions.

■ Give meticulous skin care. Check for rheumatoid nodules as well as pressure ulcers and breakdowns from immobility, vascular impairment, corticosteroid treatment, or improper splinting. Use lotion or cleansing oil, not soap, for dry skin.

■ Explain all diagnostic tests and procedures. Tell the patient to expect multiple blood samples to allow a firm diagnosis and accurate monitoring of therapy.

■ Monitor the duration, not the intensity, of morning stiffness, because duration more accurately reflects the severity of the disease. Encourage the patient to take hot showers or baths at bedtime or in the morning to reduce the need for pain medication.

■ Apply splints carefully and correctly. If the patient is in traction or wearing splints, monitor him for pressure ulcers.

■ Explain the nature of RA. Make sure that the patient and her family understand that RA is a chronic disease that requires major lifestyle changes. Emphasize that there are no miracle cures despite claims to the contrary.

■ Encourage a balanced diet, but make sure that the patient understands that special diets won't cure RA. Stress the need for weight control because obesity adds further stress to joints.

■ Urge the patient to perform activities of daily living, such as dressing and feeding herself. (Supply easy-to-open cartons, lightweight cups, and unpackaged silverware.) Allow the patient enough time to calmly perform these tasks.

■ Provide emotional support. Remember that the patient with chronic illness easily becomes depressed, discouraged, and irritable. Encourage the RA patient to discuss her fears about dependency, sexuality, body image, and self-esteem. Refer her to an appropriate social service agency as needed.

■ Discuss sexual aids: alternative positions, pain medication, and moist heat to increase mobility.

■ Provide discharge teaching and make sure that the patient knows how and when to take prescribed medication and how to recognize its adverse effects.

■ Teach the patient how to stand, walk, and sit correctly—upright and erect. Tell her to sit in chairs with high seats and armrests; she'll find it easier to get up from a chair if her knees are lower than her hips. If she doesn't own a chair with a high seat, recommend putting blocks of wood under the legs of a favorite chair. Suggest an elevated toilet seat.

■ Instruct the patient to pace daily activities, resting for 5 to 10 minutes out of each hour and alternating sitting and standing tasks. Adequate sleep is important, and so is correct sleeping posture. She should sleep on her back on a firm mattress and should avoid placing a pillow under her knees, which encourages flexion deformity.

■ Teach the patient to avoid putting undue stress on joints and to use the largest joint available for a given task; to support weak or painful joints as much as possible; to avoid positions of flexion and promote positions of extension; to hold objects parallel to the knuckles as briefly as possible; to always use her hands toward the center of her body; and to slide—not lift—objects whenever possible.

■ Enlist the aid of the occupational therapist to teach how to simplify activities and protect arthritic joints. Stress the importance of shoes with proper support.

■ Suggest dressing aids—long-handled shoehorn, reacher, elastic shoelaces, zipper-pull, and buttonhook—and helpful household items, such as easy-to-open drawers, a handheld shower nozzle, handrails, and grab bars.

■ Tell the patient to dress while sitting, if possible.

- Refer the patient to the Arthritis Foundation for more information on coping with RA.

Roseola infantum

Also called *exanthema subitum,* roseola infantum is an acute, benign, presumably viral infection. It usually affects infants and young children, typically between ages 6 months and 3 years.

Roseola affects boys and girls alike. It occurs year-round but is most prevalent in spring and fall. Overt roseola, the most common exanthem in infants younger than age 2, affects 30% of all children; inapparent roseola (febrile illness without a rash) may affect the rest.

Characteristically, it first causes a high fever and then a rash that accompanies an abrupt drop to normal temperature. (See *Incubation and duration of common rash-producing infections.*)

Human herpesvirus 6 (HHV-6) causes roseola, although similar syndromes occur with other viruses. The incubation period is 5 to 15 days.

Causes
- HHV-6; transmitted by saliva and possibly by genital secretions

Signs and symptoms
- Abruptly rising, unexplainable fever that peaks at 103° to 105° F (39.4° to 40.6° C) for 3 to 5 days and then drops suddenly; may be accompanied by seizures
- In the early febrile period, the infant possibly anorexic, irritable, and listless but doesn't seem particularly ill
- Simultaneously with an abrupt drop in temperature, a maculopapular, nonpruritic rash developing, which blanches on pressure; profuse on the infant's trunk, arms, and neck and mild on the face and legs and fading within 24 hours

Diagnostic tests
- Diagnosis usually depends on signs and symptoms.
- Causative organism is present in saliva.

Treatment
- An antipyretic is given to lower the fever.

Incubation and duration of common rash-producing infections

Infection	Incubation (days)	Duration (days)
Herpes simplex	2 to 12	7 to 21
Roseola	5 to 15	3 to 6
Rubella	6 to 18	3
Rubeola	13 to 17	5
Varicella	10 to 14	7 to 14

- An anticonvulsant is given to relieve seizures.

Nursing considerations

- Teach parents how to lower their infant's fever by giving antipyretics, keeping him in lightweight clothes, and maintaining normal room temperature.
- Stress the need for adequate fluid intake.
- Tell parents that a short febrile seizure won't cause brain damage. Explain that children with simple febrile seizures usually don't need treatment with anticonvulsants. If a seizure lasts more than 5 minutes, however, parents should seek emergency treatment.

 # Rubella

Commonly called *German measles,* rubella is an acute, mildly contagious viral disease that produces a distinctive rash and lymphadenopathy. It's most common among children ages 5 to 9, adolescents, and young adults. The period of communicability lasts from about 10 days before until 5 days after the rash appears.

Worldwide in distribution, rubella flourishes during spring (particularly in big cities), and epidemics occur sporadically. In 2005, the Centers for Disease Control and Prevention determined that the rubella virus has been eradicated in the United States; however the vaccine is still recommended since overseas travelers could bring the disease in from countries where it's still active. This disease is self-limiting, and the prognosis is excellent, except for congenital rubella, which can have disastrous consequences.

Congenital rubella syndrome occurs in 25% of infants born to women who acquire rubella during the first trimester of pregnancy; defects are rare if the in-

fection occurs after the 20th week of pregnancy. Complications in the fetus may include deafness, cataracts, microcephaly, mental retardation, congenital heart defects, and other problems. Miscarriage or stillbirth may also occur.

Causes

- Transmission of virus through contact with blood, urine, stools, or nasopharyngeal secretions of infected persons and possibly by contact with freshly contaminated articles of clothing
- Transplacental transmission (congenital rubella syndrome)

Signs and symptoms

- In children, after an incubation period of 14 to 21 days, an exanthematous, maculopapular rash that erupts abruptly
- Rash that begins on the face and spreads rapidly, sometimes covering the trunk and extremities within hours; small, red, petechial macules on the soft palate (Forschheimer spots) possibly preceding or accompanying the rash
- By the end of the second day: facial rash beginning to fade, but rash on the trunk possibly confluent and easily mistaken for scarlet fever; continuing to fade in the downward order in which it appeared
- The rash generally disappearing on the third day but possibly persisting for 4 to 5 days—sometimes accompanied by mild coryza and conjunctivitis
- Rapid appearance and disappearance of the rubella rash, distinguishing it from rubeola
- Rarely, rubella appearing without a rash
- In adolescents and adults: headache, anorexia, malaise, low-grade fever, coryza, lymphadenopathy and, sometimes, conjunctivitis (first signs and symptoms); suboccipital, postauricular,

and postcervical lymph node enlargement (hallmark of rubella)
- Low-grade fever (99° to 101° F [37.2° to 38.3° C]) that may accompany the rash but usually not after the first day of the rash; rarely, temperature reaching 104° F (40° C)

Diagnostic tests
- Cell cultures of the throat, blood, urine, and cerebrospinal fluid can confirm that the virus is present.
- Convalescent serum that shows a four-fold rise in antibody titers confirms the diagnosis.

Treatment
- Antipyretics and analgesics are given for fever and joint pain.
- Bed rest isn't necessary, but the patient should be isolated until the rash disappears.
- Immunization with live-virus vaccine RA27/3, the only rubella vaccine available in the United States, is necessary for prevention. The rubella vaccine is commonly given with measles and mumps vaccines (the MMR vaccine) at age 12 to 15 months, and a second dose during childhood.

Nursing considerations
- Make the patient with active rubella as comfortable as possible. Suggest that children be given books to read or games to play to keep them occupied.
- Explain why respiratory isolation is necessary. Make sure that the patient or his parents understand how important it is to avoid exposing pregnant women to this disease.
- Report confirmed cases of rubella to local public health officials.

When giving the rubella vaccine
- Obtain a history of allergies, especially to neomycin. If the patient is allergic to neomycin or has had a reaction to immunization in the past, check with the physician before giving the vaccine.

DRUG CHALLENGE

 If the patient is a woman of childbearing age, ask her whether she's pregnant. If she is or thinks she may be, don't give the vaccine. Warn women who receive rubella vaccine to use an effective means of birth control for at least 3 months after immunization.

- Give the vaccine at least 3 months after administration of immune globulin or blood, which could have antibodies that neutralize the vaccine.
- If the patient suffers from immunocompromise or immunodeficiency disease or is receiving immunosuppressant, radiation, or corticosteroid therapy, avoid giving him the vaccine. Instead, administer immune serum globulin to prevent or reduce infection.
- After giving the vaccine, observe the patient for signs of anaphylaxis for at least 30 minutes. Keep epinephrine 1:1,000 handy.
- Warn the patient that mild fever, slight rash, transient arthralgia (in adolescents), and arthritis (in elderly patients) are possible. Suggest aspirin or acetaminophen for fever.
- Advise the patient to apply warmth to the injection site for 24 hours after immunization (to help the body absorb the vaccine). If swelling persists after the first 24 hours, suggest a cold compress to promote vasoconstriction and prevent antigenic cyst formation.

Rubeola

Also known as *measles* or *morbilli,* rubeola is an acute, highly contagious paramyxovirus infection. Formerly a common disease, measles is seen less frequently in developed countries when childhood immunizations are widely used. It remains a very serious communicable disease among nonimmunized populations.

In temperate zones, incidence is highest in late winter and early spring. Before the availability of measles vaccine, epidemics occurred every 2 to 5 years in large urban areas. Use of the vaccine has reduced the occurrence of measles during childhood and, according to the Centers for Disease Control and Prevention, it's no longer a major public health threat in the United States. (See *Administering measles vaccine,* page 562.)

Measles remains a major cause of death in children in underdeveloped countries.

Incubation is from 10 to 14 days. Initial symptoms begin and greatest communicability occurs during a prodromal phase beginning about 11 days after exposure to the virus and lasting 4 to 5 days. Progressive signs and symptoms occur about 5 days after the appearance of Koplik's spots. (Tiny, bluish gray specks surrounded by a red halo appear on the oral mucosa opposite the molars.)

The most common complications are otitis media and diarrhea. Pneumonia and encephalitis occur less frequently. Subacute sclerosing panencephalitis (SSPE), a rare and invariably fatal complication, may develop several years after measles. SSPE is less common in patients who have received the measles vaccine.

Causes
- Transmission of paramyxovirus infection, through direct contact or contaminated airborne respiratory droplets

Signs and symptoms
Prodromal phase
- Fever
- Photophobia
- Malaise
- Anorexia
- Conjunctivitis
- Coryza
- Hoarseness
- Hacking cough
- Koplik's spots

Progressive symptoms
- Sharply rising temperature
- Sloughing of spots
- Slightly pruritic rash: starting as faint macules behind the ears and on the neck and cheeks; becoming papular and erythematous; rapidly spreading over the entire face, neck, eyelids, arms, chest, back, abdomen, and thighs; fading in same order when it reaches the feet 2 to 3 days later
- Brownish discoloration: replacing rash, disappearing in 7 to 10 days
- Temperature peaking at 103° to 105° F (39.4° to 40.6° C), with severe cough, rhinorrhea, and puffy, red eyes

Diagnostic tests
- If necessary, measles virus may be isolated from the blood, nasopharyngeal secretions, and urine during the febrile period.
- Serum antibodies appear within 3 days after onset of the rash and reach peak titers 2 to 4 weeks later.

Treatment
- The patient should receive antipyretics to control fever.

Administering measles vaccine

Generally, one bout of measles renders immunity (a second infection is extremely rare and may represent misdiagnosis); infants younger than age 4 months may be immune because of circulating maternal antibodies.

Typically, measles vaccine is given with mumps and rubella vaccine (MMR) at age 15 months. The second dose of MMR is typically administered at age 4 to 6 years.

Special considerations

■ Warn the patient or his parents that adverse effects of the vaccine include anorexia, malaise, rash, mild thrombocytopenia or leukopenia, and fever. Explain that the vaccine may produce slight reactions, usually within 7 to 10 days.
■ Ask the patient about known allergies, especially to neomycin (each dose contains a small amount). However, a patient who's allergic to eggs may receive the vaccine because it contains only minimal amounts of albumin and yolk components.
■ Avoid giving the vaccine to a pregnant woman (ask for the date of her last menstrual period). Warn a woman receiving the vaccine to avoid pregnancy for at least 3 months after vaccination.
■ Don't vaccinate children with untreated tuberculosis, immunodeficiencies, leukemia, or lymphoma or those receiving an immunosuppressant. If such children are exposed to the virus, recommend that they receive gamma globulin. (Gamma globulin won't prevent measles but will lessen its severity.)
■ Older unimmunized children who have been exposed to measles for more than 5 days may also require gamma globulin. Be sure to immunize them 3 months later.
■ Delay vaccination for 8 to 12 weeks after administration of whole blood, plasma, or gamma globulin because measles antibodies in these components may neutralize the vaccine.
■ MMR vaccine is recommended for all asymptomatic human immunodeficiency virus (HIV)-infected persons and should be considered for symptomatic HIV patients who aren't severely immunosuppressed.
■ Watch for signs of anaphylaxis for 30 minutes after vaccination. Keep epinephrine 1:1,000 handy.
■ Advise application of a warm compress to the vaccination site to facilitate absorption of the vaccine. If swelling occurs within 24 hours after vaccination, tell the patient to apply cold compresses to promote vasoconstriction and to prevent antigenic cyst formation.

■ Vaporizers and a warm environment help reduce respiratory irritation. Cough preparations and antibiotics are usually ineffective.

Nursing considerations

■ Teach parents the importance of immunizing their children against measles, and follow appropriate procedures when giving the vaccine.
■ Monitor the patient's vital signs.
■ Institute respiratory isolation precautions for 4 days after the onset of rash.
■ Administer an antipyretic as prescribed.
■ Encourage bed rest during the acute phase.
■ Darken the room if photophobia occurs.
■ Teach parents the importance of isolating the child, encouraging bed rest, and increasing fluid intake.

- Instruct the parents to report early signs and symptoms of complications, such as otitis media, pneumonia, encephalitis, bronchitis, and secondary bacterial infection.
- Follow your facility's procedures for reporting cases to local health authorities.

S

Salmonellosis

A common infection in the United States, salmonellosis is caused by gram-negative bacilli of the genus *Salmonella,* a member of the Enterobacteriaceae family. It occurs as enterocolitis, bacteremia, localized infection, typhoid, or paratyphoid fever. (See *Clinical variants of salmonellosis.*)

Nontyphoid forms usually produce mild to moderate illness with low mortality.

Typhoid, the most severe form of salmonellosis, usually lasts from 1 to 4 weeks. Mortality is about 3% in people who are treated and 10% in those untreated, usually as a result of intestinal perforation or hemorrhage, cerebral thrombosis, toxemia, pneumonia, or acute circulatory failure.

An attack of typhoid confers lifelong immunity, although the patient may become a carrier. Most typhoid patients are younger than age 30; most carriers are women older than age 50. Incidence of typhoid in the United States is increasing as more travelers return from endemic areas.

Enterocolitis and bacteremia are common (and more virulent) among infants, elderly people, and people already weakened by other infections; paratyphoid fever is rare in the United States.

Salmonellosis is 20 times more common in patients with acquired immunodeficiency syndrome. Features of the disease include an increased incidence of bacteremia, an inability to identify the infection source, and a tendency of the infection to recur after therapy is stopped. Of an estimated 1,700 serotypes of *Salmonella,* 10 cause the diseases most common in the United States; all 10 types can survive for weeks in water, ice, sewage, or food.

Causes

- Drinking water contaminated by excretions of a carrier (typhoid form)
- Fecal-oral spread (especially in children younger than age 5)
- Ingestion of contaminated or inadequately cooked or processed foods, especially eggs, chicken, turkey, and duck (nontyphoid form)

Predisposing factors

- Owning a pet turtle, lizard, or snake

Signs and symptoms

- Abdominal pain
- Fever
- Headache, increasing fever, and constipation (more common with typhoid form)
- Severe diarrhea (with enterocolitis)

Clinical variants of salmonellosis

Variant	Cause	Clinical features
Enterocolitis	Any species of nontyphoidal *Salmonella,* but usually *S. enteritidis;* incubation period of 6 to 48 hours	Mild to severe abdominal pain, diarrhea, sudden fever up to 102° F (38.9° C), nausea, vomiting; usually self-limiting but may progress to enteric fever (resembling typhoid), local abscesses (usually abdominal), dehydration, septicemia
Paratyphoid	*S. paratyphi* and *S. schottmuelleri* (formerly *S. paratyphi* B); incubation period of 3 weeks or more	Fever and transient diarrhea, generally resembles typhoid but less severe
Bacteremia	Any *Salmonella* species but most commonly *S. choleraesius;* varying incubation period	Fever, chills, anorexia, weight loss (without GI symptoms), joint pains
Localized infections	Usually follows bacteremia caused by *Salmonella* species	Site of localization determined by symptoms (osteomyelitis, endocarditis, bronchopneumonia, pyelonephritis, and arthritis)
Typhoid fever	*S. typhi* entering the GI tract and invading the bloodstream via the lymphatics, setting up intracellular sites; during this phase, infection of biliary tract leading to intestinal seeding with millions of bacilli; involved lymphoid tissues (especially Peyer's patches in ilium) enlarging, ulcerating, and becoming necrotic, resulting in hemorrhage; incubation period of usually 1 to 2 weeks	Symptoms of enterocolitis: may develop within hours of ingestion of *S. typhi,* but usually subside before onset of typhoid symptoms *1st week:* gradually increasing fever, anorexia, myalgia, malaise, headache *2nd week:* remittent fever up to 104° F (40°C) usually in the evening, chills, diaphoresis, weakness, delirium, increasing abdominal pain and distention, diarrhea or constipation, cough, moist crackles, tender abdomen with enlarged spleen, maculopapular rash (especially on abdomen) *3rd week:* persistent fever, increasing fatigue and weakness; usually subsides at end of 3rd week, although relapses possibly occurring *Complications:* intestinal perforation or hemorrhage, abscesses, thrombophlebitis, cerebral thrombosis, pneumonia, osteomyelitis, myocarditis, acute circulatory failure, chronic carrier state

Diagnostic tests

- Isolation of the organism in a culture, particularly blood (in typhoid, paratyphoid, and bacteremia) or stool (in enterocolitis, paratyphoid, and typhoid) confirms salmonellosis. Other appropriate culture specimens include urine, bone marrow, pus, and vomitus.
- Presence of *S. typhi* in stool one or more years after treatment indicates that the patient is a carrier, which is true in 3% of cases.
- Widal's test, an agglutination reaction against somatic and flagellar antigens, may suggest typhoid with a fourfold rise in titer. However, drug use or hepatic disease can also increase these titers and invalidate test results.
- Blood tests show transient leukocytosis during the 1st week of typhoidal salmonellosis, leukopenia during the 3rd week, and leukocytosis in local infection.

Treatment

- Antimicrobial therapy for typhoid, paratyphoid, and bacteremia depends on the organism's sensitivity. It may include amoxicillin (Amoxil), chloramphenicol (Chloromycetin) and, if the patient is severely toxemic, co-trimoxazole (Bactrim), ciprofloxacin (Cipro), or ceftriaxone (Rocephin).
- Localized abscesses may need surgical drainage.
- Enterocolitis requires a short course of antibiotic treatment only if it causes septicemia or prolonged fever.
- Other treatments include bed rest and replacement of fluids and electrolytes.
- Camphorated opium tincture (Paregoric), kaolin with pectin (Kapectolin), diphenoxylate hydrochloride, codeine, or small doses of morphine may be necessary to relieve diarrhea and control cramps in patients who must remain active.

Nursing considerations

- Follow standard precautions. Always wash your hands thoroughly before and after contact with the patient, and advise other facility personnel to do the same. Teach the patient to use proper handwashing technique, especially after defecating and before eating or handling food. Wear gloves and a gown when disposing of feces or fecally contaminated objects.
- Continue standard precautions until three consecutive stool cultures are negative—the first one 48 hours after antibiotic treatment ends, followed by two more at 24-hour intervals.
- Observe the patient closely for signs and symptoms of bowel perforation: sudden pain in the right lower abdominal quadrant, possibly after one or more rectal bleeding episodes; sudden fall in temperature or blood pressure; and rising pulse rate.
- During acute infection, allow the patient as much rest as possible. Raise the side rails and use other safety measures because the patient may become delirious.
- Accurately record intake and output. Maintain adequate I.V. hydration. When the patient can tolerate oral feedings, encourage high-calorie fluids such as milk shakes. Watch for constipation.
- Provide good skin and mouth care. Turn the patient frequently, and perform mild passive exercises as indicated. Apply mild heat to the abdomen to relieve cramps.
- Don't administer an antipyretic because it can mask fever and lead to hypothermia. Instead, to promote heat loss through the skin without causing shivering (which keeps fever high by vasoconstriction), apply tepid, wet towels (don't use alcohol or ice) to the patient's groin and axillae. To promote heat loss by vasodilation of peripheral blood vessels,

use additional wet towels on the arms and legs, wiping with long, vigorous strokes.

■ After draining the abscesses of a joint, provide heat, elevation, and passive range-of-motion exercises to decrease swelling and maintain mobility.

■ If the patient has positive stool cultures on discharge, tell him to use a different bathroom than other family members if possible (while he's taking an antibiotic), to wash his hands afterward, and to avoid preparing uncooked foods, such as salads, for family members.

■ To prevent salmonellosis, advise prompt refrigeration of meat and cooked foods (avoid keeping them at room temperature for a prolonged period), and teach the importance of proper hand washing. Tell the patient to avoid eating raw or under-cooked eggs, and to wash kitchen work surfaces immediately after they have had contact with raw meat. Advise those at high risk for contracting typhoid (laboratory workers, travelers) to seek vaccination.

Sarcoidosis

A multisystemic, granulomatous disorder, sarcoidosis characteristically produces lymphadenopathy, pulmonary infiltration, and skeletal, liver, eye, or skin lesions. It's most common in young adults ages 20 to 40. In the United States, sarcoidosis occurs predominantly among blacks and affects twice as many women as men.

Acute sarcoidosis usually resolves within 2 years. Chronic, progressive sarcoidosis is associated with pulmonary fibrosis and progressive pulmonary disability.

Causes
■ Unknown

Predisposing factors
■ Contact with chemicals, such as zirconium or beryllium
■ Genetic factors
■ Hypersensitivity response (possibly from a T-cell imbalance) to such agents as atypical mycobacteria, fungi, and pine pollen

Signs and symptoms
■ Initially, arthralgia (in the wrists, ankles, and elbows), fatigue, malaise, and weight loss
■ Other signs and symptoms, according to the extent and location of fibrosis:
 – Cardiovascular—arrhythmias (premature beats, bundle-branch block, or complete heart block), cardiomyopathy (rare)
 – Central nervous system (CNS)—cranial or peripheral nerve palsies, basilar meningitis, seizures, pituitary and hypothalamic lesions producing diabetes insipidus
 – Cutaneous—erythema nodosum, subcutaneous skin nodules with maculopapular eruptions, extensive nasal mucosal lesions
 – Genitourinary—hypercalciuria
 – Hepatic—granulomatous hepatitis, usually asymptomatic
 – Lymphatic—bilateral hilar and right paratracheal lymphadenopathy and splenomegaly
 – Musculoskeletal—muscle weakness, polyarthralgia, pain, punched-out lesions on phalanges
 – Ophthalmic—anterior uveitis (common); glaucoma, blindness (rare)
 – Respiratory—breathlessness, cough (usually nonproductive), substernal pain (complications in advanced pulmonary disease: pulmonary hypertension and cor pulmonale)

Diagnostic tests

- A positive Kveim-Silzbach skin test result points to sarcoidosis. When coupled with a skin biopsy at the injection site that shows discrete epithelioid cell granuloma, the test confirms the disease.
- Biopsy of the lymph node, skin, or lung reveals noncaseating granulomas with negative cultures for mycobacteria and fungi.
- Chest X-ray shows bilateral hilar and right paratracheal adenopathy with or without diffuse interstitial infiltrates; occasionally, large nodular lesions are present in lung parenchyma.
- Pulmonary function tests show decreased total lung capacity and compliance and decreased diffusing capacity.
- Arterial blood gas (ABG) analysis shows decreased partial pressure of arterial oxygen.
- Negative results for tuberculin skin test, fungal serologies, and sputum cultures for mycobacteria and fungi as well as negative biopsy cultures help rule out infection.

Treatment

- Sarcoidosis causing no symptoms requires no treatment.
- Sarcoidosis that causes ocular, respiratory, CNS, cardiac, or systemic signs and symptoms, such as fever and weight loss, requires treatment with a systemic or topical steroid, as does sarcoidosis that produces hypercalcemia or destructive skin lesions. Such therapy is usually continued for 1 to 2 years, but some patients may need lifelong therapy. Other drugs sometimes used in addition to corticosteroids include immunosuppressants, methotrexate, azathioprine (Imuran), and cyclophosphamide (Cytoxan).
- Other treatment includes a low-calcium diet and avoidance of direct exposure to sunlight in patients with hypercalcemia.

- Rarely, some individuals with irreversible organ failure require organ transplantation.

Nursing considerations

- Watch for and report complications. Be aware of abnormal laboratory results (anemia, for example) that could alter patient care.
- If the patient has arthralgia, administer an analgesic as needed. Record signs of progressive muscle weakness.
- Provide a nutritious, high-calorie diet and plenty of fluids. If the patient has hypercalcemia, suggest a low-calcium diet. Weigh the patient regularly to detect weight loss.
- Monitor the patient's respiratory function. Check chest X-rays for the extent of lung involvement; note and record bloody sputum or an increase in sputum. If the patient has pulmonary hypertension or end-stage cor pulmonale, check ABG values, watch for arrhythmias, and administer oxygen as needed.

DRUG CHALLENGE

 Because steroids may induce or worsen diabetes mellitus, perform blood glucose tests every 12 hours at the beginning of steroid therapy. Also, watch for other adverse reactions to steroids, such as fluid retention, electrolyte imbalance (especially hypokalemia), moon face, hypertension, and personality changes.

During or after steroid withdrawal (particularly in association with infection or other types of stress), watch for vomiting, orthostatic hypotension, hypoglycemia, restlessness, anorexia, malaise, and fatigue. Remember that the patient undergoing long-term or high-dose steroid therapy is vulnerable to infection.

- When preparing the patient for discharge, stress the need for compliance with prescribed steroid therapy and regular, careful follow-up examinations and treatment.

- Refer the patient with failing vision to community support and resource groups and the American Foundation for the Blind if necessary.

Scabies

An age-old skin infection, scabies results from infestation with *Sarcoptes scabiei* var. *hominis* (itch mite), which provokes a sensitivity reaction. It occurs worldwide, is predisposed by overcrowding and poor hygiene, and can be endemic.

Mites can live their entire life cycles in the skin of humans, causing chronic infection. The female mite burrows into the skin to lay her eggs, from which larvae emerge to copulate and then reburrow under the skin. The adult mite can survive without a human host for only 2 to 3 days.

Causes

- Transmission through skin or sexual contact

Signs and symptoms

- Burrows: threadlike lesions about 2 cm long, usually between fingers, on flexor surfaces of the wrists, on elbows, in axillary folds, at the waistline, on nipples in females, on genitalia in males, and on the head and neck in infants
- Itching that intensifies at night; may become generalized because of sensitization
- Lesions: usually excoriated (from intense scratching); may appear as erythematous nodules
- Secondary bacterial infection from severe excoriation due to scratching

Diagnostic tests

- Superficial scraping and examination, under a low-power microscope, of material that has been expressed from a burrow may reveal the mite, ova, or mite feces. However, excoriation or inflammation of the burrow can make such identification difficult.

Treatment

- A thin layer of pediculicide—permethrin cream (Elimite) or lindane lotion—is applied over the entire skin surface. The pediculicide is left on for 8 to 12 hours. To make certain that all areas have been treated, this application should be repeated in about 1 week.
- Other treatments include crotamiton cream (Eurax), γ-benzene hexachloride, and benzyl benzoate. Widespread bacterial infections require a systemic antibiotic such as ivermectin (Stromectol).
- Persistent pruritus (from mite sensitization or contact dermatitis) may develop from repeated use of a pediculicide rather than from continued infection. An antipruritic emollient or topical steroid can reduce itching; an intralesional steroid may resolve erythematous nodules.

Nursing considerations

- Instruct the adult patient to apply permethrin cream or lindane lotion at bedtime from the neck down, covering the entire body. The cream or lotion should be washed off in 8 to 12 hours. Contaminated clothing and linens must be washed in hot water or dry-cleaned.
- Tell the patient not to apply lindane lotion if skin is raw or inflamed. Advise him to immediately report skin irritation or a hypersensitivity reaction, to stop using the drug, and to wash it off thoroughly.
- Suggest that family members, sexual partners, and other close contacts of the

patient be checked for possible symptoms and be treated if necessary.

■ If a hospitalized patient has scabies, take steps to prevent transmission to other patients. Practice good hand-washing technique or wear gloves when touching the patient, observe wound and skin precautions for 24 hours after treatment with a pediculicide, gas autoclave blood pressure cuffs before using them on other patients, isolate linens until the patient is noninfectious, and thoroughly disinfect the patient's room after discharge.

Scoliosis

Scoliosis, a lateral curvature of the spine, may be found in the thoracic, lumbar, or thoracolumbar spinal segment. The curve may be convex to the right (more common in thoracic curves) or to the left (more common in lumbar curves). As the spine curves laterally, compensatory curves develop to maintain body balance and mark the deformity. Rotation of the vertebral column around its axis occurs and may cause rib cage deformity. Scoliosis is commonly associated with kyphosis (humpback) and lordosis (swayback). A physical examination reveals unequal shoulder heights, elbow levels, and heights of the iliac crests. Muscles on the convex side of the curve may be rounded; those on the concave side, flattened, producing asymmetry of paraspinal muscles.

Scoliosis may be functional (postural) or structural. The three types of structural scoliosis are congenital, paralytic or musculoskeletal, and idiopathic, which is the most common. Idiopathic scoliosis can be further classified as *infantile,* which affects mostly boys age 1 to 3 and causes left thoracic and right lumbar curves; *juvenile,* which affects both sexes between ages 3 and 10 and causes varying types of curvature; and *adolescent,* which generally affects girls between age 10 and achievement of skeletal maturity and causes varying types of curvature.

Causes

■ Poor posture or a discrepancy in leg lengths (functional scoliosis)
■ Deformity of the vertebral bodies (structural scoliosis)
  – Congenital defect, such as wedge vertebrae, fused ribs or vertebrae, or hemivertebrae (congenital scoliosis)
  – Asymmetrical paralysis of the trunk muscles from polio, cerebral palsy, or muscular dystrophy (paralytic or musculoskeletal scoliosis)
  – Transmission as an autosomal dominant or multifactorial trait (idiopathic scoliosis)

Signs and symptoms

■ Spinal curvature that arises in the thoracic segment, with convexity to the right, and compensatory curves (S curves) in the cervical segment above and the lumbar segment below, both with convexity to the left
■ Backache, fatigue, and dyspnea (after disease is well-established)
■ Pulmonary insufficiency (curvature may decrease lung capacity), back pain, degenerative arthritis of the spine, disk disease, and sciatica (in untreated disease)

Diagnostic tests

■ Anterior, posterior, and lateral spinal X-rays, taken with the patient standing upright and bending, determine the degree of curvature (Cobb method) and flexibility of the spine. (See *Cobb method for measuring angle of curvature.*)
■ A scoliometer can also be used to measure the angle of trunk rotation.

Treatment

- A curve of less than 25 degrees is mild and can be monitored by spinal X-rays and an examination every 3 months. An exercise program that includes sit-ups, pelvic tilts, spine hyperextension, push-ups, and breathing exercises may strengthen torso muscles and prevent curve progression. A heel lift also may help.
- A curve of 25 to 39 degrees requires management with spinal exercises and a brace. (Transcutaneous electrical nerve stimulation may be used as an alternative.)
- A brace halts progression in most cases but doesn't reverse the established curvature. Such devices passively strengthen the patient's spine by applying asymmetric pressure to skin, muscles, and ribs. Braces can be adjusted as the patient grows and can be worn until bone growth is complete.
- A curve of 40 degrees or more requires surgery (spinal fusion with instrumentation) because a lateral curve continues to progress at the rate of 1 degree per year even after skeletal maturity. Surgery corrects lateral curvature by posterior spinal fusion and internal stabilization with a Harrington rod or other fixation devices. A distraction rod on the concave side of the curve "jacks" the spine into a straight position and provides an internal splint.
- An alternative procedure, anterior spinal fusion with instrumentation, corrects curvature with vertebral staples and an anterior stabilizing cable. Some spinal fusions may require postoperative immobilization in a brace.
- Postoperatively, periodic checkups are required for several months to monitor the stability of the correction.

Cobb method for measuring angle of curvature

The Cobb method measures the angle of curvature in scoliosis.

The top vertebra in the curve (T6 in the illustration) is the uppermost vertebra whose upper face tilts toward the curve's concave side. The bottom vertebra in the curve (T12) is the lowest vertebra whose lower face tilts toward the curve's concave side.

The angle at which perpendicular lines drawn from the upper face of the top vertebra and the lower face of the bottom vertebra intersect is the angle of the curve.

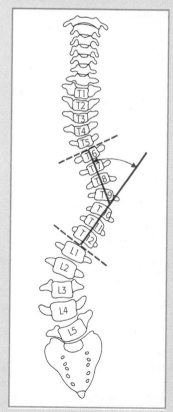

Nursing considerations

▪ Keep in mind that scoliosis affects many adolescents, who are likely to find activity limitations and treatment with orthopedic appliances distressing. Provide emotional support, along with meticulous skin and cast care, and patient teaching.

If the patient needs a brace

▪ Enlist the help of a physical therapist, a social worker, and an orthotist (orthopedic appliance specialist). Before the patient goes home, explain what the brace does and how to care for it (how to check the screws for tightness and pad the uprights to prevent excessive wear on clothing). Suggest that loose-fitting, oversized clothes be worn for greater comfort.

▪ Tell the patient to wear the brace 23 hours per day and to remove it only for bathing and exercise. Encourage the patient to lie down and rest several times a day while still adjusting to the brace.

▪ Suggest a soft mattress if a firm one is uncomfortable.

▪ To prevent skin breakdown, advise the patient not to use lotion, ointment, or powder on areas where the brace comes in contact with the skin. Instead, suggest using rubbing alcohol or tincture of benzoin to toughen the skin. Advise the patient to keep the skin dry and clean and to wear a snug T-shirt under the brace.

▪ Advise the patient to increase activities gradually and to avoid strenuous sports. Emphasize the importance of conscientiously performing prescribed exercises. Recommend swimming during the 1 hour out of the brace, but strongly warn against diving.

▪ Instruct the patient to turn the whole body, instead of just the head, when looking to the side. To make reading easier, advise holding the reading matter to look straight ahead at it instead of down. If this proves difficult, suggest prism glasses as an alternative.

If the patient needs traction or a cast before surgery

▪ Explain these procedures to the patient and his family. Remember that application of a body cast can be traumatic because it's done on a special frame and the patient's head and face are covered throughout the procedure.

▪ Check the skin around the cast edge daily. Keep the cast clean and dry and the edges of the cast "petaled" (padded). Warn the patient not to insert anything under the cast or let anything get under it and to immediately report cracks in the cast, pain, burning, skin breakdown, numbness, or odor.

▪ Before surgery, assure the patient and his family that he'll have adequate pain control after the surgery. Check sensation, movement, color, and blood supply in all extremities to detect neurovascular deficit, a serious complication following spinal surgery.

After corrective surgery

▪ Check neurovascular status every 2 to 4 hours for the first 48 hours and then several times per day. Logroll the patient often.

▪ Measure intake, output, and urine specific gravity to monitor effects of blood loss, which is commonly substantial.

▪ Monitor abdominal distention and bowel sounds.

▪ Encourage deep-breathing exercises to avoid pulmonary complications.

▪ Give an analgesic as needed, especially before activity.

▪ Promote active range-of-motion (ROM) arm exercises to help maintain muscle strength. Remember that any exercise, even brushing the hair or teeth, is helpful.

- Encourage the patient to perform quadriceps-setting, calf-pumping, and active ROM exercises of the ankles and feet.
- Watch for skin breakdown and signs of cast syndrome, such as nausea, abdominal pressure, and vague abdominal pain. Teach the patient how to recognize these signs.
- Remove antiembolism stockings for at least 30 minutes each day.
- Offer emotional support to help prevent depression, which may result from altered body image and immobility.
- If the patient is being discharged with a Harrington rod and cast and must have bed rest, arrange for a social worker and a visiting nurse to provide home care. Before discharge, make sure that the patient understands activity limitations.
- If you work in a school, screen children routinely for scoliosis during physical examinations.

Septic arthritis

A medical emergency, septic (infectious) arthritis is caused by bacterial invasion of a joint, resulting in inflammation of the synovial lining. If the organisms enter the joint cavity, effusion and pyogenesis follow, with eventual destruction of bone and cartilage. Anaerobic organisms, such as gram-positive cocci, usually infect adults and children older than age 2. *Haemophilus influenzae* commonly infects children younger than age 2.

Septic arthritis can lead to ankylosis and even fatal septicemia. However, prompt antibiotic therapy and joint aspiration or drainage cures most patients.

Causes

- Bacteria spreading from a primary site of infection, usually adjacent bone or soft tissue, through the bloodstream to a joint
- Common infecting organisms: four strains of gram-positive cocci (*Staphylococcus aureus, Streptococcus pyogenes, Streptococcus pneumoniae,* and *Streptococcus viridans*) and two strains of gram-negative cocci (*Neisseria gonorrhoeae* and *H. influenzae*); various gram-negative bacilli (*Escherichia coli, Salmonella,* and *Pseudomonas*)

Predisposing factors

- Alcoholism and older age
- Concurrent bacterial infection (of the genitourinary or upper respiratory tract, for example) or serious chronic illness (such as cancer, renal failure, rheumatoid arthritis, systemic lupus erythematosus, diabetes, or cirrhosis)
- Depressed autoimmune system or previous immunosuppressant therapy
- I.V. drug abuse
- Intra-articular injections
- Joint surgery
- Local joint abnormalities
- Recent articular trauma

Signs and symptoms

- Absence of systemic signs of inflammation (in some patients)
- Intense pain, inflammation, and swelling of the affected joint
- Low-grade fever
- Migratory polyarthritis sometimes preceding localization of the infection
- Pain in the groin, upper thigh, or buttock or referred to the knee (if bacteria invade hip)
- In the neonate or infant, voluntary immobility of the limb with the infected joint (pseudoparalysis), crying when the affected joint is moved (for example, during diaper changes), irritability, and fever

Diagnostic tests

- Arthrocentesis allows the collection of a synovial fluid specimen.
- Gram stain or culture of synovial fluid confirms the diagnosis and identifies the causative organism.
- Synovial fluid analysis shows gross pus or watery, cloudy fluid of decreased viscosity, usually with 50,000/µl or more white blood cells (WBCs), primarily neutrophils.
- Synovial fluid glucose is typically low compared with a simultaneous 6-hour postprandial blood glucose test.
- When synovial fluid culture is negative, a positive blood culture may confirm the diagnosis.
- X-rays can show typical changes as early as 1 week after initial infection—distention of joint capsules, for example, followed by narrowing of joint space (indicating cartilage damage) and erosions of bone (joint destruction).
- Radioisotope joint scan for less accessible joints (such as spinal articulations) may help detect infection or inflammation but isn't itself diagnostic.

Treatment

- Antibiotic therapy should begin promptly; it may be modified when sensitivity results become available. Medication selection requires drug sensitivity studies of the infecting organism. Bioassays or bactericidal assays of synovial fluid and bioassays of blood may confirm clearing of the infection.
- Progress is monitored through frequent analysis of joint fluid cultures, synovial fluid WBC counts, and glucose determinations.
- Rest and immobilize the affected area. The affected joint can be immobilized with a splint or traction.
- Warm compresses and elevation of the extremity help control pain.
- Needle aspiration (arthrocentesis) to remove grossly purulent joint fluid should be repeated daily until fluid appears normal.
- If cultures remain positive or the WBC count remains elevated, open surgical drainage (usually arthrotomy with lavage of the joint) may be necessary for resistant infection or chronic septic arthritis.
- Late reconstructive surgery is warranted only for severe joint damage and only after all signs of active infection have disappeared, which usually takes several months. In some cases, the recommended procedure may be arthroplasty or joint fusion.
- Prosthetic replacement remains controversial; it may worsen the infection. However, it has helped patients with damaged femoral heads or acetabula.

Nursing considerations

- Practice strict sterile technique with all procedures. Prevent contact between immunosuppressed patients and infected patients.
- Watch for signs of joint inflammation: heat, redness, swelling, pain, or drainage. Monitor the patient's vital signs and fever pattern. Remember that corticosteroids mask signs of infection.
- Check splints or traction regularly. Keep the joint in proper alignment, but avoid prolonged immobilization. Start passive range-of-motion exercises immediately, and progress to active exercises as soon as the patient can move the affected joint and put weight on it. Performing exercises for the affected joint aids the recovery process.
- Monitor pain levels and medicate accordingly, especially before exercise (remember that the pain of septic arthritis is easy to underestimate). Give analgesics and opioids for acute pain and heat or ice packs for moderate pain.

■ Carefully evaluate the patient's condition after joint aspiration. Provide emotional support throughout the diagnostic tests and procedures, which should be previously explained to the patient. Warn the patient before the first aspiration that it will be extremely painful.

■ Septic shock

Low systemic vascular resistance and elevated cardiac output characterize early septic shock. The disorder results from the body's exaggerated response to infection. This exaggerated response leads to inflammation, coagulation, and impaired fibrinolysis. Septic shock is usually a complication of another disorder or invasive procedure and has a mortality as high as 25%. Complications include disseminated intravascular coagulation (DIC), renal failure, heart failure, GI ulcers, and abnormal liver function.

Causes

■ Gram-negative bacteria: *Escherichia coli, Klebsiella, Enterobacter, Proteus, Pseudomonas,* and *Bacteroides*
■ Gram-positive bacteria: *Streptococcus pneumoniae, Streptococcus pyogenes,* and *Actinomyces*

Predisposing factors

■ Advanced age
■ Burns
■ Cirrhosis
■ Diabetes mellitus
■ Disseminated cancer
■ Hospitalization for primary infection of the genitourinary, biliary, GI, and gynecologic tracts
■ Immunodeficiency, lowered resistance from a preexisting condition
■ Prolonged antibiotic therapy
■ Recent infection
■ Recent medical or surgical procedure (transplantation of bacteria from other areas of the body through surgery, I.V. therapy, and catheters)
■ Trauma

Signs and symptoms

■ Early stage: chills, diarrhea, nausea, oliguria, prostration, sudden fever (over 101° F [38.3° C]), vomiting
■ Late stage: anuria, apprehension, hypotension, hypothermia, irritability, restlessness, tachycardia, tachypnea, thirst from decreased cerebral tissue perfusion

In infants and elderly patients

■ Altered level of consciousness
■ Hyperventilation
■ Hypotension

Diagnostic tests

■ In the early stages, arterial blood gas (ABG) analysis indicates respiratory alkalosis (low partial pressure of carbon dioxide [$Paco_2$], low or normal bicarbonate [HCO_3^-] level, and high pH).
■ As shock progresses, metabolic acidosis develops, with hypoxemia indicated by decreasing $Paco_2$ (which may increase as respiratory failure ensues) as well as decreasing partial pressure of oxygen, HCO_3^-, and pH levels.
■ Chest X-ray may reveal pneumonia or pulmonary edema.
■ These laboratory test results help support the diagnosis and determine the treatment:
 – Blood cultures isolate the organism.
 – Platelet count is decreased, and leukocytosis (15,000 to 30,000/mm^3) is found.
 – Blood urea nitrogen and creatinine levels are increased, and creatinine clearance is decreased.
 – Prothrombin time and partial thromboplastin time are abnormal.
 – Urine studies show increased specific gravity (more than 1.020) and osmolality and a decreased sodium level.

Treatment

- Remove I.V., intra-arterial, or urinary drainage catheters, and send them to the laboratory to culture for the causative organism. New catheters can be inserted in the intensive care unit.
- Immediate administration of I.V. antibiotics controls the infection. Depending on the organism, an antibiotic combination may be necessary.
- Drugs should be stopped or given in reduced doses in patients who are immunocompromised because of drug therapy.
- Administer drotrecogin alfa (Xigris) as prescribed to reduce inflammatory response.
- Insulin infusion may be prescribed to maintain blood glucose levels between 80 and 110 mg/dl. Glycemic control decreases mortality.
- Oxygen therapy should be started to maintain arterial oxygen saturation greater than 95%. Mechanical ventilation may be required if respiratory failure occurs.
- Colloid or crystalloid infusions are given to increase intravascular volume and blood pressure. If fluid resuscitation fails to increase blood pressure, a vasopressor (such as dopamine) can be started.
- Blood transfusion may be needed if the patient is anemic.

Nursing considerations

- Determine which patients are at high risk for developing septic shock. Know the signs of impending septic shock, but don't rely on technical aids to judge the patient's status. Consider any change in mental status and urine output as significant as a change in CVP.
- Maintain the patient's pulmonary, cardiac, and renal function. Carefully monitor hemodynamic parameters. Check ABG values for adequate oxygenation or gas exchange, watching for changes.

- Keep accurate intake and output records. Maintain adequate urine output (0.5 to 1 ml/kg/hour) and systolic pressure. Be careful to avoid fluid overload.
- Monitor the serum antibiotic level as indicated.
- Watch closely for complications of septic shock: DIC (abnormal bleeding), renal failure (oliguria, increased specific gravity), heart failure (dyspnea, edema, tachycardia, jugular vein distention), acute respiratory distress syndrome (tachypnea, tachycardia, poor oxygenation), GI ulcers (hematemesis, melena), and hepatic abnormalities (jaundice, hypoprothrombinemia, and hypoalbuminemia).
- Monitor the patient receiving drotrecogin alfa for signs of bleeding.

Severe combined immunodeficiency disease

Cell-mediated (T-cell) and humoral (B-cell) immunity are deficient or absent in severe combined immunodeficiency disease (SCID). This results in susceptibility to infection from all classes of microorganisms during infancy.

At least three types of SCID exist: *reticular dysgenesis*, the most severe type, in which the hematopoietic stem cell fails to differentiate into lymphocytes and granulocytes; *Swiss-type agammaglobulinemia*, in which the hematopoietic stem cell fails to differentiate into lymphocytes alone; and *enzyme deficiency*, such as adenosine deaminase (ADA) deficiency, in which the buildup of toxic products in the lymphoid tissue causes damage and subsequent dysfunction.

SCID affects more males than females; its estimated incidence is 1 in every 100,000 to 500,000 births. Most untreated patients die from infection within 1 year of birth.

Causes

- Autosomal recessive trait, although it may be X-linked
- Molecular defects, such as mutation of the kinase ZAP-70 (X-linked SCID results from a mutation of a subunit of the interleukin-2 [IL-2], IL-4, and IL-7 receptors)
- Possibly failure of the stem cell to differentiate into T and B lymphocytes
- Enzyme deficiency (less common)

Signs and symptoms

- Chronic otitis
- Extreme susceptibility to infection in the first months of life
- Failure to thrive
- Persistent oral candidiasis (sometimes with esophageal erosions)
- *Pneumocystis carinii* pneumonia: usually strikes a severely immunodeficient infant in the first 3 to 5 weeks of life; has insidious onset, with gradually worsening cough, low-grade fever, tachypnea, and respiratory distress
- Recurrent pulmonary infections (usually caused by *Pseudomonas,* cytomegalovirus, or *P. carinii*)
- Sepsis
- Viral infections (such as chickenpox)
- Watery diarrhea (associated with *Salmonella* or *Escherichia coli*)

Diagnostic tests

- Defective humoral immunity is difficult to detect before an infant is 5 months old. Before age 5 months, even normal infants have very small amounts of the serum immunoglobulins (Ig) IgM and IgA, and normal IgG levels merely reflect maternal IgG. However, severely diminished or absent T-cell number and function and lymph node biopsy showing absence of lymphocytes can confirm the diagnosis of SCID.

- Chest X-ray characteristically shows bilateral pulmonary infiltrates in infants with *P. carinii* pneumonia.

Treatment

- Histocompatible bone marrow transplant is the only satisfactory treatment available to correct immunodeficiency. Because bone marrow cells must be matched according to human leukocyte antigen and mixed leukocyte culture, the most common donors are histocompatible siblings.
- Bone marrow transplant can produce a potentially fatal graft-versus-host (GVH) reaction, so newer methods of bone marrow transplant that eliminate GVH reaction (such as lectin separation and the use of monoclonal antibodies) are being evaluated.
- Fetal thymus and liver transplants have achieved limited success.
- Administration of immune globulin may also play a role in treatment.
- Some infants with SCID have received long-term protection by being isolated in a completely sterile environment. However, this approach isn't effective if the infant already has had recurring infections.

Nursing considerations

- Monitor the infant constantly for early signs of infection; if infection develops, provide prompt and aggressive drug therapy.
- Watch for adverse reactions to medications. Avoid vaccinations, and give only irradiated blood products if the patient needs a transfusion.
- Explain all procedures, medications, and precautions to the parents.
- Although infants with SCID must remain in strict protective isolation, try to provide a stimulating atmosphere to promote growth and development. Encourage parents to visit their child often,

to hold him, and to bring him toys that can be easily sterilized.

■ Maintain a normal daily and nightly routine, and talk to the child as much as possible. If the parents can't visit, call them often to report on their infant's condition.

■ Refer parents for genetic counseling. Refer parents and siblings for psychological and spiritual counseling to help them cope with the child's inevitable long-term illness and early death.

■ For assistance in coping with the financial burden of the child's long-term hospitalization, refer the parents to social services.

Sickle cell anemia

A congenital hemolytic anemia that occurs primarily, but not exclusively, in blacks, sickle cell anemia results from a defective hemoglobin (Hb) molecule (Hb S) that causes red blood cells (RBCs) to roughen and become sickle shaped. Such cells impair circulation, resulting in chronic ill health (fatigue, dyspnea on exertion, swollen joints), periodic crises, long-term complications, and premature death. Hb electrophoresis should be done on umbilical cord blood samples at birth to screen for sickle cell disease in neonates at risk.

Sickle cell anemia is most common in tropical Africans and in people of African descent; about 1 in 10 blacks carries the abnormal gene. If two such carriers have offspring, there is a 1 in 4 (25%) chance that each child will have the disease. Overall, 1 in every 400 to 600 black children has sickle cell anemia.

The abnormal Hb S found in RBCs of patients with sickle cell anemia becomes insoluble whenever hypoxia occurs. As a result, these RBCs become rigid, rough, and elongated, forming a crescent, or sickle, shape. Such sickling can produce hemolysis (cell destruction). In addition, these altered cells tend to pile up in capillaries and smaller blood vessels, making the blood more viscous. Normal circulation is impaired, causing pain, tissue infarction, and swelling. Such blockage causes anoxic changes that lead to further sickling and obstruction.

Infection, stress, dehydration, and conditions that provoke hypoxia—strenuous exercise, high altitude, unpressurized aircraft, cold, and vasoconstrictive drugs—may all provoke periodic crises. Four types of crises can occur: vaso-occlusive, aplastic, acute sequestration, or hemolytic.

Causes

■ Homozygous inheritance of the Hb S gene, which causes substitution of the amino acid valine for glutamic acid in the B Hb chain

■ Heterozygous inheritance of the Hb S gene, resulting in sickle cell trait, usually an asymptomatic condition (see *Sickle cell trait*)

Signs and symptoms
After age 6 months

■ Aching bones
■ Cardiomegaly
■ Chest pains
■ Chronic fatigue
■ Hepatomegaly
■ Increased susceptibility to infection
■ Ischemic leg ulcers (especially around the ankles)
■ Jaundice
■ Joint swelling
■ Pallor
■ Pulmonary infarction (which may result in cor pulmonale)
■ Systolic and diastolic murmurs
■ Tachycardia
■ Unexplained dyspnea or dyspnea on exertion

Sickle cell crisis
- Hematuria
- History of recent infection, stress, dehydration, or other conditions that provoke hypoxia, such as strenuous exercise or exposure to high altitude, unpressurized aircraft, cold, or vasoconstrictive drugs
- Lethargy, listlessness, and irritability
- Pale lips, tongue, palms, and nail beds
- Severe pain
- Sleepiness with difficulty awakening
- Temperature over 104° F (40° C), or a temperature of 100° F (37.8° C) that persists for 2 or more days

Vaso-occlusive crisis
- Dark urine
- Increased jaundice
- Low-grade fever
- Severe abdominal, thoracic, muscular, or bone pain

Aplastic crisis
- Coma (possibly)
- Dyspnea
- Infection (usually viral)
- Lethargy
- Markedly decreased bone marrow activity
- Pallor
- RBC hemolysis
- Sleepiness

Acute sequestration crisis
- Hypovolemic shock and death (without treatment)
- Lethargy
- Pallor

Hemolytic crisis
- Liver congestion and hepatomegaly
- Worsening jaundice

Diagnostic tests
- Hb electrophoresis shows Hb S or other hemoglobinopathies.

Sickle cell trait

This relatively benign condition results from heterozygous inheritance of the abnormal hemoglobin S (Hb S) gene from one parent, while receiving one normal Hb gene from the other parent. Like sickle cell anemia, this condition is most common in blacks. Sickle cell trait never progresses to sickle cell anemia.

In persons with sickle cell trait (also called *carriers*), 20% to 40% of their total Hb is Hb S; the rest is normal.

Such carriers usually have no symptoms. They have normal Hb level and hematocrit and can expect a normal life span. Nevertheless, they must avoid situations that provoke hypoxia because these occasionally cause a sickling crisis similar to that in sickle cell anemia.

Genetic counseling is essential for sickle cell carriers. If two sickle cell carriers marry, each of their children has a 25% chance of inheriting sickle cell anemia.

- Blood studies show low RBC count, elevated white blood cell and platelet counts, decreased erythrocyte sedimentation rate, increased serum iron level, decreased RBC survival time, and reticulocytosis. Hb level may be low or normal.
- A lateral chest X-ray may be performed to detect "Lincoln log" deformity, where vertebrae resemble logs that form the corner of a cabin.

Treatment
- Prophylactic antibiotics are given during treatment and at follow-up, even when the patient isn't in crisis.
- If the patient's Hb level drops suddenly or if his condition deteriorates rapidly, a

Coping with sickle cell anemia

Before discharge, the patient must learn how to live with sickle cell anemia. Review with the patient and his family the need to:
■ eat a well-balanced, healthy diet
■ keep up-to-date on immunizations
■ get adequate rest
■ take all medications as prescribed
■ drink plenty of fluids
■ contact his practitioner at the first sign of infection or pain
■ keep telephone numbers for his practitioner handy
■ plan ahead for emergencies
■ contact national support groups, local groups, genetic counselors, and sickle cell treatment centers for up-to-date information on treatment and research.

transfusion of packed RBCs is needed. An iron supplement may be given if the patient's iron level is low.
■ In a sequestration crisis, treatment may include sedation, administration of analgesics, blood transfusion, oxygen administration, and large amounts of oral and I.V. fluids. A good anti-sickling agent isn't available yet; the most commonly used drug, sodium cyanate, has many adverse effects.
■ Transfusions are given to increase oxygen-carrying capacity in an effort to reduce sickling.
■ Hematopoietic cell transplantation using sibling donors has curative potential.

Nursing considerations
During a painful crisis
■ Apply warm compresses to painful areas, and cover the child with a blanket. (Never use cold compresses; this aggravates the condition.)

■ Administer an analgesic-antipyretic, such as aspirin or acetaminophen (Tylenol).
■ Encourage the patient to get plenty of bed rest, and help him sit up. If dehydration or severe pain occurs, hospitalization may be necessary.
■ Suggest biofeedback techniques, which may be helpful.
■ If the patient is an adolescent or adult male, warn him that he may have sudden, painful episodes of priapism. Explain that such episodes are common and, if prolonged, can have serious reproductive consequences. Advise the patient to report the occurrence of such episodes.

During remission
■ Advise the patient to avoid tight clothing that restricts circulation.
■ Warn against strenuous exercise, vasoconstrictive medications, cold temperatures (including drinking large amounts of ice water and swimming), unpressurized aircraft, high altitudes, and other conditions that provoke hypoxia.
■ Stress the importance of normal childhood immunizations, meticulous wound care, good oral hygiene, regular dental checkups, and a balanced diet as safeguards against infection. If a patient develops an infection, it must be treated promptly.
■ Stress the need to increase fluid intake to prevent dehydration resulting from impaired ability to concentrate urine. Tell parents to encourage their child to drink more fluids, especially in the summer, by offering milk shakes, ice pops, and eggnog.
■ Encourage normal mental and social development in the child by warning parents against being overprotective. Although the child must avoid strenuous exercise, he can enjoy most everyday activities.

- Refer parents of children with sickle cell anemia for genetic counseling to answer their questions about the risk to future offspring. Recommend screening of other family members to determine whether they're heterozygote carriers. These parents may also need psychological counseling to cope with guilty feelings. In addition, suggest they join an appropriate community support group. (See *Coping with sickle cell anemia*.)
- Women with sickle cell anemia may be a poor obstetric risk and their use of hormonal contraceptives risky. Refer these patients to a gynecologist for birth control counseling. If women with sickle cell anemia do become pregnant, they should maintain a balanced diet and take a folic acid supplement.
- During general anesthesia, make sure that the patient has optimal ventilation to prevent hypoxic crisis. Provide a preoperative transfusion of packed RBCs as needed.

Sideroblastic anemias

Sideroblastic anemias, a group of heterogenous disorders, produce a common defect—failure to use iron in hemoglobin (Hb) synthesis, despite the availability of adequate iron stores. These anemias may be hereditary or acquired; the acquired form, in turn, can be primary or secondary.

Hereditary sideroblastic anemia occurs mostly in young males. (Females are carriers and usually show no signs of disease.) This form usually responds to treatment with pyridoxine (vitamin B_6). Correction of the secondary acquired form depends on the causative disorder.

The primary acquired (idiopathic) form, known as *refractory anemia with ringed sideroblasts*, resists treatment and usually proves fatal within 10 years after onset of complications or a concomitant

disease. Most common in elderly people, this form is commonly associated with thrombocytopenia or leukopenia as part of a myelodysplastic syndrome.

Causes

- Transmission by X-linked inheritance (hereditary form)
- Normoblasts' inability to use iron to synthesize Hb, causing iron to be deposited in the mitochondria of normoblasts, which are then called *ringed sideroblasts* (primary acquired form)
- Ingestion of, or exposure to, toxins, such as alcohol and lead, or to drugs, such as isoniazid (Laniazid) and chloramphenicol (Chloromycetin) (secondary acquired form)
- Complication of rheumatoid arthritis, lupus erythematosus, multiple myeloma, tuberculosis, and severe infections (secondary acquired form)

Signs and symptoms

- Nonspecific signs and symptoms that may exist for several years before being identified: anorexia, fatigue, weakness, dizziness, pale skin and mucous membranes and, occasionally, enlarged lymph nodes
- Heart and liver failure from excessive iron accumulation in these organs, causing dyspnea, exertional angina, slight jaundice, and hepatosplenomegaly
- Increased GI absorption of iron (hereditary form)
- Additional symptoms depending on the underlying cause (secondary acquired form)

Diagnostic tests

- Microscopic examination of bone marrow aspirate, stained with Prussian blue or alizarin red dye, shows ringed sideroblasts, which confirms the diagnosis.
- Microscopic examination of blood shows hypochromic or normochromic

and slightly macrocytic red blood cells (RBCs).

- RBC precursors may be megaloblastic, with anisocytosis (abnormal variation in RBC size) and poikilocytosis (abnormal variation in RBC shape).
- Unlike iron deficiency anemia, sideroblastic anemia lowers Hb level and raises serum iron and transferrin levels. In turn, faulty Hb production raises urobilinogen and bilirubin levels.
- Platelet and leukocyte counts remain normal, but thrombocytopenia or leukopenia occasionally occurs.

Treatment
Hereditary form
- Provide high doses of pyridoxine for several weeks as ordered.

Primary acquired form
- Elderly patients with this form of the disease are less likely to improve quickly and more likely to develop serious complications. Deferoxamine may be used to treat chronic iron overload in selected patients.
- Carefully crossmatched transfusions (providing needed Hb) or high doses of androgens are effective palliative measures for some patients.
- The primary acquired form is essentially refractory to treatment and usually leads to death from acute leukemia or from respiratory or cardiac complications.
- Some patients may benefit from phlebotomy to prevent hemochromatosis. Phlebotomy increases the rate of erythropoiesis and uses up excess iron stores; thus, it reduces serum and total-body iron levels.

Secondary acquired form
- The secondary acquired form usually subsides after the causative drug or tox-

in is removed or when the underlying condition is adequately treated.
- Folic acid supplements may also be beneficial when concomitant megaloblastic nuclear changes in RBC precursors are present.

Nursing considerations
- Administer medications as needed. Teach the patient the importance of continuing prescribed therapy, even after he begins to feel better.
- Provide frequent rest periods if the patient becomes easily fatigued.
- If phlebotomy is scheduled, explain the procedure thoroughly to help reduce anxiety. If this procedure must be repeated frequently, provide a high-protein diet to help replace the protein lost during phlebotomy. Encourage the patient to follow a similar diet at home.
- Always inquire about the possibility of exposure to lead in the home (especially for children) or at work.
- Identify patients who abuse alcohol; refer them for appropriate therapy.

Silicosis

A progressive disease characterized by nodular lesions, silicosis frequently progresses to fibrosis. It's the most common form of pneumoconiosis.

Nodules result when alveolar macrophages ingest silica particles, which they're unable to process. As a result, the macrophages die and release proteolytic enzymes into the surrounding tissue. The subsequent inflammation attracts other macrophages and fibroblasts into the region to produce fibrous tissue and wall off the reaction. The resulting nodule has an onion-skin appearance when viewed under a microscope. Nodules develop adjacent to terminal and respiratory bronchioles, concentrate in the upper lobes, and are frequently accompanied by bullous changes throughout both lungs.

Silicosis can be classified according to the severity of pulmonary disease and the rapidity of its onset and progression; it usually occurs as a simple asymptomatic illness.

Acute silicosis develops after 1 to 3 years in workers exposed to very high levels of free silica (sandblasters, tunnel workers). Accelerated silicosis appears after an average of 10 years of exposure to lower levels of silica. Chronic silicosis develops after 20 or more years of exposure to lower levels of silica.

The prognosis is good, unless the disease progresses into the complicated fibrotic form, which causes respiratory insufficiency and cor pulmonale and is associated with pulmonary tuberculosis (TB). If the disease doesn't progress, minimal physiologic disturbances occur with no disability. Occasionally, however, the fibrotic response accelerates, engulfing and destroying large areas of the lung (progressive massive fibrosis or conglomerate lesions). Fibrosis may continue despite termination of exposure to dust.

Causes
- Inhalation and pulmonary deposition of respirable crystalline silica dust, mostly from quartz

Signs and symptoms
Initial stage
- May produce no signs or symptoms
- Dyspnea on exertion, commonly attributed to being "out of shape"

Progressive features
- Worsening dyspnea on exertion
- Tachypnea
- Insidious, dry cough that's most pronounced in the morning

Advanced stages
- Dyspnea on minimal exertion, worsening cough, and pulmonary hypertension, which leads to right ventricular failure and cor pulmonale
- Central nervous system changes: confusion, lethargy, and a decrease in the rate and depth of respiration as partial pressure of carbon dioxide increases

Diagnostic tests
- Auscultation may reveal decreased chest expansion, diminished intensity of breath sounds, areas of hyporesonance and hyperresonance, fine to medium crackles, and tachypnea.
- In simple silicosis, chest X-rays show small, discrete, nodular lesions distributed throughout both lung fields but typically concentrated in the upper lung zones; the hilar lung nodes may be enlarged and exhibit "eggshell" calcification.
- In complicated silicosis, chest X-rays show one or more conglomerate masses of dense tissue.
- Pulmonary function tests yield the following results:
  - Forced vital capacity (FVC) is reduced in complicated silicosis.
  - Forced expiratory volume in 1 second (FEV_1) is reduced in obstructive disease (emphysematous areas of silicosis); it's also reduced in complicated silicosis, but the ratio of FEV_1 to FVC is normal or high.
  - Maximum voluntary ventilation is reduced in restrictive and obstructive diseases.
  - Diffusing capacity of the lung for carbon monoxide is reduced when fibrosis destroys alveolar walls and obliterates pulmonary capillaries or when fibrosis thickens the alveolar capillary membrane.
- Arterial blood gas analysis shows the following:

– Partial pressure of oxygen is normal in simple silicosis; it may be significantly decreased when the patient breathes room air in the late stages of chronic or complicated disease.
– Partial pressure of carbon dioxide is normal in the early stages but may decrease because of hyperventilation; it may increase as a restrictive pattern develops, particularly if the patient is hypoxic and has severe impairment of alveolar ventilation.

Treatment

- Respiratory symptoms may be relieved through daily use of bronchodilating aerosols and increased fluid intake (at least 3 qt [3 L] daily).
- Steam inhalation and chest physiotherapy techniques, such as controlled coughing and segmental bronchial drainage with chest percussion and vibration, help clear secretions.
- In severe cases, oxygen may be administered by cannula or mask for the patient with chronic hypoxia or by mechanical ventilation if arterial oxygen can't be maintained.
- Respiratory infections require prompt administration of antibiotics.
- Treatment includes careful observation for the development of tuberculosis.

Nursing considerations

- Teach the patient to prevent infections by avoiding crowds and people with respiratory infections and by receiving influenza and pneumococcal vaccines.
- Patients with silicosis are at increased risk for developing TB. TB testing should be routine.
- Increase the patient's exercise tolerance by encouraging regular activity. Advise the patient to plan his daily activities to decrease the work of breathing; he should pace himself, rest often, and gen-erally move slowly through his daily routine.

Sjögren's syndrome

The second most common autoimmune rheumatic disorder after rheumatoid arthritis (RA), Sjögren's syndrome (SS) is characterized by diminished lacrimal and salivary gland secretion (sicca complex). SS occurs mainly in women (90% of patients); its mean age of occurrence is 50.

SS may be a primary disorder or may be associated with a connective tissue disorder, such as RA, scleroderma, systemic lupus erythematosus, or polymyositis. In some patients, the disorder is limited to the exocrine glands (glandular SS); in others, it also involves other organs, such as the lungs and kidneys (extraglandular SS).

About 50% of patients with SS have confirmed RA and a history of slowly developing sicca complex. However, some seek medical help for rapidly progressive and severe oral and ocular dryness, commonly accompanied by periodic parotid gland enlargement. Patients with SS have at least two of the following conditions: xerophthalmia, xerostomia (with a salivary gland biopsy showing lymphocytic infiltration), and an associated autoimmune or lymphoproliferative disorder.

Causes

- Unknown

Predisposing factors

- Exposure to pollen in a genetically susceptible individual
- Genetic and environmental factors
- Viral or bacterial infection

Signs and symptoms

- Ocular dryness (xerophthalmia), leading to foreign body sensation (gritty, sandy eye), redness, burning, photosensitivity, eye fatigue, itching, mucoid discharge, and the appearance of a film across the field of vision
- Oral dryness (xerostomia), leading to difficulty swallowing and talking; abnormal taste or smell sensation, or both; thirst; ulcers of the tongue, buccal mucosa, and lips (especially at the corners of the mouth); and severe dental caries
- Dryness of the respiratory tract, leading to epistaxis, hoarseness, chronic nonproductive cough, recurrent otitis media, and increased incidence of respiratory infections
- Dyspareunia and vaginal pruritus (from dryness)
- Generalized pruritus
- Fatigue
- Recurrent low-grade fever
- Arthralgia or myalgia
- Lymphadenopathy
- Interstitial pneumonitis
- Interstitial nephritis
- Raynaud's phenomenon
- Peripheral neuropathy
- Vasculitis, usually limited to the skin and characterized by palpable purpura on the legs
- Hypothyroidism
- Systemic necrotizing vasculitis (rare)

Diagnostic tests

- Blood test results are positive for antinuclear antibodies; salivary gland biopsy also yields a positive result.
- Laboratory values show elevated erythrocyte sedimentation rate in most patients, mild anemia and leukopenia in 30%, and hypergammaglobulinemia in 50%; rheumatoid factor is found in 75% to 90% of patients.
- Schirmer's tearing test and slit-lamp examination with rose Bengal dye are used to measure eye involvement.
- Salivary gland involvement is evaluated by measuring the volume of parotid saliva and by secretory sialography and salivary scintigraphy.
- A lower lip biopsy shows salivary gland infiltration by lymphocytes.

Treatment

- Mouth dryness can be relieved by using a methylcellulose swab or spray and by drinking plenty of fluids, especially at meals.
- Pilocarpine hydrochloride (Salagen) or bromhexine may be useful in treating salivary hypofunction.
- Meticulous oral hygiene is essential, including regular flossing, brushing, and fluoride treatment at home and frequent dental checkups.
- Instillation of artificial tears as often as every half hour prevents eye damage (corneal ulcerations, corneal opacifications) from insufficient tear secretion. Artificial tears, whose drops are thicker and more viscous, require less frequent application but may cause blurring or leave residue on the eyelashes.
- Some patients may also benefit from instillation of an eye ointment at bedtime or from twice daily sustained-release cellulose capsules.
- If an eye infection develops, antibiotics should be given immediately; topical steroids should be avoided.
- Parotid gland enlargement requires local heat and analgesics.
- Arthritis and arthralgia require hydroxychloroquine (Plaquenil) or nonsteroidal anti-inflammatory drugs.
- Corticosteroids are given to treat pulmonary and renal interstitial disease.
- Associated lymphoma is treated with a combination of chemotherapy, surgery, and radiation.

Nursing considerations

- Advise the patient to avoid drugs that decrease saliva production, such as atropine derivatives, antihistamines, anticholinergics, and antidepressants.
- Suggest high-protein, high-calorie liquid supplements to prevent malnutrition if mouth lesions make eating painful. Advise the patient to avoid sugar, which contributes to dental caries, and tobacco, alcohol, and spicy, salty, or highly acidic foods, which cause mouth irritation. Adequate dental hygiene after meals can also decrease the frequency of dental caries.
- Saliva flow can be stimulated by use of sugar-free, highly flavored lozenges such as lemon drops.
- Suggest the use of sunglasses to protect the patient's eyes from dust, wind, and strong light. Moisture chamber spectacles may also be helpful.
- Advise the patient to keep his face clean and to avoid rubbing his eyes because dry eyes are more susceptible to infection.
- Stress the need to humidify home and work environments to help relieve respiratory dryness. Suggest normal saline solution drops or aerosolized spray for nasal dryness. Advise the patient to avoid prolonged hot showers and baths and to use moisturizing lotions to help ease dry skin. Suggest using a vaginal lubricant.
- Refer the patient to the Sjögren's Syndrome Foundation for additional information and support.

Skull fractures

Skull fractures may be simple (closed) or compound (open) and may or may not displace bone fragments. Skull fractures are further described as linear, comminuted, or depressed. A linear fracture is a common hairline break, without displacement of structures; a comminuted fracture splinters or crushes the bone into several fragments; a depressed fracture pushes the bone toward the brain.

Because possible damage to the brain is the first concern rather than the fracture itself, a skull fracture is considered a neurosurgical condition.

In children, the skull's thinness and elasticity allow a depression without a fracture (a linear fracture across a suture line increases the possibility of epidural hematoma).

Skull fractures are also classified according to their location, such as a cranial vault fracture or a basilar fracture. A basilar fracture is located at the base of the skull and involves the cribriform plate and the frontal sinuses. Because of the danger of grave cranial complications and meningitis, basilar fractures are usually far more serious than vault fractures.

Causes

- Traumatic blow to the head

Signs and symptoms

- Scalp wounds (abrasions, contusions, lacerations, or avulsions), possibly causing profuse bleeding because the scalp contains many blood vessels, leading to hypovolemic shock if blood loss is large enough
- Signs of brain injury: agitation and irritability, loss of consciousness, changes in respiratory pattern, abnormal deep tendon reflexes (DTRs), and altered pupillary and motor response
- Persistent, localized headache
- Subdural, epidural, or intracerebral hemorrhage or hematoma, if jagged bone fragments pierce the dura mater or the cerebral cortex, which may cause hemiparesis, unequal pupils, dizziness, seizures, projectile vomiting, decreased

pulse and respiratory rates, and progressive unresponsiveness
■ Blindness, in sphenoidal fractures that damage the optic nerve
■ Unilateral deafness or facial paralysis, in temporal fractures
■ Soft-tissue swelling near the site of a vault fracture, making it hard to detect without a computed tomography (CT) scan
■ In a basilar fracture: hemorrhage from the nose, pharynx, or ears; blood under the periorbital skin ("raccoon eyes") and under the conjunctiva; and Battle's sign (supramastoid ecchymosis), sometimes with bleeding behind the eardrum; cerebrospinal fluid (CSF) or even brain tissue leaking from the nose or ears
■ Possible residual effects: seizure disorders (epilepsy), hydrocephalus, and organic brain syndrome
■ In children: headaches, giddiness, easy fatigability, neuroses, and behavior disorders
■ In elderly patients: intracranial pressure (ICP) that shows no signs until it's very high because of cortical brain atrophy, allowing more space for brain swelling under the cranium

Diagnostic tests

■ CT scan may be needed to locate the fracture (especially with vault fractures, which commonly aren't visible or palpable).
■ Neurologic examination is performed to check cerebral function (mental status and orientation to time, place, and person), level of consciousness (LOC), pupillary response, motor function, and DTRs.
■ Reagent strips are used to test the draining nasal or ear fluid for CSF. The strip will turn blue if CSF is present; it won't change in the presence of blood alone. However, the tape will turn blue also if the patient is hyperglycemic.

■ CT scan and magnetic resonance imaging reveal intracranial hemorrhage from ruptured blood vessels and swelling to assess brain damage.

Treatment
Linear fractures

■ A linear fracture usually only requires supportive treatment, including mild analgesics such as acetaminophen (Tylenol) and cleaning and debridement of any wounds after injection of a local anesthetic.
■ If the patient with a skull fracture hasn't lost consciousness, he should be observed in the emergency room for at least 4 hours. After this observation period, if vital signs are stable and if the neurosurgeon concurs, the patient can be discharged. At this time, the patient should be given an instruction sheet to follow for 24 to 48 hours of observation at home.

Vault and basilar fractures

■ More severe vault fractures, especially depressed fractures, usually require a craniotomy to elevate or remove fragments that have been driven into the brain and to extract foreign bodies and necrotic tissue, thereby reducing the risk of infection and further brain damage.
■ Other treatments for severe vault fractures include antibiotic therapy, tetanus prophylaxis and, in profound hemorrhage, blood transfusions.
■ Basilar fractures call for immediate prophylactic antibiotics to prevent the onset of meningitis from CSF leaks as well as close observation for secondary hematomas and hemorrhages. Surgery may be necessary.
■ Basilar and vault fractures commonly require I.V. or I.M. dexamethasone to reduce cerebral edema and minimize brain tissue damage.

Nursing considerations

■ Establish and maintain a patent airway; nasal airways are contraindicated in patients with possible basilar skull fractures. Intubation may be necessary.

■ Suction the patient through the mouth, not the nose, to prevent the introduction of bacteria in case a CSF leak is present.

■ Be sure to obtain a complete history of the trauma from the patient, his family, any eyewitnesses, and ambulance personnel.

■ Ask whether the patient lost consciousness and, if so, for how long. The patient will need further diagnostic tests, including a complete neurologic examination, a CT scan, and other studies.

■ Check for abnormal reflexes such as Babinski's reflex.

■ Look for CSF draining from the patient's ears, nose, or mouth. Check bed linens for CSF leaks; look for a "halo sign"—a blood-tinged spot surrounded by a lighter ring. If the patient's nose is draining CSF, wipe it—don't let him blow it. If an ear is draining, cover it lightly with sterile gauze—don't pack it.

■ Position the patient with a head injury so secretions can drain properly. Elevate the head of the bed 30 degrees if intracerebral injury is suspected.

■ Cover scalp wounds carefully with a sterile dressing; control bleeding as necessary.

■ Take seizure precautions, but don't restrain the patient. Agitated behavior may stem from hypoxia or increased ICP, so check for these symptoms. Speak in a calm, reassuring voice, and touch the patient gently. Don't make sudden, unexpected moves.

DRUG CHALLENGE

Don't give the patient opioids or sedatives because they may depress respirations, increase carbon dioxide levels, lead to increased ICP, and mask changes in the patient's neurologic status. Give acetaminophen or another mild analgesic for pain. If the patient requires a gastric tube, choose an orogastric tube if you suspect a basilar skull fracture.

If the skull fracture requires surgery

■ Obtain consent, as needed, to shave the patient's head. Explain that you're performing this procedure to provide a clean area for surgery. Type and crossmatch blood. Obtain baseline laboratory study results, such as a complete blood count, serum electrolyte studies, and urinalysis.

■ After surgery, monitor the patient's vital signs and neurologic status frequently (usually every 5 minutes until the patient is stable, and then every 15 minutes for 1 hour), watching for changes in LOC. Because skull fractures and brain injuries heal slowly, don't expect dramatic postoperative improvement.

■ Monitor intake and output frequently, and maintain patency of the indwelling urinary catheter. Take special care with fluid intake. Hypotonic fluids (even dextrose 5% in water) can increase cerebral edema. Their use should be restricted; give them only as needed.

■ If the patient is unconscious, provide parenteral nutrition. (Remember, the patient may regurgitate and aspirate food if you use a nasogastric tube for feedings.)

If the skull fracture doesn't require surgery

■ Wear sterile gloves to examine the scalp laceration. With your finger, probe the wound for foreign bodies and a palpable fracture. Gently clean lacerations and the surrounding area. Cover with sterile gauze. The patient may need suturing.

■ Provide emotional support for the patient and his family. Explain the need for procedures to reduce the risk of brain injury.

■ Before discharge, instruct the patient's family to watch closely for changes in mental status, LOC, or respirations and to relieve the patient's headache with acetaminophen. Tell them to return him to the hospital immediately if his LOC decreases, if his headache persists after several doses of mild analgesics, if he vomits more than once, or if weakness develops in his arms or legs.

■ Teach the patient and his family how to care for his scalp wound. Emphasize the need to return for suture removal and follow-up evaluation.

■ Snakebites

Poisonous snakebites are most common during summer afternoons in grassy or rocky habitats. Poisonous snakebites are medical emergencies. With prompt, correct treatment, they need not be fatal.

Causes
■ The only poisonous snakes in the United States are pit vipers (Crotalidae) and coral snakes (Elapidae).

■ Pit vipers include rattlesnakes, water moccasins (cottonmouths), and copperheads. They have a pitted depression between their eyes and nostrils and two fangs, $3/4''$ to $1 1/4''$ (2 to 3 cm) long. Because fangs may break off or grow behind old ones, some snakes may have one, three, or four fangs.

■ Because coral snakes are nocturnal and placid, their bites are less common than pit viper bites; pit vipers are also nocturnal but are more active. The fangs of coral snakes are short but have teeth behind them. Coral snakes have distinctive red, black, and yellow bands (yellow bands always border red ones), tend to bite with a chewing motion, and may leave multiple fang marks, small lacerations, and much tissue destruction.

Signs and symptoms
Pit viper bites
■ Immediate and progressively severe pain and edema (the entire extremity may swell within a few hours)
■ Local elevation in skin temperature
■ Fever
■ Skin discoloration
■ Petechiae
■ Ecchymoses
■ Blebs
■ Blisters
■ Bloody wound discharge
■ Local necrosis
■ Local and facial numbness and tingling
■ Fasciculation and twitching of skeletal muscles
■ Seizures (especially in children)
■ Extreme anxiety
■ Difficulty speaking
■ Fainting
■ Weakness
■ Dizziness
■ Excessive sweating
■ Occasional paralysis
■ Mild to severe respiratory distress
■ Headache
■ Blurred vision
■ Marked thirst
■ Impaired coagulation causing hematemesis, hematuria, melena, bleeding gums, and internal bleeding
■ Tachycardia
■ Lymphadenopathy
■ Nausea, vomiting, and diarrhea
■ Hypotension and shock
■ In severe envenomation, coma and death

Coral snakebite

- Reaction usually delayed, sometimes up to several hours
- Little or no local tissue reaction (local pain, swelling, or necrosis)
- Quick progression of neurotoxic reaction, with the following effects:
  - Local paresthesia
  - Drowsiness
  - Nausea and vomiting
  - Difficulty swallowing
  - Marked salivation
  - Dysphonia
  - Ptosis
  - Blurred vision
  - Miosis
  - Respiratory distress and possible respiratory failure
  - Loss of muscle coordination
  - Possibly, shock with cardiovascular collapse and death

Diagnostic tests

- Bleeding time and partial thromboplastin time are prolonged.
- Hemoglobin level and hematocrit are decreased.
- Platelet count is less than 200,000/mm^3.
- Urinalysis shows hematuria.
- White blood cell count is increased in victims who develop an infection. (Snake mouths typically contain gram-negative bacteria.)
- Chest X-ray shows pulmonary edema or emboli.
- Electrocardiogram (usually necessary only in patients older than age 40 with severe envenomation) may reveal tachycardia and ectopic heartbeats.
- EEG findings may be abnormal in patients with severe envenomation.

Treatment

- Prompt, appropriate first aid can reduce venom absorption and prevent severe symptoms. (See *First aid for snakebites*.)
- Antivenin may be given in life-threatening circumstances, but minor snakebites may not require this treatment.
- Watch the patient closely for signs of sensitivity and anaphylaxis. Keep emergency epinephrine on hand in case the patient develops such problems.
- Other treatments include tetanus toxoid or tetanus immune globulin; various broad-spectrum antibiotics; and, depending on the victim's respiratory status, severity of pain, and the type of snakebite, acetaminophen, codeine, morphine, or meperidine (Demerol). (Opioids are contraindicated in coral snakebites.)
- All snakebites require administration of I.V. isotonic fluids. If bleeding is severe, blood transfusions may also be needed. Antihistamines help relieve pruritus and urticaria.
- Necrotic snakebites usually need surgical debridement after 3 to 4 days.
- Intense, rapidly progressive edema requires fasciotomy within 2 to 3 hours of the bite; extreme envenomation may require amputation of the limb and subsequent reconstructive surgery, rehabilitation, and physical therapy.

Nursing considerations

- When the patient arrives at the hospital, immobilize the extremity if this hasn't already been done. If a tight tourniquet has been applied within the past hour, apply a loose tourniquet proximally and remove the first tourniquet. Release the second tourniquet gradually during antivenin administration as ordered. A sudden release of venom into the bloodstream can cause cardiorespiratory collapse, so keep emergency equipment handy.

First aid for snakebites

- If possible, identify the snake, but don't waste time trying to find it.
- Place the victim in the supine position to slow venom metabolism and absorption.
- Don't give the victim any food, beverage, or medication orally.
- Immediately immobilize the victim's affected limb below heart level, and instruct the victim to remain as quiet as possible.
- If indicated, apply a slightly constrictive band, obstructing only lymphatic and superficial venous blood flow. Apply the band about 4″ (10 cm) above the fang marks or just above the first joint proximal to the bite. The band should be loose enough to allow a finger between the band and the skin. After the band is in place, don't remove it until the victim is examined by a practitioner.

Caution: Don't apply a band if more than 30 minutes has elapsed since the bite. Keep in mind also that total constrictive band time shouldn't exceed 2 hours, nor should it delay antivenin administration.

- Never give the victim alcoholic drinks or stimulants because they speed venom absorption. Never apply ice to a snakebite because it will increase tissue damage.
- Don't excise and suction the affected area. The risk of trauma to underlying structures caused by unskilled performance of this technique is greater than the amount of venom that can be recovered.
- Transport the victim as quickly as possible, keeping him warm and quiet.

- On a flow sheet, document the patient's vital signs, level of consciousness, skin color, swelling, respiratory status, a description of the bite and surrounding area, and symptoms. Monitor his vital signs every 15 minutes, and check for a pulse in the affected limb.
- Start an I.V. line with a large-bore needle for antivenin administration. Severe bites that result in coagulotoxic signs and symptoms may require two I.V. lines—one for antivenin and one for blood products.
- Before antivenin administration, obtain a patient history of allergies and other medical problems. Perform hypersensitivity tests as ordered, and assist with desensitization as needed. During antivenin administration, keep epinephrine, oxygen, and vasopressors available

to combat anaphylaxis from horse serum.
- Give packed red blood cells, I.V. fluids and, possibly, fresh frozen plasma or platelets, as ordered, to counteract coagulotoxicity and maintain blood pressure.
- If the patient develops respiratory distress and requires endotracheal intubation or a tracheotomy, provide good tracheostomy care.
- Give an analgesic as needed. *Don't* give opioids to victims of coral snakebites. Clean the snakebite using sterile technique. Open, debride, and drain any blebs and blisters because they may contain venom. Change dressings daily.
- If the patient requires hospitalization for more than 48 hours, position him carefully to avoid contractures. Perform passive exercises until the 4th day after

the bite; after that, perform active exercises and give whirlpool treatments as ordered.
- Record signs and symptoms of progressive envenomation and when they develop. Most snakebite victims are hospitalized for only 24 to 48 hours.

Sodium imbalance

Sodium, the major cation (90%) in extracellular fluid, maintains tonicity and concentration of extracellular fluid, acid-base balance (reabsorption of sodium ions and excretion of hydrogen ions), nerve conduction and neuromuscular function, glandular secretion, and water balance.

The body requires only 2 to 4 g of sodium daily, although most people in the United States consume 6 to 10 g daily (mostly sodium chloride, as table salt) and excrete excess sodium through the kidneys and skin.

A low-sodium diet or excessive use of diuretics may cause hyponatremia (decreased serum sodium level); dehydration may induce hypernatremia (increased serum sodium level).

Causes
Hyponatremia
- Excessive GI loss of water and electrolytes from vomiting, suctioning, or diarrhea; excessive perspiration or fever; potent diuretics; or use of tap-water enemas
- Excessive drinking of water, infusion of I.V. dextrose in water without other solutes, malnutrition or starvation, and a low-sodium diet usually in conjunction with one of the other causes
- Trauma, surgery (wound drainage), and burns, which cause sodium to shift into damaged cells
- Adrenal gland insufficiency (Addison's disease)

- Hypoaldosteronism
- Cirrhosis with ascites
- Syndrome of inappropriate antidiuretic hormone (SIADH), resulting from brain tumor, stroke, pulmonary disease, or neoplasm with ectopic antidiuretic hormone (ADH) production
- Certain drugs, such as chlorpropamide (Diabinese) and clofibrate (may produce an SIADH-like syndrome)

Hypernatremia
- Decreased water intake
- Severe vomiting and diarrhea that causes water loss that exceeds sodium loss (serum sodium levels rise but overall extracellular fluid volume decreases)
- Excess adrenocortical hormones such as in Cushing's syndrome
- ADH deficiency (diabetes insipidus)
- Salt intoxication—an uncommon cause—from excessive ingestion of table salt

Signs and symptoms
- Sodium imbalance has profound physiologic effects and can induce severe central nervous system, cardiovascular, and GI abnormalities. (See *Clinical effects of sodium imbalance.*)

Diagnostic tests
- A serum sodium level of less than 135 mEq/L indicates hyponatremia.
- A serum sodium level of greater than 145 mEq/L indicates hypernatremia.

Treatment
Hyponatremia
- When possible, patients with a sodium deficit receive an oral sodium supplement. Therapy for mild hyponatremia associated with hypervolemia usually consists of restricted water intake.
- If fluid restriction alone fails to normalize serum sodium levels, demeclocycline (Declomycin) or lithium, which

Clinical effects of sodium imbalance

System	Hyponatremia	Hypernatremia
Cardiovascular	▪ Hypotension; tachycardia; with severe deficit, vasomotor collapse, thready pulse	▪ Hypertension, tachycardia, pitting edema, excessive weight gain
Central nervous	▪ Anxiety, headaches, muscle twitching and weakness, seizures	▪ Fever, agitation, restlessness, seizures
GI	▪ Nausea, vomiting, abdominal cramps	▪ Rough, dry tongue; intense thirst
Genitourinary	▪ Oliguria or anuria	▪ Oliguria
Integumentary	▪ Cold, clammy skin; decreased skin turgor	▪ Flushed skin; dry, sticky mucous membranes
Respiratory	▪ Cyanosis with severe deficiency	▪ Dyspnea, respiratory arrest, and death (from dramatic rise in osmotic pressure)

blocks ADH action in the renal tubules, can be used to promote water excretion.
▪ In extremely rare instances of severe symptomatic hyponatremia, when the serum sodium level falls below 110 mEq/L, 3% or 5% saline solution is infused. Saline infusion requires careful monitoring in an intensive care setting of venous pressure to prevent potentially fatal circulatory overload.
▪ Secondary hyponatremia is treated by correcting the underlying disorder.

Hypernatremia
▪ As ordered, administer salt-free solutions, such as dextrose in water, to return serum sodium levels to normal, followed by infusion of half-normal saline solution to prevent hyponatremia.
▪ Other measures include a sodium-restricted diet and discontinuation of drugs that promote sodium retention.

Nursing considerations
Hyponatremia
▪ Watch for extremely low serum sodium and accompanying serum chloride levels. Monitor urine specific gravity and other laboratory results. Record fluid intake and output accurately, and weigh the patient daily.
▪ During administration of isosmolar or hyperosmolar saline solution, watch closely for signs of hypervolemia (dyspnea, crackles, engorged neck or hand veins). Note conditions that may cause excessive sodium loss—diaphoresis, prolonged diarrhea or vomiting, or severe burns.
▪ Refer the patient receiving a maintenance dosage of diuretics to a dietitian for instruction about dietary sodium intake.
▪ To prevent hyponatremia, administer isosmolar solutions.

Hypernatremia
- Measure serum sodium levels every 6 hours or at least daily. Monitor the patient's vital signs for changes, especially for rising pulse rate. Watch for signs of hypervolemia, especially in the patient receiving I.V. fluids.
- Record fluid intake and output accurately, checking for body fluid loss. Weigh the patient daily.
- Obtain a drug history to check for drugs that promote sodium retention.
- Explain the importance of sodium restriction, and teach the patient how to plan a low-sodium diet. Closely monitor the serum sodium level of the high-risk patient.

▌Spinal cord defects

Various malformations of the spine—including spina bifida, meningocele, and myelomeningocele—result from defective embryonic neural tube closure during the first trimester of pregnancy. These defects usually occur in the lumbosacral area, but they're occasionally found in the sacral, thoracic, and cervical areas.

Normally, about 20 days after conception, the embryo develops a neural groove in the dorsal ectoderm. This groove rapidly deepens, and the two edges fuse to form the neural tube. By about day 23, this tube is completely closed except for an opening at each end. Theoretically, if the posterior portion of this neural tube fails to close by 4 weeks' gestation, or if it closes but then splits open from a cause such as an abnormal increase in cerebrospinal fluid (CSF) later in the first trimester, a spinal defect results.

Spina bifida occulta is the most common and least severe spinal cord defect. It's characterized by incomplete closure of one or more vertebrae without protrusion of the spinal cord or meninges.

In more severe forms of spina bifida, incomplete closure of one or more vertebrae causes protrusion of the spinal contents in an external sac or cystic lesion. In spina bifida with meningocele, this sac contains meninges and CSF. In spina bifida with myelomeningocele (meningomyelocele), this sac contains meninges, CSF, and a portion of the spinal cord or nerve roots distal to the conus medullaris.

In the United States, about 2,500 neonates each year are born with some form of spina bifida; spina bifida with myelomeningocele is less common than spina bifida occulta and spina bifida with meningocele. Incidence is highest in people of Welsh or Irish ancestry.

The prognosis varies with the degree of accompanying neurologic deficit. It's worst in patients with large open lesions, neurogenic bladders (which predispose to infection and renal failure), or total paralysis of the legs.

The prognosis is better in patients with spina bifida occulta and meningocele than in those with myelomeningocele. Many patients with these conditions can lead normal lives.

Causes
- Genetic factors
- Viruses, radiation, and other environmental factors

Signs and symptoms
Spina bifida occulta
- Depression or dimple, tuft of hair, soft fatty deposits, port wine nevi, or a combination of these abnormalities on the skin over the spinal defect
- Neurologic dysfunction (occasionally): foot weakness or bowel and bladder disturbances, especially during rapid growth phases, when the spinal cord's

ascent within the vertebral column may be impaired by its abnormal adherence to other tissues

Meningocele and myelomeningocele

- Arnold-Chiari syndrome (in which part of the brain protrudes into the spinal canal)
- Clubfoot
- Curvature of the spine
- Hydrocephalus (in about 90% of patients)
- Knee contractures
- Mental retardation
- Neurologic deficit (meningocele) (rarely)
- Permanent neurologic dysfunction, such as flaccid or spastic paralysis and bowel and bladder incontinence (myelomeningocele) depending on the level of the defect.
- Saclike structure that protrudes over the spine
- Trophic skin disturbances (ulcerations, cyanosis)

Diagnostic tests
Spina bifida occulta

- Spinal X-ray may show bone defects.
- Myelography can differentiate this condition from other spinal abnormalities, especially spinal cord tumors.

Meningocele and myelomeningocele

- Transillumination of the protruding sac may distinguish meningocele from myelomeningocele. (In meningocele, it typically transilluminates; in myelomeningocele, it doesn't.)
- In myelomeningocele, a pinprick examination of the legs and trunk shows the level of sensory and motor involvement; skull X-rays, cephalic measurements, and a computed tomography

scan demonstrate associated hydrocephalus.
- Laboratory tests in patients with myelomeningocele include urinalysis, urine cultures, and tests for renal function starting in the neonatal period and continuing at regular intervals.
- Although amniocentesis can detect only open defects, such as myelomeningocele and meningocele, this procedure is recommended for all pregnant women who have previously had children with spinal cord defects; these women are at an increased risk for having children with similar defects. If these defects are present, amniocentesis shows increased alpha fetoprotein level by 14 weeks' gestation.
- Ultrasonography can also detect or confirm the presence and extent of neural tube defects.

Treatment

- Spina bifida occulta usually requires no treatment.
- Treatment of meningocele consists of surgical closure of the protruding sac and continual assessment of growth and development.
- Treatment of myelomeningocele requires surgical repair of the sac and supportive measures to promote independence and prevent further complications. Surgery doesn't reverse neurologic deficits. A shunt may be needed to relieve associated hydrocephalus.
- If the patient has a severe spinal defect, short- and long-term treatment will require a team approach, including a neurosurgeon, orthopedist, urologist, nurse, social worker, occupational and physical therapists, and the patient's parents.
- Rehabilitation measures may include:
  - waist supports, long leg braces, walkers, crutches, and other orthopedic appliances

– diet and bowel training to manage fecal incontinence
– neurogenic bladder management to reduce urinary stasis, possibly intermittent catheterization, and anti-spasmodics, such as bethanechol (Urecholine) or propantheline (Pro-Banthine) (in severe cases, insertion of an artificial urinary sphincter or urinary diversion as a last resort to preserve kidney function).

■ Fetal surgery, typically performed at 24 to 30 weeks' gestation, may be used to correct myelomeningocele in utero, but the procedure is experimental and only performed at a few health care facilities in the United States.

Nursing considerations
Before surgical repair

■ Prevent local infection by cleaning the defect gently with sterile saline solution or other solutions. Inspect the defect often for signs of infection, and cover it with sterile dressings moistened with sterile saline solution. Don't use ointments on the defect; they may cause skin maceration.

■ Prevent skin breakdown by placing sheepskin or a foam pad under the infant. Keep skin clean, and apply lotion to knees, elbows, chin, and other pressure areas. Give antibiotics as needed.

■ Handle the infant carefully. Hold and cuddle him, but avoid placing pressure on the sac. When holding him on your lap, position him on his abdomen, and teach the parents to do the same.

■ Usually, the infant can't wear a diaper or a shirt until after surgical correction because it will irritate the sac, so keep him warm in an infant Isolette. Position him on his abdomen with the head of the bed slightly elevated to prevent contamination of the sac with urine or stools.

■ Provide adequate time for parent-child bonding if possible.

■ Measure head circumference daily, and watch for signs of hydrocephalus and meningeal irritation, such as fever or nuchal rigidity. Be sure to mark the spot so you get accurate readings.

■ Minimize contractures with passive range-of-motion exercises and casting. To prevent hip dislocation, abduct the hips with a pad between the knees or with sandbags and ankle rolls.

■ Monitor intake and output. Watch for decreased skin turgor, dryness, or other signs of dehydration. Provide meticulous skin care to genitals and buttocks to prevent infection.

■ Ensure adequate nutrition.

After surgical repair

■ Watch for hydrocephalus, which commonly follows such surgery. Measure the child's head circumference.

■ Monitor the neonate's vital signs often. Watch for signs of shock (decreased blood pressure, tachycardia, lethargy), infection (malaise, elevated temperature, alteration in feeding pattern), and increased intracranial pressure (ICP) (projectile vomiting).

■ Frequently assess the infant's fontanels. Remember that before age 2, infants don't show typical signs of increased ICP because suture lines aren't fully closed. The most revealing sign is bulging fontanels.

■ Change the dressing regularly, and watch for signs of drainage, wound rupture, or infection.

■ If leg casts have been applied to treat deformities, watch for signs that the child is outgrowing the cast. Check distal pulses to ensure adequate circulation. Petal the edges of the cast to prevent skin irritation. Use a cool-air blow-dryer to dry skin under the cast. Periodically check for foul odor and other indications of skin breakdown.

■ Help parents work through their feelings of guilt, anger, and helplessness.

■ Teach parents how to cope with their infant's problems and successfully meet long-range treatment goals. (See *Discharge teaching in spinal cord defects*.)

■ Refer parents for genetic counseling, and suggest that amniocentesis be performed in future pregnancies. For more information and names of support groups, refer parents to the Spina Bifida Association of America or other similar organizations.

■ A high percentage of children with spina bifida have latex allergy. Teach the patient about latex allergy and to avoid products that use latex as an ingredient. Give the patient a list of such products if available.

■ Teach women of childbearing age to take a daily vitamin with 400 mcg of folic acid to minimize the risk of neural tube defects.

Spinal injuries

Spinal injuries include fractures, contusions, and compressions of the vertebral column. These injuries usually result from trauma to the head or neck. The real danger lies in complications such as spinal cord damage arising from a spinal injury. (See *Complications of spinal injuries*, page 598.) Spinal fractures most commonly occur at C5, C6, and C7, T12, and L1.

Causes

■ Contact sports such as football
■ Diving into shallow water
■ Falls
■ Gunshot and stab wounds
■ Hyperparathyroidism
■ Lifting heavy objects
■ Motor vehicle accidents

Discharge teaching in spinal cord defects

Before discharge, review the following points with parents of children with spinal cord defects:

■ Teach parents how to recognize such early signs of complications as hydrocephalus, pressure ulcers, and urinary tract infections (UTIs). Also show them how to provide psychological support to the child and encourage a positive attitude.

■ Encourage parents to begin training their child in a toileting routine by age 3. Emphasize the need for increased fluid intake to prevent UTIs. Teach intermittent catheterization and conduit hygiene as needed.

■ Explain to parents how to prevent constipation and bowel obstruction. Stress the need for increased fluid intake, a high-bulk diet, exercise, and use of a stool softener (if prescribed). Teach parents to empty their child's bowel by exerting slight pressure on the abdomen, telling the child to bear down, and giving a glycerin suppository as needed.

■ Teach parents to recognize developmental lags early (a possible result of hydrocephalus). If the child does fall behind, stress the importance of follow-up IQ assessment to help plan realistic educational goals. The child may need to attend a school with special facilities. Also, stress the need for stimulation to ensure maximum mental development. Help parents plan activities appropriate to their child's age and abilities.

■ Neoplastic lesions

Signs and symptoms

■ In cervical fractures, pain that produces point tenderness; in dorsal and lumbar fractures, pain that radiates to other body areas such as the legs

- Mild paresthesia to quadriplegia and shock, with spinal cord damage, which may be delayed for several days or weeks
- Muscle spasm and back pain that worsens with movement
- Respiratory compromise with damage to C1 to C4 (also with edema at C5 to C7 expanding upward)

Diagnostic tests
- Spinal X-rays, the most important diagnostic measure, locate the fracture.
- Lumbar puncture may show increased cerebrospinal fluid pressure from a lesion or trauma in spinal compression.

- Computed tomography scan or magnetic resonance imaging can locate the spinal mass.

Treatment
- The primary treatment after spinal injury is immediate immobilization to stabilize the spine and prevent spinal cord damage; other treatment is supportive. Cervical injuries require immobilization, using sandbags on both sides of the patient's head, a hard cervical collar, or skeletal traction with skull tongs or a halo device.
- When patients show signs of spinal cord injury, high doses of methylprednisolone (Solu-Medrol) are given.

Complications of spinal injuries

The following are complications of spinal injuries: autonomic dysreflexia, spinal shock, and neurogenic shock.

Also known as *autonomic hyperreflexia,* autonomic dysreflexia is a serious medical condition that occurs after resolution of spinal shock. Emergency recognition and management is a must. Suspect autonomic dysreflexia in the patient with a history of spinal cord trauma at level T6 and above who exhibits cold or goose-fleshed skin below the lesion level, bradycardia, and hypertension. The hypertension is generally accompanied by severe, pounding headache.

Some dysreflexia is caused by noxious stimuli, most commonly a distended bladder or skin lesion. Treatment focuses on eliminating the stimulus; rapid identification and removal may avoid the need for pharmacologic control of the headache and hypertension.

Spinal shock is the loss of autonomic, reflex, motor, and sensory activity below the level of the cord lesion. It occurs secondary to damage of the spinal cord. Signs of spinal shock include flaccid paralysis, loss of deep tendon and perianal reflexes, and loss of motor and sensory function.

Until spinal shock has resolved (usually 1 to 6 weeks after injury), the extent of actual cord damage can't be assessed. The earliest indicator of spinal shock resolution is the return of reflex activity.

Neurogenic shock is a temporary loss of autonomic function below the level of injury that produces cardiovascular changes. Signs include orthostatic hypotension, bradycardia, and loss of the ability to sweat below the level of the lesion. This abnormal vasomotor response occurs secondary to disruption of sympathetic impulses from the brain stem to the thoracolumbar area and is seen most commonly in cervical cord injury.

■ Treatment of stable lumbar and dorsal fractures consists of bed rest on firm support (such as a bed board), analgesics, and muscle relaxants until the fracture stabilizes (usually 10 to 12 weeks). Later treatment includes exercises to strengthen the back muscles and a back brace or corset to provide support while walking.

■ An unstable dorsal or lumbar fracture requires a plaster cast, a turning frame and, in severe fracture, laminectomy and spinal fusion.

■ When the damage results in compression of the spinal column, neurosurgery may relieve the pressure.

■ If the cause of compression is a neoplastic lesion, chemotherapy and radiation may relieve it.

■ Surface wounds accompanying the spinal injury require tetanus prophylaxis unless the patient has had recent immunization.

Nursing considerations

■ In all spinal injuries, suspect spinal cord damage until proven otherwise.

■ During the initial assessment and X-rays, immobilize the patient on a firm surface, with sandbags on both sides of his head. Tell him not to move; avoid moving him, because hyperflexion can damage the cord.

■ If you must move the patient, get at least one other member of the staff to help you logroll him to avoid disturbing body alignment.

■ Throughout the assessment, offer comfort and reassurance. Remember, the patient's fear of possible paralysis will be overwhelming. Allow a family member who isn't too distraught to accompany the patient and talk to him quietly and calmly.

■ If the injury requires surgery, give prophylactic antibiotics. Catheterize the patient to avoid urine retention, and monitor defecation patterns to avoid impaction.

■ Explain traction methods to the patient and his family, and reassure them that traction devices don't penetrate the brain. If the patient has a halo or skull-tong traction device, clean the pin sites daily, keep his hair trimmed short, and provide analgesics for persistent headaches.

■ During traction, turn the patient often to prevent pneumonia, embolism, and skin breakdown; perform passive range-of-motion exercises to maintain muscle tone. If available, use an automatic rotational bed to facilitate turning, to avoid further spinal cord injury, and to promote adequate lung expansion.

■ Turn the patient on his side during feedings to prevent aspiration. Create a relaxed atmosphere at mealtimes.

■ Suggest appropriate diversionary activities to fill your patient's hours of immobility.

■ Watch closely for neurologic changes. Changes in skin sensation and loss of muscle strength could point to pressure on the spinal cord, possibly as a result of edema or shifting bone fragments.

■ If damage occurred to the spinal cord, involve a rehabilitation specialist as soon as possible to assist with a detailed and personal care plan.

■ Before discharge, instruct the patient about continuing analgesics or other medication, and stress the importance of regular follow-up examinations.

■ To help prevent a spinal injury from becoming a spinal cord injury, educate fire fighters, police officers, paramedics, and the general public about the proper way to handle such injuries.

Spinal neoplasms

Spinal neoplasms are tumors that are similar to intracranial tumors but that involve the spinal cord or its roots. Spinal cord tumors are rare compared with intracranial tumors (ratio of 1:4). They occur with equal frequency in men and women, with the exception of meningiomas, which usually occur in women. Spinal cord tumors can occur anywhere along the length of the cord or its roots. If untreated, they can eventually cause paralysis.

Primary spinal neoplasms originate in the meningeal coverings, the parenchyma of the cord or its roots, the intraspinal vasculature, or the vertebrae, or they may metastasize from primary tumors. These tumors may be extramedullary (occurring outside the spinal cord) or intramedullary (occurring within the cord itself).

Extramedullary tumors may be intradural (meningiomas and schwannomas), which account for 60% of all primary spinal cord neoplasms, or extradural (metastatic tumors from breasts, lungs, prostate, leukemia, or lymphomas), which account for 25% of these neoplasms.

Intramedullary tumors, or gliomas (astrocytomas or ependymomas), are comparatively rare, accounting for only about 10% of spinal neoplasms. In children, they're low-grade astrocytomas.

Extramedullary tumors produce symptoms by pressing on nerve roots, the spinal cord, and spinal vessels; intramedullary tumors, by destroying the parenchyma and compressing adjacent areas. Because intramedullary tumors may extend over several spinal cord segments, their symptoms are more variable than those of extramedullary tumors.

Causes

- Metastasis from cancers elsewhere in the body (extradural tumors)
- Possibly linked to von Recklinghausen's disease

Signs and symptoms

- Pain most severe directly over the tumor, radiating around the trunk or down the limb on the affected side, and unrelieved by bed rest
- Motor deficits: asymmetrical spastic muscle weakness, decreased muscle tone, exaggerated reflexes, positive Babinski's sign
  - Cauda equina tumors: muscle flaccidity, muscle wasting, weakness, progressive diminution in tendon reflexes
- Sensory deficits: contralateral loss of pain, temperature, and touch sensation (Brown-Séquard syndrome); less obvious to the patient than motor changes
  - Cauda equina tumors: paresthesia in the nerve distribution pathway of the involved roots
- Bladder symptoms
  - Early: incomplete emptying or difficulty with the urine stream, which is usually unnoticed or ignored
  - Late (with cord compression): urine retention
  - Cauda equina tumors: bladder and bowel incontinence from flaccid paralysis
- Constipation

Diagnostic tests

- Computed tomography scan or magnetic resonance imaging of the spine shows the location and size of the tumor or evidence of compression.
- Lumbar puncture shows clear yellow cerebrospinal fluid (CSF) as a result of increased protein levels if the flow is completely blocked. If the flow is partially blocked, protein levels rise, but CSF is only slightly yellow in proportion

to the CSF protein level. A CSF smear may show malignant cells of metastatic carcinoma.

▪ X-rays show distortions of the intervertebral foramina, changes in the vertebrae, collapsed areas in the vertebral body, and localized enlargement of the spinal canal, indicating an adjacent block.

▪ Myelography identifies the level of the tumor if it's causing partial obstruction by outlining it to show its anatomic relationship to the cord and the dura. If the obstruction is complete, the injected dye can't flow past the tumor. (This study is dangerous if cord compression is nearly complete because withdrawal or escape of CSF allows the tumor to exert greater pressure against the cord.)

▪ Radioisotope bone scan demonstrates metastatic invasion of the vertebrae by showing a characteristic increase in osteoblastic activity.

▪ Frozen section biopsy at surgery identifies the tissue type.

Treatment

▪ Laminectomy is indicated for primary tumors that produce spinal cord or cauda equina compression; it isn't usually indicated for metastatic tumors.

▪ If the tumor is slowly progressive or if it's treated before the cord degenerates from compression, symptoms are likely to disappear, and complete restoration of function is possible. In a patient with metastatic carcinoma or lymphoma who suddenly experiences complete transverse myelitis with spinal shock, functional improvement is unlikely, even with treatment, and the prognosis is poor.

▪ If the patient has incomplete paraplegia of rapid onset, emergency surgical decompression may save cord function. Steroid therapy minimizes cord edema until surgery can be performed. Partial

removal of intramedullary gliomas, followed by radiation, may alleviate symptoms for a short time.

▪ Metastatic extradural tumors can be controlled with radiation, analgesics and, in the case of hormone-mediated tumors (breast and prostate), appropriate hormone therapy.

▪ Transcutaneous electrical nerve stimulation (TENS) may control radicular pain from spinal cord tumors and is a useful alternative to opioid analgesics. In TENS, an electrical charge is applied to the skin to stimulate large-diameter nerve fibers and thereby inhibit transmission of pain impulses through small-diameter nerve fibers.

Nursing considerations

▪ On your first contact with the patient, perform a complete neurologic evaluation to obtain baseline data for planning future care and evaluating changes in his clinical status.

▪ Provide psychological support. Help the patient and his family to understand and cope with the diagnosis, treatment, potential disabilities, and necessary changes in lifestyle. Suggest appropriate support groups or organizations such as the American Cancer Society.

▪ After laminectomy, check the patient's neurologic status frequently, and watch for signs of infection. Administer analgesics, and aid the patient in early walking.

▪ Take safety precautions for the patient with impaired sensation and motor deficits. Use side rails if the patient is bedridden; if he isn't, encourage him to wear flat shoes, and remove scatter rugs and clutter to prevent falls.

▪ Make sure that the patient receives appropriate rehabilitation, including bowel and bladder retraining.

▪ Give steroids and antacids, as ordered, for cord edema after radiation therapy.

Monitor the patient for sensory or motor dysfunction, which indicates the need for more steroids.

■ Enforce bed rest for the patient with vertebral body involvement until he can safely walk; body weight alone can cause cord collapse and cord laceration from bone fragments.

■ Logroll and position the patient on his side every 2 hours to prevent pressure ulcers and other complications of immobility.

■ If the patient is to wear a back brace, make sure that he wears it whenever he gets out of bed.

Sprains and strains

A sprain is a complete or incomplete tear in the supporting ligaments surrounding a joint that usually follows a sharp twist. A strain is an injury to a muscle or tendinous attachment. A strain may be acute (an immediate result of vigorous muscle overuse or overstress) or chronic (a result of repeated overuse). A sprained ankle is the most common joint injury. Sprains and strains usually heal without surgical repair.

Causes

■ Trauma to the joint, causing the joint to move in a position it wasn't intended to move (sprain)
■ Excessive physical effort or activity, improper warming up before an activity, or poor flexibility (strain)

Signs and symptoms
Sprains
■ Ecchymosis from blood extravasating into surrounding tissues
■ Local pain (especially during joint movement)
■ Loss of mobility (possibly not until several hours after the injury)

■ Swelling

Strains
■ Sharp, transient pain (the patient may say he heard a snapping noise) and rapid swelling, followed by muscle tenderness, and then ecchymoses (acute strain)
■ Stiffness, soreness, and generalized tenderness, occurring several hours after the injury (chronic strain)

Diagnostic tests
■ X-ray rules out fractures, confirms damage to ligaments, and establishes the diagnosis.

Treatment
Sprains
■ Control of pain and swelling and immobilization of the injured joint promote healing.
■ Immediately after the injury, control swelling by elevating the joint above the level of the heart and intermittently applying ice for 12 to 48 hours. Keep a towel between the ice pack and the skin to prevent cold injuries.
■ An immobilized sprain usually heals in 2 to 3 weeks, and the patient can then gradually resume normal activities. Occasionally, however, torn ligaments don't heal properly and cause recurrent dislocation, necessitating surgical repair.
■ Some athletes may request immediate surgical repair to hasten healing; to prevent sprains, they may tape their wrists and ankles before sports activities.

Strains
■ Give analgesics and apply ice for up to 48 hours, and then apply heat.
■ Complete muscle rupture may require surgery.
■ Chronic strains usually don't need treatment; heat application, a nonsteroidal anti-inflammatory drug (such

as ibuprofen [Motrin]), or an analgesic–muscle relaxant can relieve discomfort.

Nursing considerations

- For sprains, immobilize the joint, using an elastic bandage or cast or, if the sprain is severe, a soft cast or splint. Depending on the severity of the injury, an analgesic may be necessary.
- If the patient has a sprained ankle, make sure that he receives crutch gait training. Because the patient with a sprain seldom requires hospitalization, provide patient teaching.
- Tell the patient with a sprain to elevate the joint for 48 to 72 hours after the injury (while sleeping, the joint can be elevated with pillows) and to apply ice intermittently for 12 to 48 hours.
- If an elastic bandage has been applied, teach the patient to reapply it by wrapping from below to above the injury, forming a figure-eight. For a sprained ankle, apply the bandage from the toes to midcalf. Tell the patient to remove the bandage before going to sleep and to loosen it if it causes the leg to become pale, numb, or painful.
- Instruct the patient to call if pain worsens or persists. An additional X-ray may detect a fracture that was missed originally.

▋Squamous cell carcinoma

Arising from the keratinizing epidermal cells, squamous cell carcinoma of the skin is an invasive tumor with metastatic potential. It commonly occurs in fair-skinned white men older than age 60. Outdoor employment and residence in a sunny, warm climate (southwestern United States and Australia, for example) greatly increase the risk of developing squamous cell carcinoma.

Lesions on sun-damaged skin tend to be less invasive and less likely to metastasize than lesions on unexposed skin. Notable exceptions to this tendency are squamous cell lesions on the lower lip and ears. These are almost invariably markedly invasive metastatic lesions with a generally poor prognosis.

Causes
Predisposing factors

- Overexposure to the sun's ultraviolet rays and the presence of premalignant lesions (such as actinic keratosis or Bowen's disease)
- X-ray therapy
- Ingestion of herbicides containing arsenic
- Chronic skin irritation and inflammation
- Burns or scars
- Exposure to local carcinogens, such as tar and oil
- Hereditary diseases, such as xeroderma pigmentosum and albinism
- Rarely, develops on site of smallpox vaccination, psoriasis, or chronic discoid lupus erythematosus

Signs and symptoms

- Lesions commonly on the skin of the face, ears, dorsa of the hands and forearms, and other sun-damaged areas
- Opaque, firm nodules with irregular borders, scaling, and ulceration
- Lesions that appear scaly from keratinization; most common on the face and hands
- Exophytic (outward-growing) lesions that are friable and develop chronic crusting in late stages
- Premalignant lesion that changes to squamous cell carcinoma: induration and inflammation of the preexisting lesion

- Squamous cell carcinoma that arises from healthy skin: slow-growing nodule on a firm, indurated base
- If left untreated, eventual ulceration; invasion of underlying tissues
- Metastasis to the regional lymph nodes, producing characteristic systemic symptoms of pain, malaise, fatigue, weakness, and anorexia

Diagnostic tests

- An excisional biopsy offers definitive support for a diagnosis of squamous cell carcinoma.
- Other appropriate laboratory tests depend on systemic symptoms.

Treatment

- The size, shape, location, and invasiveness of a squamous cell tumor and the condition of the underlying tissue determine the treatment method used.
- Premalignant lesions respond well to treatment. (See *Treating actinic keratoses*.)

- A deeply invasive tumor may require a combination of techniques. All the major treatment methods have excellent cure rates; the prognosis is usually better with a well-differentiated lesion than with a poorly differentiated one in an unusual location.
- Depending on the lesion, treatment may consist of:
  - surgical excision
  - curettage and electrodesiccation (for small lesions)
  - radiation therapy (usually for elderly or debilitated patients)
  - chemosurgery (for resistant or recurrent lesions).

Nursing considerations

- Keep the wound dry and clean.
- Tell the patient to use sunblock on his lips to protect the lips from sun damage.
- To prevent squamous cell carcinoma, tell the patient to avoid excessive sun exposure and wear protective clothing (hats, long sleeves).

Treating actinic keratoses

A useful drug for treating actinic keratoses, fluorouracil is available in different strengths (1%, 2%, and 5%) as a cream or solution.

Local application causes stinging and burning, followed by erythema, vesiculation, erosion, superficial ulceration, necrosis, and re-epithelialization. The 5% solution induces the most severe inflammatory response but provides complete involution of the lesions with little recurrence.

Nursing considerations

- Keep fluorouracil away from eyes, scrotum, and mucous membranes.
- Warn the patient to avoid excessive sun exposure during treatment because sun intensifies the inflammatory reaction.
- Continue application of fluorouracil until the lesions reach the ulcerative and necrotic stages (2 to 4 weeks); then consider application of a corticosteroid preparation as an anti-inflammatory.
- Adverse effects include post-inflammatory hyperpigmentation. Complete healing takes 1 to 2 months.

- Instruct the patient to periodically examine the skin for precancerous lesions and have any removed promptly.
- Advise the patient to use sunscreen containing para-aminobenzoic acid, benzophenone, and zinc oxide. He should apply these agents 30 to 60 minutes before sun exposure.

Staphylococcal infections

Staphylococci are coagulase-negative (*Staphylococcus epidermidis*) or coagulase-positive (*S. aureus*) gram-positive bacteria. Coagulase-negative staphylococci grow abundantly as normal flora on skin, but they can also cause boils, abscesses, and carbuncles. In the upper respiratory tract, they are usually nonpathogenic but can cause serious infections. Pathogenic strains of staphylococci are found in many adult carriers—usually on the nasal mucosa, axilla, or groin. Sometimes, carriers shed staphylococci, infecting themselves or other susceptible people. Coagulase-positive staphylococci tend to form pus; they cause many types of infections.

Causes
- See *Comparing staphylococcal infections,* pages 606 to 611.

Signs and symptoms
- See *Comparing staphylococcal infections,* pages 606 to 611.

Diagnostic tests
- See *Comparing staphylococcal infections,* pages 606 to 611.

Treatment
- See *Comparing staphylococcal infections,* pages 606 to 611.

Nursing considerations
- See *Comparing staphylococcal infections,* pages 606 to 611.

Staphylococcal scalded skin syndrome

A severe skin disorder, staphylococcal scalded skin syndrome (SSSS) is marked by epidermal erythema, peeling, and superficial necrosis that give the skin a scalded appearance. SSSS is most prevalent in infants ages 1 to 3 months but may develop in children; it's rare in adults.

This disease follows a consistent pattern of progression, and most patients recover fully. Mortality is 2% to 3%, with death usually resulting from complications of fluid and electrolyte loss, sepsis, and involvement of other body systems.

Causes
- Group 2 *Staphylococcus aureus,* primarily phage type 71

Predisposing factors
- Impaired immunity
- Renal insufficiency

Signs and symptoms
- Prodromal upper respiratory tract infection, possibly with concomitant purulent conjunctivitis
- Cutaneous changes that progress through three stages

Stage 1
- Erythema visible, usually around the mouth and other orifices as well as body fold areas, possibly spreading in widening circles over the entire body surface
- Skin tenderness

(*Text continues on page 612.*)

Comparing staphylococcal infections

Predisposing factors	Signs and symptoms	Diagnostic tests
Bacteremia ■ Infected surgical wounds ■ Abscesses ■ Infected I.V. or intra-arterial catheter sites or catheter tips ■ Infected vascular grafts or prostheses ■ Infected pressure ulcers ■ Osteomyelitis ■ Parenteral drug abuse ■ Source unknown (primary bacteremia) ■ Cellulitis ■ Burns ■ Immunosuppression ■ Debilitating diseases, such as chronic renal insufficiency and diabetes ■ Infective endocarditis (coagulase-positive staphylococci) and subacute bacterial endocarditis (coagulase-negative staphylococci) ■ Cancer (leukemia) or neutrophil nadir after chemotherapy or radiation	■ Fever (high fever with no obvious source in children young than age 1), shaking chills, tachycardia ■ Cyanosis or pallor ■ Confusion, agitation, stupor ■ Skin microabscesses ■ Joint pain ■ Complications: shock; acute bacterial endocarditis (in prolonged infection; indicated by new or changing systolic murmur); retinal hemorrhages; splinter hemorrhages under nails and small, tender red nodes on pads of fingers and toes (Osler's nodes); abscess formation in skin, bones, lungs, brain, and kidneys; pulmonary emboli if tricuspid valve is infected ■ Prognosis poor in patients older than age 60 or with chronic illness	■ Blood cultures (two to four samples from different sites at different times): growing staphylococci and leukocytosis (usually white blood cell [WBC] count of 12,000/µl), with shift to the left of polymorphonuclear leukocytes (70% to 90% neutrophils) ■ Urinalysis that shows microscopic hematuria ■ Erythrocyte sedimentation rate (ESR) elevated, especially in chronic or subacute bacterial endocarditis ■ Severe anemia or thrombocytopenia (possible) ■ Prolonged partial thromboplastin time and prothrombin time; low fibrinogen and platelet counts, and low factor assays; possible disseminated intravascular coagulation ■ Cultures of urine, sputum, and draining skin lesions: may identify primary infection site (chest X-rays and scans of lungs, liver, abdomen, and brain may do so as well) ■ Echocardiogram: may show heart valve vegetation

Treatment	Nursing considerations
■ Semisynthetic penicillins (oxacillin, nafcillin) or cephalosporins (cefazolin) given I.V. ■ Vancomycin I.V. for those with penicillin allergy or methicillin-resistant organism ■ Possibly, probenecid given to partially prevent urinary excretion of penicillin and to prolong blood levels ■ I.V. fluids to reverse shock ■ Removal of infected catheter or foreign body ■ Surgery	■ *S. aureus* bacteremia can be fatal within 12 hours. Stay especially alert for it in debilitated patients with I.V. catheters or in those with a history of drug abuse. ■ Administer antibiotics on time to maintain adequate blood levels, but give them slowly, using the prescribed amount of diluent, to prevent thrombophlebitis. ■ Watch for signs of penicillin allergy, especially a pruritic rash (possible anaphylaxis). Keep epinephrine 1:1,000 and resuscitation equipment handy. Monitor the patient's vital signs, urine output, and mental state for signs of shock. ■ Obtain cultures carefully, and observe for clues to the primary site of infection. Never refrigerate blood cultures; it delays identification of organisms by slowing their growth. ■ Impose wound and skin precautions if the primary site of infection is draining. Special blood precautions aren't necessary because the number of organisms present, even in fulminant bacteremia, is minimal. ■ Obtain peak and trough levels of vancomycin to determine the adequacy of treatment.

(continued)

Comparing staphylococcal infections *(continued)*

Predisposing factors	Signs and symptoms	Diagnostic tests
Pneumonia ■ Immune deficiencies, especially in elderly people and in children younger than age 2 ■ Chronic lung diseases and cystic fibrosis ■ Malignant tumors ■ Antibiotics that kill normal respiratory flora but spare *Staphylococcus aureus* ■ Viral respiratory infections, especially influenza ■ Hematogenous (blood-borne) bacteria spread to the lungs from primary sites of infections, such as heart valves, abscesses, and pulmonary emboli ■ Recent bronchial or endotracheal suctioning or intubation	■ High temperature: adults, 103° to 105° F (39.4° to 40.6° C); children, 101° F (38.3° C) ■ Cough, with purulent, yellow, or bloody sputum ■ Dyspnea, crackles, and decreased breath sounds ■ Pleuritic pain ■ In infants: mild respiratory infection that suddenly worsens: irritability, anxiety, dyspnea, anorexia, vomiting, diarrhea, spasms of dry coughing, marked tachypnea, expiratory grunting, sternal retractions, and cyanosis ■ Complications: necrosis, lung abscess, pyopneumothorax, empyema, pneumatocele, shock, hypotension, oliguria or anuria, cyanosis, loss of consciousness	■ WBC count elevated (15,000 to 40,000/mm^3 in adults; 15,000 to 20,000/mm^3 in children), with predominance of polymorphonuclear leukocytes ■ Sputum Gram stain: mostly gram-positive cocci in clusters, with many polymorphonuclear leukocytes ■ Sputum culture: mostly coagulase-positive staphylococci ■ Chest X-rays: usually patchy infiltrates ■ Arterial blood gas analysis: hypoxia and respiratory acidosis
Enterocolitis ■ Broad-spectrum antibiotics (tetracycline, chloramphenicol, or neomycin) or aminoglycosides (tobramycin, streptomycin, or kanamycin) as prophylaxis for bowel surgery or treatment of hepatic coma ■ Usually occurs in elderly people but also in neonates (associated with staphylococcal skin lesions)	■ Sudden onset of profuse, watery diarrhea usually 2 days to several weeks after start of antibiotic therapy, I.V. or by mouth ■ Nausea, vomiting, abdominal pain and distention ■ Hypovolemia and dehydration (decreased skin turgor, hypotension, fever)	■ Stool Gram stain: many gram-positive cocci and polymorphonuclear leukocytes, with few gram-negative rods ■ Stool culture: *S. aureus* ■ Sigmoidoscopy: mucosal ulcerations ■ Blood studies: leukocytosis, moderately increased blood urea nitrogen level, and decreased serum albumin level

Treatment	Nursing considerations
■ Semisynthetic penicillins (oxacillin, nafcillin) or cephalosporins given I.V. ■ Vancomycin I.V. for those with penicillin allergy or methicillin-resistant organisms ■ Isolation until sputum shows minimal numbers of *S. aureus* (about 24 to 72 hours after starting antibiotics)	■ Use masks with the isolated patient because staphylococci from lungs spread by air as well as direct contact. Use a gown and gloves only when handling contaminated respiratory secretions. Use respiratory isolation precautions. ■ Keep the door to the patient's room closed. Don't store extra supplies in his room. Empty suction bottles carefully. Place articles containing sputum, such as tissues and clothing, in a sealed plastic bag. Mark them "contaminated," and dispose of them promptly by incineration. ■ When obtaining sputum specimens, make sure that you're collecting thick sputum, not saliva. The presence of epithelial cells (found in the mouth, not lungs) indicates a poor specimen. ■ Administer antibiotics strictly on time, but slowly. Watch for signs of penicillin allergy and for signs of infection at I.V. sites. Change the I.V. site at least every 3rd day. ■ Perform frequent chest physiotherapy. Do chest percussion and postural drainage after intermittent positive-pressure breathing treatments. Concentrate on consolidated areas (revealed by X-rays or auscultation).
■ Broad-spectrum antibiotics discontinued ■ Possibly, antistaphylococcal agents, such as vancomycin, by mouth ■ Normal flora replenished with yogurt ■ Surgical debridement	■ Monitor the patient's vital signs frequently to prevent shock. Make sure that he gets plenty of fluids to correct dehydration. ■ Know serum electrolyte levels. Measure and record bowel movements when possible. Check serum chloride level for alkalosis (hypochloremia). ■ Collect serial stool specimens for Gram stain, and culture for diagnosis and for evaluating effectiveness of treatment. ■ Observe enteric precautions. ■ Consider reporting requirements, especially in a group situation such as a nursing home.

(continued)

Comparing staphylococcal infections *(continued)*

Predisposing factors	Signs and symptoms	Diagnostic tests
Osteomyelitis ■ Hematogenous organisms ■ Skin trauma ■ Infection spreading from adjacent joint or other infected tissues ■ *S. aureus* bacteremia ■ Orthopedic surgery or trauma ■ Cardiothoracic surgery ■ Usually occurs in growing bones, especially femur and tibia, of children young than age 12 ■ More common in males	■ Abrupt onset of fever—usually 101° F; shaking chills; pain and swelling over infected area; restlessness; headache ■ About 20% of children developing a chronic infection if not properly treated	■ Possible history of previous trauma to involved area ■ Positive bone and pus cultures (and blood cultures in about 50% of patients) ■ X-ray changes apparent after second or third week ■ ESR elevated with leukocyte shift to the left
Food poisoning ■ Enterotoxin produced by toxigenic strains of *S. aureus* in contaminated food (second most common cause of food poisoning in United States)	■ Anorexia, nausea, vomiting, diarrhea, and abdominal cramps 1 to 6 hours after ingestion of contaminated food ■ Subsiding of symptoms within 18 hours, with complete recovery in 1 to 3 days	■ Clinical findings sufficient ■ Stool cultures usually negative for *S. aureus*
Skin infections ■ Decreased resistance ■ Burns or pressure ulcers ■ Decreased blood flow ■ Possibly skin contamination from nasal discharge ■ Foreign bodies ■ Underlying skin diseases, such as eczema and acne ■ Common in persons with poor hygiene living in crowded quarters	■ Cellulitis—diffuse, acute inflammation of soft tissue (no drainage) ■ Pus-producing lesions in and around hair follicles (folliculitis) ■ Boil-like lesions (furuncles and carbuncles) that extend from hair follicles to subcutaneous tissues (painful, red, indurated lesions that are 0.5″ to 1″ (1 to 2 cm) in diameter with a purulent yellow discharge) ■ Small macule or skin bleb that may develop into vesicle containing pus (bullous impetigo); common in school-age children ■ Mild or spiking fever ■ Malaise	■ Clinical findings and analysis of pus cultures if sites are draining ■ Cultures of nondraining cellulitis taken from the margin of the reddened area by infiltration with 1 ml of sterile saline solution and immediate fluid aspiration

Treatment	Nursing considerations
■ Prolonged antibiotic therapy (4 to 8 weeks) ■ Vancomycin I.V. for patients with penicillin allergy or methicillin-resistant organisms	■ Identify the infected area, and mark it on the care plan. ■ Check the penetration wound from which the organism originated for evidence of present infection. ■ Severe pain may render the patient immobile. If so, perform passive range-of-motion exercises. Apply heat as needed, and elevate the affected part. (Extensive involvement may require casting until the infection subsides.) ■ Before such procedures as surgical debridement, warn the patient to expect some pain. Explain that drainage is essential for healing and that he'll continue to receive analgesics and antibiotics after surgery.
■ No treatment necessary unless dehydration becomes a problem (usually in infants and elderly); then, I.V. therapy may be necessary to replace fluids	■ Obtain a complete history of symptoms, recent meals, and other known cases of food poisoning. ■ Monitor the patient's vital signs, fluid balance, and serum electrolyte levels. ■ Check for dehydration if vomiting is severe or prolonged, and for decreased blood pressure. ■ Observe and report the number and color of stools.
■ Topical ointments; bacitracin-neomycin-polymyxin or gentamicin ■ Oral cloxacillin, dicloxacillin, or erythromycin; I.V. oxacillin or nafcillin for severe infection; I.V. vancomycin for oxacillin-resistant organisms ■ Heat application to reduce pain ■ Surgical drainage ■ Identification and treatment of sources of reinfection (nostrils, perineum) ■ Cleaning and covering the area with moist, sterile dressings	■ Identify the site and extent of infection. ■ Keep lesions clean with saline solution and peroxide irrigations as ordered. Cover infections near wounds or the genitourinary tract with gauze pads. Keep pressure off the site to facilitate healing. ■ Stay alert for the extension of skin infections. ■ Severe infection or abscess may require surgical drainage. Explain the procedure to the patient. Determine whether cultures will be taken, and be ready to collect a specimen. ■ Impetigo is contagious. Isolate the patient and alert his family. Use secretion precautions for all draining lesions.

■ Nikolsky's sign (sloughing of the skin when friction is applied)

Stage 2
■ Exfoliation occurring about 24 to 48 hours later
■ Superficial erosions and minimal crusting, generally around body orifices, possibly spreading to exposed areas of the skin
■ Eruption of large, flaccid bullae; possibly spreading to cover extensive areas of the body (in severe forms)
■ Rupture of bullae, revealing denuded skin

Stage 3
■ Drying up of affected areas, forming powdery scales
■ Scales replaced by normal skin in 5 to 7 days

Diagnostic tests
■ Results of exfoliative cytology and a biopsy aid in the differential diagnosis, ruling out erythema multiforme and drug-induced toxic epidermal necrolysis, both of which are similar to SSSS.
■ A blood culture is necessary to rule out sepsis.

Treatment
■ Systemic antibiotics treat the underlying infection.
■ Replacement measures maintain fluid and electrolyte balance to prevent dehydration.
■ Moist compresses may improve comfort, and an emollient may help keep skin moist.

Nursing considerations
■ Provide special care for the neonate, if required, including placement in a warming infant incubator to maintain body temperature and provide isolation.

■ Carefully monitor intake and output to assess fluid and electrolyte balance. In severe cases, I.V. fluid replacement may be necessary.
■ Check the infant's vital signs. Stay especially alert for a sudden rise in temperature, indicating sepsis, which requires prompt, aggressive treatment.
■ Maintain skin integrity. Remember to use strict aseptic technique to preclude secondary infection, especially during the exfoliative stage, because of open lesions.
■ To prevent friction and sloughing of the patient's skin, leave affected areas uncovered or loosely covered. Place cotton between fingers and toes that are severely affected to prevent webbing.
■ Administer warm baths and soaks during the recovery period. Gently debride exfoliated areas.
■ Reassure parents that complications are rare and that residual scars are unlikely.

Stomatitis and other oral infections

A common infection, stomatitis—inflammation of the oral mucosa—may extend to the buccal mucosa, lips, and palate. It may occur alone or as part of a systemic disease. In immunocompromised individuals, reactivation of the herpes simplex virus (HSV) infection may be frequent and severe.

There are two main types: acute herpetic stomatitis and aphthous stomatitis. Acute herpetic stomatitis is common and mild in children age 1 to 3 and is usually short-lived and easily recognized; however, it may be severe and, in neonates, may be generalized and potentially fatal.

Aphthous stomatitis is common in young girls and female adolescents. This form usually heals spontaneously, without a scar, in 10 to 14 days.

Other oral infections include gingivitis, periodontitis, Vincent's angina, and glossitis. (See *Oral infections,* pages 614 and 615.)

Causes
- HSV (acute herpetic stomatitis)
- Unclear (aphthous stomatitis)

Signs and symptoms
Acute herpetic stomatitis
- Burning mouth pain
- Swollen gums that bleed easily, tender mucous membranes
- Papulovesicular ulcers in the mouth and throat; eventually become punched-out lesions with reddened areolae, which rupture and form scales
- Submaxillary lymphadenitis
- Disappearance of pain from 2 to 4 days before healing of ulcers is complete

Aphthous stomatitis
- Burning, tingling, and slight swelling of the mucous membrane
- Single or multiple, small round ulcers with whitish centers and red borders
- Pain that lasts 7 to 10 days, with healing complete in 1 to 3 weeks

Diagnostic tests
- A smear of ulcer exudate allows identification of the causative organism.

Treatment
Acute herpetic stomatitis
- For local symptoms, management includes warm-water mouth rinses (antiseptic mouthwashes are contraindicated because they're irritating) and a topical anesthetic to relieve mouth ulcer pain.
- A course of acyclovir (Zovirax) (200 to 800 mg, five times daily for 7 to 14

days) may shorten the course and reduce postherpetic pain.
- Following a bland or liquid diet until the infection resolves may ease symptoms.
- In severe cases, I.V. fluids to maintain hydration and bed rest are needed.
- After the gums become less tender, a dentist should scale and polish the teeth and emphasize good oral hygiene.

Aphthous stomatitis
- Apply a topical anesthetic.
- Advise the patient to alleviate or prevent precipitating factors.

Nursing considerations
- Show the patient how to clean his mouth with sponges instead of a toothbrush.
- Have the patient rinse his mouth with hydrogen peroxide or normal saline to soothe irritated mucosa.
- Administer prescribed analgesics.
- If ordered, apply a topical coating or swishing agent to relieve pain.
- Soft, liquid, or pureed foods are recommended; icy cold drinks may be well tolerated.
- In severe cases, supplement oral foods with I.V. fluids or nasogastric feedings.

Streptococcal infections

Streptococci are small, spherical to ovoid gram-positive bacteria, linked together in pairs of chains. Several species occur as part of normal human flora in the respiratory, GI, and genitourinary tracts. Although researchers have identified 21 species of streptococci, three classes—groups A, B, and D—cause most infections. Organisms belonging to groups A and B beta-hemolytic streptococci are associated with a characteristic

Oral infections

Disease and causes	Signs and symptoms
Gingivitis (inflammation of the gingiva) ▪ Early sign of hypovitaminosis, diabetes, blood dyscrasias ▪ Occasionally related to use of hormonal contraceptives	▪ Inflammation with painless swelling, redness, change of normal contours, bleeding, and periodontal pocket (gum detachment from teeth)
Periodontitis (progression of gingivitis; inflammation of the oral mucosa) ▪ Early sign of hypovitaminosis, diabetes, blood dyscrasias ▪ Occasionally related to use of hormonal contraceptives ▪ Dental factors: calculus, poor oral hygiene, malocclusion (major cause of tooth loss after middle age)	▪ Acute onset of bright red gum inflammation, painless swelling of interdental papillae, easy bleeding ▪ Loosening of teeth, typically without inflammatory symptoms, progressing to loss of teeth and alveolar bone ▪ Acute systemic infection (fever, chills)
Vincent's angina (trench mouth, necrotizing ulcerative gingivitis) ▪ Fusiform bacillus or spirochete infection ▪ Predisposing factors: stress, poor oral hygiene, insufficient rest, nutritional deficiency, smoking	▪ Sudden onset: painful, superficial bleeding; gingival ulcers (rarely, on buccal mucosa) covered with a gray-white membrane ▪ Ulcers becoming punched-out lesions after slight pressure or irritation ▪ Malaise, mild fever, excessive salivation, bad breath, pain on swallowing or talking, enlarged submaxillary lymph nodes
Glossitis (tongue inflammation) ▪ Streptococcal infection ▪ Irritation or injury, jagged teeth, ill-fitting dentures, biting during convulsions, alcohol, spicy foods, smoking, sensitivity to toothpaste or mouthwash ▪ Vitamin B deficiency, anemia ▪ Skin conditions: lichen planus, erythema multiforme, pemphigus vulgaris	▪ Reddened ulcerated or swollen tongue (may obstruct airway) ▪ Painful chewing and swallowing ▪ Painful tongue without inflammation

Treatment

- Removal of irritating factors (calculus, faulty dentures)
- Good oral hygiene, regular dental checkups, vigorous chewing
- Oral or topical corticosteroids

- Scaling, root planing, and curettage for infection control
- Periodontal surgery to prevent recurrence
- Good oral hygiene, regular dental checkups, vigorous chewing

- Removal of devitalized tissue with ultrasonic cavitron
- Antibiotics (penicillin or oral erythromycin) for infection
- Analgesics as needed
- Hourly mouth rinses (equal parts hydrogen peroxide and warm water)
- Soft, nonirritating diet; rest; no smoking
- With treatment, improvement within 24 hours

- Treatment of underlying cause
- Topical anesthetic mouthwash or systemic analgesics (aspirin or acetaminophen [Tylenol]) for painful lesions
- Good oral hygiene, regular dental checkups, vigorous chewing
- Avoidance of alcohol and hot, cold, or spicy foods

pattern of human infections. Most disorders due to group D streptococcus are caused by *Enterococcus faecalis* (formerly called *Streptococcus faecalis*) or *Streptococcus bovis*.

Three states of streptococcal infection occur: carrier, acute, and delayed nonsuppurative complications. In the carrier state, the patient is infected with a disease-causing species of streptococci without evidence of infection. In the acute form, streptococci invade the tissues and cause physical symptoms. In the delayed nonsuppurative complications state, specific complications associated with streptococcal infection occur. These include the inflammatory state of acute rheumatic fever, chorea, and glomerulonephritis. If complications occur, they usually appear about 2 weeks after the acute illness, but they may be evident after a nonsymptomatic illness.

Causes
- See *Comparing streptococcal infections,* pages 616 to 623.

Signs and symptoms
- See *Comparing streptococcal infections,* pages 616 to 623.

Diagnostic tests
- See *Comparing streptococcal infections,* pages 616 to 623.

Treatment
- See *Comparing streptococcal infections,* pages 616 to 623.

Nursing considerations
- See *Comparing streptococcal infections,* pages 616 to 623.

(Text continues on page 622.)

Comparing streptococcal infections

Causes and incidence	Signs and symptoms
Streptococcus pyogenes (group A streptococcus)	
Streptococcal pharyngitis *(strep throat)* ■ Accounts for 95% of all cases of bacterial pharyngitis ■ Most common in children ages 5 to 10 from October to April ■ Spread by direct person-to-person contact via droplets of saliva or nasal secretions ■ Organism usually colonizing throats of persons with no symptoms; up to 20% of schoolchildren possible carriers; pets also possible carriers	■ After 1- to 5-day incubation period: temperature of 101° to 104° F (38.3° to 40° C), sore throat with severe pain on swallowing, beefy red pharynx, tonsillar exudate, edematous tonsils and uvula, swollen glands along the jaw line, generalized malaise and weakness, occasional abdominal discomfort ■ Up to 40% of small children having symptoms too mild for diagnosis ■ Fever abating in 3 to 5 days; nearly all symptoms subside within a week
Scarlet fever *(scarlatina)* ■ Usually follows streptococcal pharyngitis; may follow wound infections or puerperal sepsis ■ Caused by streptococcal strain that releases an erythrogenic toxin ■ Most common in children ages 2 to 10 ■ Spread by inhalation or direct contact	■ Streptococcal sore throat, fever, strawberry tongue, fine erythematous rash that blanches on pressure and resembles sunburn with goosebumps ■ Rash usually appearing first on upper chest and then spreading to neck, abdomen, legs, and arms, sparing soles and palms; flushed cheeks; pallor around mouth ■ Skin shedding during convalescence
Erysipelas ■ Occurs primarily in infants and adults older than age 30 ■ Usually follows strep throat ■ Exact mode of spread to skin unknown	■ Sudden onset, with reddened, swollen, raised lesions (skin looks like an orange peel), usually on face and scalp, bordered by areas that commonly contain easily ruptured blebs filled with yellow-tinged fluid; stinging and itching lesions on the trunk, arms, or legs usually affecting incision or wound sites ■ Other symptoms: vomiting, fever, headache, cervical lymphadenopathy, sore throat

Diagnosis	Complications	Treatment and special considerations
▪ Clinically indistinguishable from viral pharyngitis. ▪ Throat culture shows group A beta-hemolytic streptococci. (Carriers have positive throat culture.) ▪ White blood cell (WBC) count is elevated. ▪ Serology shows a fourfold rise in streptozyme titers during convalescence.	▪ Acute otitis media or acute sinusitis occurs most frequently. ▪ Rarely, bacteremic spread may cause arthritis, endocarditis, meningitis, osteomyelitis, or liver abscess. ▪ Poststreptococcal sequelae may include acute rheumatic fever or acute glomerulonephritis. ▪ Reye's syndrome may occur.	▪ Give penicillin or erythromycin, analgesics, and antipyretics as ordered. ▪ Stress the need for bed rest and isolation from others for 24 hours after antibiotic therapy begins. The patient should finish the prescription, even if symptoms subside; abscess, glomerulonephritis, and rheumatic fever can occur. ▪ Tell the patient not to skip doses and to properly dispose of soiled tissues.
▪ Characteristic rash and strawberry tongue appears. ▪ Culture and Gram stain show *S. pyogenes* from nasopharynx. ▪ Granulocytosis	▪ Although rare, complications may include high fever, arthritis, jaundice, pneumonia, pericarditis, and peritonsillar abscess.	▪ Give penicillin or erythromycin as ordered. ▪ Stress need for isolation for first 24 hours. ▪ Carefully dispose of purulent discharge. ▪ Stress the need for prompt and complete antibiotic treatment.
▪ Typical reddened lesions appear. ▪ Culture taken from edge of lesions shows group A beta-hemolytic streptococci. ▪ Throat culture is almost always positive for group A beta-hemolytic streptococci.	▪ Untreated lesions on trunk, arms, or legs may involve large body areas and lead to death.	▪ Give penicillin or erythromycin I.V. or by mouth as ordered. ▪ Give cold packs, analgesics (aspirin and codeine for local discomfort), and topical anesthetics as ordered. ▪ Prevention measures involve prompt treatment of streptococcal infections and drainage and secretion precautions.

(continued)

Comparing streptococcal infections *(continued)*

Causes and incidence	Signs and symptoms

Streptococcus pyogenes (group A streptococcus) *(continued)*

Impetigo
(streptococcal pyoderma)
- Common in poor children ages 2 to 5 in hot, humid weather; high rate of familial spread
- Predisposing factors: close contact in schools, overcrowded living quarters, poor skin hygiene, minor skin trauma
- May spread by direct contact, environmental contamination, or arthropod vector

- Small macules rapidly developing into vesicles and then becoming pustular and encrusted, causing pain, surrounding erythema, regional adenitis, cellulitis, and itching; scratching spreading infection
- Lesions commonly affecting the face, healing slowly, and leaving depigmented areas

Streptococcal gangrene
(necrotizing fasciitis)
- More common in elderly patients with arteriosclerotic vascular disease or diabetes
- Predisposing factors: surgery, wounds, skin ulcers, diabetes, peripheral vascular disease
- Spread by direct contact

- Mimics gas gangrene; within 72 hours of onset, patient showing red-streaked, painful skin lesions with dusky red surrounding tissue; Bullae with yellow or reddish black fluid developing and rupturing
- Other signs and symptoms: fever, tachycardia, lethargy, prostration, disorientation, hypotension, jaundice, hypovolemia, severe pain followed by anesthesia (due to nerve destruction)

Streptococcus agalactiae (group B streptococcus)

Neonatal streptococcal infections
- Incidence of early-onset infection (age 5 days or less): 2/1,000 live births
- Incidence of late-onset infection (age 7 days to 3 months): 1/1,000 live births
- Spread by vaginal delivery or hands of nursery staff
- Predisposing factors: maternal genital tract colonization, membrane rupture more than 24 hours before delivery, crowded nursery

- Early onset: bacteremia, pneumonia, and meningitis; mortality from 14% for neonates more than 1,500 g at birth to 61% for neonates less than 1,500 g at birth
- Late onset: bacteremia with meningitis, fever, and bone and joint involvement; mortality 15% to 20%
- Other signs and symptoms, such as skin lesions, depending on the site affected

Diagnosis	Complications	Treatment and special considerations
■ Characteristic lesions with honey-colored crust appear. ■ Culture and Gram stain of swabbed lesions show *S. pyogenes*.	■ Septicemia (rare) ■ Ecthyma, a form of impetigo with deep ulcers	■ Give penicillin I.V. or by mouth, erythromycin, or antibiotic ointments as ordered. ■ Frequently wash lesions with antiseptics, such as antibacterial soap, then thoroughly dry. ■ Isolate patient with draining wounds. ■ Prevention measures include good hygiene and proper wound care.
■ Culture and Gram stain usually show *S. pyogenes* from early bullous lesions and commonly from blood.	■ Extensive necrotic sloughing ■ Bacteremia, metastatic abscesses, and death ■ Thrombophlebitis, when lower extremities are involved	■ Immediate, wide, deep surgery of all necrotic tissues is required. ■ High-dose penicillin I.V. is given. ■ Good preoperative skin preparation and sterile surgical and suturing technique is required.
■ Group B streptococcus is isolated from blood, cerebrospinal fluid (CSF), or skin. ■ Chest X-ray shows massive infiltrate similar to that of respiratory distress syndrome or pneumonia.	■ Overwhelming pneumonia, sepsis, and death	■ Give penicillin or ampicillin and an aminoglycoside I.V. as ordered. ■ Patient isolation is unnecessary unless open draining lesion is present, but careful hand washing is essential. If draining lesion is present, take drainage and secretion precautions.

(continued)

Comparing streptococcal infections *(continued)*

Causes and incidence	Signs and symptoms
Streptococcus agalactiae (group B streptococcus) *(continued)*	
Adult group B streptococcal infection ■ Most adult infections occurring in postpartum women, usually in the form of endometritis or wound infection following cesarean section ■ Incidence of group B streptococcal endometritis: 1.3/1,000 live births	■ Fever, malaise, uterine tenderness ■ Change in lochia
Streptococcus pneumoniae (group D streptococcus)	
Pneumococcal pneumonia ■ Accounts for 70% of all cases of bacterial pneumonia ■ More common in men, elderly people, Blacks, and Native Americans, in winter and early spring ■ Spread by air and contact with infective secretions ■ Predisposing factors: trauma, viral infection, underlying pulmonary disease, overcrowded living quarters, chronic diseases, immunodeficiency	■ Sudden onset with severe shaking chills, temperature of 102° to 105° F (38.9° to 40.6° C), bacteremia, cough (with thick, scanty, blood-tinged sputum) accompanied by pleuritic pain ■ Malaise, weakness, and prostration (common) ■ Tachypnea, anorexia, nausea, and vomiting (less common) ■ Severity of pneumonia usually due to host's cellular defenses, not bacterial virulence
Otitis media ■ About 76% to 95% of all children getting otitis media at least once; *S. pneumoniae* causing half of these cases	■ Ear pain, ear drainage, hearing loss, fever, lethargy, irritability ■ Other possible symptoms: vertigo, nystagmus, tinnitus
Meningitis ■ Can follow bacteremic pneumonia, mastoiditis, sinusitis, skull fracture, or endocarditis ■ Mortality (30% to 60%) highest in infants and in elderly patients	■ Fever, headache, nuchal rigidity, vomiting, photophobia, lethargy, coma, wide pulse pressure, bradycardia

Diagnosis	Complications	Treatment and special considerations
■ Group B streptococcus is isolated from blood or infection site.	■ Bacteremia followed by meningitis or endocarditis	■ Give ampicillin or penicillin I.V. as ordered. ■ Carefully observe for symptoms of infection following delivery. ■ Take drainage and secretion precautions.
■ Gram stain of sputum shows gram-positive diplococci; culture shows *S. pneumoniae*. ■ Chest X-ray shows lobular consolidation in adults; bronchopneumonia in children and in elderly patients. ■ WBC count is elevated. ■ Blood cultures are commonly positive for *S. pneumoniae*.	■ Pleural effusion in 25% of patients ■ Pericarditis (rare) ■ Lung abscess (rare) ■ Bacteremia ■ Disseminated intravascular coagulation ■ Death, if bacteremia is present ■ Hearing loss if attacks recur	■ Give penicillin or erythromycin I.V. or I.M. as ordered. ■ Monitor and support respirations as needed. Record sputum color and amount. ■ Prevent dehydration. ■ Avoid sedatives and opioids to preserve the cough reflex. ■ Carefully dispose of all purulent drainage. (Respiratory isolation is unnecessary.) Advise high-risk patients to receive vaccine and to avoid infected persons.
■ Fluid is found in middle ear. ■ *S. pneumoniae* is isolated from aspirated fluid if necessary.	■ Persistent hearing deficits, seizures, hemiparesis, or other nerve deficits ■ Encephalitis	■ Give amoxicillin or ampicillin and analgesics as ordered. ■ Tell the patient to report a lack of response to therapy after 72 hours.
■ *S. pneumoniae* is isolated from CSF or blood culture. ■ CSF cell count and protein level are increased; CSF glucose level is decreased. ■ Computed tomography scan of head is performed. ■ EEG is performed.	■ Embolization ■ Pulmonary infarction ■ Osteomyelitis	■ Give penicillin I.V. or chloramphenicol as ordered. ■ Monitor the patient closely for neurologic changes. ■ Watch for symptoms of septic shock, such as acidosis and tissue hypoxia.

(continued) |

Comparing streptococcal infections (continued)

Causes and incidence	Signs and symptoms

Streptococcus pneumoniae (group D streptococcus)

Causes and incidence	Signs and symptoms
Endocarditis ▪ Group D streptococci (enterococci) causing 10% to 20% of all bacterial endocarditis ▪ Most common in elderly patients and in those who abuse I.V. substances ▪ Typically follows bacteremia from an obvious source, such as a wound infection or an I.V. insertion site infection ▪ Most cases subacute	▪ Weakness, fatigability, weight loss, fever, night sweats, anorexia, arthralgia, splenomegaly, new systolic murmur

Stroke

Stroke is a sudden impairment of cerebral circulation in one or more blood vessels supplying the brain. Stroke interrupts or diminishes oxygen supply and commonly causes serious damage or necrosis in brain tissues.

The sooner circulation returns to normal after a stroke, the better the chances are for complete recovery. However, about half of those who survive a stroke remain permanently disabled and experience a recurrence within weeks, months, or years.

Stroke is the third most common cause of death in the United States today and the most common cause of neurologic disability. It affects 500,000 people each year; half of them die as a result.

Strokes are classified according to their course of progression. The least severe is the transient ischemic attack (TIA), or little stroke, which results from a temporary interruption of blood flow, usually in the carotid and vertebrobasilar arteries. A progressive stroke, or stroke-in-evolution (thrombus-in-evolution), begins with slight neurologic deficit and worsens in a day or two. In a completed stroke, neurologic deficits are maximal at onset and don't progress.

Causes
▪ Embolism
▪ Hemorrhage
▪ Thrombosis

Risk factors
▪ Arrhythmias
▪ Atherosclerosis
▪ Cardiac or myocardial enlargement
▪ Cigarette smoking
▪ Diabetes mellitus
▪ Electrocardiogram changes
▪ Family history of stroke
▪ Gout
▪ High serum triglyceride level
▪ Hormonal contraceptives
▪ Hypertension
▪ Lack of exercise
▪ Orthostatic hypotension
▪ Rheumatic heart disease
▪ TIAs

Diagnosis	Complications	Treatment and special considerations
▪ Anemia, increased erythrocyte sedimentation rate and serum immunoglobulin level, and positive blood culture for group D streptococcus may be found. ▪ Echocardiogram shows vegetation on valves.	▪ Embolization ▪ Pulmonary infarction ▪ Osteomyelitis	▪ Give penicillin for *Streptococcus bovis* (nonenterococcal group D streptococci) as ordered. ▪ Give penicillin or ampicillin and an aminoglycoside for enterococcal group D streptococci as ordered.

Signs and symptoms

▪ Variable signs and symptoms, depending on the artery affected (and, consequently, the portion of the brain it supplies), severity of damage, and extent of collateral circulation that develops to help the brain compensate for decreased blood supply

▪ Left hemisphere stroke: symptoms on the right side of the body

▪ Right hemisphere stroke: symptoms on the left side of the body

▪ Stroke that causes cranial nerve damage: signs of cranial nerve dysfunction on the same side as the hemorrhage

▪ Symptoms usually classified according to the artery affected:

– middle cerebral artery: aphasia, dysphasia, visual field cuts, and hemiparesis on the affected side (more severe in the face and arm than in the leg)

– carotid artery: weakness, paralysis, numbness, sensory changes, and visual disturbances on the affected side; altered level of consciousness; bruits; headaches; aphasia; and ptosis

– vertebrobasilar artery: weakness on the affected side, numbness around the lips and mouth, visual field cuts, diplopia, poor coordination, dysphagia, slurred speech, dizziness, amnesia, and ataxia

– anterior cerebral artery: confusion, weakness and numbness (especially in the leg) on the affected side, incontinence, loss of coordination, impaired motor and sensory functions, and personality changes

– posterior cerebral arteries: visual field cuts, sensory impairment, dyslexia, coma, and cortical blindness

▪ Symptoms also classified as premonitory, generalized, or focal

– Premonitory (rare): drowsiness, dizziness, headache, and mental confusion

– Generalized: headache, vomiting, mental impairment, seizures, coma, nuchal rigidity, fever, and disorientation

– Focal (such as sensory and reflex changes): reflect the site of hemorrhage or infarction and may worsen

Diagnostic tests

- Computed tomography (CT) scan shows evidence of hemorrhagic stroke immediately but may not show evidence of thrombotic infarction for 48 to 72 hours.
- Magnetic resonance imaging may help identify ischemic or infarcted areas and cerebral swelling.
- Positron emission tomography can quantify cerebral blood flow. Single-photon emission tomography, CT perfusion, and magnetic resonance perfusion techniques report relative blood flow and are research tools.
- Ophthalmoscopy may show signs of hypertension and atherosclerotic changes in retinal arteries.
- Angiography outlines blood vessels and pinpoints atherosclerotic plaques, vessel occlusion, or the rupture site.
- EEG helps to localize the damaged area.
- Other baseline laboratory studies include urinalysis, coagulation studies, complete blood cell count, serum osmolality, and electrolyte, glucose, triglyceride, creatinine, and blood urea nitrogen levels.

Treatment

- Early medical diagnosis of the type of stroke coupled with new drug treatments can greatly reduce the long-term disability secondary to ischemia.
- Surgery performed to improve cerebral circulation for patients with thrombotic or embolic stroke includes an endarterectomy (the removal of atherosclerotic plaque from the inner arterial wall) or a microvascular bypass (the surgical anastomosis of an extracranial vessel to an intracranial vessel).
- Medications useful in treating stroke include:
  – alteplase (Activase) (recombinant tissue plasminogen activator), effective in emergency treatment of embolic stroke (See *Restoring ischemic brain tissue with alteplase.*) (Patients with embolic or thrombotic stroke who aren't candidates for alteplase [3 to 6 hours post-stroke] should receive aspirin, warfarin [Coumadin], or heparin.)
  – long-term use of aspirin or ticlopidine (Ticlid), used as antiplatelet agents to prevent recurrent stroke
  – anticoagulants (heparin, warfarin), which may be required to treat crescendo TIAs not responsive to antiplatelet drugs
  – antihypertensives, antiarrhythmics, and antidiabetics, which may be used to treat risk factors associated with recurrent stroke.

Nursing considerations
Early supportive therapy

- Frequently assess the patient's neurologic status, using the National Institutes of Health (NIH) Stroke Scale to determine deficits. (See *Using the NIH Stroke Scale,* pages 626 and 627.)
- If the patient received alteplase, monitor him for signs of hemorrhage.
- Monitor blood pressure frequently; give labetalol (Trandate) for hypertension. If labetalol is ineffective, nitroprusside may be needed for severe hypertension.
- Remember that because autoregulation is disrupted in patients with stroke, it's necessary to maintain perfusion higher than the usual blood pressure.
- Use acetaminophen (Tylenol) and hypothermia blankets to control fever.
- Maintain a patent airway and oxygenation status; intubate and ventilate the patient as needed.
- Monitor blood glucose levels.
- Monitor electrocardiogram results, and treat arrhythmias as early as possible.
- If the patient develops a headache, administer an analgesic.

Ongoing care

- Watch for signs and symptoms of pulmonary emboli, such as chest pain, shortness of breath, dusky color, tachycardia, fever, and changed sensorium. If the patient is unresponsive, monitor his blood gas levels often, looking for increased partial pressure of carbon dioxide or decreased partial pressure of arterial oxygen.
- Watch for signs of other complications, such as infection, cerebral edema, hydrocephalus, seizures, aspiration pneumonia, deep vein thrombosis, pressure ulcers, urinary tract infections, contractures, and subluxation.
- Offer the urinal or bedpan every 2 hours. If the patient is incontinent, he may need an indwelling urinary catheter, but this should be avoided, if possible, because of the risk of infection.
- Ensure adequate nutrition. Check the patient's gag reflex before offering small oral feedings of semisolid foods. (A speech pathologist should assess the patient to determine his needs and specific feeding strategies for dysphagia.) Place the food tray within the patient's visual field. If oral feedings aren't possible, insert a nasogastric tube.
- To prevent aspiration pneumonia, position the patient in an upright, lateral position to allow secretions to drain. Turn the patient frequently.
- Position the patient and align his extremities correctly to prevent external rotation. Use high-topped sneakers to prevent footdrop when the patient is sitting up and his feet are on the floor. Avoid subluxation of the affected shoulder through proper support and positioning.
- Provide range-of-motion exercises throughout the day. Consult a physical therapist for additional positioning and transfer strategies and splinting devices.

Restoring ischemic brain tissue with alteplase

The phrase *time is brain* highlights the need to treat stroke as an emergency. Brain tissue can't tolerate loss of blood supply for long. During this critical time, a thrombolytic enzyme, alteplase (Activase) (recombinant tissue plasminogen activator), can be effective in restoring blood flow.

When blood flow stops, an infarct occurs almost immediately. However, cells in the ischemic area (the penumbra, which surrounds the infarct) can maintain metabolism for 3 to 6 hours poststroke, creating a "therapeutic window." Interventions, such as alteplase, indirectly interrupt the ischemic cascade (a complex process involving protein synthesis, altered glucose use, loss of intercellular calcium, increased intracellular sodium, cellular swelling [edema], and death) to help maintain cell function and minimize the extent of permanent damage.

Research into the use of neuroprotective agents that directly protect the penumbra is under way. It appears that calcium channel blockers may also act to protect ischemic brain tissue.

- Consult a physical therapist, an occupational therapist, and a speech therapist for short- and long-term rehabilitative care goals. A multidisciplinary approach is necessary to help minimize long-term disability. Deficits can include motor weakness, coordination and balance problems, diminished corneal reflex, visual field deficits, dysarthria, dys-

(*Text continues on page 628.*)

Using the NIH Stroke Scale

Evaluate the patient's neurologic status by administering the stroke scale items in the order listed. Record his performance after each category is assessed.

Category	Description	Score	Baseline date/time score	Date/ time score
			7/15/07 1100	
1a. Level of consciousness (LOC)	Alert	0		
	Drowsy	1		
	Stuporous	2	1	
	Coma	3		
1b. LOC questions (Month, age)	Answers both correctly	0	0	
	Answers one correctly	1		
	Incorrect	2		
1c. LOC commands (Open/close eyes, make fist, let go)	Obeys both correctly	0	1	
	Obeys one correctly	1		
	Incorrect	2		
2. Best gaze (Eyes open—patient follows examiner's finger or face.)	Normal	0	0	
	Partial gaze palsy	1		
	Forced deviation	2		
3. Visual (Introduce visual stimulus/threat to patient's visual field quadrants.)	No visual loss	0	1	
	Partial hemianopia	1		
	Complete hemianopia	2		
	Bilateral hemianopia	3		
4. Facial palsy (Show teeth, raise eyebrows, and squeeze eyes shut.)	Normal	0	2	
	Minor	1		
	Partial	2		
	Complete	3		
5a. Motor arm—left (Elevate extremity to 90 degrees and score drift/movement.)	No drift	0	4	
	Drift	1		
	Can't resist gravity	2		
	No effort against gravity	3		
	No movement	4		
	Amputation, joint fusion (explain)	9		
5b. Motor arm—right (Elevate extremity to 90 degrees and score drift/movement.)	No drift	0	0	
	Drift	1		
	Can't resist gravity	2		
	No effort against gravity	3		
	No movement	4		
	Amputation, joint fusion (explain)	9		

Using the NIH Stroke Scale *(continued)*

Category	Description	Score	Baseline Date/time score	Date/ time score
6a. Motor leg—left (Elevate extremity to 30 degrees and score drift/movement.)	No drift Drift Can't resist gravity No effort against gravity No movement Amputation, joint fusion (explain)	0 1 2 3 4 9	4	
6b. Motor leg—right (Elevate extremity to 30 degrees and score drift/movement.)	No drift Drift Can't resist gravity No effort against gravity No movement Amputation, joint fusion (explain)	0 1 2 3 4 9	0	
7. Limb ataxia (Finger-nose, heel down shin)	Absent Present in one limb Present in two limbs	0 1 2	0	
8. Sensory (Pinprick to face, arm, trunk, and leg—compare side to side.)	Normal Partial loss Severe loss	0 1 2	2	
9. Best language (Name items; describe a picture and read sentences.)	No aphasia Mild to moderate aphasia Severe aphasia Mute	0 1 2 3	1	
10. Dysarthria (Evaluate speech clarity by patient repeating listed words.)	Normal articulation Mild to moderate dysarthria Near to unintelligible or worse Intubated or other physical barrier	0 1 2 9	1	
11. Extinction and inattention (Use information from previous testing to identify neglect or double simultaneous stimuli testing.)	No neglect Partial neglect Complete neglect	0 1 2	0	
		Total	17	

Individual Administering Scale: _H. Hareson, RN_

phasia, impaired memory and concentration, and pain.

- Establish and maintain communication with the patient. If he's aphasic, set up a simple method of communicating basic needs. Remember to phrase your questions so he can answer using this system. Repeat yourself quietly and calmly, and use gestures, if necessary, to help him understand. Even the unresponsive patient can hear, so don't say anything in his presence you wouldn't want him to hear and remember.
- Provide psychological support. Set realistic short-term goals. Involve the patient's family in his care when possible, and explain his deficits and strengths.
- Establish rapport with the patient. Spend time with him, and provide a means of communication. Simplify your language, asking questions that can be answered with a yes or no whenever possible. Don't correct his speech or treat him like a child. Remember that building rapport may be difficult because of mood changes that may result from brain damage or as a reaction to being dependent.
- If necessary, teach the patient to comb his hair, dress, and wash. With the aid of a physical therapist and an occupational therapist, obtain appliances, such as walking frames, hand bars for the toilet, and ramps as needed.
- If speech therapy is indicated, encourage the patient to begin as soon as possible and follow through with the speech therapist's suggestions.
- To reinforce teaching, involve the patient's family in all aspects of rehabilitation. With their cooperation and support, devise realistic discharge goals, and let them help decide when the patient can return home.
- Before discharge, warn the patient and his family to report premonitory signs or symptoms of stroke, such as severe

headache, drowsiness, confusion, and dizziness. Emphasize the importance of regular follow-up visits.

- If aspirin has been prescribed to minimize the risk of embolic stroke, tell the patient to watch for GI bleeding related to ulcer formation. Make sure that the patient realizes that he can't substitute acetaminophen for aspirin.

▌Syndrome of inappropriate antidiuretic hormone

Excessive release of antidiuretic hormone (ADH) disturbs fluid and electrolyte balance in syndrome of inappropriate antidiuretic hormone secretion (SIADH). The excessive ADH causes an inability to excrete dilute urine, retention of free water, expansion of extracellular fluid volume, and hyponatremia.

SIADH occurs secondary to diseases that affect the osmoreceptors (supraoptic nucleus) of the hypothalamus. The prognosis depends on the underlying disorder and response to treatment.

Causes

- Central nervous system disorders: brain tumor or abscess, stroke, head injury, and Guillain-Barré syndrome
- Drugs: chlorpropamide (Diabinese), vincristine, cyclophosphamide (Cytoxan), carbamazepine (Tegretol), metoclopramide (Reglan), and morphine
- Miscellaneous conditions: psychosis and myxedema
- Neoplastic diseases, such as pancreatic and prostatic cancer, Hodgkin's disease, and thymoma
- Pulmonary disorders: pneumonia, tuberculosis, lung abscess, positive-pressure ventilation, and small cell carcinoma of the lung

Signs and symptoms
- Edema (rare)
- Muscle weakness
- Seizures and coma (possibly)
- Restlessness
- Weight gain despite anorexia, nausea, and vomiting

Diagnostic tests
- Serum osmolality is less than 280 mOsm/kg of water, and serum sodium level is less than 123 mEq/L.
- Urine osmolality is greater than plasma osmolality.
- Urine sodium secretion is high (more than 20 mEq/L), without diuretics.
- Renal function test results are normal, with no evidence of dehydration.

Treatment
- Symptomatic treatment begins with restricted water intake (500 to 1,000 ml/day).
- With severe water intoxication, administration of 200 to 300 ml of 3% to 5% saline solution may be necessary to raise the serum sodium level.
- When possible, treatment should include correction of the underlying cause of SIADH.
- If SIADH results from cancer, success in alleviating water retention may be obtained by surgical resection, irradiation, or chemotherapy.
- If fluid restriction is ineffective, demeclocycline (Declomycin) may be helpful by blocking the renal response to ADH.

Nursing considerations
- Closely monitor and record intake and output, vital signs, and daily weight. Watch the patient's serum sodium level.
- Observe for restlessness, irritability, seizures, heart failure, and unresponsiveness resulting from hyponatremia and water intoxication.

- To prevent water intoxication, explain to the patient and his family why he must restrict his intake.

Syphilis

A chronic, infectious, sexually transmitted disease, syphilis begins in the mucous membranes as chancres (small, fluid-filled lesions) and quickly becomes systemic, spreading to nearby lymph nodes and the bloodstream. This disease, when untreated, is characterized by progressive stages: primary, secondary, latent, and late (formerly called *tertiary*).

The primary and secondary stages of syphilis have a high incidence among urban populations, especially in people ages 15 to 39, drug users, and those infected with the human immunodeficiency virus (HIV).

Untreated syphilis leads to crippling or death, but the prognosis is excellent with early treatment.

Causes
- Infection with the spirochete *Treponema pallidum*
- Transmission through sexual contact during the primary, secondary, and early latent stages of infection
- Prenatal transmission from an infected mother to her fetus (see *Prenatal syphilis,* page 630)

Signs and symptoms
Primary syphilis (after 3-week incubation period)
- One or more painless chancres, which erupt on the genitalia or anus, fingers, lips, tongue, nipples, tonsils, or eyelids; starting as papules and then eroding; with indurated raised edges and clear bases

Prenatal syphilis

A woman can transmit syphilis transplacentally to her unborn child throughout pregnancy. This type of syphilis is commonly called *congenital,* but prenatal is a more accurate term. Approximately 50% of infected fetuses die before or shortly after birth. The prognosis is better for those who develop overt infection after age 2.

Signs and symptoms

The neonate with prenatal syphilis may appear healthy at birth but usually develops characteristic lesions—vesicular, bullous eruptions, usually on the palms and soles—weeks later. Shortly afterward, a maculopapular rash similar to that in secondary syphilis may erupt on the face, mouth, genitalia, palms, or soles. Condylomata lata commonly occur around the anus.

Lesions may erupt on the mucous membranes of the mouth, pharynx, and nose. When the infant's larynx is affected, his cry becomes weak and forced. If the nasal mucous membranes are involved, he may also develop nasal discharge, which can be slight and mucopurulent or copious with blood-tinged pus.

Visceral and bone lesions, liver or spleen enlargement with ascites, and nephrotic syndrome may also develop.

Late prenatal syphilis becomes apparent after age 2; it may be identifiable through blood studies or may cause unmistakable syphilitic changes: screwdriver-shaped central incisors, deformed molars or cusps, thick clavicles, saber shins, bowed tibias, nasal septum perforation, eighth cranial nerve deafness, and neurosyphilis.

Diagnosis

In the neonate with prenatal syphilis, Venereal Disease Research Laboratory titer, if reactive at birth, stays the same or rises, indicating active disease. The infant's titer drops in 3 months if the mother has received effective prenatal treatment. An absolute diagnosis necessitates a dark-field examination of umbilical vein blood or lesion drainage.

Treatment

An infant with abnormal cerebrospinal fluid (CSF) may be treated with I.M. or I.V. aqueous crystalline penicillin G or I.M. aqueous penicillin G procaine. An infant with normal CSF may be treated with a single injection of penicillin G benzathine.

When caring for a child with prenatal syphilis, record the extent of the rash, and watch for signs of systemic involvement, especially laryngeal swelling, jaundice, and decreasing urine output.

■ Chancres commonly overlooked in women because they develop internally on cervix or vagina
■ Disappearance of chancres after 3 to 6 weeks, even when untreated
■ Regional lymphadenopathy (unilateral or bilateral)

Secondary syphilis

■ Development of symmetrical mucocutaneous lesions and general lymphataneous lesions and general lymphadenopathy within a few days or up to 8 weeks after the onset of initial chancres
■ Rash: macular, papular, pustular, or nodular; lesions of uniform size, well defined, and generalized
■ Macules: usually erupt in moist warm areas (perineum, scrotum, vulva, or between rolls of fat on the trunk) as well as on the arms, palms, soles, face, and scalp and then enlarge and erode, pro-

ducing highly contagious, pink or gray-ish white lesions (condylomata lata)
- Clearing of rash without treatment
- Mild constitutional symptoms: headache, malaise, anorexia, weight loss, nausea, vomiting, sore throat and, possibly, slight fever
- Alopecia possible, with or without treatment; usually temporary
- Brittle, pitted nails

Latent syphilis
- Renders body capable of producing a reactive serologic test result for syphilis
- No signs or symptoms in early latent stage
- Early latent stage considered conta-gious because infectious lesions may reappear for up to first 4 years
- No signs or symptoms from late latent stage until death in about two-thirds of patients (late-stage symptoms occur in the rest)

Late syphilis
- Final, destructive, but noninfectious stage of the disease: has three subtypes, any or all of which may affect the pa-tient: late benign syphilis, cardiovascular syphilis, and neurosyphilis
- Lesions of late benign syphilis (called *gummas*):
  – solitary chronic, superficial nodules or deep, granulomatous lesions; asym-metrical, painless, and indurated
  – developing 1 to 10 years after infec-tion
  – may appear on the skin, bones (espe-cially leg bones), mucous membranes, upper respiratory tract, and organs
  – in liver, may cause epigastric pain, tenderness, enlarged spleen, and ane-mia
  – in upper respiratory tract, may cause perforation of the nasal septum or the palate

– in severe cases, may destroy bones or organs, eventually resulting in death
- Cardiovascular syphilis:
  – developing about 10 years after the initial infection in about 10% of pa-tients with late, untreated syphilis
  – causing fibrosis of elastic tissue of the aorta and leads to aortitis; most com-mon in the ascending and transverse sections of the aortic arch
  – may be asymptomatic or may cause aortic regurgitation or aneurysm
- Neurosyphilis:
  – developing in about 8% of patients with late, untreated syphilis and ap-pearing 5 to 35 years after infection
  – causing meningitis and widespread central nervous system damage that may include general paresis, personali-ty changes, and arm and leg weakness

Diagnostic tests
- Identifying *T. pallidum* from a lesion on a dark-field examination provides im-mediate diagnosis of syphilis. This method is most effective when moist le-sions are present, such as in primary, secondary, and prenatal syphilis.
- The fluorescent treponemal antibody-absorption test identifies antigens of *T. pallidum* tissue, ocular fluid, cere-brospinal fluid (CSF), tracheobronchial secretions, and exudate from lesions. This is the most sensitive test available for detecting syphilis in all stages. After the result becomes reactive, it remains so permanently.
- Other appropriate procedures include:
  – Venereal Disease Research Laboratory (VDRL) slide test and rapid plasma reagin test detect nonspecific antibod-ies. Both tests, if positive, become re-active within 1 to 2 weeks after the primary lesion appears or 4 to 5 weeks after the infection begins.
  – CSF examination identifies neuro-syphilis when the total protein level is

above 40 mg/dl, VDRL slide test is reactive, and CSF cell count exceeds 5 mononuclear cells/mm^3.

Treatment
- Administration of penicillin I.M. is the treatment of choice.
- For early syphilis, treatment may consist of a single injection of penicillin G benzathine I.M.
- Syphilis of more than 1 year's duration should be treated with penicillin G benzathine I.M.
- Nonpregnant patients who are allergic to penicillin may be treated with oral tetracycline or doxycycline (Vibramycin) for 15 days for early syphilis and for 30 days for late infections. Tetracycline is contraindicated in pregnant women.
- Nonpenicillin therapy for latent or late syphilis should be used only after neurosyphilis has been excluded.
- Patients who receive treatment must abstain from sexual contact until the syphilis sores are completely healed.
- Rashes from secondary syphilis will clear up without treatment.

Nursing considerations
- Stress the importance of completing the course of therapy even after symptoms subside. Instruct those infected to inform their partners that they should be tested and, if necessary, treated.
- Check for a history of drug sensitivity before administering the first dose.
- Practice standard precautions.
- In secondary syphilis, keep lesions clean and dry. If they're draining, dispose of contaminated materials properly.
- In late syphilis, provide symptomatic care during prolonged treatment.
- In cardiovascular syphilis, check for signs of decreased cardiac output (decreased urine output, hypoxia, and decreased sensorium) and pulmonary congestion.

- In neurosyphilis, regularly check the patient's level of consciousness, mood, and coherence. Watch for signs of ataxia.
- Urge patients to seek VDRL testing after 3, 6, 12, and 24 months to detect possible relapse. Patients treated for latent or late syphilis should receive blood tests at 6-month intervals for 2 years.
- Be sure to report all cases of syphilis to local public health authorities. Urge the patient to inform sexual partners of his infection so that they can receive treatment also.
- Refer the patient and his sexual partners for HIV testing.

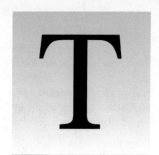

Tay-Sachs disease

Tay-Sachs disease, also known as *GM₂ gangliosidosis,* is the most common of the lipid storage diseases; it strikes people of Eastern European Jewish (Ashkenazi) ancestry about 100 times more often than the general population. It results from a congenital deficiency of the enzyme hexosaminidase A, which is necessary for metabolism of gangliosides, water-soluble glycolipids found primarily in central nervous system (CNS) tissues. Without hexosaminidase A, accumulating lipid pigments distend and progressively destroy and demyelinate CNS cells. Tay-Sachs disease is characterized by progressive mental and motor deterioration and is usually fatal before age 5, although some with hexosaminidase A deficiency have lived to adolescence and adulthood.

Causes
- Autosomal recessive disorder (enzyme hexosaminidase A deficiency)

Signs and symptoms
- Apathy
- Ataxia
- Blindness
- Deafness
- Decerebrate rigidity
- Difficulty turning over
- Exaggerated Moro reflex in the neonate
- Generalized paralysis
- Inability to grasp objects
- Inability to sit up or lift head
- Neck, trunk, arm, and leg muscle weakness
- Progressive motor retardation
- Progressive vision loss
- Pupils dilated and unresponsive to light
- Recurrent bronchopneumonia after age 2
- Response only to loud sounds
- Seizures
- Spasticity

Diagnostic tests
- Serum analysis shows deficient hexosaminidase A levels.
- Ophthalmologic examination shows optic nerve atrophy and a distinctive cherry-red spot on the retina that supports the diagnosis. (The cherry-red spot may be absent in the juvenile form.)
- A blood test evaluating hexosaminidase A levels can identify carriers.
- Amniocentesis or chorionic villus sampling can detect hexosaminidase A deficiency in the fetus.

Treatment
- Nutritional supplements may be given by tube feedings.
- Suctioning and postural drainage are used to remove pharyngeal secretions.
- Skin care helps prevent pressure ulcers in bedridden children.
- Mild laxatives relieve neurogenic constipation.
- Anticonvulsants usually fail to prevent seizures.

Nursing considerations
- If the parents care for their child at home, teach them how to do suctioning, postural drainage, and tube feeding. Also teach them how to provide good skin care to prevent pressure ulcers.
- Consult with social services to assist the family with care or placement of the child.
- Because the parents of an affected child may feel excessive stress or guilt because of the child's illness and the emotional and financial burden it places on them, refer them for psychological counseling, if indicated.
- Refer the parents for genetic counseling, and stress the importance of amniocentesis in future pregnancies. Refer siblings for screening to determine whether they're carriers. If they are carriers and are adults, refer them for genetic counseling, but stress that both parents must be carriers to transmit the disease to their offspring.
- For more information on this disease, refer parents to the National Tay-Sachs and Allied Diseases Association.

▌Tendinitis and bursitis

A painful inflammation of tendons and of tendon-muscle attachments to bone, tendinitis usually occurs in the shoulder rotator cuff, hip, Achilles tendon, or hamstring. Bursitis is a painful inflammation of one or more of the bursae—closed sacs that are lubricated with small amounts of synovial fluid that facilitate the motion of muscles and tendons over bony prominences. Bursitis usually occurs in the subdeltoid, olecranon, trochanteric, calcaneal, or prepatellar bursae.

Causes
Bursitis
- Musculoskeletal disease (rheumatoid arthritis, gout)
- Recurring trauma

Chronic bursitis
- Attacks of acute bursitis
- Infection
- Repeated trauma

Septic bursitis
- Bacterial invasion of skin over the bursa
- Wound infection

Tendinitis
- Abnormal body development
- Hypermobility
- Musculoskeletal disorder (rheumatic diseases, congenital defects)
- Postural misalignment
- Trauma such as strain during sports activity

Signs and symptoms
Bursitis
- Inflammation
- Irritation
- Limited movement
- Sudden or gradual pain
- Symptoms variable with site

Hip bursitis
- Pain when crossing the legs

Prepatellar bursitis (housemaid's knee)

- Pain when climbing stairs

Subdeltoid bursitis

- Impaired arm abduction

Tendinitis

- Localized pain, severe at night
- Pain (from acromion to deltoid muscle insertion) with abduction (50 and 130 degrees)
- Proximal weakness
- Restricted shoulder movement, especially abduction
- Shoulder pain aggravated by heat
- Swelling

Diagnostic tests

- X-rays may be normal at first in tendinitis but later show bony fragments, osteophyte sclerosis, or calcium deposits.
- Computed tomography scan and magnetic resonance imaging (MRI) have replaced X-ray and even arthrography of the shoulder as diagnostic tools. An MRI will usually identify tears, partial tears, inflammation, or tumor but can't reveal irregularities of the tendon sheath itself. Arthrography is usually normal in tendinitis, with occasional small irregularities on the undersurface of the tendon.
- Arthrocentesis detects microorganisms and other causes of inflammation if joint infection is suspected.
- Localized pain and inflammation and a history of unusual strain or injury 2 to 3 days before onset of pain are the bases for diagnosing bursitis. During early stages, X-rays are usually normal, except in calcific bursitis, in which X-rays may show calcium deposits.

Treatment

- Rest the joint by immobilization with a sling, splint, or cast.

- Administer systemic analgesics.
- Apply cold or heat.
- A mixture of a corticosteroid and an anesthetic, such as lidocaine, generally provides immediate pain relief. Extended-release injections of a corticosteroid, such as triamcinolone or prednisolone, offer longer pain relief.
- Treatment also includes oral anti-inflammatories.
- Fluid removal by aspiration may be indicated.
- Physical therapy is used to preserve motion and prevent frozen joints (improvement usually follows in 1 to 4 weeks).
- For calcific tendinitis, apply ice packs; rarely, surgical removal of calcium deposits is necessary.
- Long-term control of chronic bursitis and tendinitis may require changes in lifestyle to prevent recurring joint irritation.

Nursing considerations

- Assess the severity of pain and the range of motion to determine the treatment's effectiveness.
- Before injecting corticosteroids or local anesthetics, ask the patient about drug allergies.

DO'S & DON'TS

 Before intra-articular injection, scrub the patient's skin thoroughly with povidone-iodine or a comparable solution, and shave the injection site, if necessary. After the injection, massage the area to ensure penetration through the tissue and joint space. Apply ice intermittently for about 4 hours to minimize pain. Avoid applying heat to the area for 2 days.

- Provide patient teaching as indicated. (See *Tendinitis and bursitis tips,* page 636.)

Testicular cancer

Malignant testicular tumors primarily affect young to middle-age men; they are the most common solid tumor in this age-group. Lifetime risk of testicular cancer is about 1 in 300. (In children, testicular tumors are rare.) Most testicular tumors originate in gonadal cells. About 40% are seminomas—uniform, undifferentiated cells resembling primitive gonadal cells. The rest are nonseminomas—tumor cells showing various degrees of differentiation. Testicular cancer accounts for less than 1% of all male cancer deaths. Testicular cancer spreads through the lymphatic system to the para-aortic, iliac, and mediastinal lymph nodes and may metastasize to the lungs, liver, viscera, and bone. The prognosis varies with the cell type and disease stage. When treated with surgery and radiation, almost all patients with localized disease survive beyond 5 years.

Causes
■ Unknown

Predisposing factors
■ Cryptorchidism (even when surgically corrected)
■ Exposure to certain chemicals
■ Family history of testicular cancer
■ Infection with human immunodeficiency virus
■ Mother's use of diethylstilbestrol during pregnancy

Signs and symptoms
■ Abdominal mass
■ Cough
■ Fatigue
■ Firm, painless, smooth testicular mass
■ Gynecomastia
■ Hemoptysis
■ Lethargy
■ Nipple tenderness
■ Pallor
■ Sense of testicular heaviness
■ Shortness of breath
■ Ureteral obstruction
■ Weight loss

Diagnostic tests
■ Mass may be detected during self-examination or testicular palpation during a routine physical examination.
■ Transillumination can distinguish a tumor (which doesn't transilluminate) from a hydrocele or spermatocele (which does).
■ Excretory urography detects ureteral deviation resulting from para-aortic lymph node involvement.
■ Computed tomography scanning can detect metastases, as can lymphangiography, ultrasonography, and magnetic resonance imaging.

- Serum alpha-fetoprotein and beta-human chorionic gonadotropin levels, indicators of testicular tumor activity, provide a baseline for measuring response to therapy and determining the prognosis.
- Surgical excision and biopsy of the tumor and testis permits histologic verification of the tumor cell type—essential for effective treatment. Inguinal exploration determines the extent of nodal involvement.

Treatment
- Surgical procedures include orchiectomy and retroperitoneal node dissection. Most surgeons remove just the testis, not the scrotum (to allow for a prosthetic implant). Hormone replacement therapy may be needed after bilateral orchiectomy.
- The retroperitoneal and homolateral iliac nodes may receive radiation after removal of a seminoma. All positive nodes receive radiation after removal of a nonseminoma. Patients with retroperitoneal extension receive prophylactic radiation to the mediastinal and supraclavicular nodes.
- Chemotherapy is most effective for late-stage seminomas and most nonseminomas when used for recurrent cancer after orchiectomy and removal of the retroperitoneal lymph nodes.
- Chemotherapy (high-dose) and radiation followed by autologous bone marrow transplantation may help unresponsive patients.

Nursing considerations
- Develop a treatment plan that addresses the patient's psychological and physical needs.

Before orchiectomy
- Reassure the patient that sterility and impotence need not follow unilateral or-

chiectomy, that synthetic hormones can restore hormonal balance, and that most surgeons don't remove the scrotum. In many cases, a testicular prosthesis can correct anatomic disfigurement.

After orchiectomy
- For the first day after surgery, apply an ice pack to the scrotum and provide analgesics.
- Check for excessive bleeding, swelling, and signs of infection.
- Provide a scrotal athletic supporter to minimize pain during ambulation.

During chemotherapy
- Give antiemetics, as needed, for nausea and vomiting. Encourage small, frequent meals to maintain oral intake despite anorexia due to chemotherapy.
- Establish a mouth care regimen and check for stomatitis. Watch for signs of myelosuppression.

DRUG CHALLENGE

 If the patient receives vinblastine, assess for signs and symptoms of neurotoxicity (peripheral paresthesia, jaw pain, and muscle cramps). If he receives cisplatin (Platinol-AQ), check for ototoxicity.

▌Tetanus

Tetanus, also known as *lockjaw*, is an acute exotoxin-mediated infection caused by the anaerobic, spore-forming, gram-positive bacillus *Clostridium tetani*. Usually, such infection is systemic; less commonly, it's localized. Tetanus is fatal in up to 60% of nonimmunized people, usually within 10 days of onset. Complications include atelectasis, pneumonia, pulmonary emboli, acute gastric ulcers, flexion contractures, and cardiac arrhythmias. When symptoms develop within 3 days after exposure, the prognosis is poor. After *C. tetani* enters the body, it causes local infection and tissue necrosis. It produces toxins that spread to central nervous system tissue. Tetanus occurs worldwide, but it's more prevalent in agricultural regions and developing countries. It's one of the most common causes of neonatal deaths in developing countries, where neonates of unimmunized mothers are delivered under nonsterile conditions. In such neonates, the unhealed umbilical cord is the portal of entry.

Causes
- Burns
- Minor wounds
- Puncture wound contaminated by soil, dust, or animal excreta containing *C. tetani*

Signs and symptoms
Generalized (systemic)
- Arched-back rigidity (opisthotonos)
- Boardlike abdominal rigidity
- Cyanosis with convulsions
- Grotesque, grinning expression called risus sardonicus
- Hyperactive deep tendon reflexes
- Intermittent tonic convulsions
- Locked jaw (trismus)
- Low-grade fever
- Marked muscle hypertonicity
- Painful, involuntary muscle contractions
- Profuse sweating
- Sudden death by asphyxiation
- Tachycardia

Neonatal
- Excessive crying
- Irritability
- Nuchal rigidity
- Poor sucking at 3 to 10 days after birth
- Progression to total inability to suck

Diagnostic tests
- Diagnosis frequently rests on clinical features and a history of trauma and no previous tetanus immunization.
- Blood cultures and tetanus antibody tests are commonly negative.
- One-third of patients have a positive wound culture.
- Cerebrospinal fluid pressure may rise above normal.

Treatment
- Within 72 hours after a puncture wound, a patient with no previous history of tetanus immunization first requires tetanus immune globulin (TIG) or tetanus antitoxin to confer temporary protection.
- Active immunization with tetanus toxoid is required. (A patient who hasn't received tetanus immunization within 10 years needs a booster injection of tetanus toxoid.)
- Debridement ensures that the source of the toxin has been removed.
- Airway maintenance is started as necessary.
- Muscle relaxants, such as diazepam (Valium), decrease muscle rigidity and spasm. A neuromuscular blocker may be needed, if muscle relaxants don't relieve muscle contractions.
- The patient with tetanus also requires high-dose antibiotics (penicillin I.V. or an alternative).

Nursing considerations
For the patient with a puncture wound
- Thoroughly clean the injury site with 3% hydrogen peroxide, and check the patient's immunization history. Record the cause of injury. If it's a dog bite, report the case to local public health authorities.
- Before giving penicillin and TIG, antitoxin, or toxoid, obtain an accurate his-

tory of allergies to immunizations or penicillin. If the patient has a history of allergies, keep epinephrine 1:1,000 and resuscitative equipment available.
■ Stress the importance of maintaining active immunization with a booster dose of tetanus toxoid every 10 years.

After tetanus develops
ACTION STAT!

 Maintain an adequate airway and ventilation. Suction often and watch for signs of respiratory distress. Keep emergency airway equipment on hand because the patient may require artificial ventilation or oxygen administration. Insert an artificial airway, if necessary, to prevent tongue injury and maintain the airway during spasms.

■ Maintain an I.V. line for medications and emergency care if necessary.
■ Monitor electrocardiography frequently for arrhythmias. Accurately record intake and output, and check the patient's vital signs often.
■ Turn the patient frequently to prevent pressure sores and pulmonary stasis.
■ Because even minimal external stimulation provokes muscle spasms, keep the patient's room dark and quiet. Warn visitors not to upset or overly stimulate the patient.
■ If urinary retention develops, insert an indwelling urinary catheter.
■ Give muscle relaxants and sedatives, as ordered, and schedule patient care to coincide with heaviest sedation.
■ Provide adequate nutrition to meet the patient's increased metabolic needs; provide nasogastric feedings or total parenteral nutrition, as ordered.

▌Thrombocytopenia

The most common cause of hemorrhagic disorders, thrombocytopenia is characterized by a deficiency of circulating platelets. Because platelets play a vital role in coagulation, this disease poses a serious threat to hemostasis. The prognosis is excellent in drug-induced thrombocytopenia if the offending drug is withdrawn; in such cases, recovery may be immediate. Otherwise, the prognosis depends on response to treatment of the underlying cause. (See *Precautions in thrombocytopenia,* page 640.)

Causes
■ Acquired or congenital
■ Decreased or defective production of platelets in the marrow (such as occurs in leukemia, aplastic anemia, or toxicity with certain drugs)
■ Drugs (nonsteroidal anti-inflammatory agents, sulfonamides, histamine blockers, alkylating agents, heparin, alcohol, or antibiotic chemotherapeutic agents)
■ Idiopathic
■ Increased destruction outside the marrow caused by an underlying disorder (such as cirrhosis of the liver, disseminated intravascular coagulation, or severe infection)
■ Platelet loss
■ Sequestration (hypersplenism, hypothermia)
■ Transient form possibly following viral infections (Epstein-Barr virus or infectious mononucleosis)

Signs and symptoms
■ Abrupt onset of petechiae or ecchymoses in the skin
■ Bleeding into any mucous membrane
■ Hemorrhage
■ Large blood-filled bullae in the mouth
■ Loss of consciousness
■ Malaise, fatigue, weakness

DO'S & DON'TS

Precautions in thrombocytopenia

Do's

■ If the patient must receive long-term steroid therapy, teach him to watch for and report cushingoid symptoms (acne, moon face, hirsutism, buffalo hump, hypertension, girdle obesity, thinning arms and legs, glycosuria, and edema). Emphasize that steroid doses must be discontinued gradually.

■ Teach the patient to recognize and report signs and symptoms of bleeding, such as tarry stools, coffee-ground vomitus, epistaxis, menorrhagia, and gingival or urinary tract bleeding.

Don'ts

■ Warn the patient to avoid all forms of aspirin and other drugs that impair coagulation. Teach him how to recognize aspirin or ibuprofen compounds on labels of over-the-counter remedies.

■ Advise the patient to avoid straining while defecating or coughing because both can lead to increased intracranial pressure, possibly causing cerebral hemorrhage in the patient with thrombocytopenia. Provide a stool softener to prevent constipation.

■ If thrombocytopenia is drug-induced, stress the importance of avoiding the offending drug.

■ Shortness of breath
■ Tachycardia

Diagnostic tests

■ Coagulation tests reveal a decreased platelet count (in adults, < 100,000/mm^3), prolonged bleeding time, and normal prothrombin time and partial thromboplastin time. Platelet-associated antibodies may be present.

■ If increased destruction of platelets is causing thrombocytopenia, bone marrow studies will reveal a greater number of megakaryocytes (platelet precursors) and shortened platelet survival (several hours or days rather than the usual 7 to 10 days).

Treatment

■ Give corticosteroids or immune globulin to increase platelet production.
■ Correct the underlying cause.
■ Remove the offending agents in drug-induced thrombocytopenia.
■ Platelet transfusions are helpful in treating complications of severe hemor-

rhage and may be used to stop episodic abnormal bleeding.
■ Splenectomy is necessary when the cause is platelet destruction.

Nursing considerations

■ Protect the patient from trauma. Keep the side rails up, and pad them if possible. Promote the use of an electric razor and a soft toothbrush. Avoid invasive procedures, such as venipuncture or urinary catheterization, if possible. When venipuncture is unavoidable, be sure to exert pressure on the puncture site for at least 20 minutes or until the bleeding stops.

■ Monitor platelet count as ordered; 1- to 2-hour post–platelet transfusion count may be done to assess response.

■ Test stool for guaiac, and urine and emesis for blood.

■ Watch for bleeding (petechiae, ecchymoses, surgical or GI bleeding, and menorrhagia).

- During periods of active bleeding, keep the patient on strict bed rest, if necessary.
- When administering platelet concentrate, remember that platelets are extremely fragile, so infuse them quickly. Don't give platelets to a patient with a fever, because fever destroys blood products.

DO'S & DON'TS

 During platelet transfusion, monitor the patient for a febrile reaction (flushing, chills, fever, headache, tachycardia, hypertension). Human leukocyte antigen–typed platelets may prevent a febrile reaction.

DRUG CHALLENGE

 A patient with a history of minor reactions may benefit from acetaminophen (Tylenol) and diphenhydramine (Benadryl) before platelet transfusion. During steroid therapy, monitor fluid and electrolyte balance, and watch for infection, pathologic fractures, and mood changes.

Thrombophlebitis

An acute condition characterized by inflammation and thrombus formation, thrombophlebitis may occur in deep (intermuscular or intramuscular) or superficial (subcutaneous) veins. Deep vein thrombophlebitis (DVT) affects small veins and is frequently progressive, leading to pulmonary embolism, a potentially lethal complication. Superficial thrombophlebitis is usually self-limiting and rarely leads to pulmonary embolism. Thrombophlebitis commonly begins with localized inflammation alone (phlebitis), but such inflammation rapidly provokes thrombus formation.

Rarely, venous thrombosis develops without associated inflammation of the vein (phlebothrombosis).

Causes
Deep vein thrombophlebitis
- Accelerated blood clotting
- Endothelial damage
- Idiopathic
- Reduced blood flow

Predisposing factors
- Childbirth
- Hormonal contraceptives (estrogens)
- Prolonged bed rest
- Surgery
- Trauma

Superficial thrombophlebitis
- Chemical irritation (extensive use of I.V. route for medications and diagnostic tests)
- Infection
- I.V. drug abuse
- Trauma

Signs and symptoms
Deep vein thrombophlebitis
- Chills
- Fever
- Malaise
- Positive Homans' sign (pain on dorsiflexion of the foot)
- Severe pain
- Swelling and cyanosis of the affected arm or leg

Superficial thrombophlebitis
- Heat
- Induration along the length of the affected vein
- Lymphadenitis with extensive involvement
- Pain
- Rubor
- Swelling
- Tenderness

Diagnostic tests

- Doppler ultrasonography is used to identify reduced blood flow to a specific area and any obstruction to venous flow, particularly in iliofemoral DVT.
- Plethysmography shows decreased circulation distal to the affected area; it's more sensitive than ultrasonography in detecting DVT.
- Phlebography can show filling defects and diverted blood flow and usually confirms the diagnosis.
- Elevated D-dimer results indicate an abnormally high level of fibrin degradation products, reflective of significant clot formation and breakdown in the body; however, it doesn't reveal location or cause.
- Diagnosis of superficial thrombophlebitis is based on physical examination (redness and warmth over the affected area, a palpable vein, and pain during palpation or compression).

Treatment

- Symptomatic measures include bed rest, with elevation of the affected arm or leg; warm, moist soaks to the affected area; and analgesics.

Deep vein thrombophlebitis

- Antiembolism stockings are applied before the patient gets out of bed (after the acute episode subsides).
- Anticoagulants (initially, heparin; later, warfarin [Coumadin]) prolong clotting time.

DRUG CHALLENGE

 The full anticoagulant dose must be discontinued during any operative period because of the risk of hemorrhage. After some types of surgery, especially major abdominal or pelvic operations, prophylactic doses of anticoagulants may reduce the risk of DVT and pulmonary embolism.

- For lysis of acute, extensive deep vein thrombosis, treatment should include streptokinase (Streptase) or urokinase (Abbokinase).
- In complete venous occlusion, ligation, vein plication, or clipping may be done.
- Embolectomy and insertion of a vena caval umbrella or filter may also be done.

Superficial thrombophlebitis

- Medications may include an anti-inflammatory such as indomethacin (Indocin), aspirin, or ibuprofen (Motrin).
- Application of antiembolism stockings, warm compresses, and elevation of the patient's leg may be beneficial.

Nursing considerations

- Enforce bed rest, and elevate the patient's affected arm or leg. If you plan to use pillows for elevating the leg, place them so they support the entire length of the affected leg to prevent possible compression of the popliteal space.
- Apply warm soaks to increase circulation to the affected area and to relieve pain and inflammation. Give analgesics to relieve pain.
- Measure and record the circumference of the affected arm or leg daily, and compare this measurement to the other arm or leg. To ensure accuracy and consistency of serial measurements, mark the skin over the area and measure at the same spot daily.
- Administer heparin I.V. with an infusion monitor or pump to control the flow rate if necessary. Measure partial thromboplastin time regularly for the patient receiving heparin therapy, and prothrombin time and International

Normalized Ratio (INR) for the patient receiving warfarin (therapeutic anticoagulation values for both are 1½ to 2 times control values, and INR is 2 to 3 times control values).

Drug challenge

 Watch for signs and symptoms of bleeding, such as coffee-ground vomitus, ecchymoses, and black, tarry stools. Encourage the patient to use an electric razor and to avoid medications that contain aspirin unless prescribed.

- Stay alert for signs of pulmonary embolism (crackles, dyspnea, hemoptysis, sudden changes in mental status, restlessness, and hypotension).
- Emphasize the importance of follow-up blood studies to monitor anticoagulant therapy.
- If the patient is being discharged on heparin therapy, teach him or his family how to give subcutaneous injections. If he requires further assistance, arrange for a visiting nurse.
- Tell the patient to avoid prolonged sitting or standing to help prevent recurrence.
- Teach the patient how to properly apply and use antiembolism stockings. Tell him to report complications such as cold, blue toes.
- To prevent thrombophlebitis in the high-risk patient, perform range-of-motion exercises while he's on bed rest, use intermittent pneumatic calf massage during lengthy surgical or diagnostic procedures, apply antiembolism stockings postoperatively, and encourage early ambulation.

▌Thyroid cancer

Thyroid cancer occurs in all age-groups, especially in people who have had radia-tion treatment to the neck area. Papillary and follicular carcinomas are most common and are usually associated with prolonged survival. Papillary carcinoma metastasizes slowly. Follicular carcinoma is less common but more likely to recur and metastasize to the regional nodes and through blood vessels into the bones, liver, and lungs. Medullary carcinoma originates in the parafollicular cells derived from the last branchial pouch and contains amyloid and calcium deposits. It can produce calcitonin, histaminase, corticotropin (producing Cushing's syndrome), and prostaglandin E_2 and F_3 (producing diarrhea). This rare form of thyroid cancer is familial, associated with pheochromocytoma, and completely curable when detected before it causes symptoms. Untreated, it progresses rapidly. Seldom curable by resection, giant and spindle cell cancer (anaplastic tumor) resists radiation and metastasizes rapidly.

Causes
- Genetic—medullary thyroid carcinoma (possibly)

Predisposing factors
- Chronic goiter
- Familial predisposition
- Prolonged thyrotropin stimulation (through radiation or heredity)
- Radiation exposure

Signs and symptoms
- Anorexia
- Diarrhea
- Dysphagia
- Dyspnea
- Hard nodule in an enlarged thyroid gland
- Hoarseness
- Hypothyroidism (low metabolism, mental apathy, and sensitivity to cold)
- Irritability

- Pain on palpation
- Painless nodule
- Palpable lymph nodes with thyroid enlargement
- Symptoms of distant metastasis
- Thyrotoxicosis (sensitivity to heat, restlessness, and hyperactivity)
- Vocal cord paralysis

Diagnostic tests

- The first clue to thyroid cancer is usually an enlarged, palpable node in the thyroid gland, neck, lymph nodes of the neck, or vocal cords.
- Fine needle biopsy detects cancer cells.
- Thyroid scan differentiates functional nodes (rarely malignant) from hypofunctional nodes (commonly malignant); in thyroid cancer, the scintiscan shows a "cold," nonfunctioning nodule.
- Computed tomography scan, ultrasonography, and serum calcitonin assay diagnose medullary cancer. Calcitonin assay is a reliable clue to silent medullary carcinoma.

Treatment

- Treatment may include one or a combination of the following:
  - Total or subtotal thyroidectomy, with modified node dissection (bilateral or homolateral) is performed on the side of the primary cancer (papillary or follicular cancer)
  - Total thyroidectomy and radical neck excision (for medullary or anaplastic cancer)
  - Radioisotope (^{131}I) therapy with external radiation or alone
  - Adjunctive thyroid suppression, with exogenous thyroid hormones suppressing thyrotropin production, and simultaneous administration of a beta-adrenergic blocker such as propranolol

(Inderal), which increases the patient's tolerance of surgery and radiation
  - Chemotherapy using doxorubicin (Rubex) for symptomatic, widespread metastasis

Nursing considerations

- Before surgery, tell the patient to expect temporary voice loss or hoarseness lasting several days after surgery.
- The patient will most likely require thyroid hormone replacement therapy after surgery.

Postoperative care

- When the patient regains consciousness, keep him in semi-Fowler's position, with his head neither hyperextended nor flexed, to avoid pressure on the suture line. Support the patient's head and neck with sandbags and pillows; when you move him, continue this support with your hands.
- After monitoring the patient's vital signs, check his dressing, neck, and back for bleeding. If he complains that the dressing feels tight, loosen it.
- Check serum calcium levels daily; hypocalcemia may develop if parathyroid glands are removed.

ACTION STAT!

 Watch for and report other complications, including: hemorrhage and shock (elevated pulse rate and hypotension), tetany (carpopedal spasm, twitching, and seizures), thyroid storm (high fever, severe tachycardia, delirium, dehydration, and extreme irritability), and respiratory obstruction (dyspnea, crowing respirations, and retraction of neck tissues).

- Keep a tracheotomy set and oxygen equipment handy in case of respiratory obstruction. Use a continuous air humidifier in the patient's room until his chest is clear.

- The patient may need I.V. fluids or a soft diet, but he may be able to tolerate a regular diet within 24 hours of surgery.

Thyroiditis

Inflammation of the thyroid gland occurs as autoimmune thyroiditis (long-term inflammatory disease), postpartum thyroiditis (silent thyroiditis), subacute granulomatous thyroiditis (self-limiting inflammation), Riedel's thyroiditis (rare, invasive fibrotic process), and miscellaneous thyroiditis (acute suppurative, chronic infective, and chronic noninfective). Autoimmune thyroiditis causes inflammation and lymphocytic infiltration (Hashimoto's thyroiditis); it commonly occurs in females, with peak incidence in middle age, and is the most prevalent cause of spontaneous hypothyroidism.

Causes
Autoimmune thyroiditis
- Antibodies to thyroid antigens
- Glandular atrophy
- Graves' disease

Postpartum thyroiditis
- Occurs within 1 year after delivery

Subacute granulomatous thyroiditis
- Adenovirus infection
- Coxsackievirus infection
- Influenza
- Mumps

Riedel's thyroiditis
- Unknown (rare)

Miscellaneous thyroiditis
- Actinomycosis
- Bacterial invasion (in acute suppurative form)
- Other infectious agents (in chronic infective form)
- Sarcoidosis and amyloidosis (in chronic noninfective form)
- Syphilis
- Tuberculosis (TB)

Signs and symptoms
Autoimmune thyroiditis
- Usually asymptomatic
Postpartum thyroiditis
- Usually asymptomatic

Subacute granulomatous thyroiditis
- Dysphagia
- Follows upper respiratory tract infection or a sore throat
- Moderate thyroid enlargement
- Painful and tender thyroid

Riedel's thyroiditis
- Compressed trachea or esophagus
- Enlarged thyroid
- Firm thyroid
- Tissue replaced by hard, fibrous tissues

Miscellaneous thyroiditis
- Fever
- Pain
- Reddened skin over the gland
- Tenderness

Diagnostic tests
- High titers of thyroglobulin and microsomal antibodies present in serum confirm autoimmune thyroiditis.
- Elevated erythrocyte sedimentation rate, increased thyroid hormone levels, and decreased thyroidal radioactive iodine uptake confirm subacute granulomatous thyroiditis.
- An elevated white blood cell count accompanying physical symptoms suggests chronic infective thyroiditis.

Treatment

- Drug therapy includes levothyroxine (Synthroid) for hypothyroidism.
- Analgesics and anti-inflammatories may be given for mild subacute granulomatous thyroiditis.
- Propranolol (Inderal) is administered for transient hyperthyroidism.
- Steroids may be indicated for severe episodes of acute inflammation.
- Suppurative thyroiditis requires antibiotic therapy.
- A partial thyroidectomy may be necessary to relieve tracheal or esophageal compression in Riedel's thyroiditis.

Nursing considerations

- Before treatment, obtain a patient history to identify underlying diseases that may cause thyroiditis, such as TB or a recent viral infection.
- Check the patient's vital signs, and examine his neck for unusual swelling, enlargement, or redness.
- Provide a liquid diet if the patient has difficulty swallowing, especially when due to fibrosis. If the neck is swollen, measure and record the circumference daily to monitor progressive enlargement.
- In suppurative thyroiditis, administer antibiotics, and report and record elevations in temperature.
- Instruct the patient to watch for and report signs of hypothyroidism (lethargy, restlessness, sensitivity to cold, forgetfulness, and dry skin)—especially if he has Hashimoto's thyroiditis, which commonly causes hypothyroidism.
- Check for signs of thyrotoxicosis (nervousness, tremor, and weakness), which usually occur in subacute thyroiditis.
- After thyroidectomy, check the patient's vital signs every 15 to 30 minutes until his condition stabilizes.

- Assess dressings frequently for excessive bleeding. Watch for signs of airway obstruction, such as difficulty talking or increased swallowing; keep tracheotomy equipment handy.

▌Thyrotoxicosis

Thyrotoxicosis is a metabolic imbalance that results from thyroid hormone overproduction or thyroid hormone overrelease from the gland. The most common form of thyrotoxicosis is Graves' disease, which increases thyroxine (T_4) production, enlarges the thyroid gland (goiter), and causes multiple system changes. (See *Other forms of thyrotoxicosis.*)

With treatment, the patient can lead a normal life. In a person with inadequately treated thyrotoxicosis, stress—including stress triggered by surgery, infection, toxemia of pregnancy, and diabetic ketoacidosis—can precipitate thyroid storm. Thyroid storm—an acute, severe exacerbation of thyrotoxicosis—is a medical emergency that may

Other forms of thyrotoxicosis

Varied forms of thyrotoxicosis may include the following:

Toxic adenoma

This small, benign nodule in the thyroid gland secretes thyroid hormone and is a common cause of thyrotoxicosis. The cause of toxic adenoma is unknown. Signs and symptoms are essentially similar to those of Graves' disease, except that toxic adenoma doesn't induce ophthalmopathy, pretibial myxedema, or acropachy.

The presence of adenoma is confirmed by iodine 131 (^{131}I) uptake and a thyroid scan, which show a single hyperfunctioning nodule suppressing the rest of the gland. Treatment includes ^{131}I therapy or surgery to remove the adenoma after antithyroid drugs achieve a euthyroid state.

Toxic multinodular goiter

Common in the elderly, this form of thyrotoxicosis involves thyroid hormone overproduction by one or more autonomously functioning nodules within a diffusely enlarged gland.

Thyrotoxicosis factitia

This form of thyrotoxicosis results from a chronic ingestion of thyroid hormone for thyrotropin suppression in patients with thyroid carcinoma, or from thyroid hormone abuse by persons who are trying to lose weight.

Functioning metastatic thyroid carcinoma

This rare disease causes excess thyroid hormone production.

TSH-secreting pituitary tumor

A pituitary tumor that secretes thyroid-stimulating hormone (TSH) causes thyroid hormone overproduction.

Subacute thyroiditis

This is a virus-induced granulomatous inflammation of the thyroid, producing transient thyrotoxicosis with fever, pain, pharyngitis, and thyroid gland tenderness.

Silent thyroiditis

Self-limiting, silent thyroiditis is a transient form of thyrotoxicosis, with histologic thyroiditis but no inflammatory symptoms.

cause life-threatening cardiac, hepatic, or renal consequences.

Causes

- Endocrine abnormalities (coexists with diabetes mellitus, thyroiditis, and hyperparathyroidism)
- Excessive dietary intake of iodine
- Genetic factors (autosomal recessive)
- Immunologic factors (production of autoantibodies)
- Stress

Signs and symptoms
Graves' disease

- Enlarged thyroid (goiter)
- Exophthalmos
- Frequent bowel movements
- Heat intolerance
- Nervousness
- Palpitations
- Sweating
- Tremor
- Weight loss despite increased appetite

Systemic signs and symptoms

- Cardiovascular system: tachycardia, widened pulse pressure, cardiomegaly,

increased cardiac output and blood volume, visible point of maximal impulse, paroxysmal supraventricular tachycardia and atrial fibrillation, systolic murmur at the left sternal border, and full, bounding pulse
- Central nervous system: difficulty in concentrating, excitability or nervousness, emotional instability and mood swings, and fine tremor, shaky handwriting, and clumsiness
- Eyes: exophthalmos, diplopia, increased tearing, and occasional inflammation of conjunctivae, corneas, or eye muscles
- GI system: excessive oral intake with weight loss, nausea and vomiting, increased defecation, soft stools or diarrhea, and liver enlargement
- Musculoskeletal system: weakness (especially in proximal muscles), fatigue, and muscle atrophy; paralysis; and acropachy (soft-tissue swelling, accompanied by underlying bone changes where new bone formation occurs)
- Reproductive system: in females, oligomenorrhea or amenorrhea, decreased fertility, and a higher incidence of spontaneous abortions; in males, gynecomastia; in both sexes, diminished libido
- Respiratory system: dyspnea on exertion and at rest
- Skin, hair, and nails: smooth, warm, flushed skin; fine, soft hair; premature graying and increased hair loss; friable nails and onycholysis (distal nail separated from the bed); thickened skin; and accentuated hair follicles, raised red patches of skin that are itchy and sometimes painful, with occasional nodule formation

Thyroid storm
- Coma
- Delirium
- Extreme irritability

- Hypertension
- Tachycardia
- Temperature up to 106° F (41.1° C)
- Vomiting

Diagnostic tests
- Radioimmunoassay shows increased serum T_4 and triiodothyronine (T_3) levels.
- Thyroid scan reveals increased uptake of radioactive iodine 131 (^{131}I). This test is contraindicated if the patient is pregnant.
- Thyrotropin-releasing hormone (TRH) stimulation test indicates thyrotoxicosis if the thyroid-stimulating hormone (TSH) level fails to rise within 30 minutes after the administration of TRH. TRH testing is rarely necessary due to highly sensitive TSH assays.
- Ultrasonography confirms subclinical ophthalmopathy.

Treatment
- Therapy with antithyroid drugs is used for children, young adults, pregnant females, and patients who refuse surgery or ^{131}I treatment. Antithyroid drugs are also used to correct the thyrotoxic state in preparation for ^{131}I treatment or surgery. Thyroid hormone antagonists include propylthiouracil and methimazole (Tapazole), which block thyroid hormone synthesis.

DRUG CHALLENGE

Although hypermetabolic symptoms subside within 4 to 8 weeks after antithyroid drug therapy begins, the patient must continue the medication for 6 months to 2 years.

- Propranolol (Inderal) is given to manage tachycardia and other peripheral effects of excessive hypersympathetic activity.

- During pregnancy, antithyroid medication should be kept at the minimum dosage required to keep maternal thyroid function within the high-normal range until delivery and to minimize the risk of fetal hypothyroidism. (See *Congenital thyrotoxicosis*.) Propylthiouracil is the preferred agent for the pregnant patient.

- The treatment of choice for patients not planning to have children is a single oral dose of ^{131}I. In most patients, hypermetabolic symptoms diminish 6 to 8 weeks after such treatment. However, some patients may require a second dose of ^{131}I.

- Subtotal (partial) thyroidectomy, which decreases the thyroid gland's capacity for hormone production, is indicated for patients whose thyrotoxicosis has repeatedly relapsed after drug therapy or patients who refuse or aren't candidates for ^{131}I treatment.

DRUG CHALLENGE

 Preoperatively, the patient may receive iodides (Lugol's solution or saturated solution of potassium iodide), antithyroid drugs, and high doses of propranolol to help prevent thyroid storm. If euthyroidism isn't achieved, surgery should be delayed, and antithyroid drugs and propranolol should be administered to decrease the risk of systemic side effects such as cardiac arrhythmias caused by thyrotoxicosis. After surgery, patients require regular medical supervision for the rest of their lives because they usually develop hypothyroidism, sometimes as long as several years after treatment.

- Treatment for ophthalmopathy includes local application of topical medications but may require high doses of corticosteroids. A patient with severe exophthalmos that causes pressure on the

Congenital thyrotoxicosis

Most neonates of hyperthyroid mothers are born with mild, transient thyrotoxicosis, caused by placental transfer of thyroid-stimulating immunoglobulins. Neonatal thyrotoxicosis may necessitate treatment with antithyroid drugs and propranolol (Inderal) for 2 to 3 months.

Because thyrotoxicosis sometimes worsens in the puerperal period, continuous control of maternal thyroid function is essential. About 3 to 6 months postpartum, antithyroid drug administration can be gradually tapered and thyroid function reassessed.

Mothers shouldn't breast-feed during treatment with antithyroid drugs because this can cause neonatal hypothyroidism.

optic nerve may require external-beam radiation therapy or surgical decompression to lessen pressure on the orbital contents.

- Treatment for thyroid storm includes administration of an antithyroid drug, such as PTU, I.V. propranolol to block sympathetic effects, a corticosteroid to inhibits production of T_3 and T_4, and an iodide to block the release of thyroid hormone.

- Supportive measures include administering nutrients, vitamins, fluids, and sedatives.

Nursing considerations

- Monitor serum electrolytes, and check periodically for hyperglycemia and glycosuria.

- Carefully monitor cardiac function if the patient is elderly or has coronary artery disease. If the heart rate is more than 100 beats/minute, check his blood pressure and pulse rate often.

■ If the patient is pregnant, tell her to watch closely during the first trimester for signs of spontaneous abortion (spotting, occasional mild cramps) and report such signs immediately.

■ The patient with dyspnea is most comfortable sitting upright or in high Fowler's position.

■ Remember, severe thyrotoxicosis may produce bizarre behavior, such as extreme nervousness, emotional instability, and mood swings ranging from occasional outbursts to overt psychosis. Reassure the patient and his family that such behavior will probably subside with treatment. Provide sedatives as necessary, and encourage the patient to verbalize his feelings about body image changes.

■ If iodide is part of the treatment, mix it with milk, juice, or water to prevent GI distress, and give it through a straw to prevent tooth discoloration.

DRUG CHALLENGE

 Give preparations containing iodine only after antithyroid drugs have been started. Otherwise, the iodine is used by the already overactive gland to make more thyroid hormone and worsen the toxic state.

■ Watch for signs of thyroid storm (tachycardia, hyperkinesis, fever, vomiting, and hypertension).

■ Check intake and output carefully to ensure adequate hydration and fluid balance.

■ Monitor temperature. If the patient has a high fever, reduce it with appropriate hypothermic measures.

■ If the patient has exophthalmos or another ophthalmopathy, suggest eye patches to protect his eyes from dryness at night. Moisten the conjunctivae often

with isotonic eyedrops. Instruct him to report symptoms of decreased visual acuity.

■ Avoid excessive palpation of the thyroid to help prevent thyroid storm.

After thyroidectomy

■ Check for respiratory distress, and keep a tracheotomy tray at the patient's bedside.

ACTION STAT!

 Watch for evidence of hemorrhage into the neck such as a tight dressing with no blood on it. Change dressings and perform wound care; check the back of the dressing for drainage. Keep the patient in semi-Fowler's position, and support his head and neck with sandbags to ease tension on the incision.

■ Check for dysphagia or hoarseness, which may result from laryngeal nerve injury.

■ Watch for signs of hypoparathyroidism (tetany, numbness), a complication that results from accidental removal of the parathyroid glands during surgery.

■ Stress the importance of regular medical follow-up after discharge because hypothyroidism may develop from 2 to 4 weeks postoperatively.

DRUG CHALLENGE

 Drug and ^{131}I therapy require careful monitoring and comprehensive patient teaching. After ^{131}I therapy, tell the patient not to expectorate or cough freely because his saliva is radioactive for 24 hours. Stress the need for repeated measurement of serum T_4 levels. Be sure that the patient understands that he must not resume antithyroid drug therapy.

Instruct the patient to take medications with meals to minimize GI distress and to avoid over-the-counter cough preparations because many contain iodine.

■ Watch the patient taking propranolol for signs of hypotension (dizziness and decreased urine output). Tell him to rise slowly after sitting or lying down to prevent orthostatic hypotension.

■ Instruct the patient receiving antithyroid drugs or ^{131}I therapy to report symptoms of hypothyroidism.

 # Tonsillitis

Inflammation of the tonsils, or tonsillitis, can be acute or chronic. The uncomplicated acute form usually lasts 4 to 6 days and commonly affects children ages 5 to 10. The presence of proven chronic tonsillitis justifies tonsillectomy, the only effective treatment. Tonsils tend to hypertrophy during childhood and atrophy after puberty.

Causes
■ Bacteria
■ Infection with group A beta-hemolytic streptococci (most common)
■ Oral anaerobes
■ Viruses

Signs and symptoms
Acute tonsillitis
■ Chills
■ Constant urge to swallow
■ Constricted feeling at the back of the throat
■ Dysphagia
■ Fever
■ Headache
■ Malaise
■ Mild to severe sore throat
■ Muscle and joint pain

■ Pain (frequently referred to the ears)
■ Refusal to eat (in children)
■ Swelling and tenderness of the lymph glands in the submandibular area

Chronic tonsillitis
■ Frequent attacks of acute tonsillitis
■ Purulent drainage in the tonsillar crypts
■ Recurrent sore throat
■ Signs of obstruction (from tonsillar hypertrophy or peritonsillar abscess)

Diagnostic tests
■ Diagnostic confirmation requires a thorough throat examination that reveals generalized inflammation of the pharyngeal wall, swollen tonsils that exude white or yellow follicles, purulent drainage when pressure is applied to the tonsillar pillars, and possible edematous and inflamed uvula.
■ Throat culture may determine the infecting organism and indicate appropriate antibiotic therapy.
■ Leukocytosis is also usually present.
■ Needle biopsy helps differentiate cellulitis from abscess.

Treatment
■ Tonsillitis caused by bacterial infection requires antibiotics; when the causative organism is group A beta-hemolytic streptococcus, penicillin is the drug of choice.
■ Most oral anaerobes respond to penicillin.
■ Additional treatment includes rest, adequate fluid intake, and acetaminophen (Tylenol) or aspirin for pain.

 To prevent complications, continue antibiotic therapy for the full prescribed course.

- Chronic tonsillitis or the development of complications (obstructions from tonsillar hypertrophy, peritonsillar abscess) may require a tonsillectomy, but only after the patient has been free from tonsillar or respiratory tract infections for 3 to 4 weeks.

Nursing considerations

- Despite dysphagia, urge the patient to drink plenty of fluids, especially if he has a fever. Offer a child ice cream and flavored drinks and ices.
- Suggest gargling to soothe the throat, unless it exacerbates pain.
- Make sure the patient and his parents understand the importance of completing the prescribed course of antibiotic therapy.
- Before a tonsillectomy, explain to the adult patient that a local anesthetic prevents pain but allows a sensation of pressure during surgery. Warn the patient to expect considerable throat discomfort and some bleeding postoperatively. For the pediatric patient, keep your explanation simple and nonthreatening. Show the child the operating and recovery rooms, and briefly explain the hospital routine. Most facilities allow one parent to stay with the child.

DRUG CHALLENGE

Advise the patient not to take aspirin or medications containing aspirin for 7 to 10 days before surgery to decrease the risk of bleeding. Aspirin and medications containing aspirin are also contraindicated postoperatively.

- Postoperatively, maintain a patent airway. To prevent aspiration, place the patient on his side.

ACTION STAT!

Monitor the patient's vital signs frequently, and check for bleeding. Stay alert for excessive bleeding, increased pulse rate, dropping blood pressure, or frequent swallowing.

- After the patient is fully alert and the gag reflex has returned, allow him to drink water. Encourage oral intake with cool liquids and advance to a soft, bland diet as tolerated; avoid citrus juices and highly spiced foods.
- Encourage the patient to ambulate and to take frequent deep breaths to prevent pulmonary complications. Give pain medication as needed.
- Before discharge, provide the patient or his parents with written instructions on home care. Tell the patient to expect a white scab to form in the throat 5 to 10 days postoperatively and to report bleeding, ear discomfort, or a fever that lasts longer than 3 days.
- Instruct the patient to avoid coughing or excessive clearing of the throat, which can irritate the throat and cause increased bleeding.
- Tell the patient that blood-tinged mucus is normal for 5 to 7 days after surgery.

▎Toxic shock syndrome

An acute bacterial infection, toxic shock syndrome (TSS) is caused by toxin-producing, penicillin-resistant strains of *Staphylococcus aureus* and *Streptococcus pyogenes*. It's associated with use of tampons (mostly super-absorbent types) in females and with skin wounds. Both provide entry for the organism via traumatized areas. Major complications include persistent neuropsychological abnormalities, mild renal failure, a rash, and cyanotic arms and legs.

Causes

- Infection with *S. aureus* or *S. pyrogenes*

Predisposing factors

- Abscesses
- Barrier contraceptive devices (diaphragms and sponges)
- Menstruating females who use tampons
- Osteomyelitis
- Recent childbirth
- Recent surgery

Signs and symptoms

- Conjunctival hyperemia
- Decreased level of consciousness
- Deep red rash, especially on the palms and soles; later desquamates
- Diarrhea
- Fever over 104° F (40° C)
- Headache
- Intense myalgia
- Rigors
- Severe hypotension
- Vaginal hyperemia and discharge
- Vomiting

Diagnostic tests

- Isolation of the infecting organism from vaginal discharge or lesions helps support the diagnosis. TSS is typically diagnosed when the patient has the following signs and symptoms:
  - fever of 102° F (38.9° C) or higher
  - hypotension (including fainting or dizziness on standing)
  - involvement of at least three organ systems
  - shedding of skin, especially on palms and soles, 1 to 2 weeks after onset of illness
  - widespread red, flat rash

Treatment

- The patient should receive I.V. antibiotics, such as cephalosporins (cefditoring,

ceftazidime, ceftizoxime), clindamycin, oxacillin, nafcillin, and methicillin.
- To reverse shock, replace fluids with I.V. saline solution and colloids.
- Shock that doesn't respond to fluids may necessitate the use of pressor agents such as dopamine.
- Dialysis may be necessary for kidney dysfunction.
- I.V. immunoglobulin may also be considered for severe cases.

Nursing considerations

- Monitor the patient's vital signs frequently.
- Administer antibiotics slowly and strictly on time. Be sure to watch for signs of penicillin allergy.
- Check the patient's fluid and electrolyte balance.
- Obtain specimens for culture of *S. aureus*.
- Tell the patient to avoid using tampons, as appropriate.

Toxoplasmosis

One of the most common infectious diseases, toxoplasmosis results from infection with the protozoa *Toxoplasma gondii*. Occurring worldwide, it's less common in cold or hot, arid climates and at high elevations. It usually causes localized infection but may produce significant generalized infection, especially in immunodeficient patients or neonates. Congenital toxoplasmosis, characterized by lesions in the central nervous system, may result in stillbirth or serious birth defects.

Causes

T. gondii transmitted by:
- fecal-oral contamination from infected cats
- ingestion of tissue cysts in raw or undercooked meat

■ transplacental transmission from an infected mother

Signs and symptoms
Congenital toxoplasmosis
Initial

■ Cerebral calcification
■ Fever
■ Hepatosplenomegaly
■ Hydrocephalus or microcephalus
■ Jaundice
■ Lymphadenopathy
■ Rash
■ Retinochoroiditis
■ Seizures
■ Stillbirth (if acquired in the first trimester of pregnancy)

Months or years later
■ Blindness
■ Epilepsy
■ Mental retardation
■ Strabismus

Acquired toxoplasmosis
Localized infection

■ Fatigue
■ Fever
■ Headache
■ Lymphadenopathy
■ Malaise
■ Myalgia
■ Sore throat

Generalized infection

■ Delirium
■ Diffuse maculopapular rash (except on the palms, soles, and scalp)
■ Encephalitis
■ Fever
■ Headache
■ Hepatitis
■ Myocarditis
■ Pneumonitis
■ Polymyositis
■ Seizures
■ Vomiting

Diagnostic tests

■ Isolation of *T. gondii* in mice after their inoculation with specimens of body fluids, blood, and tissue or *T. gondii* antibodies in such specimens confirms toxoplasmosis.

Treatment

■ Acute disease is treated with sulfonamides and pyrimethamine (Daraprim) for 4 to 6 weeks; and possibly, folinic acid to control pyrimethamine's adverse effects.

■ In patients who also have acquired immunodeficiency syndrome (AIDS), treatment continues indefinitely. A patient with AIDS who can't tolerate sulfonamides may receive clindamycin instead.

- Clindamycin is the primary treatment in ocular toxoplasmosis.

Nursing considerations

- Advise the patient to seek follow-up care.
- Report all cases of toxoplasmosis to your local public health department.
- When caring for patients with toxoplasmosis, monitor drug therapy carefully and emphasize thorough patient teaching to prevent complications and control spread of the disease. (See *Avoiding toxoplasmosis.*)

DRUG CHALLENGE

 Because sulfonamides cause blood dyscrasias and pyrimethamine depresses bone marrow, closely monitor the patient's hematologic values.

- If the patient is pregnant, she should have a friend or family member change her cat's litter box daily. If she must do it herself, she should wear gloves and wash her hands immediately afterward. Diligent hand washing is important because the parasite found in cat feces can infect a person a few days after being passed.

■ Trigeminal neuralgia

Also called *tic douloureux,* trigeminal neuralgia is a painful disorder of one or more branches of the fifth cranial (trigeminal) nerve that produces paroxysmal attacks of excruciating facial pain precipitated by stimulation of a trigger zone. The pain of trigeminal neuralgia is probably produced by an interaction or short-circuiting of touch and pain fibers. Trigeminal neuralgia can subside spontaneously, with remissions lasting from several months to years.

Causes

- Afferent reflex phenomenon (centrally, or more peripherally in the sensory root)
- Compression of the nerve root by posterior fossa tumors, middle fossa tumors, or vascular lesions (subclinical aneurysm)
- Herpes zoster
- Multiple sclerosis

Signs and symptoms

- Pain
  - Searing or burning
  - Occurring in lightning-like jabs and lasting from 1 to 15 minutes (usually 1 to 2 minutes) in an area innervated by one of the divisions of the trigeminal nerve, primarily the superior mandibular or maxillary division
  - Rarely affecting more than one division, and seldom the first division (ophthalmic) or both sides of the face
  - Affects the second (maxillary) and third (mandibular) divisions of the trigeminal nerve equally
  - Attacks characteristically following stimulation of a trigger zone, usually by a light touch to a hypersensitive area, such as the tip of the nose, the cheeks, or the gums
  - Attacks possibly following eating, smiling, talking, drinking hot or cold beverages, or exposure to draft, heat, or cold
  - Variable frequency of attacks (from many times per day to several times per month or year)
  - Absence of pain between attacks (typically; constant, dull ache in some patients)
- No impairment of sensory or motor function (indeed, sensory impairment implies a space-occupying lesion as the cause of pain)
- Patient attempting to avoid pain
  - May splint the affected area

– May hold his face immobile when talking
– May leave the affected side of his face unwashed and unshaven
– May protect his face with a coat or shawl

Diagnostic tests

- The patient's pain history is the basis for diagnosis because trigeminal neuralgia produces no objective clinical or pathologic changes.
- Skull X-rays, computed tomography (CT) scanning, and magnetic resonance imaging rule out tumors and sinus or tooth infections.

Treatment

- Oral administration of antiepileptic drugs, such as carbamazepine (Tegretol) or phenytoin (Dilantin), may relieve or prevent pain.
- Opioids may be helpful during an acute pain episode.
- If these nonsurgical treatments fail, percutaneous electrocoagulation of nerve rootlets under local anesthesia is the treatment of choice for permanent relief.
- Percutaneous radio-frequency procedure, which causes partial root destruction and relieves pain, and microsurgery for vascular decompression (using guided CT) of the trigeminal nerve are additional treatments.

Nursing considerations

- Observe and record the characteristics of each attack, including the patient's protective mechanisms.
- Provide adequate nutrition in small, frequent meals at room temperature.

DRUG CHALLENGE

 If the patient is receiving carbamazepine, watch for cutaneous and hematologic reactions (ery-

thematous and pruritic rashes, urticaria, photosensitivity, exfoliative dermatitis, leukopenia, agranulocytosis, eosinophilia, aplastic anemia, thrombocytopenia) and, possibly, urine retention and transient drowsiness.

- For the first 3 months of carbamazepine therapy, complete blood count and liver function should be monitored weekly and then monthly thereafter. Warn the patient to immediately report fever, sore throat, mouth ulcers, easy bruising, or petechial or purpuric hemorrhage.

DRUG CHALLENGE

 Fever, sore throat, mouth ulcers, easy bruising, or petechial or purpuric hemorrhage may signal thrombocytopenia or aplastic anemia and may require discontinuation of drug therapy.

- If the patient is receiving phenytoin, also watch for adverse effects, including ataxia, skin eruptions, gingival hyperplasia, and nystagmus.
- After resection of the first division of the trigeminal nerve, tell the patient to avoid rubbing his eyes and using aerosol spray. Advise him to wear glasses or goggles outdoors and to blink often.
- After surgery to sever the second or third division, tell the patient to avoid hot foods and drinks, which could burn his mouth, and to chew carefully to avoid biting his mouth.
- Advise the patient to place food in the unaffected side of his mouth when chewing, to brush his teeth and rinse his mouth often, and to see a dentist twice per year to detect cavities. (Cavities in the area of the severed nerve won't cause pain.)
- After surgical decompression of the root or partial nerve dissection, check

the patient's neurologic and vital signs often.

- Provide emotional support, and encourage the patient to express his fear and anxiety. Promote independence through self-care and maximum physical activity. Reinforce natural avoidance of stimulation (air, heat, and cold) of trigger zones (lips, cheeks, and gums).
- Refer the patient to a pain clinic as necessary.

Tuberculosis

An acute or chronic infection caused by *Mycobacterium tuberculosis,* tuberculosis (TB) is characterized by pulmonary infiltrates, formation of granulomas with caseation, fibrosis, and cavitation. People living in crowded, poorly ventilated conditions are most likely to become infected. In patients with strains that are sensitive to the usual antitubercular agents, the prognosis is excellent with correct treatment. However, in those with strains that are resistant to two or more of the major antitubercular agents, mortality is 50%. After exposure to *M. tuberculosis,* roughly 5% of infected people develop active TB within 1 year; in the remainder, microorganisms cause a latent infection. The host's immune system usually controls the tubercle bacillus by killing it or walling it up in a tiny nodule (tubercle); the bacillus may lie dormant for years and later reactivate and spread. The disease is twice as common in males as in females and four times as common in nonwhites as in whites. Incidence is highest in people who live in crowded, poorly ventilated, unsanitary conditions, such as prisons, tenement houses, and homeless shelters. Those at higher risk for disease progression or reactivation of dormant disease include infants, the elderly, and individuals who are immunocompromised

(such as those with acquired immunodeficiency syndrome [AIDS], those undergoing chemotherapy, or transplant recipients taking antirejection medications).

Causes

- Exposure to *M. tuberculosis* transmitted by droplet nuclei

Reactivation risk factors

- AIDS
- Gastrectomy
- Hodgkin's disease
- Leukemia
- Silicosis
- Treatment with corticosteroids or immunosuppressants
- Uncontrolled diabetes mellitus

Signs and symptoms

- Anorexia
- Fatigue
- Low-grade fever
- Night sweats
- Weakness
- Weight loss

In reactivation

- Chest pain
- Cough that produces mucopurulent sputum
- Crepitant crackles, bronchial breath sounds, wheezes, and whispered pectoriloquy on auscultation
- Dullness over the affected area indicating consolidation or pleural fluid (on chest percussion)
- Hemoptysis (occasionally)

Diagnostic tests

- Chest X-ray, a tuberculin skin test, and sputum smears and cultures confirm the presence of *M. tuberculosis.*
- Chest X-ray shows nodular lesions, patchy infiltrates (mainly in the upper lobes), cavity formation, scar tissue, and

calcium deposits; however, it may not be able to distinguish active from inactive TB.

- Tuberculin skin test detects exposure to TB. Intermediate-strength purified protein derivative or 5 tuberculin units (0.1 ml) are injected intradermally on the forearm. The test results are read in 48 to 72 hours; a positive reaction (induration of greater than or equal to 10 mm, depending on risk factors) develops 2 to 10 weeks after infection in active and inactive TB. However, severely immunosuppressed patients may never develop a positive reaction.
- Stains and cultures (of sputum, cerebrospinal fluid, urine, drainage from abscess, or pleural fluid) show heat-sensitive, nonmotile, aerobic, acid-fast bacilli.
- Computed tomography scanning or magnetic resonance imaging allow the evaluation of lung damage or confirm a difficult diagnosis.
- Bronchoscopy may be performed if the patient can't produce an adequate sputum specimen.

Treatment

- Treatment includes antitubercular therapy with daily oral doses of isoniazid, rifampin, and pyrazinamide (and sometimes ethambutol [Myambutol]) for at least 6 months. Longer courses may be required for patients with AIDS or for those who respond slowly. After 2 to 4 weeks, the disease generally is no longer infectious. The patient can resume his normal lifestyle while taking medication.
- Patients with atypical mycobacterial disease or drug-resistant TB may require treatment with second-line drugs, such as capreomycin, streptomycin, para-aminosalicylic acid, cycloserine, amikacin (Amikin), and quinolone drugs.

Nursing considerations

- Isolate the infectious patient in a quiet, well-ventilated room until he's no longer contagious.
- Teach the patient to cough and sneeze into tissues and to dispose of all secretions properly. Place a covered trash can nearby or tape a waxed bag to the side of the bed for used tissues.
- Instruct the patient to wear a mask when outside his room. Visitors and hospital personnel should wear masks when they're in the patient's room.
- Remind the patient to get plenty of rest and to eat balanced meals. If the patient is anorexic, urge him to eat small meals throughout the day. Record weight weekly.

Drug challenge

 Stay alert for adverse effects of medications. Because isoniazid sometimes leads to hepatitis or peripheral neuritis, monitor aspartate aminotransferase and alanine aminotransferase levels. To prevent or treat peripheral neuritis, give pyridoxine (vitamin B_6). If the patient receives ethambutol, watch for optic neuritis; if it develops, discontinue the drug. If he receives rifampin, watch for hepatitis and purpura. Also observe the patient for other complications such as hemoptysis.

- Emphasize the importance of regular follow-up examinations, and instruct the patient and his family concerning the signs and symptoms of recurring TB.
- Advise people who have been exposed to infected patients to receive tuberculin tests and, if necessary, chest X-rays and prophylactic isoniazid.

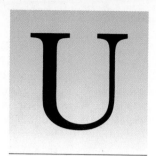

Ulcerative colitis

An inflammatory condition that affects the surface of the colon, ulcerative colitis causes friability and erosions with bleeding. The disease usually begins in the rectal area and may extend through the entire bowel. Less frequently, it extends into the splenic flexure, or more proximally extends upward into the entire colon. It rarely affects the small intestine, except for the terminal ileum. Severity ranges from a mild, localized disorder to a fulminant disease that may lead to a perforated colon, progressing to peritonitis and toxemia.

Causes
- Autoimmune response (possibly)
- Exacerbated or triggered by stress

Signs and symptoms
- Anemia
- Ankylosing spondylitis
- Arthritis
- Bloody diarrhea
- Cholangiocarcinoma
- Cirrhosis
- Coagulation defects
- Episcleritis
- Erythema nodosum on the face and arms
- Fecal urgency
- Hypovolemia
- Impaired nutrition
- Intermittent bleeding and mucus production
- Left lower quadrant pain relieved by defecation
- Loss of muscle mass
- Pericholangitis
- Peritonitis
- Pyoderma gangrenosum on the legs and ankles
- Sclerosing cholangitis
- Strictures, pseudopolyps, stenosis, and perforated colon
- Tenesmus
- Thromboembolic events
- Toxemia
- Uveitis

Diagnostic tests
- Sigmoidoscopy establishes the diagnosis by demonstrating increased mucosal friability, decreased mucosal detail, edema, and erosions.
- Biopsy can help confirm the diagnosis.
- Colonoscopy may be used to determine the extent of the disease and to evaluate the areas of stricture and pseudopolyps. Colonoscopy shouldn't be performed during an acute episode because of the risk of perforation.
- Stool specimen analysis reveals blood, pus, and mucus but no pathogenic organisms.

Treatment

- The goals of treatment are to control inflammation, replace nutritional losses and blood volume, and prevent complications.
- Supportive treatment includes I.V. fluid replacement, dietary therapy, bed rest, and medications.
- Total parenteral nutrition (TPN) rests the intestinal tract, decreases stool volume, and restores positive nitrogen balance.
- The patient with moderate signs and symptoms may receive Ensure or another brand of elemental feeding to provide adequate nutrition with minimal bowel stimulation.
- Blood transfusions or iron supplements may be necessary to correct anemia.
- Medications to control inflammation include corticotropin and adrenal corticosteroids, such as prednisone, prednisolone, and hydrocortisone; sulfasalazine, which has anti-inflammatory and antimicrobial properties; and mesalamine, given rectally or orally.
- Surgery, the treatment of last resort, is recommended for patients who have toxic megacolon or who fail to respond to drugs and supportive measures. Surgery may include proctocolectomy with ileostomy; total colectomy and ileorectal anastomosis (requires observation of the remaining rectal stump for any signs of cancer or colitis); pouch ileostomy (Kock pouch or continent ileostomy), or an ileoanal reservoir (a two-step procedure that preserves the anal sphincter and provides the patient with a reservoir made from the ileum and attached to the anal opening.

Nursing considerations

- Accurately record intake and output, particularly the frequency and volume of stools.
- Watch for signs and symptoms of dehydration and electrolyte imbalances, specifically of hypokalemia (muscle weakness, paresthesia) and hypernatremia (fever, tachycardia, flushed skin, and dry tongue).
- Monitor hemoglobin and hematocrit levels, and transfuse as ordered.
- Provide good mouth care for the patient who's allowed nothing by mouth.
- After each bowel movement, thoroughly clean the skin around the rectum.

DRUG CHALLENGE

 Watch for adverse effects of prolonged corticosteroid therapy (moon face, hirsutism, edema, and gastric irritation). Be aware that such therapy may mask infection.

- If the patient needs TPN, change dressings, assess for inflammation at the insertion site, and check blood glucose every 6 hours.
- Take precautionary measures if the patient is prone to bleeding. Watch closely for signs of complications, such as a perforated colon and peritonitis (fever, severe abdominal pain, abdominal rigidity and tenderness, and cool, clammy skin), and toxic megacolon (abdominal distention, decreased bowel sounds).
- Prepare the patient for surgery, and provide teaching related to the care of an ileostomy. Consult the enterostomal therapy nurse for preoperative teaching and stoma marking. Provide bowel preparation as ordered.
- After surgery, provide education regarding ostomy care as well as psychological support. Arrange for the patient to consult an enterostomal therapy nurse.
- Keep the nasogastric tube patent. After removal of the tube, provide a clear liq-

uid diet. Gradually advance to a low-residue diet as tolerated.

■ After a proctocolectomy and ileostomy, provide education regarding ostomy care. Wash the skin around the stoma with soapy water and dry it thoroughly. Apply karaya powder around the base of the stoma to prevent irritation and provide a tight seal. Cut an opening in the ring to fit over the stoma, and secure the pouch to the skin. Empty the pouch when it's one-third full.

■ After a pouch ileostomy, uncork the catheter every hour to allow contents to drain. After 10 to 14 days, gradually increase the length of time the catheter is left corked until it can be opened every 3 hours. Then remove the catheter and reinsert it every 3 to 4 hours for drainage. Teach the patient how to insert the catheter and how to take care of the stoma.

■ Encourage the patient to have regular physical examinations.

Urinary tract infection, lower

Cystitis and urethritis, the two forms of lower urinary tract infection (UTI), are nearly 10 times more common in females than in males. Lower UTI is also a prevalent bacterial disease in children, with girls also most commonly affected. In men and in children of either sex, lower UTIs are usually related to anatomic or physiologic abnormalities and therefore require extremely close evaluation. UTIs typically respond readily to treatment, but recurrence and resistant bacterial flare-up during therapy are possible.

Causes

■ Ascending infection by a single gram-negative enteric bacterium (*Escherichia coli, Klebsiella, Proteus, Enterobacter, Pseudomonas,* or *Serratia*)

■ Simultaneous infection with multiple pathogens

Predisposing factors

■ Benign prostatic hyperplasia
■ Bowel incontinence
■ Catheterization
■ Cystoscopy
■ Diabetes
■ History of analgesic or reflux nephropathy
■ Immobility or decreased mobility
■ Incomplete emptying of the bladder (in elderly patients)
■ Indwelling urinary catheter
■ Lack of adequate fluids
■ Pregnancy
■ Prostatitis
■ Urethral strictures

Signs and symptoms

■ Abdominal pain or tenderness over the bladder area
■ Chills
■ Cramps or bladder spasms
■ Dysuria
■ Feeling of warmth during urination
■ Fever
■ Flank pain
■ Hematuria
■ Itching
■ Low back pain
■ Malaise
■ Nausea, vomiting
■ Nocturia
■ Urethral discharge in males (possibly)
■ Urinary frequency
■ Urinary urgency

Diagnostic tests

■ Characteristic signs and symptoms and a microscopic urinalysis showing red blood cell and white blood cell counts greater than 10 per high-power field suggest lower UTI.

Treating and preventing urinary tract infections

The following measures can help your patients treat urinary tract infections and prevent recurrences.

Treatment

■ Explain the nature and purpose of antimicrobial therapy. Emphasize the importance of completing the prescribed course of therapy or, with long-term prophylaxis, of adhering strictly to the ordered dosage.

■ Recommend taking nitrofurantoin macrocrystals (Macrobid) with milk or a meal to prevent GI distress. If therapy includes phenazopyridine, warn the patient that this drug may turn his urine red-orange.

■ Urge the patient to drink at least eight glasses of water per day. Stress the need to maintain a consistent fluid intake of about 2,000 ml/day. More or less than this amount may alter the effect of the prescribed antimicrobial.

■ Tell the patient that fruit juices, especially cranberry juice, and oral doses of vitamin C may help acidify urine and enhance the action of the medication.

■ Suggest warm sitz baths for relief from perineal discomfort.

Prevention

To prevent recurrent infections in men, urge prompt treatment of predisposing conditions such as chronic prostatitis.

To prevent recurrent infections in women, teach the patient to:

■ carefully wipe the perineum from front to back and to clean it thoroughly with soap and water after defecation

■ void immediately after sexual intercourse

■ drink plenty of fluids

■ routinely avoid postponing urination. Recommend frequent comfort stops during long car trips, and stress the need to empty the bladder completely.

■ A clean-catch, midstream urine specimen revealing a bacterial count of more than 100,000/ml confirms the diagnosis. Lower counts don't necessarily rule out infection, especially if the patient is voiding frequently, because bacteria require 30 to 45 minutes to reproduce in urine. Careful midstream, clean-catch collection is preferred to catheterization, which can reinfect the bladder with urethral bacteria.

■ Sensitivity testing determines the appropriate therapeutic antimicrobial agent.

■ Voiding cystoureterography or excretory urography may disclose congenital anomalies that predispose the patient to recurrent UTIs.

Treatment

■ Appropriate antimicrobials are the treatment of choice for most initial lower UTIs. A 7- to 10-day course of antibiotic therapy is standard, but recent studies suggest that a single dose of an antibiotic or a 3- to 5-day antibiotic regimen may be sufficient to render the urine sterile. After 3 days of antibiotic therapy, urine culture should show no organisms.

■ If the urine isn't sterile after 3 days of antibiotic therapy, bacterial resistance has probably occurred, making the use of a different antimicrobial necessary.

■ Single-dose antibiotic therapy with amoxicillin or co-trimoxazole may be effective in females with an acute, uncomplicated UTI. A urine culture taken 1 to 2 weeks later indicates whether the infection has been eradicated.

- Recurrent infections due to infected renal calculi, chronic prostatitis, or a structural abnormality may necessitate surgery; prostatitis also requires long-term antibiotic therapy. In patients without these predisposing conditions, long-term, low-dosage antibiotic therapy is the treatment of choice.

Nursing considerations

- Teach the female patient how to clean the perineum properly and keep the labia separated during voiding to collect a clean-catch, midstream urine specimen. Explain that an uncontaminated midstream specimen is essential for accurate diagnosis.
- Watch for GI disturbances from antimicrobial therapy.
- Teach the patient how to prevent and treat UTIs. (See *Treating and preventing urinary tract infections.*)
- Collect all urine samples for culture and sensitivity testing carefully and promptly.

▌Urticaria and angioedema

Urticaria and angioedema are commonly present in allergic reactions. Urticaria, also known as *hives,* is an episodic, usually self-limited skin reaction characterized by local dermal wheals surrounded by an erythematous flare. Angioedema, another dermal eruption, involves additional skin layers (including subcutaneous tissue) and produces deeper, larger wheals (usually on the hands, feet, lips, genitals, and eyelids) and a more diffuse swelling of loose subcutaneous tissue. Urticaria and angioedema can occur simultaneously, but angioedema may last longer. Nonallergic urticaria and angioedema are related to histamine release after external physical stimuli.

Causes

- Dermographism urticaria (develops after stroking or scratching the skin): varying pressure (tight clothing); aggravated by scratching
- Allergy to drugs, foods, insect stings, or inhaled particles, such as animal dander and cosmetics
- Binding of immunoglobulin (Ig) G or IgM, resulting in complement activation
- Collagen vascular diseases
- Connective tissue diseases such as systemic lupus erythematosus
- External physical stimuli (cold, heat, water, or sunlight)
- IgE-induced release of mediators from cutaneous mast cells
- Localized or secondary infections such as respiratory infection
- Neoplastic diseases such as Hodgkin's disease
- Psychogenic diseases

Signs and symptoms

- Angioedema: nonpitting swelling of deep subcutaneous tissue (eyelids, lips, genitalia, and mucous membranes); nonpruritic (possibly, burning and tingling)
- Cholinergic urticaria: tiny, blanched wheals surrounded by erythematous flares
- Distinct, raised, evanescent dermal wheals surrounded by erythematous flares
- Lesions of varying sizes

Diagnostic tests

- Skin testing, an elimination diet, and a food diary (recording time and amount of food eaten and circumstances) can pinpoint provoking allergens.
- Recurrent angioedema without urticaria, along with a familial history, points to hereditary angioedema. Decreased serum levels of C1, C2, and C4 inhibitors confirm this diagnosis.

Treatment

- After the triggering stimulus has been removed, urticaria usually subsides in a few days. (Drug reactions may persist until the drug is no longer in the bloodstream.)
- During desensitization, progressively larger doses of specific antigens (determined by skin testing) are injected intradermally.
- Diphenhydramine (Benadryl) or another antihistamine can ease itching and swelling in every kind of urticaria, although they may induce drowsiness.
- Corticosteroid therapy may be necessary for some patients.

Nursing considerations

- Maintain a patent airway if an allergic reaction is severe.
- Monitor the patient's vital signs, cardiac rate and rhythm, and respiratory depth and quality.
- Administer medications and monitor the patient for adverse effects.
- Position the patient for comfort.
- An accurate patient history can help determine the cause of urticaria. Such a history should include:
  – drug history, including over-the-counter preparations (vitamins, aspirin, and antacids)
  – frequently ingested foods (strawberries, milk products, and fish)
  – environmental influences (pets, carpet, clothing, soap, inhalants, cosmetics, hair dye, and insect bites and stings).
- Be supportive during allergy testing; provide teaching and information about the procedure.
- Provide patient education on avoiding allergens, as appropriate.

Uterine cancer

Cancer of the endometrium, or uterine cancer, is the most common female reproductive cancer. It typically afflicts postmenopausal females between ages 50 and 60. It's uncommon between ages 30 and 40 and rare before age 30. Most premenopausal females who develop uterine cancer have a history of anovulatory menstrual cycles or another hormonal imbalance. Generally, uterine cancer is an adenocarcinoma that metastasizes late, usually from the endometrium to the cervix, ovaries, fallopian tubes, and other peritoneal structures. It may spread to distant organs, such as the lungs and the brain, through the blood or the lymphatic system. Lymph node involvement can also occur. Less common uterine tumors include adenoacanthoma, endometrial stromal sarcoma, lymphosarcoma, mixed mesodermal tumors (including carcinosarcoma), and leiomyosarcoma.

Causes
Predisposing factors

- Abnormal uterine bleeding
- Diabetes
- Estrogen therapy (controversial)
- Familial tendency
- History of atypical endometrial hyperplasia
- Hypertension
- Low fertility index and anovulation
- Obesity

Signs and symptoms

- Discharge: watery and blood-streaked initially; gradually becoming more bloody
- Pain and weight loss (in advanced cancer)
- Persistent and unusual premenopausal bleeding
- Postmenopausal bleeding

- Uterine enlargement

Diagnostic tests

- Endometrial, cervical, or endocervical biopsy results confirm the presence of cancer cells. Fractional dilatation and curettage is used to identify the problem when the disease is suspected but the endometrial biopsy result is negative.
- The following tests are performed for baseline data and staging:
  – blood studies, urinalysis, and electrocardiography
  – chest X-ray or computed tomography scan
  – complete physical examination proctoscopy or barium enema studies (if bladder and rectal involvement are suspected)
  – Schiller's test staining of the cervix and vagina.

Treatment

- Surgery generally involves total abdominal hysterectomy, bilateral salpingo-oophorectomy or, possibly, omentectomy with or without pelvic or para-aortic lymphadenectomy.
- When the tumor isn't well differentiated, intracavitary or external radiation (or both), given 6 weeks before surgery, may inhibit recurrence and lengthen survival time.
- Hormonal therapy using tamoxifen (Nolvadex) produces a 20% to 40% response rate, and may be given as a second-line treatment.
- Chemotherapy, including both cisplatin and doxorubicin, as well as others is usually tried when other treatments have failed.

Nursing considerations
Before surgery

- Reinforce previous teaching about the surgery, and explain routine tests, such as repeated blood tests the morning after surgery, and postoperative care.
- If the patient is premenopausal, inform her that removal of her ovaries will induce menopause.

After surgery

- Measure fluid contents of the blood drainage system every 8 hours. Stay alert for drainage that exceeds 400 ml in 8 hours.
- If the patient has received subcutaneous heparin, continue administration until she's fully ambulatory again.
- Check the patient's vital signs every 4 hours. Watch for signs of complications, such as bleeding, abdominal distention, severe pain, wheezing, or other breathing difficulties. Provide analgesics.
- Regularly encourage the patient to breathe deeply and cough to help prevent complications. Promote the use of an incentive spirometer once every waking hour to help keep lungs expanded.

Internal radiation therapy

- Explain that internal radiation usually requires a 2- to 3-day hospital stay, bowel preparation, a povidone-iodine vaginal douche, a clear-liquid diet, and nothing taken by mouth as ordered before the implantation. Mention that internal radiation also requires an indwelling urinary catheter.
- Tell the patient that if the procedure is performed in the operating room, she will receive a general anesthetic. She'll be placed in a dorsal position, with her knees and hips flexed and her heels resting in footrests. If the radioactive source isn't implanted in the operating room, it may be implanted by a member of the radiation team while the patient is in her room. She'll require a private room.
- Encourage the patient to limit movement while the radioactive source is in place. If necessary, administer a sedative,

such as diazepam (Valium), to help her relax and remain still. If she prefers, elevate the head of the bed slightly. Make sure she can reach everything she needs (call bell, telephone, water) without stretching or straining.

■ Assist the patient in range-of-motion arm exercises (leg exercises and other body movements could dislodge the implanted radioactive source). Organize the time you spend with the patient to minimize your exposure to radiation.

■ Check the patient's vital signs every 4 hours; watch for skin reactions, vaginal bleeding, abdominal discomfort, or evidence of dehydration.

■ Inform visitors of safety precautions and hang a sign listing these precautions on the patient's door.

External radiation therapy

■ Teach the patient and her family about the therapy before it begins. Tell the patient that treatment is usually given 5 days a week for 6 weeks. Warn her not to scrub body areas marked with indelible ink for treatment because it's important to direct treatment to exactly the same area each time.

■ Administer antidiarrheal medication to minimize diarrhea, a possible adverse effect of pelvic radiation.

■ To minimize skin breakdown and reduce the risk of skin infection, tell the patient to keep the treatment area dry, to avoid wearing clothes that rub against the area, and to avoid using heating pads, alcohol rubs, or any skin creams.

■ Teach the patient how to use a vaginal dilator to prevent vaginal stenosis and to facilitate vaginal examinations and sexual intercourse.

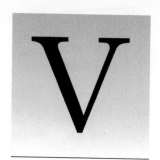

Valvular heart disease

In valvular heart disease, three types of mechanical disruption can occur: stenosis, or narrowing, of the valve opening; incomplete closure of the valve; or valve prolapse. They can result from such disorders as endocarditis (most common), congenital defects, and inflammation, and they can lead to heart failure. (See *Forms of valvular heart disease,* pages 668 to 671.)

Aortic insufficiency
- Blood flowing back into the left ventricle during diastole and causing fluid overload in the ventricle, which dilates and hypertrophies
- Excess volume causing fluid overload in the left atrium and, finally, the pulmonary system
- Left-sided heart failure and pulmonary edema (eventually)

Aortic stenosis
- Increased left ventricular pressure attempting to overcome the resistance of the narrowed valvular opening
- Added workload increasing the demand for oxygen, and diminishing cardiac output, causing poor coronary artery perfusion, ischemia of the left ventricle, and left-sided heart failure

Mitral insufficiency
- Blood from the left ventricle flowing back into the left atrium during systole and causing the atrium to enlarge to accommodate the backflow
- Dilation of the left ventricle to accommodate the increased blood volume from the atrium and compensate for diminishing cardiac output
- Ventricular hypertrophy and increased end-diastolic pressure resulting in increased pulmonary artery pressure, eventually leading to left-sided and right-sided heart failure

Mitral stenosis
- Narrowing of the valve by valvular abnormalities, fibrosis, or calcification, thereby obstructing blood flow from the left atrium to the left ventricle
- Increase of left atrial volume and pressure and dilation of the chamber
- Greater resistance to blood flow causing pulmonary hypertension, right ventricular hypertrophy, and right-sided heart failure
- Inadequate filling of the left ventricle, producing low cardiac output

Mitral valve prolapse
- Anatomic prolapse accompanied by signs and symptoms unrelated to the valvular abnormality

(Text continues on page 671.)

Forms of valvular heart disease

Causes and incidence	Clinical features	Diagnostic measures
Aortic insufficiency ■ Results from rheumatic fever, syphilis, hypertension, endocarditis, or may be idiopathic ■ Associated with Marfan syndrome ■ Most common in males ■ Associated with ventricular septal defect, even after surgical closure	■ Dyspnea, cough, fatigue, palpitations, angina, syncope ■ Pulmonary vein congestion, heart failure, pulmonary edema (left-sided heart failure), "pulsating" nail beds (Quincke's pulse) ■ Rapidly rising and collapsing pulses (pulsus biferiens), cardiac arrhythmias, wide pulse pressure in severe regurgitation ■ Auscultation that reveals an S_3 and a diastolic blowing murmur at the left sternal border ■ Palpation and visualization of apical impulse in chronic disease	■ Cardiac catheterization: reduction in arterial diastolic pressures, aortic insufficiency, other valvular abnormalities, and increased left ventricular end-diastolic pressure ■ X-ray: left ventricular enlargement, pulmonary vein congestion ■ Echocardiography: left ventricular enlargement, alterations in mitral valve movement (indirect indication of aortic valve disease), and mitral thickening ■ Electrocardiography: sinus tachycardia, left ventricular hypertrophy, and left atrial hypertrophy in severe disease
Aortic stenosis ■ Results from congenital aortic bicuspid valve (associated with coarctation of the aorta), congenital stenosis of valve cusps, rheumatic fever, or atherosclerosis in elderly people ■ Most common in males	■ Dyspnea on exertion, paroxysmal nocturnal dyspnea, fatigue, syncope, angina, palpitations ■ Pulmonary vein congestion, heart failure, pulmonary edema (left-sided heart failure) ■ Diminished carotid pulses, decreased cardiac output, cardiac arrhythmias; may have pulsus alternans ■ Auscultation that reveals a systolic murmur heard at base or in carotids and, possibly, an S_4	■ Cardiac catheterization: pressure gradient across valve (indicating obstruction), increased left ventricular end-diastolic pressures ■ X-ray: valvular calcification, left ventricular enlargement, and pulmonary vein congestion ■ Echocardiography: thickened aortic valve and left ventricular wall, possibly coexistent with mitral valve stenosis ■ Electrocardiography: left ventricular hypertrophy

Forms of valvular heart disease *(continued)*

Causes and incidence	Clinical features	Diagnostic measures
Mitral insufficiency • Results from rheumatic fever, hypertrophic cardiomyopathy, mitral valve prolapse, myocardial infarction, severe left-sided heart failure, or ruptured chordae tendineae • Associated with other congenital anomalies such as transposition of the great arteries • Rare in children without other congenital anomalies	• Orthopnea, dyspnea, fatigue, angina, palpitations • Peripheral edema, jugular vein distention, hepatomegaly (right-sided heart failure) • Tachycardia, crackles, pulmonary edema • Auscultation that reveals a holosystolic murmur at the apex, possible split S_2, and an S_3	• Cardiac catheterization: mitral insufficiency with increased left ventricular end-diastolic volume and pressure, increased atrial pressure and pulmonary artery wedge pressure (PAWP), and decreased cardiac output • X-ray: left atrial and ventricular enlargement, pulmonary venous congestion • Echocardiography: abnormal valve leaflet motion, left atrial enlargement • Electrocardiography: may show left atrial and ventricular hypertrophy, sinus tachycardia, and atrial fibrillation
Mitral stenosis • Results from rheumatic fever (most common cause) • Most common in females • May be associated with other congenital anomalies	• Dyspnea on exertion, paroxysmal nocturnal dyspnea, orthopnea, weakness, fatigue, palpitations • Peripheral edema, jugular vein distention, ascites, hepatomegaly (right-sided heart failure in severe pulmonary hypertension) • Crackles, cardiac arrhythmias (atrial fibrillation), signs of systemic emboli • Auscultation that reveals a loud S_1 or opening snap and a diastolic murmur at the apex	• Cardiac catheterization: diastolic pressure gradient across valve; elevated left atrial and pulmonary artery wedge pressures (PAWP > 15 mm Hg) with severe pulmonary hypertension and pulmonary artery pressures; elevated right-sided heart pressure, decreased cardiac output; and abnormal contraction of the left ventricle • X-ray: left atrial and ventricular enlargement, enlarged pulmonary arteries, and mitral valve calcification • Echocardiography: thickened mitral valve leaflets, left atrial enlargement • Electrocardiography: left atrial hypertrophy, atrial fibrillation, right ventricular hypertrophy, and right axis deviation

(continued)

Forms of valvular heart disease *(continued)*

Causes and incidence	Clinical features	Diagnostic measures
Mitral valve prolapse ■ Cause unknown. Researchers speculate that metabolic or neuroendocrine factors cause constellation of signs and symptoms. ■ Most commonly affects young females but may occur in both sexes and in all age-groups	■ May produce no signs ■ Chest pain, palpitations, headache, fatigue, exercise intolerance, dyspnea, light-headedness, syncope, mood swings, anxiety, panic attacks ■ Auscultation that typically reveals a mobile, mid-systolic click, with or without a mid-to-late systolic murmur	■ Two-dimensional echocardiography: prolapse of mitral valve leaflets into left atrium ■ Color-flow Doppler studies: mitral insufficiency ■ Resting electrocardiography: ST-segment changes, biphasic or inverted T waves in leads II, III, or aV_F ■ Exercise electrocardiography: evaluates chest pain and arrhythmias
Pulmonic insufficiency ■ May be congenital or may result from pulmonary hypertension ■ May rarely result from prolonged use of pressure monitoring catheter in the pulmonary artery	■ Dyspnea, weakness, fatigue, chest pain ■ Peripheral edema, jugular vein distention, hepatomegaly (right-sided heart failure) ■ Auscultation that reveals a diastolic murmur in pulmonic area	■ Cardiac catheterization: pulmonary insufficiency, increased right ventricular pressure, and associated cardiac defects ■ X-ray: right ventricular and pulmonary arterial enlargement ■ Electrocardiography: right ventricular or right atrial enlargement
Pulmonic stenosis ■ Results from congenital stenosis of valve cusp or rheumatic heart disease (infrequent) ■ Associated with other congenital heart defects such as tetralogy of Fallot	■ Asymptomatic or symptomatic with dyspnea on exertion, fatigue, chest pain, syncope ■ May lead to peripheral edema, jugular vein distention, hepatomegaly (right-sided heart failure) ■ Auscultation that reveals a systolic murmur at the left sternal border and a split S_2 with a delayed or absent pulmonic component ■ Dyspnea and fatigue	■ Cardiac catheterization: increased right ventricular pressure, decreased pulmonary artery pressure, and abnormal valve orifice ■ Electrocardiography: may show right ventricular hypertrophy, right axis deviation, right atrial hypertrophy, and atrial fibrillation

Forms of valvular heart disease *(continued)*

Causes and incidence	Clinical features	Diagnostic measures
Tricuspid insufficiency ▪ Results from right-sided heart failure, rheumatic fever and, rarely, trauma and endocarditis ▪ Associated with congenital disorders	▪ May lead to peripheral edema, jugular vein distention, hepatomegaly, and ascites (right-sided heart failure) ▪ Auscultation that reveals a possible S_3 and a systolic murmur at the lower left sternal border that increases with inspiration	▪ Right heart catheterization: high atrial pressure, tricuspid insufficiency, and decreased or normal cardiac output ▪ X-ray: right atrial dilation, right ventricular enlargement ▪ Echocardiography: systolic prolapse of tricuspid valve, right atrial enlargement ▪ Electrocardiography: right atrial or right ventricular hypertrophy, atrial fibrillation
Tricuspid stenosis ▪ Results from rheumatic fever ▪ May be congenital ▪ Associated with mitral or aortic valve disease ▪ Most common in females	▪ May be symptomatic with dyspnea, fatigue, and syncope ▪ Possibly peripheral edema, jugular vein distention, hepatomegaly, and ascites (right-sided heart failure) ▪ Auscultation that reveals a diastolic murmur at the lower left sternal border that increases with inspiration	▪ Cardiac catheterization: increased pressure gradient across valve, increased right atrial pressure, decreased cardiac output ▪ X-ray: right atrial enlargement ▪ Echocardiography: leaflet abnormality, right atrial enlargement ▪ Electrocardiography: right atrial hypertrophy, right or left ventricular hypertrophy, and atrial fibrillation

▪ One or both valve leaflets protruding into the left atrium

Pulmonic insufficiency
▪ Blood ejected into the pulmonary artery during systole flowing back into the right ventricle during diastole, causing fluid overload in the ventricle, ventricular hypertrophy and, finally, right-sided heart failure

Pulmonic stenosis
▪ Obstructed right ventricular outflow causing right ventricular hypertrophy

▪ Right-sided heart failure (eventually)

Tricuspid insufficiency
▪ Incompetent tricuspid valve causing blood to flow back into the right atrium during systole, decreasing blood flow to the lungs and the left side of the heart
▪ Decreasing cardiac output
▪ Eventual fluid overload in the right side of the heart, possibly leading to right-sided heart failure

Tricuspid stenosis

- Obstructed blood flow from the right atrium to the right ventricle causing the right atrium to dilate and hypertrophy
- Right-sided heart failure and increased pressure in the vena cava (eventually)

Causes

- See *Forms of valvular heart disease,* pages 668 to 671.

Signs and symptoms

- See *Forms of valvular heart disease,* pages 668 to 671.

Diagnostic tests

- See *Forms of valvular heart disease,* pages 668 to 671.

Treatment

- The nature and severity of associated symptoms determine treatment for a patient with valvular heart disease.
- A cardiac glycoside, a low-sodium diet, a diuretic, a vasodilator, and an angiotensin-converting enzyme inhibitor are used to treat patients with left-sided heart failure.
- Anticoagulants prevent thrombus formation around diseased or replaced valves and may not be necessary with tissue valve replacements.
- Prophylactic antibiotics are required before and after surgery or dental care.
- Some patients may require valvuloplasty.
- If the patient has severe signs and symptoms that can't be managed medically, open heart surgery using cardiopulmonary bypass for valve replacement is indicated.
- Valve replacement may be the treatment of choice for some valvular heart diseases, such as severe aortic insufficiency.
- Supplemental oxygen may be necessary for acute episodes.

Nursing considerations

- Watch closely for signs of heart failure or pulmonary edema and for adverse effects of drug therapy.
- Teach the patient about dietary restrictions, medications, and the importance of consistent follow-up care.
- If the patient undergoes surgery, watch for hypotension, arrhythmias, and thrombus formation. Monitor his vital signs, arterial blood gas values, intake, output, daily weight, blood chemistries, chest X-rays, and pulmonary artery catheter readings.

Vancomycin intermediately resistant *Staphylococcus aureus*

Vancomycin intermediately resistant *Staphylococcus aureus* (VISA) is a mutation of a bacterium that's easily spread by direct person-to-person contact. It occurs in patients who previously received multiple courses of vancomycin for methicillin-resistant *S. aureus* (MRSA) infections. Another mutation, vancomycin-resistant *S. aureus* (VRSA) is fully resistant to vancomycin. Patients most at risk for resistant organisms include:

- those with a history of taking vancomycin, third-generation cephalosporins, or antibiotics targeted at anaerobic bacteria such as *Clostridium difficile*
- patients with indwelling urinary or central venous catheters
- elderly patients, especially those with prolonged or repeated hospital admissions
- patients with cancer or chronic renal failure
- patients undergoing cardiothoracic or intra-abdominal surgery or organ transplants
- patients with wounds with an opening to the pelvic or intra-abdominal area, in-

cluding surgical wounds, burns, and pressure ulcers

■ patients with enterococcal bacteremia, commonly associated with endocarditis

■ patients exposed to contaminated equipment or to a patient with the infecting microbe.

Causes

■ Vancomycin-resistant enterococcus (VRE) and MRSA: an infected or colonized patient or a colonized health care worker (VISA and VRSA thought to be colonized in a similar method)

■ Contact between the patient and caregiver

■ Contact between patients

■ Contact with contaminated surfaces such as an overbed table

Signs and symptoms

■ None

Diagnostic tests

■ The causative agent may be found incidentally when culture results show the organism. Someone with no signs or symptoms of infection is considered colonized if VISA or VRSA can be isolated from stools or a rectal swab.

Treatment

■ No single antibiotic is currently available to combat VISA or VRSA.

■ The practitioner may opt not to treat an infection at all. Instead, he may stop all antibiotics and simply wait for normal bacteria to repopulate and replace the strain. Combinations of various drugs may also be used, depending on the infection's source.

■ A colonized patient is placed in contact isolation until culture-negative or discharged. Colonization can last indefinitely; no protocol has been established for the length of time a patient should remain in isolation.

■ In 1996, the Centers for Disease Control and Prevention and the Hospital Infection Control Practices Advisory Committee proposed a two-level system of precautions to simplify isolation for resistant organisms.

– The first level calls for standard precautions, which incorporate features of universal blood and body fluid precautions and body substance isolation precautions to be used for all patient care.

– The second level calls for transmission-based precautions, implemented when a particular infection is suspected.

Nursing considerations

■ Hand washing before and after care of the patient is crucial.

■ Use an antiseptic soap such as chlorhexidine; bacteria have been cultured from workers' hands after they've washed with milder soap.

DO'S & DON'TS

 Use contact isolation precautions when in contact with the patient. Provide a private room and dedicated equipment for the patient. Disinfect the environment. Change gloves when contaminated or when moving from a "dirty" area of the body to a clean one. Don't touch potentially contaminated surfaces, such as a bed or bed stand, after removing gown and gloves.

■ Be particularly prudent in caring for a patient with an ileostomy, colostomy, or draining wound that isn't contained by a dressing.

■ Instruct family and friends to wear protective garb when they visit the patient, and teach them how to dispose of it.

- Provide teaching and emotional support to the patient and his family.
- Consider grouping infected patients together; thereby having the same nursing staff care for them (known as *cohorting*).
- Don't place equipment used on the patient on the bed or the bed stand; wipe it with appropriate disinfectant before leaving the room.
- Ensure judicious and careful use of antibiotics.
- Instruct patients to take antibiotics for the full prescription period, even if they begin to feel better.

Vancomycin-resistant enterococcus

Vancomycin-resistant enterococcus (VRE) is a mutation of a very common bacterium that's spread easily by direct person-to-person contact. Facilities in more than 40 states have reported VRE, with rates as high as 14% in oncology units of large teaching facilities. Patients most at risk for contracting VRE include:

- patients who are immunosuppressed or those with severe underlying disease
- patients with a history of taking vancomycin, third-generation cephalosporins, or antibiotics targeted at anaerobic bacteria such as *Clostridium difficile*
- patients with indwelling urinary or central venous catheters
- elderly patients, especially those with prolonged or repeated hospital admissions
- patients with malignancies or chronic renal failure
- patients undergoing cardiothoracic or intra-abdominal surgery or organ transplants
- patients with wounds with an opening to the pelvic or intra-abdominal area, including surgical wounds, burns, and pressure ulcers

- patients with enterococcal bacteremia, commonly associated with endocarditis
- patients exposed to contaminated equipment or to a VRE-positive patient.

Causes

- Contact with a colonized health care worker or an infected or colonized patient
- Contact with contaminated surfaces such as an overbed table

Signs and symptoms

- None

Diagnostic tests

- Someone with no signs or symptoms of infection is considered colonized if VRE can be isolated from stools or a rectal swab. When colonized, a patient is more than 10 times as likely to become infected with VRE—for example, through a breach in the immune system.

Treatment

- Because no single antibiotic currently available can eradicate VRE, the practitioner may opt not to treat an infection. Instead, he may stop all antibiotics and wait for normal bacteria to repopulate and replace the VRE strain.
- Combinations of various drugs may also be used, depending on the infection's source.

Nursing considerations

- Hand washing before and after care of the patient is crucial.
- Use an antiseptic soap such as chlorhexidine; bacteria have been cultured from workers' hands after they've washed with milder soap.

Do's & Don'ts

 Use contact isolation precautions when in contact with the patient. Provide a private room and dedicated equipment for the patient to prevent transmission of VRE to other patients. Disinfect the environment. Change gloves when contaminated or when moving from a "dirty" area of the body to a clean one. Don't touch potentially contaminated surfaces, such as a bed or bed stand, after removing gown and gloves.

- Be particularly prudent in caring for a patient with an ileostomy, colostomy, or draining wound that isn't contained by a dressing.
- Instruct family and friends to wear protective garb when they visit the patient, and teach them how to dispose of it.
- Provide teaching and emotional support to the patient and his family.
- Consider grouping infected patients together and having the same nursing staff care for them (known as *cohorting*).
- Don't place equipment used on the patient on the bed or the bed stand; wipe it with appropriate disinfectant before leaving the room.
- Ensure judicious and careful use of antibiotics.
- Instruct patients to take antibiotics for the full prescription period, even if they begin to feel better.

▌Varicella

Varicella, also called *chickenpox,* is a common, acute, and highly contagious infection caused by the herpesvirus varicella zoster (VZ), the same virus that, in its latent stage, causes herpes zoster (shingles). It can occur at any age, but it's most common in children ages 5 to 9 years. The varicella vaccine is effective in preventing varicella in up to 90% of recipients. The American Academy of Pediatrics recommends the vaccine for all children and for adolescents and adults who haven't had varicella. It's unknown how the vaccine affects shingles.

Causes

- Congenital varicella: infants whose mothers had acute infections in their first or early second trimester (possibly)
- Transmitted by direct contact (primarily with respiratory secretions; less commonly with skin lesions) and respiratory droplets

Signs and symptoms

- Anorexia
- Fever (slight)
- Hypoplastic deformity and scarring of a limb, retarded growth, and central nervous system and eye manifestations (with congenital varicella)
- Lesions and a high fever lasting longer than 7 days (patients who are immunocompromised)
- Malaise
- Rash:
  - crops of small, erythematous macules on the trunk or scalp progressing to papules followed by clear vesicles on an erythematous base (the so-called "dewdrop on a rose petal")
  - clouding and breakage of vesicles; formation of scabs
  - spreading to the face and, rarely, to the extremities
  - new vesicles forming for 3 to 4 days
- Severe pruritus, which may lead to infection, scarring, impetigo, furuncles, and cellulitis
- Shallow ulcers on mucous membranes of the mouth, conjunctivae, and genitalia (occasionally)

Complications

- Acute myositis
- Arthritis
- Bleeding disorders
- Fulminating encephalitis (Reye's syndrome)

- Hepatitis
- Myocarditis
- Nephritis
- Pneumonia

Diagnostic tests

- Varicella is diagnosed by characteristic signs and symptoms and usually doesn't require laboratory tests.
- The virus can be isolated from vesicular fluid within the first 3 to 4 days of the rash.
- Serum contains antibodies 7 days after onset of symptoms.
- Serologic testing is useful in differentiating rickettsial pox from varicella.

Treatment

- Chickenpox requires airborne and contact precautions until all vesicles have crusted over. Children can go back to school, however, if just a few scabs remain because, at this stage, varicella is no longer contagious. Congenital varicella requires no isolation.
- Local (such as calamine lotion) or systemic antipruritics help relieve itching.
- Cool bicarbonate of soda baths may also provide relief from itching.
- Diphenhydramine (Benadryl) or another antihistamine may be given for itching.
- Acyclovir (Zovirax) is the antiviral drug of choice to shorten the duration of symptoms.
- Antibiotics aren't necessary unless bacterial infection develops.

DRUG CHALLENGE

 Salicylates are contraindicated in children because of their link to Reye's syndrome.

- Patients who are immunocompromised may need special treatment. When given up to 72 hours after exposure to chickenpox, varicella-zoster im-

mune globulin may provide passive immunity. I.V. acyclovir may slow vesicle formation, speed skin healing, and control the systemic spread of infection.

Nursing considerations

- Teach the child and his family how to apply topical antipruritic medications correctly. Stress the importance of good hygiene.
- Tell the patient not to scratch the lesions. However, because the need to scratch may be overwhelming, parents should trim the child's fingernails or tie mittens on his hands.
- Warn parents to watch for and immediately report signs of complications. Severe skin pain and burning may indicate a serious secondary infection and require prompt medical attention.
- To help prevent varicella, don't admit a child exposed to varicella to a unit that contains children who receive immunosuppressant agents or who have leukemia or immunodeficiency disorders.
- A vulnerable child who has been exposed to varicella should receive VZ immune globulin to lessen its severity.

Variola

Variola, or smallpox, is an acute, highly contagious infectious disease caused by the poxvirus variola. Although naturally occurring smallpox has been eradicated, variola virus preserved in laboratories remains a potential source of infection, however unlikely. In response to bioterrorism concerns, smallpox vaccination has been offered to members of the military, health department officials, first responders, and key health care providers. Should a bioterrorism event involving smallpox occur or be suspected, vaccination programs can be initiated.

Variola developed in three major forms: variola major (classic smallpox), which carried a high mortality; variola minor, a mild form that occurred in unvaccinated people and resulted from a less virulent strain; and varioloid, a mild variant that occurred in previously vaccinated people who had only partial immunity.

Causes

- Exposure through inhalation (in a terrorist attack)
- Transmitted directly by dried scales of virus-containing lesions
- Transmitted directly by respiratory droplets
- Transmitted indirectly through contact with contaminated linens or other objects

Signs and symptoms

- Incubation period of 10 to 14 days
- Abrupt onset of chills (and possible seizures in children)
- High fever (above 104° F [40° C])
- Headache
- Backache
- Severe malaise
- Vomiting (especially in children)
- Marked prostration
- Violent delirium, stupor, or coma (occasionally)
- 2 days after onset: increased severity of symptoms
- 3 days after onset: patient begins to feel better
- Sore throat and cough along with lesions on the mucous membranes of the mouth, throat, and respiratory tract
- Skin lesions progressing from macular to papular, vesicular, and pustular (pustules may be as large as 8 mm in diameter)
- Increase in temperature and return of early symptoms during pustular stage
- 10 days after onset: rupture of pustules followed by drying and formation of scabs
- 1 to 2 weeks after onset: desquamation of the scabs with intense pruritus, commonly resulting in permanently disfiguring scars
- About 14 days after onset: subsiding of symptoms
- Diffuse dusky appearance over the patient's face and upper chest (in fatal cases)
- Death due to encephalitic manifestations, extensive bleeding from any or all orifices, or secondary bacterial infections

Diagnostic tests

- Although variola is readily recognizable—especially during an epidemic or after a known contact—the most conclusive diagnostic test is a variola virus culture isolated from an aspirate of vesicles and pustules.
- Other laboratory tests include microscopic examination of smears from lesion scrapings and complement fixation to detect virus or virus antibodies in the patient's blood.

Treatment

- Patients with variola require hospitalization with strict droplet and contact precautions.
- Antimicrobial therapy is used to treat bacterial complications.
- Symptomatic treatment of lesions consists of administering antipruritics and is started during the pustular stage.
- If the smallpox vaccination is given within 1 to 4 days of exposure to the disease, it may prevent illness or lessen symptoms. Treatment once the disease has started is limited.

Nursing considerations
- Monitor the patient's vital signs, intake, and output.
- Monitor the patient's response to medications.
- Provide oxygenation as ordered; maintain a patent airway.
- Provide skin care as ordered.
- Maintain isolation.
- If smallpox is suspected, the state health department should be notified immediately.

Vascular retinopathies

Vascular retinopathies are noninflammatory retinal disorders that result from interference with the blood supply to the eyes. Types of vascular retinopathy are central retinal artery occlusion, central retinal vein occlusion, diabetic retinopathy, and hypertensive retinopathy. When one of the arteries maintaining blood circulation in the retina becomes obstructed, the diminished blood flow causes visual deficits.

Causes
- Diabetic retinopathy: diabetes
- Hypertensive retinopathy: prolonged hypertensive disease

Central retinal artery occlusion
- Unknown
- Atherosclerosis
- Conditions that slow blood flow, such as carotid occlusion and heart valve vegetation
- Embolism
- Infection

Central retinal vein occlusion
- Atherosclerosis
- Diabetes
- External compression of the retinal vein
- Generalized and localized infections
- Glaucoma
- Granulomatous diseases
- Thrombosis
- Trauma

Signs and symptoms
Central retinal artery occlusion
- Sudden, painless, unilateral vision loss (partial or complete)
- Following amaurosis fugax or transient episodes of unilateral loss of vision lasting from a few seconds to minutes (possibly)
- Typically, permanent vision loss
- Spontaneous resolution within hours with partial regaining of vision in some patients

Central retinal vein occlusion
- Reduced visual acuity, allowing perception of only hand movement and light
- Painless (except with resulting secondary neovascular glaucoma—uncontrolled proliferation of weak blood vessels)
- Secondary glaucoma within 3 to 4 months after occlusion (5% to 20% of patients)

Nonproliferative diabetic retinopathy
- No symptoms (some patients)
- Fluid leakage into the macular region causing significant loss of central visual acuity (necessary for reading and driving) and diminished night vision

Proliferative diabetic retinopathy
- Vitreous hemorrhage with corresponding sudden vision loss

Diagnosing vascular retinopathies

In vascular retinopathies, diagnosis varies, depending on the type of retinopathy.

Central retinal artery occlusion

- History reveals sudden vision loss.
- External examination reveals a marked afferent pupillary defect.
- Ophthalmoscopy reveals narrowed retinal arterioles, "boxcarring" or segmentation of the blood column in the arterioles, and may reveal whitening of the retina around the disk (caused by a decreased blood supply) and a cherry-red spot in the macula.
- Physical examination may reveal elevated blood pressure.
- Erythrocyte sedimentation rate may detect giant cell arteritis.
- Doppler ultrasound provides carotid artery evaluation.
- Echocardiogram and Holter monitoring reveal clots from vegetations on a heart valve.
- Fluorescein angiography confirms the diagnosis.

Central retinal vein occlusion

- Ophthalmoscopy (direct or indirect) shows retinal hemorrhages, retinal vein engorgement, white patches among hemorrhages, and edema around the disk.
- History may reveal the use of hormonal contraceptives or diuretics or a sudden loss of monocular vision.

- Physical examination may detect elevated blood pressure and reveal the underlying cause.

Diabetic retinopathy

- Indirect ophthalmoscopy shows retinal changes such as microaneurysms (earliest change), retinal hemorrhages and edema, venous dilation and beading of the vessel, exudates, and vitreous hemorrhage. New blood vessel growth, which leaks lipids and causes edema, and microinfarcts of the nerve fiber layer may also occur.
- Fluorescein angiography shows fluorescein leakage from new blood vessels and differentiates microaneurysms from true hemorrhages.
- History reveals long-standing diabetes and decreased vision.

Hypertensive retinopathy

- Ophthalmoscopy (direct or indirect) shows changes in arteriovenous crossing; cottonwool spots; flame-shaped, silver-wire appearance of narrowed arterioles; nicking of veins where arteries cross them (arteriovenous nicking); hard exudates (lipid deposits); "macular star," flame-shaped hemorrhages; retinal edema; arterial microaneurysms; and swelling of the optic nerve head (disk edema).
- Physical examination detects elevated blood pressure.
- History reveals decreased vision, occipital headache, and hypertension.

- Macular distortion
- Retinal detachment

Hypertensive retinopathy

- Blurred vision
- Mild, prolonged disease: eventual visual defects

- Severe, prolonged disease: eventual blindness

Diagnostic tests

- Appropriate diagnostic tests depend on the type of vascular retinopathy. (See *Diagnosing vascular retinopathies*.)

- The diagnostic testing process always includes determination of visual acuity and ophthalmoscopic examination.

Treatment
Central retinal artery occlusion

- No treatment is known to control central retinal artery occlusion. Treatment focuses on attempting to release the occlusion into the peripheral circulation.
- To reduce intraocular pressure, treatment includes eyeball massage with a Goldman-type goniolens and, possibly, anterior chamber paracentesis after anesthetizing the surface with topical cocaine 2% to 4% drops, acetazolamide (Diamox) 500 mg I.V., and inhalation of carbogen (95% oxygen and 5% carbon dioxide) to improve retinal oxygenation.

DRUG CHALLENGE

Because inhalation therapy may be given hourly for up to 48 hours, the patient should be hospitalized so his vital signs can be monitored.

- If the patient is young, the source of the occlusion may be the heart. Echocardiography may be necessary. Treatment in this case is to heparinize the patient.

Central retinal vein occlusion

- Aspirin may be given due to its mild anticoagulant properties.
- Laser photocoagulation can reduce the risk of neovascular glaucoma for some patients whose eyes have widespread capillary nonperfusion.

Diabetic retinopathy

- Careful control of blood glucose levels during the first 5 years of the disease may reduce the severity of retinopathy or delay its onset.

- For the patient with microaneurysms, therapy should include frequent eye examinations (three or four times yearly) to monitor the condition. For a child with diabetes, therapy should include an annual eye examination by an ophthalmologist.
- Treatment for proliferative diabetic retinopathy is laser photocoagulation, which cauterizes the leaking blood vessels, thereby eliminating the cause of the edema. Laser treatment may be focal (aimed at new blood vessels) or panretinal (placing burns throughout the peripheral retina).
- Despite treatment, neovascularization doesn't always regress, and vitreous hemorrhage, with or without retinal detachment, may follow. Vitrectomy is the treatment of choice for vitreous hemorrhage to restore vision.

Hypertensive retinopathy
- Blood pressure is controlled with appropriate drugs, diet, and exercise.

Nursing considerations
ACTION STAT!

Arrange for immediate ophthalmologic evaluation when a patient complains of sudden, unilateral vision loss. Blindness may be permanent if treatment is delayed.

- Be sure to monitor the patient's blood pressure if he complains of an occipital headache and blurred vision.
- Administer acetazolamide I.V. During inhalation therapy, monitor the patient's vital signs carefully. Stop therapy if blood pressure fluctuates or if he develops arrhythmias or becomes disoriented.
- Encourage the patient with diabetes to comply with the prescribed regimen.
- For a patient with hypertensive retinopathy, stress the importance of

complying with antihypertensive therapy.

Vasculitis

A broad spectrum of disorders, vasculitis is characterized by inflammation and necrosis of blood vessels. Its clinical effects depend on the vessels involved and reflect tissue ischemia caused by blood flow obstruction. The prognosis is also variable. For example, hypersensitivity vasculitis is usually a benign disorder limited to the skin, but more extensive polyarteritis nodosa can be rapidly fatal. Vasculitis can occur at any age, except for mucocutaneous lymph node syndrome, which occurs only during childhood. Vasculitis may be a primary disorder or secondary to other disorders, such as rheumatoid arthritis or systemic lupus erythematosus.

Causes

- History of serious infectious disease, such as hepatitis B or bacterial endocarditis
- High-dose antibiotic therapy
- Excessive circulating antigens, which trigger the formation of soluble antigen antibody complexes (type III hypersensitivity reaction)
- Formation of autoantibodies directed at the body's cellular and extracellular proteins (a type II hypersensitivity reaction)
- Cell-mediated (T cell) immune response
- Exposure to allergens (type I hypersensitivity reaction)

Signs and symptoms

See *Types of vasculitis*, pages 682 to 685.

Diagnostic tests

See *Types of vasculitis*, pages 682 to 685.

Treatment

- Treatment in primary vasculitis minimizes irreversible tissue damage associated with ischemia.
- Treatment may involve removing an offending antigen (antigenic drugs, food, and other environmental substances) or use of an anti-inflammatory or an immunosuppressant.
- Drug therapy in primary vasculitis usually involves low-dose oral cyclophosphamide (Cytoxan) with daily corticosteroids. In rapidly fulminant vasculitis, the cyclophosphamide dosage may be increased.
- Prednisone should be given in divided doses for 7 to 10 days, with consolidation to a single morning dose by 2 to 3 weeks.
- When the vasculitis appears to be in remission or when prescribed cytotoxic drugs take full effect, corticosteroids are tapered down to a single daily dose and then to an alternate-day schedule for 3 to 6 months, after which steroids are slowly discontinued.
- In secondary vasculitis, treatment focuses on the underlying disorder.

Nursing considerations

- Assess for dry nasal mucosa in patients with Wegener's granulomatosis. Instill nose drops to lubricate the mucosa and diminish crusting, or irrigate nasal passages with warm normal saline solution.
- Monitor the patient's vital signs. Use a Doppler ultrasonic flowmeter, if available, to auscultate blood pressure in the patient with Takayasu's arteritis, whose peripheral pulses are frequently difficult to palpate.
- Monitor intake and output. Check daily for edema. Keep the patient well hydrated (3 L/day) to reduce the risk of hemorrhagic cystitis associated with cyclophosphamide therapy.

(Text continues on page 684.)

Types of vasculitis

Type	Vessels involved	Peak age at onset (years)	Male:female ratio
Allergic angiitis and granulomatosis (Churg-Strauss syndrome)	Small- to medium-sized arteries and small vessels (arterioles, capillaries, and venules), mainly of the lungs, kidneys, and other organs	40 to 60	2:1
Behçet's syndrome	Small vessels, primarily of the mouth and genitalia but also of the eyes, skin, joints, GI tract, and central nervous system	20 to 25	1:1
Henoch-Schönlein purpura	Small vessels (arterioles, venules, and capillaries), especially of the skin and GI tract	5 to 20	1:1
Hypersensitivity vasculitis	Small vessels, especially of the skin	30 to 50	1:1
Microscopic polyangiitis	Small- to medium-sized arteries and small vessels (arterioles, capillaries, and venules) of the lungs and kidneys (different from PAN in that smaller vessels are involved)	40 to 60	1:1
Mucocutaneous lymph node syndrome (Kawasaki disease)	Small- to medium-sized vessels, primarily of the lymph nodes; may progress to involve coronary arteries	1 to 5	1:1
Polyarteritis nodosa (PAN)	Small- to medium-sized arteries throughout body. Lesions tend to be segmental, occur at bifurcations and branchings of arteries, and spread distally to arterioles. In severe cases, lesions circumferentially involve adjacent veins. They don't involve arterioles or venules.	40 to 60	2:1

Signs and symptoms	Diagnosis
Resembles PAN with hallmark of severe pulmonary involvement	History of asthma. Eosinophilia, increased serum immunoglobulin (IgE); tissue biopsy shows granulomatous inflammation with eosinophilic infiltration.
Recurrent oral ulcers, eye lesions, genital lesions, and cutaneous lesions	History of symptoms.
Abdominal pain, bloody diarrhea, palpable purpura, and maculopapular rash	History of symptoms; may see elevated serum IgA. Tissue biopsy shows leukocytoclastic vasculitis.
Palpable purpura, papules, nodules, vesicles, bullae, ulcers, or chronic or recurrent urticaria	History of exposure to antigen, such as a microorganism or drug. Tissue biopsy shows leukocytoclastic angiitis, usually in postcapillary venules.
Fever, pulmonary congestion, hemoptysis, hematuria, abnormal urine sediment, weight loss, malaise	Usually involves lung and kidneys, elevated erythrocyte sedimentation rate (ESR); 50% are positive for perinuclear ANCA. Tissue biopsy shows necrotizing vasculitis without immune deposits or granuloma formation.
Fever, nonsuppurative cervical adenitis, edema, congested conjunctivae, erythema of oral cavity, lips, and palms, and desquamation of fingertips; may progress to arthritis, myocarditis, pericarditis, myocardial infarction, and cardiomegaly.	History of symptoms; elevated ESR. Tissue biopsy shows intimal proliferation and infiltration of vessel walls with mononuclear cells. Echocardiography is necessary.
Hypertension, abdominal pain, myalgia, headache, arthralgia, weakness, weight loss, mononeuropathy or polyneuropathy	History of symptoms. Elevated blood urea nitrogen and serum creatinine levels, elevated ESR, leukocytosis, anemia, thrombocytosis, depressed C3 complement, rheumatoid factor > 1:60, circulating immune complexes. Tissue biopsy shows necrotizing vasculitis and immune deposits.

(continued)

Types of vasculitis *(continued)*

Type	Vessels involved	Peak age at onset (years)	Male:female ratio
Takayasu's arteritis (aortic arch syndrome)	Medium- to large-sized arteries, particularly the aortic arch and its branches and, possibly, the pulmonary artery	15 to 25	1:9
Temporal arteritis	Medium- to large-sized arteries, most commonly branches of the carotid artery; involvement may skip segments	60 to 75	1:3
Wegener's granulomatosis	Medium- to large-sized vessels of the upper and lower respiratory tract and kidneys; may also involve small arteries and veins	40 to 50	1:1

▪ Provide emotional support to help the patient and his family cope with an altered body image—the result of the disorder or its therapy. (For example, Wegener's granulomatosis may cause saddle nose; steroids, weight gain; and cyclophosphamide, alopecia.)

DRUG CHALLENGE

Monitor the patient's white blood cell count during cyclophosphamide therapy to prevent severe leukopenia.

Volvulus

A twisting of the intestine at least 180 degrees on its mesentery, volvulus results in blood vessel compression and ischemia. It usually occurs in a bowel segment with a mesentery long enough to twist. The most common area, particularly in adults, is the sigmoid colon; the small bowel is a common site in children. Other common sites include the stomach and cecum.

Causes
▪ Unknown
▪ Adhesion
▪ Anomaly of rotation
▪ Chronic constipation (in children and elderly people)
▪ Ingested foreign body
▪ Meconium ileus (in cystic fibrosis)

Signs and symptoms
▪ Abdominal pain
▪ Absence of bowel movements

Signs and symptoms	Diagnosis
Malaise, pallor, nausea, night sweats, arthralgia, anorexia, weight loss, pain or paresthesia distal to affected area, bruits, loss of distal pulses, syncope and, if carotid artery is involved, diplopia and transient blindness; may progress to heart failure or stroke	Decreased hemoglobin (Hb) level, leukocytosis, positive lupus erythematosus cell preparation, and elevated ESR. Arteriography shows calcification and obstruction of affected vessels. Tissue biopsy shows inflammation of adventitia and intima of vessels and thickening of vessel walls.
Fever, myalgia, jaw claudication, vision changes, headache (associated with polymyalgia rheumatica syndrome)	Decreased Hb level; elevated ESR; tissue biopsy shows panarteritis with infiltration of mononuclear cells, giant cells within vessel wall (seen in 50% of patients), fragmentation of internal elastic lamina, and proliferation of intima.
Fever, pulmonary congestion, cough, malaise, anorexia, weight loss, mild to severe hematuria	Tissue biopsy shows necrotizing vasculitis with granulomatous inflammation. Leukocytosis, elevated ESR, IgA, and IgG; low titer rheumatoid factor; circulating immune complexes; antineutrophil cytoplasmic antibody in more than 90% of patients. Renal biopsy shows focal segmental glomerulonephritis.

- Cramps
- Failure to pass flatus
- Nausea and vomiting

Complications
- Ischemia
- Perforation
- Peritonitis
- Shock
- Strangulation

Diagnostic tests
- Physical examination may reveal a distended abdomen and tenderness.
- Abdominal X-rays may show multiple distended bowel loops and a large bowel without gas. In midgut volvulus, abdominal X-rays may be normal. Computed tomography scanning may be helpful for diagnosis.
- In cecal volvulus, barium from a barium enema fills the colon distal to the section of cecum; in sigmoid volvulus, barium may twist to a point and, in adults, take on an "ace of spades" configuration.
- White blood cell count shows more than 15,000/mm^3 in strangulation and more than 20,000/mm^3 in bowel infarction.

Treatment
- For children with midgut volvulus, treatment is surgical.
- For adults with sigmoid volvulus, a flexible sigmoidoscopy examination is performed to check for infarction, and nonsurgical treatment includes reduction by careful insertion of a sigmoido-

scope or a long rectal tube to deflate the bowel.

- Success of nonsurgical reduction results in expulsion of flatus and immediate relief from abdominal pain.
- If the bowel is distended but viable, surgery consists of detorsion (untwisting); a necrotic bowel warrants exploratory laparostomy and resection.

Nursing considerations

- After surgical correction of volvulus, monitor the patient's vital signs, watching for fever (a sign of sepsis) and tachycardia and hypotension (signs of septic shock).
- Carefully monitor fluid intake and output (including stools), electrolyte values, and complete blood count. Be sure to measure and record drainage from the nasogastric (NG) tube and drains.
- Encourage frequent coughing and deep breathing.
- Reposition the patient every 2 hours. Encourage ambulation on the day of surgery.
- Keep dressings clean and dry. Record excessive or unusual drainage. Following dressing removal, assess for erythema and wound separation.
- When bowel sounds and peristalsis return, begin oral feedings with clear liquids, as ordered. Before removing the NG tube, clamp it for a trial period, and watch for abdominal distention, nausea, or vomiting. Advance to a regular diet, as tolerated.
- Reassure the patient and his family, and explain all diagnostic procedures. If the patient is a child, encourage parents to participate in their child's care to minimize the stress of hospitalization.

von Willebrand's disease

A hereditary bleeding disorder, von Willebrand's disease is characterized by prolonged bleeding time, moderate deficiency of clotting factor VIII (antihemophilic factor [AHF]), and impaired platelet function. This disease commonly causes bleeding from the skin or mucosal surfaces and, in females, excessive uterine bleeding. Bleeding may range from mild, causing no symptoms, to severe, potentially fatal hemorrhage. The prognosis, however, is usually good.

Causes

- Hereditary form: autosomal dominant trait
- Acquired form: cancer and immune disorders
- Defective platelet function characterized by:
  - decreased agglutination and adhesion at the bleeding site
  - reduced platelet retention when filtered through a column of packed glass beads
  - diminished ristocetin-induced platelet aggregation

Signs and symptoms

- Bleeding from the gums
- Easy bruising
- Epistaxis
- Sporadic bleeding episodes (may bleed excessively after one dental extraction but not after another)
- Severe forms of this disease may cause:
  - GI bleeding
  - hemorrhage after laceration or surgery
  - massive soft tissue hemorrhage and bleeding into joints (rare)
  - menorrhagia

Diagnostic tests

- A positive family history and characteristic bleeding patterns and laboratory values help establish the diagnosis.
- Typical laboratory data include:
  - prolonged bleeding time (over 6 minutes)
  - slightly prolonged partial thromboplastin time (over 45 seconds)
  - absent or reduced levels of factor VIII–related antigens, and low factor VIII activity level
  - defective in vitro platelet aggregation (using the ristocetin coagulation factor assay test)
  - normal platelet count and normal clot retraction.

Treatment

- The aims of treatment are to shorten bleeding time by local measures and to replace factor VIII (and, consequently, von Willebrand's factor [vWF]) by infusion of cryoprecipitate or blood fractions that are rich in factor VIII.
- During bleeding and before surgery, I.V. infusion of cryoprecipitate or fresh frozen plasma (in quantities sufficient to raise factor VIII levels to 50% of normal) shortens bleeding time.
- Desmopressin given parenterally or intranasally is effective in raising serum levels of vWF by enhancing cellular release of stored factor VIII.

Nursing considerations

- Care should include local measures to control bleeding and patient teaching to prevent bleeding, unnecessary trauma, and complications.
- After surgery, monitor bleeding time for 24 to 48 hours, and watch for signs of new bleeding.
- During a bleeding episode, elevate the bleeding site and apply cold compresses and gentle pressure.

- Refer parents of affected children for genetic counseling.
- Advise the patient to seek medical attention after even minor trauma and before all surgery to determine whether replacement of blood components is necessary.
- Tell the patient to watch for signs of hepatitis for 6 weeks to 6 months after transfusion.
- Warn the patient against using aspirin and other drugs that impair platelet function.
- Advise the patient who has a severe form of von Willebrand's disease to avoid contact sports.
- Encourage the patient to wear a medical identification bracelet at all times.

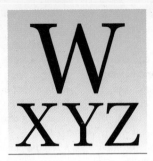

West Nile encephalitis

Part of a family of vector-borne diseases that also includes malaria, yellow fever, and Lyme disease, West Nile encephalitis is an infectious disease that primarily causes inflammation of the brain (encephalitis). It's caused by the West Nile virus, a flavivirus commonly found in humans, birds, and other vertebrates in Africa, West Asia, and the Middle East. In temperate areas, West Nile encephalitis occurs mainly in the late summer or early fall. In southern climates with milder temperatures, West Nile encephalitis can occur year-round. All persons living in endemic areas carry a risk of contracting West Nile encephalitis, but persons older than age 50 or those with compromised immune systems have the greatest risk.

Causes
- Bite of an infected mosquito (primarily the *Culex* species)

Signs and symptoms

Mild infection
- Body aches
- Fever
- Headache
- Skin rash
- Swollen lymph glands

Severe infection
- Coma
- Convulsions
- Disorientation
- Headache
- High fever
- Neck stiffness
- Paralysis
- Stupor
- Tremors

Diagnostic tests
- For immunoglobulin M antibody capture, enzyme-linked immunosorbent assay (ELISA) is the test of choice for rapid definitive diagnosis, especially when performed with acute serum or cerebrospinal fluid specimens.

Treatment
- Treatment is supportive and includes:
  – I.V. fluids
  – fever control
  – respiratory support.
- No vaccine exists at present to prevent the transmission of West Nile virus.

Nursing considerations
- Maintain I.V. fluids; monitor intake and output.
- Use fever control methods as ordered; these may include such measures as antipyretics and the use of a hypothermia blanket.

- Maintain a patent airway; provide oxygenation as ordered and monitor for effect.
- Use universal precautions when handling body fluids and blood.
- Report suspected cases of West Nile encephalitis to the state's Department of Health.

Prevention and risk reduction

- Advise patients to stay indoors at dawn, at dusk, and in early evening.
- Suggest wearing long-sleeved shirts and long pants whenever outdoors.
- Instruct patients to apply insect repellent containing N,N-diethyl-meta-toluamide (DEET) sparingly to exposed skin and clothing; an effective repellent contains 20% to 30% DEET. DEET in high concentrations (greater than 30%) can cause adverse effects, particularly in children; avoid the use of these products.

Wounds, open trauma

Open trauma wounds (abrasions, avulsions, crush wounds, lacerations, missile injuries, and punctures) are injuries that commonly result from accidental injury or acts of violence.

Signs and symptoms

- Vary with the specific type of wound
- Signs of underlying peripheral nerve damage:
  – Imedian nerve—numbness in the tip of the index finger; inability to place the forearm in the prone position; weak forearm, thumb, and index finger flexion
  – Iperoneal nerve—footdrop, inability to extend the foot or big toe
  – Iradial nerve—weak forearm dorsiflexion, inability to extend the thumb in a hitchhiker's sign
  – sciatic and tibial nerves—paralysis of the ankles and toes, footdrop, weakness in the leg, numbness in the soles
  – ulnar nerve—numbness in the tip of the little finger, clawing of the hand

Diagnostic tests

- A thorough physical examination of the patient reveals traumatic wounds.
- In all open wounds, assess the extent of injury, the patient's vital signs, his level of consciousness (LOC), obvious skeletal damage, local neurologic deficits, and his general condition.
- Obtain an accurate history of the injury from the patient or witnesses, including such details as the mechanism and time of injury and any treatment already provided.
- If the injury involved a weapon, notify the police.
- If a head injury is suspected, a computed tomography scan should be obtained to rule out underlying central nervous system involvement.
- Specific testing is required of the underlying organs suspected in involvement of the injury (such as echocardiography and electrocardiography with cardiac involvement).
- In those with suspected nerve involvement, electromyography, nerve conduction, and electrical stimulation tests can provide more detailed information about possible peripheral nerve damage.

Treatment

- For all types of traumatic wounds, treatment includes stabilizing the airway, breathing, and circulation and immobilizing the victim if you suspect spinal injuries. (For types of wounds and specific management, see *Managing open trauma wounds,* pages 690 to 692.)
- If hemorrhage occurs, stop bleeding by applying direct pressure on the

(*Text continues on page 693.*)

Managing open trauma wounds

Type	Clinical actions
Abrasion ■ Open surface wounds (scrapes) of the epidermis and possibly the dermis, resulting from friction; nerve endings exposed ■ Diagnosis based on scratches, reddish welts, bruises, pain, and history of friction injury	■ Obtain a history to distinguish injury from second-degree burn. ■ Clean the wound gently with topical germicide, and irrigate it. Too vigorous scrubbing of abrasions increases tissue damage. ■ Remove all imbedded foreign objects. Apply a local anesthetic if cleaning is very painful. ■ Apply a light, water-soluble antibiotic cream to prevent infection. ■ If the wound is severe, apply a loose protective dressing that allows air to circulate. ■ Give tetanus prophylaxis if necessary.
Avulsion ■ Complete tissue loss that prevents approximation of wound edges, resulting from cutting, gouging, or complete tearing of skin; frequently affects nose tip, earlobe, fingertip, and penis ■ Diagnosis based on full-thickness skin loss, hemorrhage, pain, and history of trauma; X-ray required to rule out bone damage; complete blood count (CBC) before surgery	■ Check the patient's history for bleeding tendencies and use of anticoagulants. ■ Record the time of injury to help determine whether tissue is salvageable. Preserve tissue (if available) in cool saline solution for a possible split-thickness graft or flap. ■ Control hemorrhage with pressure, an absorbable gelatin sponge, or topical thrombin. ■ Clean the wound gently, irrigate it with saline solution, and debride it if necessary. Cover with a bulky dressing. ■ Tell the patient to leave the dressing in place until return visit, to keep the area dry, and to watch for signs of infection (pain, fever, redness, swelling). ■ Give analgesics and tetanus prophylaxis if necessary.

Managing open trauma wounds *(continued)*

Type	Clinical actions

Crush wound

- Heavy falling object splitting skin, causing necrosis along split margins and damage to tissue underneath; may look like a laceration.
- Diagnosis based on history of trauma, edema, hemorrhage, massive hematomas, damage to surrounding tissues (fractures, nerve injuries, loss of tendon function), shock, pain, and history of trauma; X-rays required to determine extent of injury to surrounding structures; CBC and electrolyte count also required

- Check the patient's history for bleeding tendencies and use of anticoagulants.
- Clean open areas gently with soap and water.
- Control hemorrhage with pressure and a cold pack.
- Apply a dry, sterile bulky dressing; wrap the entire extremity in a compression dressing.
- Immobilize the injured extremity, and encourage the patient to rest. Monitor his vital signs, and check peripheral pulses and circulation often.
- Give tetanus prophylaxis if necessary.
- A severe injury may require I.V. infusion of lactated Ringer's or saline solution with a large-bore catheter as well as surgical exploration, debridement, and repair.

Laceration

- Open wound, possibly extending into deep epithelium, resulting from penetration with a sharp object or from a severe blow with a blunt object
- Diagnosis based on hemorrhage, torn or destroyed tissues, pain, and history of trauma
- Treatment dependent on site, age, and contamination of laceration

- Check the patient's history for bleeding tendencies and use of anticoagulants.
- Clean wound gently with saline solution.
- Apply pressure and elevate the injured extremity to control hemorrhage.
- Determine the approximate time of injury and estimate the amount of blood lost.
- Assess for neuromuscular, tendon, and circulatory damage.
- Administer tetanus prophylaxis and antibiotic therapy as prescribed.
- If sutures are required, stress the need for follow-up care and suture removal.

(continued)

Managing open trauma wounds *(continued)*

Type	Clinical actions
Missile injury ■ High-velocity tissue penetration such as a gunshot wound ■ Diagnosis based on entry and possibly exit wounds, signs of hemorrhage, shock, pain, and history of trauma; X-rays, CBC, and electrolyte levels required to assess extent of injury and estimate blood loss	■ Check the patient's history for bleeding tendencies and use of anticoagulants. ■ Control hemorrhage with pressure, if possible. If the injury is near vital organs, use large-bore catheters to start two I.V. lines, using lactated Ringer's solution, normal saline solution, or blood transfusions for volume replacement. Prepare for possible exploratory surgery. ■ Maintain a patent airway, and monitor for signs of hypovolemia, shock, and cardiac arrhythmias. Check the patient's vital signs and neurovascular response often. ■ Cover a sucking chest wound during exhalation with petroleum gauze and an occlusive dressing. ■ Clean the wound gently with saline solution or water (after visualization by police); debride as necessary. ■ If damage is minor, apply a dry, sterile dressing. ■ Administer tetanus prophylaxis, if needed. ■ Obtain X-rays to detect retained fragments. ■ If possible, determine the caliber of the weapon. ■ Report the injury to the police.
Puncture wound ■ Small-entry wounds that probably damage underlying structures, resulting from sharp, pointed objects ■ Diagnosis based on hemorrhage (rare), deep hematomas (in chest or abdominal wounds), ragged wound edges (in bites), small-entry wound (in very sharp object), pain, and history of trauma; X-rays can detect retention of injuring object	■ Check the patient's history for bleeding tendencies and use of anticoagulants. ■ Obtain a description of the injury, including force of entry. ■ Assess the extent of the injury. ■ Don't remove impaling objects until the injury has been completely evaluated. (If the eye is injured, call an ophthalmologist immediately.) ■ Thoroughly clean the injured area with soap and water. Irrigate all minor wounds with saline solution after removing a foreign object.

wound and, if necessary, on arterial pressure points.

■ If the wound is on an extremity, elevate it if possible.

■ Don't apply a tourniquet except in a life-threatening hemorrhage. If you must do so, be aware that resulting lack of tissue perfusion could require limb amputation.

■ If the wound is due to gunshot, stab, abuse, or other type of maltreatment, follow police protocol and preserve all evidence as ordered (usually in paper bags). Don't clean gunpowder from the skin (wound, fingers, or otherwise) until directed by the police.

■ Give tetanus prophylaxis if needed.

Nursing considerations

■ Frequently assess vital signs in patients with major wounds.

ACTION STAT!

 Stay alert for a 20 mm Hg drop in blood pressure and a 20-beat increase in pulse (compare the patient's blood pressure and pulse taken when he's sitting with those taken when he's lying down), increased respiratory rate, decreasing LOC, thirst, and cool, clammy skin—these indicate blood loss and hypovolemic shock.

■ Give oxygen as ordered.

■ Send blood samples to the laboratory for typing and crossmatching, complete blood count (including hematocrit and hemoglobin level), and prothrombin time and partial thromboplastin time.

■ Prepare the patient for surgery, if needed.

■ As much as possible, tell the patient about the procedures that he'll undergo (even if he appears unconscious) and provide reassurance.

■ Start I.V. lines, using two large-bore catheters, and infuse lactated Ringer's solution, normal saline solution, or whole blood, as ordered.

■ Insert a central venous pressure line, and place the patient in a modified V position (with his head flat and his legs elevated). If the modified V position doesn't help, the Trendelenburg position may be an alternative.

Rare diseases

Disease	Description
Addison-Schilder disease: adrenoleukodystrophy	Adrenal atrophy and diffuse degeneration of the brain in infancy or adolescence; characterized by loss of myelin and progressive loss of cerebral function, leading to spasticity, optic neuritis, blindness, and dementia
Alport's syndrome	Hereditary nephritis characterized by recurrent gross or microscopic hematuria; associated with deafness, albuminuria, and progressive azotemia
American trypanosomiasis: Chagas' disease	Febrile parasitic illness prevalent in Central and South America; cardiomyopathy may occur; megaesophagus and megacolon may develop many years later; can be severe and sometimes fatal in children
Arc-welders' disease: siderosis	Benign pneumoconiosis that can occur in iron ore miners, welders, metal grinders, and polishers from the inhalation and retention of iron
Armstrong's disease: lymphocytic choriomeningitis	Form of meningitis, usually occurring in adults ages 20 to 40 during fall and winter; usually asymptomatic or mild, although myocarditis and severe meningoencephalitis can occur; can spread to fetus with congenital infection, resulting in hydrocephalus
Ataxia telangiectasia: Louis-Bar's syndrome	Progressive, severe ataxia with telangiectasia of the face, earlobes, and conjunctivae; chronic recurrent sinopulmonary infections occur; ataxia usually occurs before age 2 but may not develop until as late as age 9; degree of immunodeficiency determines rate of deterioration
Basal cell carcinoma of the eye	Common extraorbital cancer affecting the eyelid, conjunctivae, and cornea
Behr's disease: degeneration of the macula retinae	Familial spastic paraplegia with or without optic atrophy; hyperactive deep tendon reflexes and sensory disturbances in adolescents and adults
Berylliosis: beryllium poisoning and beryllium disease	Systemic granulomatous disorder that's a form of pneumoconiosis with dominant pulmonary manifestations; two forms: acute nonspecific pneumonitis and chronic noncaseating granulomatous disease with interstitial fibrosis; death may result from respiratory failure and cor pulmonale
Bouillaud's syndrome: rheumatic endocarditis	Manifests as a heart murmur of either mitral or aortic insufficiency; pericarditis and heart failure are seen in severe cases

Cause	Treatment
Transmitted as X-linked recessive disorder	Symptomatic and supportive treatment; bone marrow transplant in boys; adrenal hormones; fatal in 1 to 10 years
Transmitted as X-linked autosomal trait	Supportive and symptomatic; antibiotic therapy for infection; antihypertensive therapy; protein-restricted diet; dialysis or renal transplant; avoidance of ototoxic drugs
Trypanosoma cruzi transmitted by insect; can also be transmitted through the transfusion of blood donated by a person who's infected	Nifurtimox or benznidazole in acute phase; supportive treatment in chronic phase
Inhalation and retention of iron after exposure to iron oxide fumes and dust	Supportive and symptomatic treatment; limiting or preventing exposure to iron dust or fumes with approved industrial respirators prevents progression of this disease
Infection caused by lymphocytic chorio-meningitis virus (a member of the family *Arenaviridae*) that follows exposure to food or dust contaminated by an infected common house mouse	Supportive and symptomatic treatment; infection can be prevented by careful hand washing (although mode of transmission may be airborne); corticosteroids and ribavirin may be considered in some cases
Transmitted as autosomal recessive disorder; a genetic mutation found in the ATM gene	Supportive treatment with early, aggressive antibiotic therapy to prevent or control recurrent infections; immune globulin; fetal thymus transplant or histocompatible bone marrow transplant
Unknown, but predisposing factors include exposure to sunlight, radiation, chemicals, and other carcinogens	Surgery; possibly radiation therapy
Hereditary form of cerebellar ataxia	No confirmed treatment; vitamin B therapy is sometimes indicated
Inhalation or absorption of beryllium; severity depends on amount inhaled or absorbed	Beryllium ulcer requires excision or curettage; acute form requires prompt corticosteroid therapy, oxygen and, possibly, mechanical ventilation; chronic form is treated with corticosteroids
Delayed sequel to pharyngeal infection by group B streptococci	Although no cure available, a course of penicillin should still be given to eliminate group A streptococci; additionally, supportive therapy to reduce morbidity and mortality

Disease	Description
Breisky's disease: kraurosis vulvae	Vulval atrophy and dryness of skin and mucous membranes, causing shrinkage of the vaginal outlet; histopathologically identical to lichen sclerosis
Brown-Symmers disease	Acute serous encephalitis in children
Budd-Chiari syndrome	Hepatic vein obstruction that impairs blood flow out of the liver, producing massive ascites and hepatomegaly; may be acute or chronic
Cat-scratch fever: cat-scratch disease	Subacute self-limiting disease characterized by a primary local lesion and regional lymphadenopathy; more common in children and young adults in contact with cats (90% of cases); disseminated form, bacillary angiomatosis, found in people who are immunocompromised, such as those infected with the human immunodeficiency virus
Central core disease: Shy-Magee syndrome	Rare muscle disease in which severe hypotonia causes weakness and arrests motor development in infancy; lack of oxidative enzymes in central core of each muscle fiber is diagnostic
Charcot-Marie-Tooth disease	Neuropathic (peroneal) muscular atrophy characterized by progressive weakness of the distal muscles of the arms and feet; most common form of the muscular dystrophies
Chédiak-Higashi syndrome	Characterized by morphological changes in granulocytes that impair the ability to respond to chemotaxis and to digest or kill invading organisms; associated with partial albinism
Chester's disease: cerebrotendinous xanthomatosis	Form of leukodystrophy indicated by excessive accumulation of lipids in the long bones; results in progressive cerebellar ataxia, dementia, mental retardation, spinal cord paresis, tendon xanthomas, and cataracts
Chiari-Frommel syndrome	Postpartum condition marked by uterine atrophy, persistent lactation, galactorrhea, prolonged amenorrhea, and low levels of urinary estrogen and gonadotropin
Cockayne's syndrome	Hereditary syndrome consisting of dwarfism with retinal atrophy and deafness; associated with progeria, prognathism, mental retardation, photosensitivity, and accelerated atherosclerosis
Conradi-Hunermann syndrome: dysplasia epiphysealis punctata	Abnormal development of the secondary bone-forming center, marked by depressions or pinpoint structures

Cause	Treatment
Probable hypoestrogen	Surgery
Viral pathogens (rabies, measles, mumps, rubella, influenza)	Supportive care; control of intracranial pressure; correction of metabolic problems, disseminated intravascular coagulation, bleeding, renal failure, pulmonary emboli, and pneumonia; invariably fatal
Any condition or medication that obstructs blood flow from hepatic veins; acute form due to acute thrombosis of main hepatic vein or inferior vena cava; chronic due to fibrosis of intrahepatic veins	Surgery to shunt hepatic blood flow and remove obstruction; if congenital, transcardiac membranectomy or percutaneous stent placement for patients with inferior vena cava web; liver transplant may be recommended for patients with marked hepatocellular dysfunction
Bartonella henoele; flea-borne transmission to kittens creates a feline reservoir for the disease	Symptomatic treatment; if patient is ill, can use ciprofloxacin, doxycycline, co-trimoxazole, erythromycin, cefoxitin, cefotaxime, mezlocillin, aminoglycosides, or antimycobacterials
Transmitted as autosomal dominant trait	Symptomatic and supportive treatment; genetic testing is available; recognition of this disease is important because patients with it have a well-established predisposition for malignant hyperthermia during anesthesia
Transmitted as autosomal dominant trait	Supportive treatment, including counseling, braces for foot drop, or orthopedic surgery to stabilize the foot and treat fractures
Transmitted as autosomal recessive trait; mutations found in CHS1 gene	Vigorous early treatment with antimicrobials and surgical drainage; large doses of vitamin C
Transmitted as autosomal recessive trait that causes disturbances of lipid metabolism	Chenodeoxycholic acid to arrest and reverse progression of disease
Possibly pituitary dysfunction or tumor	Treatment of underlying illness; bromocriptine to prevent osteoporosis
Transmitted as autosomal recessive trait	Effective treatment unknown; symptomatic treatment, establishment of protective environment
Transmitted as autosomal dominant and X-linked dominant trait	Supportive treatment ensuring adequate calcium intake

Disease	Description
Cystinuria	Inborn error of amino acid transport in the kidneys and intestine that allows excessive urinary excretion of cystine and other dibasic amino acids; results in recurrent cystine renal calculi
Dengue: breakbone or dandy fever	Acute febrile disease with myalgia and arthralgia; endemic during the warmer months in the tropics and subtropics; rarely fatal unless it progresses to hemorrhagic shock syndrome
Eales disease: peripheral neovascular retinopathy	Condition marked by recurrent hemorrhages into the retina and vitreous; mainly affects males in the second and third decades of life; most cases spontaneous and unilateral; some cases associated with trauma or stress, but also occurs after awakening
Economo's disease: lethargic encephalitis	Epidemic encephalitis marked by increasing languor, apathy, and drowsiness, progressing to lethargy; accompanied by ophthalmoplegia; usually occurs in winter
Elevator disease	Form of occupational pneumoconiosis affecting people who work in grain elevators
Eosinophilic endomyocardial disease: Löffler's endocarditis, Loeffler's endocarditis	Form of progressive endocarditis denoted by a highly increased number of eosinophilic granulocytes in the blood; fibrosis and thickening of the endocardium occur; cardiomegaly and heart failure may be present
Epstein-Barr virus: mononucleosis	Classic heterophil-positive infectious mononucleosis, occasionally complicated by neurologic diseases, such as encephalitis or transverse myelitis
Erysipeloid	Acute, self-limiting skin infection most common in butchers, farmers, cooks, fishermen, and others who handle infected material; may progress to infective endocarditis or affect other body systems if primary lesions aren't treated
Erythrasma	Superficial, bacterial skin infection that usually affects the skin folds, especially in the groin, axillae, and toe webs
Eulenberg's disease: paramyotonia congenita, Thomsen's disease	Slowly progressive disease of skeletal muscles; similar to muscular dystrophy; muscle stiffness in hands, legs, and eyelids is most prominent manifestation
Fabry's disease	Renal disorder that produces malfunctions of the proximal renal tubules, leading to hyperkalemia, hypernatremia, glycosuria, phosphaturia, aminoaciduria, uricosuria, bicarbonate wasting and retarded growth and development, and rickets

Cause	Treatment
Transmitted as autosomal recessive trait	Supportive treatment, including increasing fluid intake, sodium bicarbonate administration, alkaline-ash diet, and penicillamine; surgical removal of calculi
Group B arborviruses transmitted by the female *Aedes* mosquito	Symptomatic treatment; nonaspirin analgesics; I.V. fluid replacement; complete bed rest
Etiology unknown	Treatment of underlying causes
Pathogen not clearly identified, but may be arthropod-borne virus or sequela of influenza, rubella, varicella, or vaccinia	Symptomatic treatment, including appropriate antibiotics for secondary infection
Inhalation of dust particles, causing irritation and inflammation of respiratory tract	Avoidance of exposure to dust
Unknown	Suppression of eosinophilia with prednisolone or hydroxyurea; digoxin; diuretics; medical and surgical therapy for cardiac complications should be used as indicated
Epstein-Barr virus	Symptomatic treatment; generally benign course
Erysipelothrix rhusiopathiae (insidiosa) transmitted by contact with infected animals	Penicillin or erythromycin in combination with rifampin if the patient has penicillin allergy; the patient with the systemic form may need valve replacement surgery or other surgery depending on the organ involved
Corynebacterium minutissimum	Topical antibiotics; treatment with oral erythromycin or tetracycline often produces quick resolution; antibacterial soap to prevent recurrence
Transmitted as autosomal dominant trait	Treatment with quinine sulfate, procainamide, tocainide, mexiletine, or phenytoin may help
Transmitted as X-linked recessive trait	Symptomatic treatment with low-dose phenytoin or carbamazepine for pain in hands and feet; metoclopramide or nutritional supplement for GI hyperactivity; enzyme replacement therapy

Disease	Description
Fanconi's syndrome: de Toni-Fanconi syndrome	Disorder of fat storage related to a deficiency of enzyme alpha-galactosidase A; characterized by glycolipid accumulation in body tissues; results in clouding of the cornea, burning sensations of hands and feet, small raised purple blemishes on the skin, impaired arterial circulation, and renal and GI involvement
Fifth disease: erythema infectiosum	Contagious disease characterized by rose-colored eruptions diffused over the skin, usually starting on the cheeks; mainly affects children ages 4 to 10; infection in a patient who's pregnant can cause fetal hydrops and increase the risk of fetal death in the first half of pregnancy
Fish-skin disease: ichthyosis vulgaris	Condition of dry and scaly skin resembling fish skin; several forms, including vulgaris and lamellar
Fleischner's disease	Inflammation of bone and cartilage affecting the middle phalanges of the hand
Gerlier's disease: endemic paralytic vertigo, paralyzing vertigo	Nervous system disorder marked by pain, vertigo, paresis, and muscle contractions
Glioma of the optic nerve	Slow-growing tumor that causes progressive vision loss
Glossopharyngeal neuralgia	Disease of the ninth cranial (glossopharyngeal) nerve that produces paroxysms of pain in the ear, posterior pharynx, base of the tongue, or jaws; sometimes accompanied by syncope
Glucose-6-phosphate dehydrogenase (G6PD) deficiency	Deficiency of the red blood cell enzyme G6PD, which causes anemia; common in people of African or Mediterranean descent
Habermann's disease	Sudden onset of a polymorphous skin eruption of macules, papules, and occasionally vesicles, with hemorrhage
Hagner's disease	Obscure bone disease resembling acromegaly; associated with increased soft-tissue growth after puberty, increased metabolic rate, and increased sweating and sebaceous activity
Hemangioma of the eye	In children, tumors not encapsulated, grow quickly in the first year, and then regress by about age 7; in adults, tumors encapsulated
Hemochromatosis: bronze diabetes, Recklinghausen-Applebaum disease	Disorder characterized by iron overload in parenchymal cells, leading to cirrhosis, diabetes, cardiomegaly with heart failure and arrhythmias, and increased skin pigmentation

Cause	Treatment
If diagnosed as a child, may be congenital; if diagnosed as an adult, considered acquired and may be secondary to Wilson's disease, cystinosis, galactosemia, or exposure to a toxins as in heavy metal poisoning	Symptomatic treatment with replacement therapy, vitamin D for rickets, and aluminum hydroxide for hyperphosphatemia; treatment of underlying cause for acquired form; dialysis as necessary
Human parvovirus B19, probably transmitted by respiratory tract	Symptomatic treatment; screening of donated blood, which might prevent transfusion-related transmission; transfusion if aplastic crisis; immune globulin I.V. if immunocompromised; intra-arterial blood transfusion if fetal hydrops present
Hereditary form is an autosomal dominant genetic disorder; acquired form seen in adulthood usually associated with internal disease such as malignancy	Alphahydroxy acids (lactic, glycolic, or pyruvic acids) to help hydrate the skin; removal of scales by keratolytics; propylene glycol; topical retinoids; treatment of underlying systemic condition for acquired form
Unknown	Anti-inflammatory agents (including steroids in severe cases); analgesics
Disease of the internal ear from pressure of cerumen on the drum membrane	Symptomatic treatment, including scopolamine to combat nausea
Unknown	Surgical excision; radiation therapy
Unknown	Surgery; carbamazepine, phenytoin
Transmitted as an X-linked trait	Avoidance of known oxidant drugs, including primaquine, salicylates, sulfonamides, nitrofurans, phenacetin, naphthalene
Virus resembling smallpox	Supportive treatment, possibly isolation
Growth hormone-secreting tumors that develop after puberty	Treatment of cardiovascular complications; surgery and irradiation (proton beam or heavy particle treatment and supravoltage) for large tumors
Unknown	Surgical excision for adults; no treatment for children
Erythropoietic disorders, hepatic disorders that increase iron absorption, autosomal recessive inheritance	Phlebotomy to remove excess iron; chelating agents such as deferoxamine

Disease	Description
Hemoglobin C-thalassemia disease	Simultaneous heterozygosity for hemoglobin C and thalassemia; characterized by mild hemolytic anemia and persistent splenomegaly
Hutchinson-Gifford disease: progeria	Premature old age marked by small stature, wrinkled skin, and gray hair, with attitude and appearance of old age in very young children
Iceland disease: epidemic neuromyasthenia, benign myalgic encephalomyelitis	Marked by headaches, muscle pain, low-grade fever, lymphadenopathy, fatigue, and paresthesia; outbreaks occur in summer, usually in young women
Interstitial cystitis	Inflammation of the bladder wall occurring most often in women and marked by urinary frequency and urgency and abdominal, urethral, or vaginal pain; dyspareunia possibly also occurring; urine cultures and urinalysis are normal; cystoscopic examination revealing pinpoint hemorrhages on distended bladder wall
Isambert's disease: tuberculosis laryngitis	Acute miliary tuberculosis of the larynx and pharynx
Jaffee-Lichtenstein disease: cystic osteofibromatosis	Form of polyostotic fibrous dysplasia marked by an enlarged medullary cavity with a thin cortex, which is filled with fibrous tissue (fibroma)
Jaksch's syndrome: anemia pseudoleukemia infantum, Jaksch's anemia, van Jaksch's syndrome	Syndrome of anisocytosis, peripheral red blood cell immaturity, leukocytosis, and hepatosplenomegaly that usually occurs in children younger than age 3
Jansen's disease: metaphyseal dysostosis	Skeletal abnormality with nearly normal epiphyses in which the metaphyseal tissues are replaced by masses of cartilage
Keratosis pilaris: keratosis follicularis, Darier's disease	Skin condition marked by formation of horny plugs in the orifices of hair follicles; lesions appearing primarily on the lateral aspects of the upper arms, thighs, and buttocks; may also occur on face; more severe in the winter months
Kienböck's disease: lunatomalacia	Slowly progressive osteochondrosis of the semilunar (carpal lunate) bone from avascular necrosis
Köhler's bone disease: tarsal scaphoiditis, epiphysitis juvenilis	Osteochondrosis of the tarsal navicular bone in children, occurring at about age 5
Kugelberg-Welander syndrome: type III spinal muscular atrophy	Slowly progressive muscular atrophy resulting from lesions of the anterior horns of the spinal cord; usual onset in preschool or adolescent years

Cause	Treatment
Hereditary and congenital	Supportive treatment, including transfusions for severe anemia and folate therapy
Unknown	No known treatment
Probably infection but possibly psychosocial phenomenon	Symptomatic treatment
Unknown	Symptomatic treatment (anti-inflammatory drugs, antispasmodics, antihistamines, and muscle relaxants)
Mycobacterium tuberculosis	Tuberculostatic agents
May be a lipoid granuloma	Symptomatic and supportive treatment; surgery
Malnutrition, chronic infection, malabsorption, hemoglobinopathies	Treatment of underlying causes
Unknown	Surgery
Genetic follicular disease but may be transmitted as autosomal dominant trait	No specific therapy; keratolytic lotions to prevent cracking, drying, and skin breakdown possibly useful
Degenerative process precipitated by trauma	Anti-inflammatories and immobilization of wrist for several months (if ineffective, surgery)
Unknown but trauma suspected	Protection of foot from excessive use or trauma; if pain is severe, plaster cast may be required for 6 to 8 weeks; oral analgesics as needed; complete spontaneous recovery may occur
Transmitted as autosomal recessive or dominant trait	Supportive treatment with physical therapy; bracing or special appliances may help; normal life span probable

Disease	Description
Larsen's disease: Sinding-Larsen and Johanssen syndrome, Larsen-Johansson disease, patellar chondropathy	Accessory center of ossification within the patella, associated with flat facies and short metacarpals
Lenegre's disease	Acquired complete heart block
Leptospirosis	Infectious disease that causes meningitis, hepatitis, nephritis, or febrile disease; may be mild (anicteric) or severe (icteric or Weil's disease)
Lesch-Nyhan syndrome	Disorder of purine metabolism marked by behavioral problems that include cognitive dysfunction and aggressive and impulsive behaviors; also includes self-injurious behaviors, spasticity, hyperuricemia, and excessive uricaciduria
Little's disease: cerebral palsy	Form of cerebral spastic paralysis and stiffness of the limbs associated with muscle weakness, seizures, bilateral athetosis, and mental deficiencies
Ludwig's angina	Infection of the sublingual and submandibular spaces characterized by brawny induration of the submaxillary region, edema of the sublingual floor of the mouth, and elevation of the tongue
Macroglobulinemia: Waldenström's macroglobulinemia	Malignant neoplastic disease of plasma and lymphoid cells that produces immunoglobulin M antibodies; may produce no symptoms or diverse signs and symptoms
Malignant melanoma of the eye	Malignant tumor stemming from the melanocytes in the uvea, retina, or iris
Maple syrup urine disease	Enzyme defect in the metabolism of the branched chain amino acids, resulting in mental and physical retardation, reflex changes, feeding difficulties, characteristic odor of urine and perspiration, seizures, and death; four clinical phenotypes: classic, intermediate, intermittent, and thiamine-responsive
Medullary cystic disease: familial juvenile nephronophthisis	Congenital renal disorder marked by cyst formation, primarily in the medulla and the corticomedullary junction, with insidious onset of uremia that causes death between ages 4 and 14

Cause	Treatment
Unknown	Supportive treatment; surgery
Primary sclerodegeneration of the conduction system	Artificial pacemaker; supportive treatment
Bacteria of genus *Leptospira* transmitted by contact with water, soil, food, or vegetation contaminated with urine from an infected lower mammal	Doxycycline or ampicillin
Defective enzyme transmitted by female carriers as X-linked recessive trait	Allopurinol to control urine and sedimentation; baclofen and benzodiazepines for spasticity; symptomatic and supportive treatment, such as behavioral modification and medications for behavior treatment; few patients live beyond age 40 and most die suddenly
Congenital, resulting from birth trauma, fetal anoxia, or maternal illness during pregnancy	Preventive measures; symptomatic treatment
Causative bacteria include many gram-negative and anaerobic organisms, streptococci, and staphylococci	Significant airway obstruction may require tracheotomy; high doses of penicillin G given I.V., sometimes in combination with other drugs; incision and drainage to relieve pressure in affected tissues
Unknown but genetic predisposition suspected	Plasmapheresis for hyperviscosity; chemotherapy; interferon alpha; asymptomatic patients need no specific therapy
Unknown, but excessive exposure to sunlight is a risk factor	Laser or radiation therapy; chemotherapy; surgical excision; eye enucleation
Decarboxylation of the corresponding α-ketoacids by the branched-chain α-keto acid dehydrogenase components; transmitted as autosomal recessive trait	Supportive treatment; controlled intake of branched chain amino acids; peritoneal dialysis, hemodialysis, or both; one form is responsive to early initiation of thiamine
Transmitted as autosomal recessive or dominant trait	Symptomatic treatment: erythropoietin for anemia, recombinant growth hormone for growth retardation, peritoneal dialysis or hemodialysis; transplantation

Disease	Description
Megaloblastic anemia	Folic acid or vitamin B_{12} deficiency that alters the nucleic acid production needed for erythrocyte maturation in bone marrow
Milroy's disease: congenital lymphedema	Chronic lymphatic obstruction causing lymphedema of the legs; sometimes associated with edema of the arms, trunk, and face
Morton's neuroma: metatarsalgia, forefoot neuroma	Pain over the ball of the foot, especially left plantar surface distally
Myelosclerosis	Sclerosis of the spinal cord; obliteration of the normal marrow cavity by the formation of small spicules of bone
Nezelof syndrome	Primary immunodeficiency disease characterized by absent T-cell function and variable B-cell function, with fairly normal immunoglobulin levels and little or no specific antibody production; failure to thrive and increased susceptibility to infection typical; usually fatal as a result of sepsis
Niemann-Pick disease: sphingomyelin lipidosis	Lipid storage disorder resulting in abnormal accumulation of sphingomyelin in reticuloendothelial cells; most common in people of Ashkenazi Jewish ancestry; occurs in five different phenotypes, each with slightly different symptoms but characterized by pulmonary infiltrates, brownish skin, and sea blue histiocytes
Norrie's disease: atrophia bulborum hereditaria; retinal dysplasia	Bilateral blindness from absence of retinal ganglion cells; associated with cataracts, bilateral leukokoria, micro-ophthalmia, and mental retardation; represents inherited form of persistent hyperplastic primary vitreous
Nystagmus	Recurring, involuntary eyeball movement that may be jerking or pendular
Olivopontocerebellar atrophy	Progressively deteriorating neurologic disease marked by ataxia, dysarthria, and an action tremor that develops late in middle life; usually normal deep tendon reflexes; associated with occasional rigidity and other extrapyramidal signs

Cause	Treatment
Cobalamin (vitamin B_{12}) deficiency, secondary to pernicious anemia and folate deficiency, resulting from poor diet, sprue, pregnancy, or antifolate medication	Folic acid or vitamin B_{12} supplementation
Congenital and hereditary; transmitted as autosomal dominant trait	Microsurgery to rechannel lymph flow; supportive care; compression stockings
Repeated injury	Supportive, orthopedic shoes; analgesics; perineural injections of long-acting corticosteroids with local anesthetics; arch support or orthotics; surgical excision if needed
Unknown	Antibiotics for actinomycetoma (streptomycin, co-trimoxazole, amikacin, rifampin, minocycline); itraconazole or ketoconazole for eumycetoma from fungi; surgery for affected tissue or amputation if bone is involved
May be transmitted as autosomal recessive trait	Symptomatic treatment (usually includes antibiotics for infection and monthly treatment with immune globulin or fresh frozen plasma infusions); bone marrow transplantation
Transmitted as autosomal recessive trait	Supportive and symptomatic treatment; possibly liver transplantation in an infant with type A
Transmitted as X-linked trait	No known treatment
May be congenital or acquired; jerking nystagmus results from excessive stimulation of the vestibular apparatus in the inner ear, lesions of the brain stem or cerebellum, drugs and alcohol toxicity, and congenital neurologic disorder; pendular nystagmus results from improper transmission of visual impulses to the brain in the presence of corneal opacification, high astigmatism, congenital cataract, or congenital anomalies of optic disk or bilateral macular lesions	Correction of the underlying cause if possible; eyeglasses for vision disturbances
Transmitted as autosomal dominant trait	No definitive therapy; death usually follows aspiration pneumonia secondary to loss of cough reflex

Disease	Description
Opitz's disease	Thrombophlebitic splenomegaly
Paracoccidioidomycosis: South American blastomycosis	Fungal infection of the skin, lungs, mucous membranes, lymphatics, and viscera, seen primarily in the tropical forests of South America and Mexico
Pelizaeus-Merzbacher disease: sudanophilic leukodystrophy	Hyperplastic centrolobular sclerosis marked by nystagmus, ataxia, tremors, choreoathetotic movements, parkinsonian facies, and mental deterioration; begins early in life and occurs primarily in males
Pemphigus	Chronic blistering disease that causes superficial and deep lesions; pemphigus vulgaris, most common form of this disease, can be fatal
Progressive multifocal leukoencephalopathy	Demyelination of the white substance of the brain, producing sensory aphasia, cortical blindness, deafness, weakness, spasticity of the limbs and, eventually, complete paralysis, dementia, and coma; primarily affects patients who are immunosuppressed
Q fever	Rickettsial disease with acute and chronic stages, affecting respiratory as well as GI and cardiac systems
Refsum's disease: type IV hereditary sensorimotor neuropathy	Defect in metabolism of phytanic acid, marked by chronic polyneuritis, retinitis pigmentosa, and cerebellar signs (mild ataxia) with persistent elevation of protein levels in cerebrospinal fluid
Retinoblastoma	Most common intraocular cancer in children, arising from retinal gum cells; white pupil (leukokoria), poorly aligned eyes (strabismus), or a red and painful eye may be first indications
Rhabdomyosarcoma	Malignant tumors of muscle; areas affected include genitourinary tract, extremities, trunk, and retroperitoneum; in children, head and neck soft tissue sarcoma most common
Richter's syndrome	Chronic lymphocytic leukemia that evolves into an aggressive lymphoma
Rickettsialpox	Mild self-limiting zoonotic febrile illness characterized by a papulovesicular skin rash at the location of a tick bite
Strabismus: squint, heterotropia, cross-eye	Eye malalignment due to the absence of normal, parallel, or coordinated eye movement
Tangier disease	Deficiency of high-density-lipoproteins in the serum with storage of cholesterol esters in the tonsils causing orange-yellow tonsillar hyperplasia, and in the liver and spleen, causing hepatosplenomegaly

Cause	Treatment
Thrombosis of the splenic vein	Symptomatic and supportive treatment, including anti-coagulation therapy
Paracoccidioides brasiliensis	Ketoconazole, itraconazole, fluconazole; amphotericin B given I.V. for extremely ill patients
Familial transmission as an X-linked recessive trait, caused by mutations of the PLP gene located on the long arm of the X chromosome (Xq 22)	No specific treatment; supportive care, such as physical therapy, orthotics, and antispasticity agents; severely affected patients need airway protection and anticonvulsant therapy
Autoimmune disorder; occasionally caused by reaction to such medications as penicillamine, captopril, carbidopa, and levodopa	Corticosteroids, immunosuppressants; antibiotics for secondary skin infections; plasmapheresis; dapsone for pemphigus foliaceus
Common human polyomavirus, JC virus	Symptomatic and supportive treatment
Inhalation of infected particles by *Coxiella burnetii;* considered category B agent for biologic warfare	Appropriate antibiotic therapy (doxycycline or chloramphenicol); possibly valve replacement
Transmitted as autosomal recessive trai	Symptomatic and supportive treatment; therapeutic plasma exchange; transplantation of α-hydroxylase containing tissue
Transmitted as autosomal dominant trait (deletion of q14 band of chromosome 13)	Radiotherapy, chemotherapy-based multimodality therapy, or cryotherapy; enucleation
Unknown	Radiation therapy; surgical excision
Clonal evolution of original leukemia	Chemotherapy for the lymphoma
Rickettsia akari transmitted by bites of mites carried by infected rodents	Chloramphenicol, doxycycline, ciprofloxacin, levofloxacin; supportive care
May be inherited; nonhereditary risk factors include trauma and vision problems	Depends on type, but may include patching, prescriptive lenses, surgery, eye exercises
Transmitted as autosomal recessive metabolic disorder	Dependent on symptoms; may include heart surgery, removal of organs, or gene therapy

Disease	Description
Toxocariasis: visceral larva migrans	Chronic, frequently mild syndrome common in children involving roundworm migration from the intestine to various organs and tissues (visceral larva migrans); characterized by hepatosplenomegaly, eosinophilia, cough, difficulty sleeping, abdominal pain, and behavioral problems; ocular larva migrans can also occur, resulting in decreased vision, red eye or leukokoria (white pupil), retinal detachment, and vision loss
Trench fever: Wolhynia fever, shin bone fever, His-Werner disease, quintan fever	Fever with bone pain of the tibia, neck, and back, worsening with attacks; conjunctivitis, rash, splenomegaly, and hepatomegaly may also occur
Tropical sprue	GI disorder that causes atrophy of the small intestine, resulting in malabsorption, malnutrition, and folic acid deficiency; characterized by bulky, pale, frothy stools with increased fecal fat and macrocytic anemia; occurs mainly in Puerto Rico, Cuba, Haiti, Dominican Republic, and India
Typhus, endemic: murine, rat or flea typhus	Mild form of typhus causing systemic illness characterized by fever, headache, rash, and myalgia
Typhus, epidemic: European, classic, or louse-borne typhus	Acute systemic illness that may lead to death; signs and symptoms include severe headache, high fever, myalgia, chills, hypotension, delirium, and rash
Typhus, scrub: Japanese river or flood fever, tsutsugamushi fever	Acute systemic disease occurring almost exclusively in the western Pacific, Japan, and Southeast Asia
Tyrosinemia	*Hereditary form:* results in liver failure and renal tubular failure, hypoglycemia, rickets, darkening of the skin, and mild mental retardation; occasionally causes liver cancer *Transient form:* usually occurs in premature neonates; marked by elevation of blood tyrosine levels
Volkmann's disease: Volkmann's deformity	Deformity of the hand, fingers, or wrist caused by injury to the muscles of the forearm
von Hippel-Lindau disease: cerebroretinal angiomatosis	Phakomatosis characterized by angiomatosis of the retina, cerebellum, spinal cord and, less commonly, cysts of the pancreas, kidneys, and other viscera; onset usually in third decade and marked by symptoms of retinal or cerebral tumors
Wegner's disease: Bednar-Parrot disease, Parrot's pseudoparalysis	Pseudoparalysis from osteochondrotic separation of the epiphyses; onset most common in first weeks of life and seldom after 3 months

Cause	Treatment
Ingestion of *Toxocara* larvae, usually from dirt or sand; risk factors include eating without handwashing and living with or raising dogs and cats	Thiabendazole or mebendazole; albendazole; diethyl-carbamazine; ocular surgery
Bartonella quintana transmitted by body lice	Doxycycline, ceftriaxone, tetracycline, analgesics, anti-pyretics; delousing with lindane or other pediculicides; valve surgery if endocarditis occurs
Unknown	Tetracycline or oxytetracycline; folic acid and vitamin B_{12}
Rickettsia typhi transmitted by bites of in-fected fleas or lice or by inhalation of contaminated flea feces	Tetracycline, doxycycline, or chloramphenicol; anal-gesics; antipyretics
Rickettsia prowazekii transmitted by *Pediculus humanus trichiura*	Tetracycline, doxycycline, or chloramphenicol; anal-gesics; antipyretics; delousing with lindane or other pediculicide
Rickettsia tsutsugamushi transmitted by mite larvae	Chloramphenicol or tetracycline (Resistance to doxycy-cline and chloramphenicol has appeared in northern Thailand.)
Autosomal recessive trait resulting in ex-cess of tyrosine in blood and urine; gene maps to band 15q23-q25 identify 30 distinct mutations	Tyrosine and phenylalanine restriction; nitisinone (a ty-rosine degradation inhibitor); genetic counseling; liver transplantation is last resort
Trauma	Surgery
Transmitted as autosomal dominant trait	Early surgical intervention
Congenital syphilis	Effective treatment of syphilis during pregnancy; after delivery, neonate is also treated for syphilis

Disease	Description
Werdnig-Hoffmann disease: spinal muscular atrophy	Progressive degeneration of anterior horn cells and bulbar motor nuclei in a fetus or neonate; type 1 is most severe, as neonates are born with weak thin muscles and breathing problems; type 2 has less severe symptoms during early infancy, but becomes progressively weaker until the infant's death; type 3 is the least severe form, with signs and symptoms appearing after age 2 (weakening becomes more profound as the patient ages, but survival may be into early adulthood)
Whipple's disease: intestinal lipodystrophy, lipophagia granulomatosis	GI malabsorption disorder characterized by chronic diarrhea and progressive wasting, with skin pigmentation and polyarthralgia
Wilms' tumor: congenital nephroblastoma, embryonal adenomyosarcoma	Malignant mixed tumors of the kidneys, primarily affecting children; major signs—abdominal mass, enlarged abdomen, hypertension, vomiting, and hematuria
Yaws: frambesia tropica	Chronic relapsing infection characterized by highly contagious primary and secondary cutaneous lesions and noncontagious tertiary lesions, as well as systemic signs and symptoms; primarily occurs in Africa, Asia, South America, and Oceania—where overcrowding and poor sanitation prevail in warm, humid tropical regions
Yellow fever	Flavivirus infection that causes sudden illness accompanied by fever, slow pulse rate, and headache, nausea, and vomiting; endemic in tropical Africa and Central and South America

Cause	Treatment
Transmitted as autosomal recessive trait	Symptomatic and supportive treatment, including physiotherapy and bracing; airway clearance is a priority due to secretions
Tropheryma whippelii	Appropriate antibiotic therapy; supportive therapy with fluid and electrolyte replacement; iron, folate, vitamin D, and magnesium supplementation
Wilms' tumor recessive oncogen WT_1 at 11p15 locus	Nephrectomy; radiation therapy; chemotherapy
Treponema pertenue	Penicillin G benzathine, tetracycline, or erythromycin; after single penicillin injection, early lesions become noninfectious in 24 hours; tissue damage occurring later in yaws is irreversible
Flavivirus transmitted by *Haemagogus* mosquitoes in South America and *Aedes africanus* in Africa; the mosquitoes bite monkeys, which act as hosts for the virus, then the mosquitos bite humans, transmitting the disease	Supportive treatment for fluid volume and maintenance of normothermia; yellow fever vaccine; prevention of gastric bleeding with histamine-2 antagonists

Selected references

ACC Atlas of Pathophysiology, 2nd ed. Philadelphia: Lippincott Williams & Wilkins, 2005.

Anderson, M.L. "Atopic Dermatitis—More than a Simple Skin Disorder," *Journal of the American Academy of Nurse Practitioners* 17(7):249-55, July 2005.

Bauldoff, G.S., and Diaz, P.T. "Improving Outcomes for COPD Patients," *Nurse Practitioner* 31(8):26-28, 33-43, August 2006.

Boe, K., and Tillotson, E.A. "Encouraging Sun Safety for Children and Adolescents," *Journal of School Nursing* 22(3):136-41, June 2006.

Bunting-Perry, L.K. "Palliative Care in Parkinson's Disease: Implications for Neuroscience Nursing," *Journal of Neuroscience Nursing* 38(2):106-13, April 2006.

Carusone, S.C., et al. "A Clinical Pathway for Treating Pneumonia in the Nursing Home: Part I: The Nursing Perspective," *Journal of the American Medical Director's Association* 7(5):271-78, June 2006.

Diagnostic and Statistical Manual of Mental Disorders, Fourth Edition, Text Revision. Washington, D.C.: American Psychiatric Publishing, 2000.

Diseases: A Nursing Process Approach to Excellent Care, 4th ed. Philadelphia: Lippincott Williams & Wilkins, 2006.

Fickert, N.A. "Taking a Closer Look at Acute Otitis Media in Kids," *Nursing* 36(4):20-21, April 2006.

Fowler, S., and Newton, L. "Complementary and Alternative Therapies: The Nurse's Role," *Journal of Neuroscience Nursing* 38(4):261-64, August 2006.

Frith, M., and Harmon, C.B. "Acne Scarring: Current Treatment Options," *Dermatology Nursing* 18(2):139-42, April 2006.

Gallimore, D. "Understanding the Drugs Used During Cardiac Arrest Response," *Nursing Times* 102(23):24-26, June 2006.

Gedaly-Duff, V., et al. "Pain, Sleep Disturbance, and Fatigue in Children with Leukemia and Their Parents: A Pilot Study," *Oncology Nursing Forum* 33(3):641-46, May 2006.

Gorse, G.J., et al. "Impact of a Winter Respiratory Virus Season on Patients with COPD and Association with Influenza Vaccination," *Chest* 130(4):1109-16, October 2006.

Handbook of Diseases, 3rd ed. Philadelphia: Lippincott Williams & Wilkins, 2004.

Harrell, J.S., et al. "Changing Our Future: Obesity and the Metabolic Syndrome in Children and Adolescents," *Journal of Cardiovascular Nursing* 21(4):322-30, July-August 2006.

Hart, E.S., et al. "Broken Bones: Common Pediatric Fractures—Part I," *Orthopedic Nursing* 25(4):251-56, July-August 2006.

Hodgson, I. "Empathy, Inclusion and Enclaves: The Culture of Care of People with HIV/AIDS and Nursing Implications," *Journal of Advanced Nursing* 55(3):283-90, August 2006.

Isaksson, A.K., and Ahlstrom, G. "From Symptom to Diagnosis: Illness Experience of Multiple Sclerosis Patients," *Journal of Neuroscience Nursing* 38(4):229-37, August 2006.

Jacobson, C. "Tools for Teaching Arrhythmias: Wide QRS Beats and Rhythms," *Advanced Critical Care Nursing* 17(3):353-58, July-September 2006.

Kasim, K.M., et al. "Comparison of Intramuscular and Intradermal Applications of Hepatitis B Vaccine in Hemodialysis Patients," *Renal Failure* 28(7):561-65, 2006.

Kasper, D.L., et al. *Harrison's Principles of Internal Medicine,* 16th ed. New York: McGraw-Hill Book Co., 2005.

Lachat, M.F., et al. "HIV and Pregnancy: Considerations for Nursing Practice," *MCN American Journal of Maternal Child Nursing* 31(4):233-40, July-August 2006.

Laskowski-Jones, L. "First Aid for Burns," *Nursing* 36(1):41-43, January 2006.

Luthy, K.E., et al. "Safety of Live-Virus Vaccines for Children with Immune Deficiency," *Journal of the American Academy of Nurse Practitioners* 18(10):494-503, October 2006.

Managing Chronic Disorders. Philadelphia: Lippincott Williams & Wilkins, 2006.

McNally, P.R. *GI/Liver Secrets,* 3rd ed. Philadelphia: Hanley & Belfus, Inc., 2006.

Michael, K.M., and Shaughnessy, M. "Stroke Prevention and Management in Older Adults," *Journal of Cardiovascular Nursing* 21(5 Suppl 1):S21-26, September-October 2006.

Myers, L.B., and Horn, S.A. "Adherence to Chest Physiotherapy in Adults with Cystic Fibrosis," *Journal of Health Psychology* 11(6):915-26, December 2006.

Nettina, S.M. *Lippincott Manual of Nursing Practice,* 8th ed. Philadelphia: Lippincott Williams & Wilkins, 2005.

Nolan, S. "Traumatic Brain Injury: A Review," *Critical Care Nursing Quarterly* 28(2): 188-94, April-June 2005.

Nurse's 5-Minute Clinical Consult: Diseases. Philadelphia: Lippincott Williams & Wilkins, 2007.

Nurse's Quick Check: Diseases. Philadelphia: Lippincott Williams & Wilkins, 2004.

Nursing2007 Drug Handbook, 27th ed. Philadelphia: Lippincott Williams & Wilkins, 2007.

O'Boyle, C., et al. "Public Health Emergencies: Nurses' Recommendations for Effective Actions," *AAOHN Journal* 54(8): 347-53, August 2006.

O'Sullivan, J., and McCabe, J.T. "Migraine Development, Treatments, Research Advances, and Anesthesia Implications," *AANA Journal* 74(1):61-69, February 2006.

Odagiri, T. "Preparedness and International Contribution on H5N1 Highly Pathogenic Avian Influenza and Pandemic-Influenza," *Uirusu: Journal of Virology* 56(1): 77-84, June 2006.

Phillips, D. "Aortic Stenosis: A Review," *AANA Journal* 74(4):309-15, August 2006.

Professional Guide to Diseases, 8th ed. Philadelphia: Lippincott Williams & Wilkins, 2005.

Rebmann, T. "Defining Bioterrorism Preparedness for Nurses: Concept Analysis," *Journal of Advanced Nursing* 54(5):623-32, June 2006.

Reiss, G., et al. "*Escherichia Coli* O157:H7 Infection in Nursing Homes: Review of Literature and Report of Recent Outbreak," *Journal of the American Geriatric Society* 54(4):680-84, April 2006.

Roebuck, H.L., and Siegel, M.T. "The ABCs of Melanoma Recognition," *Nurse Practitioner* 31(6):11-13, June 2006.

Sargent, S., and Martin, W. "Renal Dysfunction in Liver Cirrhosis," *British Journal of Nursing* 15(1):12-16, January 2006.

Schack-Nielsen, L., and Michaelsen, K.F. "Breast Feeding and Future Health," *Current Opinion in Clinical Nutrition and Metabolic Care* 9(3):289-96, May 2006.

Simpson, T., and Ivey, J. "Pediatric Management Problems: GERD," *Pediatric Nursing* 31(3):214-15, May-June 2005.

Spollett, G. "Promoting Continuing Education in Diabetes Management," *Endocrine Practitioner* 12 Suppl 3:68-71, July-August 2006.

Stockwell, J. "Endometriosis: Clinical Assessment and Medical Management," *Advance for Nurse Practitioners* 14(1):43-45, January 2006.

Strategies for Managing Multisystem Disorders. Philadelphia: Lippincott Williams & Wilkins, 2006.

Tanaka, M., and Kazuma, K. "Ulcerative Colitis: Factors Affecting Difficulties of Life and Psychological Well Being of Patients in Remission," *Journal of Clinical Nursing* 14(1):65-73, January 2005.

Thomas, S.A., et al. "Quality of Life and Psychological Status of Patients with Implantable Cardioverter Defibrillators," *American Journal of Critical Care* 15(4): 389-98, July 2006.

Tierney, L., et al. *Current Medical Diagnosis & Treatment,* 43rd ed. New York: McGraw-Hill Book Co., 2004.

Tweddale, C.J. "Trauma During Pregnancy," *Critical Care Nursing Quarterly* 29(1): 53-67, January-March 2006.

Woodgate, R.L. "Siblings' Experiences with Childhood Cancer: A Different Way of Being in the Family," *Cancer Nursing* 29(5):406-14, September-October 2006.

Yildiz, B., et al. "Bell's Palsy and Hepatitis Infection," *Pediatrics International* 48(5): 493-94, October 2006.

Young, F. "Syphilis: Still with Us, So Watch Out!" *Journal of Family Health Care* 16(3):77-81, 2006.

Index

i refers to an illustration; t refers to a table.

i refers to an illustration; t refers to a table.

D

E

i refers to an illustration; t refers to a table.

F

G

i refers to an illustration; t refers to a table.

i refers to an illustration; t refers to a table.

i refers to an illustration; t refers to a table.

N

---

i refers to an illustration; t refers to a table.

i refers to an illustration; t refers to a table.

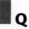

Q

R

---

i refers to an illustration; t refers to a table.

S

---

i refers to an illustration; t refers to a table.

i refers to an illustration; t refers to a table.